Library of Congress Cataloging-in-Publication Data
Main entry under title:

Valvular heart disease.

Includes index.
1. Heart—Valves—Diseases. I. Greenberg, Barry H.
II. Murphy, Edward, MD. [DNLM: 1. Heart Valve
Diseases. WG 260 v21512]
RC685.V2V35 1986 616.1′25 85-28454
ISBN 0-88416-472-1

Published by:
PSG PUBLISHING COMPANY, INC.
545 Great Road
Littleton, Massachusetts 01460

Printed in the United States of America.

International Standard Book Number: 0-88416-472-1

Library of Congress Catalog Card Number: 85-28454

Last digit is print number: 9 8 7 6 5 4 3 2 1

VALVULAR HEART DISEASE

Edited by

Barry H. Greenberg, MD
Associate Professor of Medicine
Division of Cardiology
The Oregon Health Sciences University
Portland, Oregon

and

Edward Murphy, MD
Associate Professor of Medicine
Division of Cardiology
The Oregon Health Sciences University and
Portland Veterans Administration Hospital
Portland, Oregon

PSG Publishing Company, Inc.
Littleton, Massachusetts

To our families

Contributors

J. David Bristow, MD
Professor of Medicine
Director of Cardiovascular Research and Training
Division of Cardiology
Oregon Health Sciences University
Portland, Oregon

Bruce Brundage, MD
Chief, Cardiology Section
University of Illinois
Chicago, Illinois

Randolph C. Byrd, MD
Assistant Professor of Medicine
Division of Cardiology
San Francisco General Hospital
San Francisco, California

Melvin Cheitlin, MD
Professor of Medicine
Department of Cardiology
San Francisco General Hospital
Department of Cardiology
San Francisco, California

Henry DeMots, MD
Chief, Cardiology Section, VA Medical Center
Head, Division of Cardiology, OHSU
VA Medical Center
Portland, Oregon

Barry Greenberg, MD
Associate Professor of Medicine
Director, CCU
Division of Cardiology
Oregon Health Sciences University
Portland, Oregon

Henry Issenberg, MD
Assistant Professor of Pediatrics
Department of Pediatrics
Montefiore Medical Center
Bronx, New York

Dean Keriakes, MD
Fellow in Cardiology
University of California
San Francisco, California

Sidney Levitsky, MD
Chief, Cardiothoracic Surgery
Professor of Surgery
University of Illinois
Chicago, Illinois

John McAnulty, MD
Professor of Medicine
Director, Cardiac Catheterization Lab
Division of Cardiology
Oregon Health Sciences University
Portland, Oregon

Dan G. McNamara, MD
Chief of Pediatric Cardiology
Texas Children's Hospital
Houston, Texas

Gerald Marx, MD
Assistant Professor of Pediatrics (Cardiology)
Department of Pediatrics
University of Arizona
Health Sciences Center
Tuscon, Arizona

Barry Massie, MD
Associate Professor of Medicine
VA Medical Center
San Francisco, California

James Metcalfe, MD
Professor of Medicine
Director of Heart Research Laboratory
Oregon Health Sciences University
Portland, Oregon

Mark Morton, MD
Assistant Professor of Medicine
Division of Cardiology
Oregon Health Sciences University
Portland, Oregon

Edward Murphy, MD
Associate Professor of Medicine
Oregon Health Sciences University
Director, CCU
VA Medical Center
Division of Cardiology
Portland, Oregon

Ali Nusrat, MD
Resident in Medicine
University of California
San Francisco, California

George Pantely, MD
Associate Professor of Medicine
Director, ECG Lab
Division of Cardiology
Oregon Health Sciences University
Portland, Oregon

Kirk Peterson, MD
Director, Cardiac Catheterization Laboratory
University of California
San Diego, California

Tom Ports, MD
Associate Professor of Medicine
Director, Cardiac Catheterization Laboratory
University of California
Medical Center
San Francisco, California

Stuart Rich, MD
Associate Professor of Medicine
Associate Chief, Section of Cardiology
University of Illinois
Chicago, Illinois

David Schwartz, MD
Associate Director of Cardiology
Division of Cardiology
Children's Hospital Medical Center
Cincinnati, Ohio

Jeffrey Shanes, MD
Assistant Professor of Medicine
Cardiology Section
University of Illinois
Chicago, Illinois

Contents

Preface **ix**

1 **The Heart in Pressure Overload 1**
Mark J. Morton

2 **Volume Overload: Effects on the Heart 12**
Kirk L. Peterson

3 **Evaluation of the Patient With Valvular Heart Disease 24**
J. David Bristow

4 **Congenital Lesions of the Tricuspid Valve 32**
David Schwartz

5 **Acquired Tricuspid Valve Disease 46**
Bruce Brundage, Stuart Rich, Sidney Levitsky, and Jeffrey G. Shanes

6 **Pulmonic Valve Disease 58**
Henry J. Issenberg

7 **Congenital Mitral Valve Disease 77**
Gerald R. Marx

8 **Mitral Valve Disease 92**
Melvin D. Cheitlin and Randolph C. Byrd

9 **Congenital Anomalies of the Aortic Valve 123**
Dan G. McNamara

10 **Acquired Aortic Valve Disease 147**
Barry Greenberg

11 **Multivalvular Heart Disease 174**
Henry DeMots

12 **Effects of Pregnancy in Patients with Valvular Heart Disease 183**
James Metcalfe and John McAnulty

13 **Interaction of Coronary Artery Disease and Valvular Heart Disease 192**
George A. Pantely

14 **The Role of Exercise Measurements in the Evaluation of Valvular Heart Disease 204**
Ali Nusrat and Barry M. Massie

15 **Emergencies in Valvular Heart Disease 215**
Dean J. Kereiakes and Thomas A. Ports

16 **Endocarditis 234**
Randolph C. Byrd and Melvin D. Cheitlin

17 **Prosthetic Cardiac Valves 261**
Edward S. Murphy

Index **283**

Preface

Valvular heart disease is one of the most challenging and exciting areas of medicine. We believe this is so because it is an area where the clinician is compelled to combine a thorough medical history and physical examination with an understanding of the pathophysiology of volume and pressure overload, and then integrate this with the natural history of the specific valve disease being evaluated. In addition, the clinician must be able to interpret a variety of invasive and noninvasive tests and design and supervise the most effective patient management.

With the development of valve replacement surgery over the past three decades, both the natural history of the patient with a valve lesion and the role of the clinician in that process have been dramatically and irrevocably altered. It is not an overestimate to state that valve replacement has enabled tens and even hundreds of thousands of persons around the world to live longer and more normal lives. Concurrently, the physician's role has evolved from that in which he is mainly an observer to one in which he takes an active role in determining the course of the disease by deciding when valve replacement should be undertaken. To assist him in this new role, a variety of tests (both invasive and noninvasive) are available to provide a plethora of numbers and pictures describing cardiac structure and function. However, to make rational decisions about interventions in patients with valvular lesions, the physicians must be able to assess the value of the tests and to integrate the information that they provide with our knowledge of pathophysiology and natural history.

The book is constructed to assist physicians in evaluating patients with valvular heart disease. We begin with reviews of the effects of volume and pressure overload on the heart and follow with an overview of principles in the evaluation of the patient. Subsequent chapters deal with specific valve lesions. The interaction of multiple valve lesions, the association of valve disease with coronary disease, exercise, pregnancy, endocarditis, or other emergencies are so complex and often confusing, that separate chapters are devoted to each topic. We conclude with a chapter reviewing prosthetic valve disease.

Each of our contributors has previously made important contributions to the understanding of valvular heart disease and, like ourselves, are students of the discipline. We are grateful that they have taken the time and care to produce outstanding chapters. We also thank our teachers and coworkers, especially Drs K. Chatterjee, M. Cheitlin, SH Rahimtoola, and JD Bristow for their insight and encouragement. In addition, we would like to thank Kathy Elkins, John Davis, and Marie Watkins for their thoroughness and precision in preparation of the manuscripts. We thank our publisher for their enthusiasm, guidance, and patience.

We hope this book will assist physicians in the management of patients. Most of all, we hope this book can be used to benefit the patients themselves.

Edward Murphy, M.D.
Barry Greenberg, M.D.

CHAPTER 1
The Heart in Pressure Overload

Mark J. Morton

The impact of pressure overload lesions caused by valvular heart disease is best understood by reviewing the normal and pathophysiologic reactions of the myocardium to increased systolic pressure. Geometric considerations in the intact heart must be blended with an understanding of how individual sarcomeres function. Acute responses to increased pressure are modified by subsequent myocardial hypertrophy in chronic pressure overload. The hypertrophy process itself should be examined. The variability of responses of different cardiac chambers to pressure overload needs to be explained. The detection of, and determination of the etiology of pump dysfunction in long-standing severe pressure overload is clinically important. Finally, reversal of compensatory mechanisms after correction of systolic pressure overload can be demonstrated.

GEOMETRIC CONSIDERATIONS

When heart muscle contracts, the amount of blood expelled from a chamber will be determined by the end-diastolic volume (or muscle length) and the ejection fraction (or extent of shortening). What determines end-diastolic muscle length and systolic extent of shortening must be understood before tackling an intact cardiac chamber. Basic concepts central to developments in the following sections can be reviewed in a comprehensive textbook of cardiac physiology.[1]

Muscle Strip

The contractile elements (which constitute about 50% of the volume of heart muscle) are assumed to be fully extensible in diastole. This assumption may not be correct in the presence of severe ischemia.[2] However, the importance of ischemic prolongation of relaxation or contracture to pressure overload lesions is uncertain. Accordingly, we will assume that the diastolic length of, for example, a papillary muscle (Figure 1-1) will be determined by its unstressed length, the force applied to the muscle, the cross-sectional area of the muscle, and the passive stress-strain relationship of the tissue. Sarcolemma and intercellular connective tissue are the presumptive sites for the latter parameter. The diastolic length of the muscle in turn will determine the length of the freely extensible contractile elements. It is of note that physiologic diastolic filling pressures in normal hearts produce diastolic sarcomere lengths near the apex of the active length-tension curve. The factors determining the length of the sarcomere at end-diastole are then, the force per unit area (stress) and the stress-strain relationship of the muscle. As will be discussed later, proliferation of connective tissue during chronic severe pressure loading may importantly alter the stress-strain relationship of cardiac muscle.

Shortening of our hypothetical papillary muscle will be related to end-diastolic sarcomere length (Starling's law) and inversely related to the systolic force per unit area against which the muscle shortens. In isotonically contracting papillary muscles, systolic force or afterload is easy to understand since the muscle simply elevates a weight on a pulley. In this preparation, for a given end-diastolic length (preload) and contractility, rate and extent of shortening are inversely related to the systolic force per unit area (afterload).[3] A slight correction of area

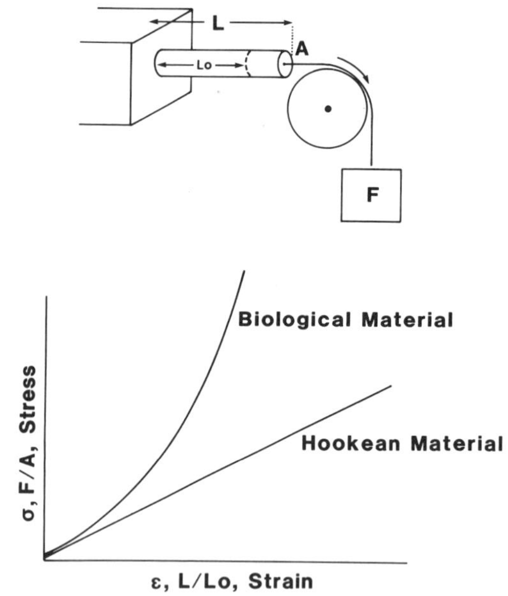

Figure 1-1 The diastolic length of a cardiac muscle strip is determined by the unstressed length (Lo), the force extending the muscle normalized for muscle cross-sectional area (F/A), and the intrinsic stiffness of the muscle. The relationship between L/Lo (Strain) and F/A (Stress) for cardiac muscle is not linear and responds like other biologic materials. The instantaneous slope of this relationship $d\sigma/d\varepsilon$ is called the elastic modulus. Elastic modulus can be approximated by $E = k\sigma + c$ where k and c are constants. From this equation, we see that cardiac muscle becomes progressively stiff as stress increases.

would have to be made to account for muscle thickening during shortening.

Cardiac Chamber

In a muscle strip, diastolic stress determines length, and systolic stress negatively relates to shortening. The same principles should apply to the muscle in a cardiac chamber except that geometry and the auxotonic nature (increasing then decreasing stress) of cardiac contraction make the transfer of these concepts difficult. For simplicity, we will use a thin-wall sphere to approximate a cardiac chamber (Figure 1-2). For an isotropic material (elastic properties independent of orientation), stress in a thin-wall sphere can be readily approximated by knowing transmural pressure (P), radius (r), and wall thickness (h).

$$\sigma = Pr/2h \qquad (1)$$

Diastole End-diastolic volume (EDV) then should be a function of the unstressed volume of

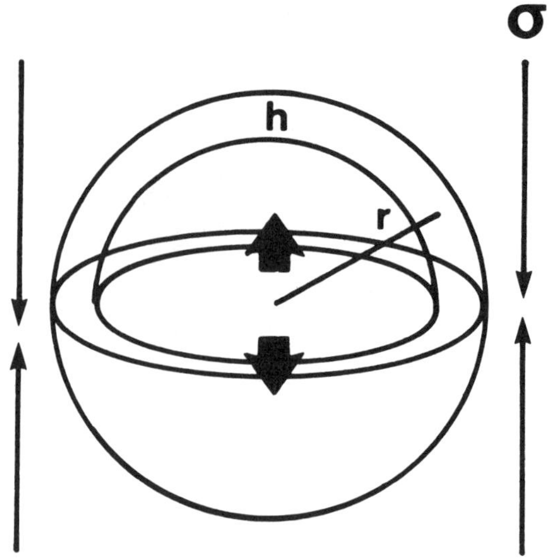

Figure 1-2 In equilibrium, a sphere with pressure P, mean radius r, wall thickness h and circumferential wall stress σ will have equal, opposed forces separating and holding the hemispheres together:

$$P\pi(r - h/2)^2 = \sigma 2\pi rh$$

For $r \gg h/2$ (thin wall assumption)

$$P\pi r^2 = \sigma 2\pi rh \quad \text{and} \quad \sigma = Pr/2h$$

the chamber (V_o) (corresponding to Lo in Figure 1-1), the diastolic wall stress $f(\sigma)$, and the material properties of the muscle (E) as defined by elastic modulus-stress relationship (equation 2). Wall stress, in turn will depend on transmural pressure, and the radius/wall thickness ratio (r/h) (equation 1). For example, wall stress will be increased by lengthening of radius or elevations of pressure but decreased by thickening of the wall. The critical interaction between transmural pressure and r/h ratio in determining wall stress cannot be overemphasized and is essential to understanding compensation for systolic pressure overload.

$$EDV = V_o + f(\sigma) \cdot f(1/E) \qquad (2)$$

In pressure overload, unstressed volume is probably not affected until quite late in the disease. Hypertrophy, however, reduces the radius/wall thickness ratio. Myocardial fibrosis, a possible consequence of pressure overload, may elevate E for a given level of stress. The effect of these alterations on diastolic pressure–volume relations may be quite dramatic. Substantial transmural pressure may be required to fill hypertrophied chambers. The elevated filling pressure is necessary to offset both the reduced r/h ratio and the increased stiffness associated with fibrosis. The circulation must maintain high filling pressures in pressure overload because of the important role that preload plays in determining shortening.

Systole Stroke volume is the important analogue of muscle shortening in a cardiac chamber. Since muscle shortening is inversely related to systolic stress, stroke volume should be and is importantly affected by systolic pressure, and the r/h ratio, the determinants of wall stress.[4] Unlike the isotonically contracting papillary muscle, cardiac chamber muscle contracts auxotonically because pressure rises and then falls and r/h ratio decreases steadily during ejection.

If systolic pressure is increased, and other factors remain constant, systolic wall stress will increase, and rate and extent of shortening will be reduced. The net effect will be a reduction of stroke volume. A pressure–volume loop for a cardiac cycle is shown in Figure 1-3. Increased systolic pressure results in increased end-systolic volume; stroke volume is reduced. However, circulatory homeostasis can be restored by increasing end-diastolic volume. Now, end-systolic volume can remain increased, but the difference between end-diastolic volume and end-systolic volume, stroke volume, will be normal. This mechanism of matching afterload with preload is important for the maintenance of circulatory homeostasis.[5] However, this mechanism is not capable of compensating for the magnitude of pressure loading present in valvular heart disease. End-systolic pressure and volume are linearly related at constant contractility.[6] End-diastolic pressure–volume relations are curvilinear and pressure rises steeply at volumes much above normal. In Figure 1-3, we can see that further increases in systolic pressure will result in reduced stroke volume and filling pressures that might cause congestion in organs upstream.

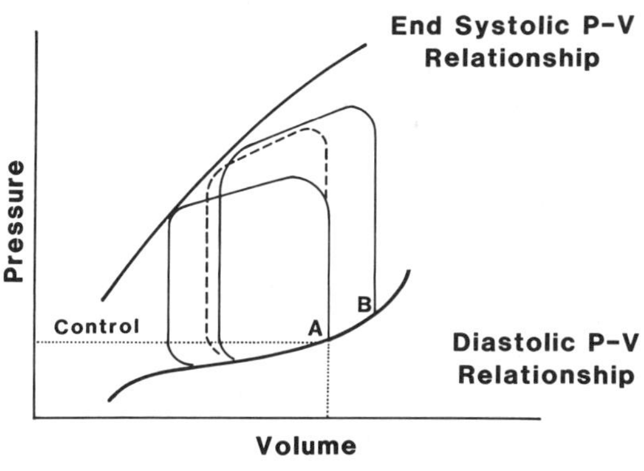

Figure 1-3 A continuous pressure–volume loop is shown at constant contractility. Increased systolic pressure (—) results in increased end-systolic volume and stroke volume (SV) falls (SV = end-diastolic volume minus end-systolic volume). The normal compensation for this reduced stroke volume is an increase in end-diastolic volume from control to loop B which returns stroke volume to normal. Because end-diastolic pressure rises rapidly at volumes much above control, this mechanism is poorly suited for long-term maintenance of pumping capacity in pressure overload.

It is not surprising that a second more effective mechanism has evolved for dealing with pressure loading. Returning to equation (1), we see that wall stress would be normalized despite increased pressure if r/h ratio could be kept proportionately low. This could be achieved by increasing muscle mass. Hypertrophy, enlargement of individual muscle cells, is the long-term mechanism by which heart muscle compensates for systolic pressure loading. Investigations of chronically instrumented animals subjected to aortic constriction have documented the acute and long-term responses of the left ventricle to pressure loading.[7] Unstressed chamber volume remains relatively constant while wall thickness is increased. Because systolic wall stress is normalized, muscle shortening can remain normal despite substantial increases in systolic pressure. Chamber stroke volume can remain normal. In the absence of pathologic hypertrophy, the only drawback to this compensatory mechanism will be the higher filling pressures required to overcome the reduced r/h ratio at end diastole.

CARDIAC MUSCLE HYPERTROPHY

Increased muscle mass is the most readily recognized feature of the cardiac adaptation to pressure overload. The mechanism for increased mass, however, may limit importantly the extent to which this adaptation may be utilized. The number of myocardial muscle cells is probably fixed shortly after birth. Increased cardiac mass during growth must therefore largely derive from increased cell size (hypertrophy). Further increases in cardiac mass in the adult subjected to pressure overload must come from even further increases in cell size. The physiology and biochemistry of hypertrophy have been the subject of several recent reviews.[8–10]

Stimulus for Hypertrophy

Experiments with isolated working hearts and cardiac muscle support systolic loading as an important stimulus for hypertrophy.[8] Within one hour of pressure loading, mRNA synthesis is increased. Increased protein synthesis follows in another two hours. In papillary muscles, protein synthesis is much greater during electrically stimulated isometric contraction than during passive stretch. Likewise, elevated calcium levels increase contractility and amplitude of contraction but not protein synthesis. Thus, increased systolic loading rapidly turns on the genetic machinery of the myocyte for the production of new contractile proteins.

The precise stimulus for hypertrophy in the intact circulation is uncertain and remains the goal of many current investigations. Although it is intellectually attractive to imagine that the myocardium could recognize increased systolic wall stress and transduce mechanical information to protein synthesis to normalize the stress through hypertrophy, other signals may be important. Laks suggested that norepinephrine was the mediator for myocardial hypertrophy.[11] More recently, Simpson et al demonstrated that specific agonism of α-receptors on cultured myocytes produced increased cell volume and protein content.[12] Nichols et al showed that hypertrophy due to experimental coarctation was inhibited by the absence of the adrenal cortex but not the adrenal medulla.[13] It is therefore possible that both hormonal and local mechanical factors interact to control myocardial cell size and mass.

Myocardial Constituents in Hypertrophy

Successful hypertrophy would normalize systolic stress for each myofibril; accordingly, contractile protein synthesis is the dominant feature biochemically and morphologically of hypertrophy. To keep pace with the increased energy expenditure per cell, mitochondria and capillaries must also proliferate. Limitation of hypertrophy as a successful compensatory mechanism could reside either with the failure to synthesize adequate contractile protein or with inadequate expansion of the energy supply system, or both.

Contractile Proteins The rapid accumulation of contractile proteins following afterload stress appears to be due to increased synthesis rather then reduced degredation. In some experimental models, the adenosine triphosphatase (ATPase) activity of cardiac myosin has been altered during hypertrophy.[10] Subsequent investigation identified three myosin isoenzymes which could be separated by electrophoretic mobility. Importantly, the myosin isoenzymes had ATPase activities which varied by as much as 200%. Genetic control of cardiac function in response to stress could be reasonably hypothesized and tested. Despite the attractiveness of these findings in laboratory animal models of hypertrophy, their relevance to human pathophysiology has not been demonstrated. Specimens of human cardiac muscle obtained at the time of cardiac surgery for clinically important volume or pressure overload have not shown significant alterations in myosin isoenzyme content.[14] Alterations of systolic function in human pressure overload are probably not due to biochemical abnormalities of the contractile proteins.

Mitochondria Shortly after pressure loading (less than three days) mitochondrial volume increases relative to contractile protein. Thereafter, the ratio of mitochondria to contractile protein decreases and falls below control values.[8] The role of decreased relative mitochondrial volume in human pressure overload is unclear, but the potential for reduced energy supply is present.

Interstitial Tissue Myocardial interstitial space is composed primarily of blood vessels and connective tissue. In sharp contrast to myocytes, blood vessel and connective tissue nuclei take up tritiated thymidine following afterload stress indicating hyperplasia.[8] A proportional increase in myocardial blood vessels and connective tissue would be expected during myocardial hypertrophy if functional integrity were to be maintained. Such is not the case. The diminished functional reserve of the vascular bed in ventricular hypertrophy is examined in detail in chapter 13.

Fibrosis, mainly due to increased deposition of subendocardial collagen, is a common finding in experimental hypertrophy and in human valvular heart disease. However, the stimulus for excessive collagen deposition is unknown. Substantial ventricular hypertrophy can be produced without fibrosis in experiments with gradual afterloading of the ventricle.[14] On the other hand rapid loading of the ventricle may produce subendocardial ischemia.[15] This happens because subendocardial oxygen supply is outstripped by demand. Filling pressure increases to offset increased afterload. High filling pressure, increased systolic mural pressure, and a relatively lower vasodilator reserve in the subendocardium all add to this process which is further described in chapter 13. Tissue hypoxia and acidosis ensue. Tissue acidosis or hypoxia may be the critical features which promote myocyte loss and proliferation of collagen.[17] The importance of the rate of loading is understandable if these factors are causative.

There appear to be important limits to the hypertrophy process. As alluded to above, rapid loading of the myocardium may damage the tissue. However, even progressive loading, characteristic of human valvular lesions, cannot be compensated for indefinitely. The innexorable increase in myocyte size necessitated by the expanding contractile protein mass reduces the surface area/volume ratio of the cell. At the same time, the diffusion distance to the interior of the cell is increasing. Eventually, reduced coronary reserve, unfavorable diffusion geometry, and a relative reduction of mitochondria will produce the same inadequate metabolic environment that exists with acute pressure loading. Decreased contractility and finally myocardial cell death and fibrosis ensue.

CARDIAC FUNCTION IN CLINICAL PRESSURE OVERLOAD LESIONS

Diastolic Function

The clinical evaluation of diastolic function is in rapid evolution.[18] Although subject to future refinement, much can be learned from clinical studies at this time. The important diastolic parameter for the patient is the filling pressure that is required to produce stroke volume. Filling pressures are frequently increased and a source of morbidity both before and to a lesser extent after surgical treatment of pressure overload lesions. Understanding the mechanisms for increased filling pressure is therefore desirable.

One source of elevated filling pressure is unrelated to diastolic function; it is reduced systolic function. As reviewed earlier, circulatory homeostasis in the presence of reduced shortening will be maintained (or will attempt to maintain) with increased preload. In the ventricle, this is effected by increasing end-diastolic volume and therefore end-diastolic pressure. The diastolic properties may not be altered; rather, we move sharply up the curvilinear relationship between pressure and volume. Filling pressures rise even further during exercise if contractility does not increase normally or afterload is excessive. Both are observed in pressure overload lesions.

The diastolic abnormalities of ventricular muscle which raise left ventricular end-diastolic pressure are hypertrophy and increased intrinsic muscle stiffness. Prolonged relaxation has been demonstrated in hypertrophied ventricles, but the clinical importance of this phenomenon to elevated filling pressures remains to be demonstrated.[19] Further definition of the causes of increased intrinsic muscle stiffness is needed. However, fibrosis with increased collagen deposition appears to play an important role. The separation of the effects of wall thickening and muscle stiffness is accomplished by assessment of diastolic pressure–volume relations and ventricular geometry and wall thickness, and then calculation of muscle stiffness from stress-strain relationships.[20] It is important to distinguish between chamber stiffness and intrinsic muscle stiffness. Chamber stiffness is affected both by operating filling pressure, geometry, and intrinsic muscle stiffness.

Peterson et al examined diastolic pressure–volume relations in patients with aortic stenosis.[21] Through geometric modeling, they were able to determine whether increased left ventricular end-diastolic pressure was due to reduced r/h ratio (hypertrophy) or increased muscle stiffness, or both. Those patients with both reduced r/h ratio and increased stiffness had much higher filling pressures. One patient with hypertrophy and increased stiffness was studied after valve replacement. Diastolic pressure was reduced both because of increased r/h ratio (reversal of hypertrophy) and reduced muscle stiffness. This interesting observation suggests that increased intrinsic myocardial stiffness is not invariably related to irreversible myocardial fibrosis. On the other hand, left ventricular end-diastolic pressure (LVEDP) remained mildly increased at rest in this subject. Hess et al have obtained specimens of left ventricular myocardium before and after aortic valve replacement.[22] Myocardium was stained for collagen and graded according to the amount of fibrosis which was present. Analysis of diastolic pressure–volume relations was performed in the same patients. Interestingly, the amount of fibrosis present on the tissue specimen did not necessarily predict increased intrinsic stiffness of the myocardium. However after valve replacement for aortic stenosis, regression of hypertrophy was associated with increased relative fibrosis and myocardial stiffness.[22]

Further studies of the reversibility of diastolic abnormalities of the ventricle after removal of outflow obstruction are needed. It would be desirable to intervene in outflow obstruction prior to the point of irreversible increases in myocardial stiffness. The techniques for quantifying diastolic function, though laborious, are available and should continue to be applied prospectively to this problem. There may be a role for myocardial biopsy. Finally, techniques of studying diastolic function which do not include pressure measurement but rely on rate of filling during diastole, eg, radionuclide ventriculography, should be applied to this problem.

Systolic Function

The clinical quantification of systolic function in outflow obstruction is every bit as complex as the study of diastolic function. For the patient, the important factors are the stroke volume and the price (filling pressure) that must be paid to get it. Generally, the circulation will attempt to preserve cardiac output despite important abnormalities of systolic or diastolic ventricular function. The short-term compensatory mechanisms will be increased filling pressure, elevated heart rate, and augmented sympathetic tone. On the other hand, successful cardiac adaptation to pressure loading through hypertrophy will normalize afterload and preserve systolic function. Other compensatory mechanisms are not necessary.

How do we characterize systolic function in pressure overload? Muscle shortening during systole necessitates expulsion of blood and therefore is central to the characterization of systolic function. We previously reviewed the concepts that muscle shortening will depend on preload, afterload, and contractility. Obviously, the number of contractile elements in series will influence the absolute amount of shortening and we must accordingly normalize shortening for the dimension at end diastole. The shortening fraction can also be expressed in volumetric terms as the stroke volume normalized for end-diastolic volume, or ejection fraction. Normalized velocities of shortening or ejection are also clinically useful. These ejection phase indices of ventricular function are relatively insensitive to changes in preload, but accurately track changes in contractility and afterload.[1]

For the patient with severe pressure overload and normal ejection phase indices of function, the clinician can safely assume that contractility is normal. It is now clear from laboratory investigations that substantial ventricular hypertrophy does not necessarily impair the intrinsic strength of cardiac contraction.[23] Assessment of ventricular geometry and wall thickness by two-dimensional echocardiography or angiography with simultaneous intraventricular pressure measurement in humans with normal ejection fraction should demonstrate that wall stress or afterload has been normalized by the hypertrophy process. It is unlikely that reduced contractility will adversely affect the surgical outcome for that patient in the absence of a surgical catastrophe.

Evaluation of the patient with reduced ejection phase indices of function and severe pressure overload is more complicated. Either contractility may be reduced for reasons previously discussed, or afterload may be too high or both. Reduced contractility is usually not reversible and its presence increases surgical risk and leaves residual ventricular dysfunction if surgery is successful. Pressure overload lesions, although chronic problems, are progressive, and progression of severity of aortic stenosis has been demonstrated.[24,25] Gorlin's formula states that the area of a stenotic valve is proportional to the flow rate across the valve and inversely proportional to the square root of the pressure drop across the valve. Small decrements in area of severely stenotic orifices will therefore require huge increases in the pressure gradient to sustain flow. It is not surprising then that the hypertrophy process may be outstripped by progressive increases in ventricular pressure. When the pressure increase exceeds the compensatory reduction in r/h ratio, wall stress will rise (afterload) and shortening will fall. Now, circulatory homeostasis will be threatened and the short-term compensatory mechanisms will be called upon. The increase in filling pressure which ensues is self-defeating in the long run. As the ventricle expands in diastole, the wall becomes thinner because of the conservation of mass. Radius/wall thickness ratio increases sharply and wall stress climbs further; shortening is further depressed. This vicious cycle is rapidly terminated by upstream organ congestion, circulatory collapse, or death. The relatively brief and unpredictable survival of patients with severe symptomatic aortic stenosis is at least in part due to this process.

Reduced ejection phase indices of function may therefore be due to inadequate hypertrophy. Calculation of wall stress from assessments of ventricular geometry, wall thickness, and pressure should show that afterload (wall stress) is abnormally high. This hypothesis has been tested in patients with severe aortic stenosis by Gunther and Grossman[26] and later by Carabello et al.[27] A tight negative correlation between ejection fraction and mean systolic circumferential stress was demonstrated. Patients with shortening which was less than predicted for the degree of afterload were thought to also have reduced contractility.

It may be quite important to differentiate between reduced contractility and inadequate hypertrophy. Three of four patients thought to have poor contractility and severe aortic stenosis died in the operative or perioperative period while the lone survivor had a poor functional result.[27] The patients with inadequate hypertrophy to account for reduced ejection fraction did well. These results need to be confirmed but appear to follow logically from our understanding of how the heart works in pressure overload.

A different approach has been utilized that estimates contractility directly. From high-fidelity pressure tracings, the first derivative of pressure with respect to time can be obtained (dP/dt). The theory that allows this type of index of contractility to be used is as follows.[1]

During isovolumic contraction, before the aortic valve opens, the myocardium is assumed to be contracting isometrically. Therefore, pressure and stress are linearly related and contractile element shortening will be linearly related to dP/dt/P. The maximum velocity of contractile element shortening at 0 load (V_{max}) is thought to reflect the intrinsic contractile state of the myocardium. Extrapolation back to 0 load can be avoided by selecting certain points on the curve relating dP/dt/P to P. Unfortunately, these indices of contractility have their limitations. The most important is that they fall as end-diastolic pressure increases, a common finding in severe pressure overload. Nevertheless, Mirsky et al were able to accurately predict postoperative ejection fraction in patients with aortic valve disease from $(dP/dt/P)_{max}$.[28] Huber et al used a similar index to study patients with aortic stenosis.[29] They found decreased contractility in 25 of 76 patients. Importantly, they concluded that decreased contractility in severe aortic stenosis was as important a contributor to poor ejection performance as inadequate hypertrophy with excessive afterload.

It is clear that we need a simple, reliable method for determining the contractile state of the ventricle in pressure overload. Ejection phase indices such as ejection fraction are simple to obtain (radioisotope or contrast left ventriculography) but are affected by inadequate hypertrophy. Isovolumic pressure indices require sophisticated intraventricular pressure transducers and are still subject to substantial criticism. Some might consider the precise quantification of ventricular contractility in severe aortic stenosis moot. Most patients will be symptomatic and will be offered surgery.[30] Nevertheless, as surgical techniques, myocardial preservation, and valvular prostheses continue to improve, it will be increasingly attractive to relieve outflow obstruction *before* irreversible damage to myocardial function has occurred. Simple techniques for tracking left ventricular contractility in pressure overload are not at hand.

ATRIAL CONTRIBUTION IN PRESSURE OVERLOAD

The adaptations of the atria to pressure overload have not been examined as thoroughly as those of the ventricles. We know only that the walls become thicker and dimensions are mildly increased. Hemodynamic changes related to atrial function are well characterized and are critical to circulatory homeostasis in pressure overload.[31,32] In animals with normal circulatory physiology, mean left atrial pressure and left ventricular end-diastolic pressure are not different by more than a few millimeters mercury over a wide range of filling pressures.[33] The significance of this finding is that loss of effective atrial contraction, eg, with atrial fibrillation or atrioventricular dissociation, will not markedly alter filling pressures or stroke volume providing heart rate is controlled. This is not true with left ventricular hypertrophy. Left ventricular end-diastolic pressure is consistently greater than mean left atrial pressure when atrial contraction (A-wave) assists in filling a functionally stiff left ventricle. The booster pump function of the left atrium in aortic stenosis therefore allows stroke volume to be generated at a much lower average atrial pressure than the increased LVEDP would require without atrial hypertrophy.

The critical role of atrial transport function in severe aortic stenosis is frequently evidenced by the sudden deterioration of patients with the onset of atrial fibrillation or junctional rhythm. At the instant atrial contraction is lost, LVEDP falls to approximately mean left atrial pressure. The loss of stroke volume may average 40%.[32] Circulatory homeostasis will attempt to be preserved by the usual mechanisms. Mean left atrial pressure will be increased to restore stroke volume. Unfortunately, the mean left atrial pressure necessary to maintain stroke volume will frequently lead to pulmonary congestion or edema. Ineffective increases in mean left atrial pressure may leave stroke volume and cardiac output low and result in hypotension.

DIFFERENCES BETWEEN RIGHT AND LEFT VENTRICULAR RESPONSES TO PRESSURE OVERLOAD

The responses of the right and left ventricle to pressure loading in the adult are clearly different. The right ventricle fails when pulmonary artery pressure reaches systemic levels in, for example, primary pulmonary hypertension or mitral stenosis. Transposition of the great arteries corrected by interatrial baffle procedures provides an example of right ventricular function in the presence of systemic pressures from birth. The right ventricle does not fail in this setting.[34] Nevertheless, right ventricular ejection fraction is mildly reduced and exercise function is abnormal. Patients with congenitally "corrected" transposition have similar deficits suggesting that the surgical procedure or preoperative hypoxic damage are not causative. When the right ventricle is loaded in utero, eg, with congenital pulmonic stenosis, right ventricular ejection fraction may be above normal in childhood despite suprasystemic pressures.[35] The disparate responses above suggest that the timing of right ventricular loading may determine importantly the functional outcome.

We can speculate why the timing of right ventricular loading might have an important effect on the ventricle's response. In utero, both hyperplasia and hypertrophy of myocytes affect growth of the ventricles.[36] After birth, systolic loading of the right ventricle normally drops (decreased pressure/volume ratio) while left ventricular loading increases (loss of low resistance placental circuit). It is assumed that the striking differences between postnatal right and

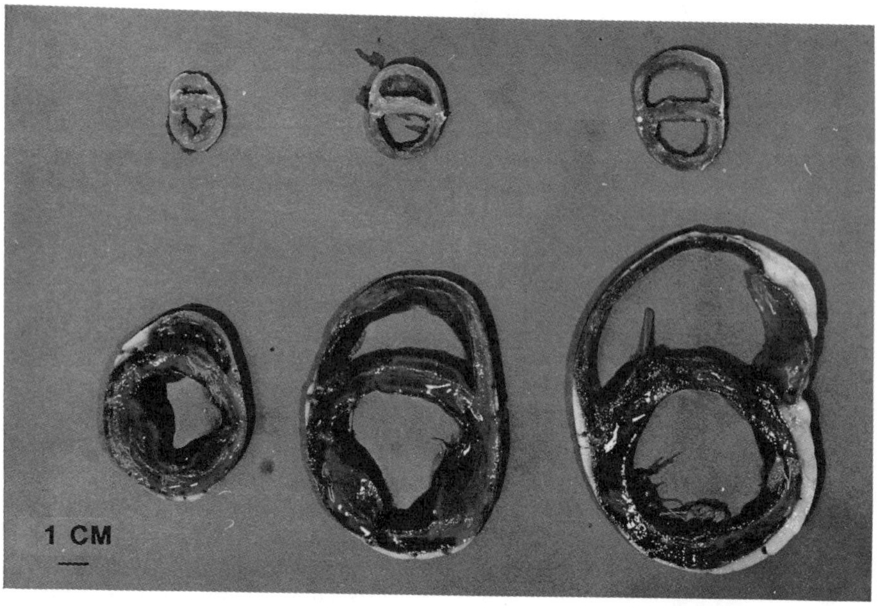

Figure 1-4 Cross sections of mature fetal (top) and adult (bottom) sheep hearts were taken at equidistant intervals along the major axis. The view is from the apex; anterior is to the left. The hearts were fixed following potassium arrest at 5 mmHg distending pressure in the fetal right and left ventricles and adult right ventricle. The adult left ventricle was maintained at 10 mmHg. The shapes of the fetal and adult ventricles are similar despite different in vivo loading conditions. The thickness of the fetal right and left ventricular free walls is the same reflecting the common arterial pressure facing the ventricles in utero. In the adult, the right ventricular (RV) free wall is relatively thin and the septum bulges into the RV cavity. (Specimens were provided by C. Wright Pinson, MD, Oregon Health Sciences University, Portland).

left ventricular masses are due to these changes in loading. In the rat, differential growth rates of the right and left ventricle in the postnatal period are achieved chiefly by greater myocyte division in the left than in the right ventricle.[37] Shortly, myocyte hyperplasia ceases and further enlargement of the ventricles occurs through hypertrophy. The left ventricular wall, then, is composed of both more and larger cells than the right ventricle as growth continues. Assuming that cell size is an important limiting factor in the hypertrophy process, the left ventricle will have a greater potential maximum mass than the right ventricle because of its greater number of cells. With equal geometry, the ventricle with the greater mass will be able to maintain performance at higher levels of systolic pressure.

The right ventricle may also be at a disadvantage because of its geometry. The anterior placement of the pulmonic valve and its separation from the tricuspid valve by the conus arteriosus gives the right ventricular free wall a much larger radius of curvature than the left ventricular free wall (Figure 1-4). Since the radius/wall thickness ratio will be an important determinant of function, even massive degrees of right ventricular hypertrophy may not allow the right ventricle to achieve the pressures generated in severe aortic stenosis. With these factors in mind, we can rationalize why the right ventricle in the adult responds poorly to pressure loading.

In contrast, the fetal ventricle retains the ability for hyperplasia. Perhaps congenital lesions such as pulmonic stenosis prepare the right ventricle in utero for the subsequent necessary increase in mass by stimulating a larger number of myocytes. Geometry might also be favorably affected. Volumetric analysis of children with pulmonic stenosis has shown reductions of right ventricular end-diastolic volume.[38] The capacity for adaptation to pressure loading might be intermediate at birth. At this time, some potential for hyperplasia and shape change might be present. The ability of the right ventricle to sustain systemic pressures after birth with transposition of the great arteries with only mild functional abnormalities is consistent with this hypothesis. The speculative nature of this discussion cannot be overemphasized. The need for more information in this interesting area is obvious.

REGRESSION OF HYPERTROPHY

Sudden relief of experimental aortic constriction might be comparable to valve replacement for severe aortic stenosis. In the animal model, the hypertrophied ventricle has supernormal function when faced with the sudden reduction in afterload.[6] Calculated wall stress falls to levels below normal. The stage is set for reversal of compensatory mechanisms. Elevated filling pressure drops because a lower preload will be needed to produce stroke volume. Hypertrophy might be reversed if low wall stress signals that process. Reversal of hypertrophy will further lower filling pressures by increasing r/h ratio.

Reversal of hypertrophy has been shown in multiple clinical and experimental studies of pressure loading and its relief. It is therefore taken for granted that unloading will cause regression of hypertrophy. Cooper and Tomanek have shown that even without previous hypertrophy, unloading ventricular muscle causes a rapid reduction in cell size.[39] Thus, cardiac muscle is in dynamic equilibrium determined largely by loading conditions.

To what extent will central hemodynamics and cardiac morphology return to normal after the relief of pressure overload? From experimentally induced pressure loading, we know that if unloading occurs before the onset of heart failure, hemodynamics and morphology return to normal.[40,41] This appears to be the case in the pediatric population relieved of severe pulmonic or aortic stenosis in childhood.[34] On the other hand, experimental animals with heart failure did not regain normal function and morphology. There appears to be a transition from reversible to less reversible cardiac change in pressure loading. This concept is easy to accept since the cardiac hypertrophy process is a normal, adaptive physiologic mechanism. The extent to which pathologic increases in intrinsic muscle stiffness and reduction of contractility relate to irreversibility of hypertrophy are unknown. Nevertheless, at the boundaries, we see that hearts with preserved function have complete regression of hypertrophy and those with obviously impaired function have residual abnormalities after unloading.

With human valve replacement for relief of obstruction, several other factors are operative. Probably the most important is myocardial preservation at the time of valve replacement. The thick, hypertrophied ventricle can ill afford additional ischemic insult or high oxygen demands associated with rapid heart rates, inotropic stimulation, or dilation. Nevertheless, the necessities of surgical practice may impose all of these stresses on myocardial integrity. The recent widespread adoption of hypothermic arrest of the ventricle during valve replacement appears to be a large step toward reducing myocardial damage. Continued research to improve myocardial preservation at surgery is necessary.

The effective areas of valve prostheses are substantially less than the normal valves they replace.[42] Accordingly, some patients will have mild to moderate obstruction to outflow after valve replacement. Although substantial improvement in this setting could be projected for patients with severe stenosis, complete regression of hypertrophy would be unlikely. Coronary artery disease, disease of other valves, or of the conduction system also may affect myocardial function after valve replacement and prevent a return to normal hemodynamics and morphology.

Unloading damaged ventricles is desirable even though normalization of hemodynamics or morphology may not be expected. Reduced afterload improves function despite residual abnormalities. Reduced filling pressure with improved cardiac output corroborates subjective functional improvement in these patients.[30,43] Nevertheless, poor surgical outcomes or death occur in patients with severe aortic stenosis and evidence of substantial myocardial dysfunction. Those patients with both low ejection fraction (< 0.25) and low gradients (< 25 mmHg) were at highest risk in the study of Carabello et al.[27]

REFERENCES

1. Braunwald E, Ross J Jr, Sonnenblick EH (eds): *Mechanisms of Contraction of the Normal and Failing Heart.* Boston, Little Brown & Co, 1976.
2. Weisfeldt ML, Armstrong P, Scully HE, et al: Incomplete relaxation between beats after myocardial hypoxia and ischemia. *J Clin Invest* 1974; 53:1626–1636.
3. Sonnenblick EH: Force-velocity relations in mammalian heart muscle. *Am J Physiol* 1962; 202:931–939.
4. Burns JW, Covell JW, Ross J Jr: Mechanics of isotonic left ventricular contractions. *Am J Physiol* 1973;224:725–732.
5. Ross J Jr: Afterload mismatch and preload reserve: A conceptual framework for the analysis of ventricular function. *Prog Cardiovas Dis* 1976; 28:255–264.
6. Sasayama S, Ross J Jr, Franklin D, et al: Adaptations of the left ventricle to chronic pressure overload. *Circ Res* 1976;38:172–178.
7. Sugo H, Sagawa K, Shoukas AA: Load independence of the instantaneous pressure–volume ratio of the canine left ventricle and effects of epinephrine and heart rate on the ratio. *Circ Res* 1973;32:314–322.
8. Wikman-Coffelt J, Parmley WW, Mason DT: The cardiac hypertrophy process: Analyses of factors determining pathological vs physiological development. *Circ Res* 1979;45:697–707.
9. Schreiber SS, Evans CD, Oratz M, et al: Protein synthesis and degredation in cardiac stress. *Cir Res* 1981;48:601–611.
10. Zak R: Cardiac hypertrophy: Biochemical and cellular relationships. *Hosp Pract* 1983;18:85–97.
11. Laks MM: Norepinephrine, the producer of myocardial cellular hypertrophy and/or necrosis and/or fibrosis. *Am Heart* J 1977;94:394–399.
12. Simpson P, McGrath A, Savion S: Myocyte hypertrophy in neonatal rat heart cultures and its regulation by serum and by catecholamines. *Circ Res* 1982;51:787–801.
13. Nichols JR, Clancy RL, Gonzalez NC: Role of adrenals on development of pressure-induced myocardial hypertrophy. *Am J Physiol* 1983;244 (suppl 13):244:H224–H238.
14. Mercadier JJ, Bouveret P, Gorza L, et al: Myosin isoenzymes in normal and hypertrophied human ventricular myocardium. *Circ Res* 1983;53:52–62.
15. Serizawa T, Mirsky I, Carabello BA, et al: Diastolic myocardial stiffness in gradually developing left ventricular hypertrophy in dog. *Am J Physiol* 1982;242 suppl 11:H633–H637.
16. Buckberg GD, Fixler DE, Archie JP, et al: Experimental subendocardial ischemia in dogs with normal coronary arteries. *Circ Res* 1972; 30:67–81.
17. Bishop SP, Melsen LR: Myocardial necrosis, fibrosis and DNA synthesis in experimental cardiac hypertrophy induced by sudden pressure overload. *Circ Res* 1976;39:238–245.
18. Glantz SA, Parmley WW: Factors which affect the diastolic pressure–volume curve. *Circ Res* 1980; 42:171–180.
19. Eickhorn P, Grimm J, Koch R, et al: Left ventricular relaxation in patients with left ventricular hypertrophy secondary to aortic valve disease. *Circulation* 1982;65:1395–1404.
20. Mirsky I: Assessment of passive elastic stiffness of cardiac muscle: Mathematical concepts, physiologic and clinical consideration, directions of future research. *Prog Cardiovas Dis* 1976; 18:277–308.
21. Peterson KL, Tsuji J, Johnson A, et al: Diastolic left ventricular pressure–volume and stress-strain relations in patients with valvular aortic stenosis and left ventricular hypertrophy. *Circulation* 1978; 58:77–89.
22. Hess OM Ritter M, Schneider, J, et al: Diastolic stiffness and myocardial structure in aortic valve disease before and after valve replacement. *Circulation* 1984;69:855–865.
23. Julian FJ, Morgan DL, Moss RL, et al: Myocyte growth without physiological impairment in gradually induced rat cardiac hypertrophy. *Circ Res* 1981;49:1300–1310.
24. Cheitlin MD, Gertz EW, Brundage BH, et al: Rate of progression of severity of valvular stenosis in the adult. *Am Heart J* 1979;98:689–700.
25. Wagner S, Selzer A: Patterns of progression of

aortic stenosis: A longitudinal hemodynamical study. *Circulation* 1982;65:709–712.
26. Gunther S, Grossman W: Determinants of ventricular function in pressure-overload hypertrophy in man. *Circulation* 1979;59:679–688.
27. Carabello BA, Green LH, Grossman W, et al: Hemodynamic determinants of prognosis of aortic valve replacement in critical aortic stenosis and advanced congestive heart failure. *Circulation* 1980;62:42–48.
28. Mirsky I, Henschke C, Hess OM, et al: Prediction of postoperative performance in aortic valve disease. *Am J Cardiol* 1981;48:295–303.
29. Huber D, Grimm J, Koch R, et al: Determinants of ejection performance in aortic stenosis. *Circulation* 1981;64:126–134.
30. Smith N, McAnulty JH, Rahimtoola SH: Severe aortic stenosis with impaired left ventricular function and clinical heart failure: Results of valve replacement. *Circulation* 1978;58:255–264.
31. Braunwald E, Frahm CJ: Studies on Starling's law of the heart IV. Observations on the hemodynamic function of the left atrium in man. *Circulation* 1961;24:633–642.
32. Stott DK, Marpole DGF, Bristow JD, et al: The role of left atrial transport in aortic and mitral stenosis. *Circulation* 1970;41:1031–1041.
33. Mitchell JH, Gilmore JP, Sarnoff SJ: The transport function of the atrium: factors influencing the relation between mean left atrial pressure and left ventricular end diastolic pressure. *Am J Cardiol* 1962;9:237–247.
34. Parrish MD, Graham TP, Bender HW, et al: Radionuclide angiographic evaluation of right and left ventricular function during exercise and after repair of transposition of the great arteries: comparison with normal subjects and patients with congenitally corrected transposition. *Circulation* 1983;67:178–183.
35. Graham TP: Ventricular performance in adults after operation for congenital heart disease. *Am J Cardiol* 1982;50:612–620.
36. Zak R, Kizer A, Bugaisky L: Cardiac hypertrophy: Its characteristics as a growth process. *Am J Cardiol* 1979;44:941–946.
37. Anserva P, Olivetti C, Loud AV: Morphometric study of early postnatal development in the left and right ventricular myocardium of the rat. *Circ Res* 1980;46:495–512.
38. Makoto N, Marks RA, Isabel-Jones J, et al: Right and left ventricular volume characteristics in children with pulmonary stenosis and intact ventricular septum. *Circulation* 1976;53:884–890.
39. Cooper G IV, Tomanek RJ: Load regulation of the structure, composition and function of mammalian myocardium. *Circ Res* 1982; 50:788–798.
40. Cooper G IV, Satava RM, Harrison CE, et al: Normal myocardial function and energetics after reversing pressure overload hypertrophy. *Am J Physiol* 1974;226:1158–1165.
41. Coulson RL, Yazdanfar S, Rubio E, et al: Recuperative potential of cardiac muscle following relief of pressure overload hypertrophy and right ventricular failure in the cat. *Circ Res* 1977; 40:41–49.
42. Rahimtoola SH: The problem of valve prosthesis-patient mismatch. *Circulation* 1978;58:20–24.
43. Pantely GA, Morton MJ, Rahimtoola SH: Effects of successful uncomplicated valve replacement on ventricular hypertrophy volume and performance in aortic stenosis and in aortic incompetence. *J Thorac Cardiovas Surg* 1978;75:383–391.

CHAPTER 2
Volume Overload: Effects on the Heart

Kirk L. Peterson

Volume overload of the heart is a pathophysiologic state and refers to a repetitive, beat-by-beat excess in filling volume at rest of one or more of the four cardiac chambers. The excess in filling volume is caused most commonly by leakage of an atrioventricular or semilunar valve but may also be a consequence of a congenital or acquired connection(s) between a left and right heart chamber, between the aorta and pulmonary artery, between the aorta and a right or left heart chamber, or between a large systemic artery and vein [Table 2-1]. An increase in absolute circulating blood volume, as observed in patients with morbid exogenous obesity, or the increase in cardiac chamber volumes seen in response to sustained exercise conditioning, might also be considered volume overload states by the above definition; however, the alterations in heart structure and function observed here are considered physiologic rather than pathophysiologic adaptations. Appropriate to the theme of this book, the primary emphasis in this chapter will be on the alterations seen with valvular lesions of the heart.

Table 2-1
Causes of Volume Overload (Chamber(s) Affected)

1. *Leakage of Atrioventricular or Semilunar Valves*
   a. Aortic regurgitation (LV)
   b. Mitral regurgitation (LV, LA)
   c. Pulmonic regurgitation (RV)
   d. Tricuspid regurgitation (RV, RA)
2. *Congenital or Acquired Connection(s) Between Left and Right Sides of Heart*
   a. Atrial septal defect (LA, RA, RV)
   b. Partial anomalous pulmonary veins (RA, RV)
   c. Ventricular septal defect (LV, LA, RV)
   d. Patent ductus arteriosus (LA, LV)
   e. Aortic sinus of Valsalva–right ventricular fistula (RV, LA, LV)
3. *Systemic Arteriovenous Fistula*
   a. Aortoinferior vena cava (RA, RV, LA, LV)

LV = left ventricle, LA = left atrium, RV = right ventricle, RA = right atrium

GROSS AND ULTRASTRUCTURAL ADAPTATIONS OF CARDIAC CHAMBER MORPHOLOGY TO VOLUME OVERLOAD

Of the four cardiac chambers, the left ventricle has been most extensively studied in relation to its adaptations to a volume overload state. This priority stems from its relative importance to maintenance of an adequate systemic cardiac output, its accessibility by both noninvasive and invasive techniques for functional assessment, and the ease with which it can be geometrically modeled. Study of the left atrium is facilitated by its elliptical shape and smooth borders, but it is relatively inaccessible for selective angiographic or echocardiographic measurements of its pressure and volume. Chamber pressure can be measured readily within the right ventricle, but its irregular geometric shape and indistinct endocardial borders inhibit accurate volume measurements. The right atrium again is accessible for pressure and volume measurements, but its physiologic importance to maintenance of cardiac output is small compared to the function of the left-sided cardiac chambers.

Volume overload of a cardiac chamber gives rise to an increase in chamber work (the integral of instantaneous developed pressure × stroke volume) due primarily to an increase in stroke volume. Enlargement of cardiac myocytes (hypertrophy) is noted as a consequence, although the exact stimulus to this morphologic adaptation is not fully understood. It is now well accepted that hypertrophy serves to maintain afterload (forces resisting shortening or wall stress) within relatively normal limits and to preserve a normal extent of chamber shortening per unit of internal chamber circumference.

For the left ventricle the pattern of hypertrophy for a volume overload state is characterized by preservation of the ratio of wall thickness to radius (or mass to volume) despite the significant increase in chamber size. This pattern of increased myocardial mass has come to be known as "eccentric" hypertrophy since the heart enlarges to the left in the overall thorax, thus becoming eccentric with respect to other structures of the chest. By comparison, pressure-overload hypertrophy is notable for a normal or slightly reduced end-diastolic volume, an increase in the ratio of wall thickness to chamber radius, and no appreciable increase in the eccentricity of the heart within the thorax. This pattern is commonly referred to as "concentric" hypertrophy. In either type of hypertrophy the stimulus(i) which initiates and perpetuates the increase in muscle mass and myofiber size is unknown. Protein synthesis is known to be quite sensitive to hemodynamic conditions, but the biochemical links between increased chamber work and synthesis of contractile protein remain obscure. Moreover, little is understood about the mechanisms by which hypertrophy regresses once a pathologic loading state is relieved (see below).

Left Ventricle

As the left ventricle is subjected to a volume overload, progressive dilatation or an increase in the end-diastolic volume occurs irrespective of the underlying cause. In the two relevant valvular lesions (mitral or aortic regurgitation) there are some differences in the geometric remodeling of the chamber; with mitral valve leakage, the normally elliptical chamber assumes a more spherical shape whereas with aortic valve leakage the enlarged left ventricle retains a relatively normal elliptical shape until decompensation occurs.[1–4] Despite these differences in geometry, the modest initial increase in size in acute volume overload is thought to be caused by the Frank-Starling mechanism with an increase in sarcomere end-diastolic stretch from approximately 1.9 to 2.1–2.2 μm. An increase in sarcomere length of this magnitude is not sufficient to account for a two- to threefold increase in end-diastolic volume as is commonly noted in *chronic* mitral or aortic regurgitation. Other adaptations must occur which involve either reorientation of myofibers, myofiber slippage, or serial replication of sarcomeres. Based on animal models of left ventricular volume overload, it appears that all three of the latter mechanisms are operative.[5–7]

Using a large aortoinferior vena caval shunt to create a volume load on all four cardiac chambers, it has been shown that the myocardial fibers lose their predominant minor axis circumferential orientation and shift toward a more longitudinal direction. This shift in the fundamental fiber orientation contrasts with that seen in a pressure overload state where the left ventricular wall thickens proportionately more and fiber angles do not apparently shift as long as the ventricular chamber does not dilate.

Along with fiber orientation, there also is rather convincing experimental evidence that the increase in size and length of myofibers in chronic volume overload is due at least in part to sarcomere slippage. As shown in Figure 2-1, volume overloaded dog hearts (with end-diastolic volume measurements approximately twice control and which were potassium-arrested to insure diastolic arrest) demonstrated maintenance of sarcomere lengths of 2.2 μm, but loss of Z-line registry by electron microscopy, ie, myofiber slippage.[7] Biopsies of volume-overloaded human hearts, taken at the time of cardiac surgery, can likewise show loss of organized sarcomere orientation, although the random time of the cardiac cycle during which the biopsies are taken makes the phenomena of sarcomere and myofiber slippage difficult to assess.

Left Atrium

During either chronic mitral or aortic regurgitation, there is noted an increase in the overall size (volume) of the left atrium. With leakage of the mitral valve this is secondary to an increase in systolic filling (antegrade and retrograde) from the pulmonary veins and left ventricle, respectively, as well as to increased resistance to diastolic filling of the left ventricle. By contrast, in aortic valve leakage the left atrium itself does not receive an augmented amount of blood during ventricular systole, but, nevertheless, the chamber dilates and exhibits an increase in both active and passive extent of shortening. Pre-

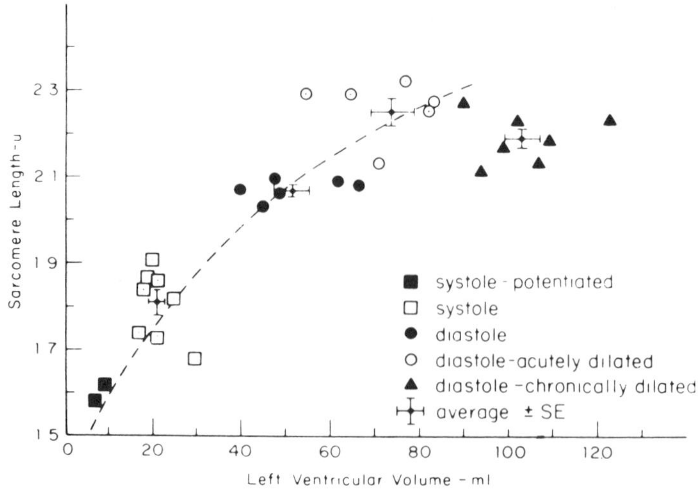

Figure 2-1A Plot of sarcomere length (μm) *v* left ventricular volume (mL) in normal canine left ventricle arrested in systole (squares), normal diastole (solid circles), after acute dilatation (open circles), and after chronic dilatation (closed triangles). Volume overload was created by a large arteriovenous shunt. Reproduced with permission of the authors and the American Heart Association.[7]

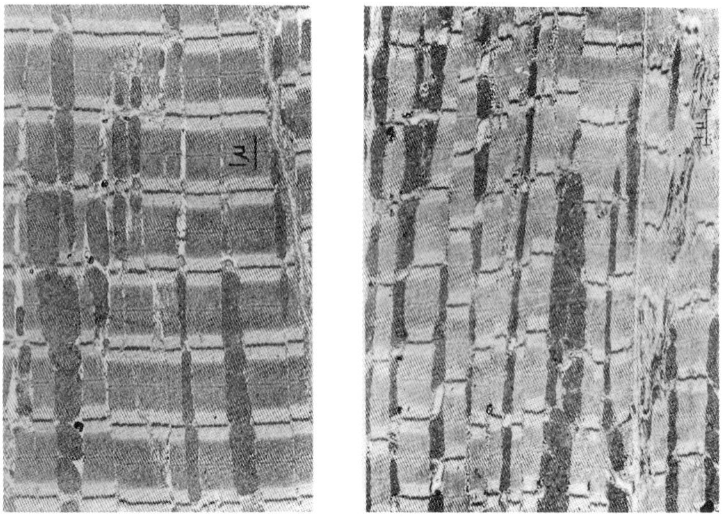

B Electron photomicrographs of a normal diastolic canine left ventricle fixed acutely at an elevated end-diastolic pressure (left), and a chronically dilated diastolic left ventricle (right). Note that with chronic dilatation there is loss of Z-line registry (myofibril slippage) and elongation and angulation of the transverse tubular system. Reproduced with permission of the authors and the American Heart Association.[7]

sumably, the stimulus to left atrial dilatation is related to the diastolic properties of the left ventricle and the resistance to filling which the left atrium encounters once the mitral valve opens.[8] That the left atrium can increase its overall extent of shortening in response to acute volume loading has been demonstrated in the instrumented dog.[9,10]

Usually, the left atrium, as it enlarges in response to a volume overload of the left heart, remains relatively spherical. The mechanisms which explain the overall increase in chamber size are not well defined, although presumably there is again stretching of elastic elements in the wall, replication of sarcomeres, and a certain amount of myofiber rearrangement.

Right Ventricle, Right Atrium

The right ventricle and right atrium also dilate in response to isolated volume overload of the right heart, eg, tricuspid regurgitation, pulmonic regurgitation. The percentage increase in right ventricular size can be comparable to that seen with lesions affecting the left side of the heart. Similarly, tricuspid regurgitation can give rise to a massively dilated right atrial chamber. It is of interest that a pressure or volume overload imposed on the right ventricle from birth stimulates growth of the right ventricular comparable to that of the left ventricle and signs of right ventricular failure seldom appear. If, on the other hand, a mature right ventricle is subjected to a volume or pressure overload, the performance of the chamber is less assured. It seems that with age the right ventricular myocardium loses some of its capacity to hypertrophy, becomes remarkably sensitive to afterload, and exhibits a reduced extent of shortening in the face of this increased load.

MYOCARDIAL CONTRACTILITY AND VOLUME-OVERLOAD HYPERTROPHY

Extensive investigations have been carried out both in isolated muscle and the whole heart in an effort to understand the effects of both concentric and eccentric hypertrophy on myocardial function. Early studies of cat papillary muscles harvested from the right ventricle 6 weeks after pulmonary artery banding suggested that pressure-overload hypertrophy was associated with depression of contractility.[11] A subsequent investigation, using a nearly identical protocol but harvesting the papillary muscle after 24 weeks, suggested that contractility had recovered.[12] By contrast, papillary muscle studies in experimental animals exposed to various types of relatively acute volume overload, eg, aortocaval fistula, aortic regurgitation, mitral regurgitation, atrial septal defect, have suggested that myocardial contractility remains normal in the face of a relatively acute volume overload.[13–15]

The effects of various types of volume overload on isovolumic and ejection phase indices of left ventricular myocardial contractility have been studies extensively. Isovolumic indices (peak dP/dt, V_{max}, peak V_{ce},) are limited by a significantly shortened period of isovolumic contraction in either of the two common volume overload lesions, mitral or aortic regurgitation. For example, peak dP/dt, a measure independent of an assumed muscle model, did not appear to change appreciably as the left ventricle adapted over 4 weeks to acutely imposed mitral regurgitation in the awake, instrumented dog (Figure 2-2). Over this same time period, while the left ventricular regurgitant fraction equaled 0.40 to 0.50 and the end-diastolic volume increased progressively, the ejection fraction increased significantly.

Similarly, when ejection phase dynamics were studied in the instrumented dog before and after production of a fistula between the aorta and inferior vena cava, resulting in progressive left ventricular dilatation and moderate left ventricular hypertrophy without clinical evidence of heart failure, the length-active tension relation remained essentially normal. Following chronic adjustment to the shunt, the mean velocity of circumferential fiber shortening usually remained normal, although in some dogs with very large shunts and signs of congestive heart failure, this index became depressed.[16]

These findings have been taken to indicate that the development of eccentric hypertrophy (sarcomeres added in both parallel and in series with maintenance of a normal ratio of wall thickness to radius or mass to volume) allows the volume-overload heart to deliver an increased stroke volume at a normal level of contractility using a normal extent of shortening of each individual sarcomere. The increase in number of sarcomeres, in addition to the use of reserve preload at the sarcomere level, allows the delivery of more external work. Thus, there is little evidence to support the notion that a relatively acute or subacute volume overload of the left ventricle is associated with depression of myocardial contractility.

In man, however, long-standing mitral or aortic regurgitation is not infrequently associated with depressed left ventricular function which is irreversible and worsens post correction of the valve leakage.[17,18] Moreover, identification of depressed myocardial contractility preoperatively can be problematic due to the complex afterload conditions which are operative during mitral or aortic regurgitation.[15] Patients with mitral regurgitation may have a deceptively high left ventricular ejection fraction due to the

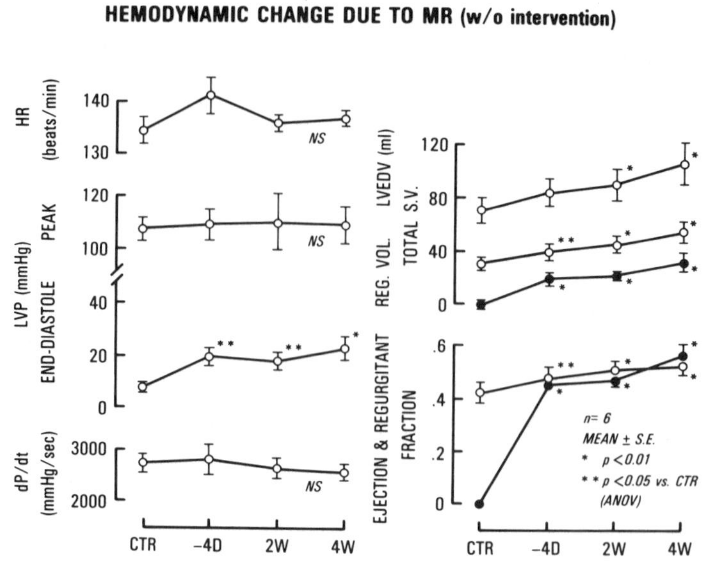

Figure 2-2 Plot of hemodynamic changes (HR = heart rate, LVP = left ventricular pressure, dP/dt = peak first derivative of LVP, LVEDV = left ventricular end-diastolic volume, S.V. = stroke volume, reg. vol. = regurgitant volume) before (CTR) and sequentially thereafter from four days to 4 weeks after induction of mitral regurgitation (MR) in chronically instrumented dogs. See text for discussion.

enhanced unloading into the left atrium and pulmonary veins where impedance to ejection is low. Similarly, in aortic regurgitation, the left ventricle begins to eject into the aorta at a relatively lower pressure, again providing some measure of unloading to the ventricle compared to the normal physiologic state. Thus, it is recognized that a normal ejection fraction may be observed in the presence of significant, long-standing mitral or aortic valvular regurgitation despite impairment of the contractile state. Once the ejection fraction or mean velocity of circumferential fiber shortening becomes depressed, despite the favorable afterload conditions, one can then assume that myocardial contractility is depressed.

The challenge in aortic or mitral regurgitation is to devise constructs which allow appreciation of depressed contractility before the traditional extent and speed of shortening indices become abnormal. In recent years, Suga et al[19] and Sagawa[20] in the isolated heart, Mahler et al[21] in the instrumented dog, and Grossman et al[22] in man have described the utility of the end-systolic pressure–volume and stress-volume relations as unique descriptors of myocardial contractility independent of the effects of preload and encompassing the effects of afterload. Under experimental conditions, as the preload, or end-diastolic volume, of the left ventricle increases over a physiologic range in response to an increase in afterload, the chamber ejects down to an end-systolic pressure–volume coordinate which is either upon or very close to a linear relation (Figure 2-3A). This function can be described by its slope (E_{max}) and volume intercept at a pressure of zero (V_o). Similarly, if end-diastolic volume, or preload, is held constant and afterload is acutely augmented, left ventricular percent shortening (ejection fraction) diminishes until ultimately an isovolumetric contraction occurs (Figure 2-3B). The end-systolic pressure–volume coordinates continue to fall on a linear relation. However, if myocardial contractility increases acutely, the linear end-systolic pressure–volume relation shifts upward (V_o decreases) and the slope steepens (E_{max} increases). Conversely, as contractility diminishes acutely, the end-systolic relation shifts downward and to the right (V_o increases, E_{max} decreases) (Figure 2-3C). During *chronic* changes in systolic loading conditions, eg aortic valvular stenosis, the ventricular wall hypertrophies: under these circumstances systolic pressure is no longer an accurate reflection of afterload, and it is necessary to assess the end-systolic relation using a stress-volume, rather than a pressure–volume, loop.

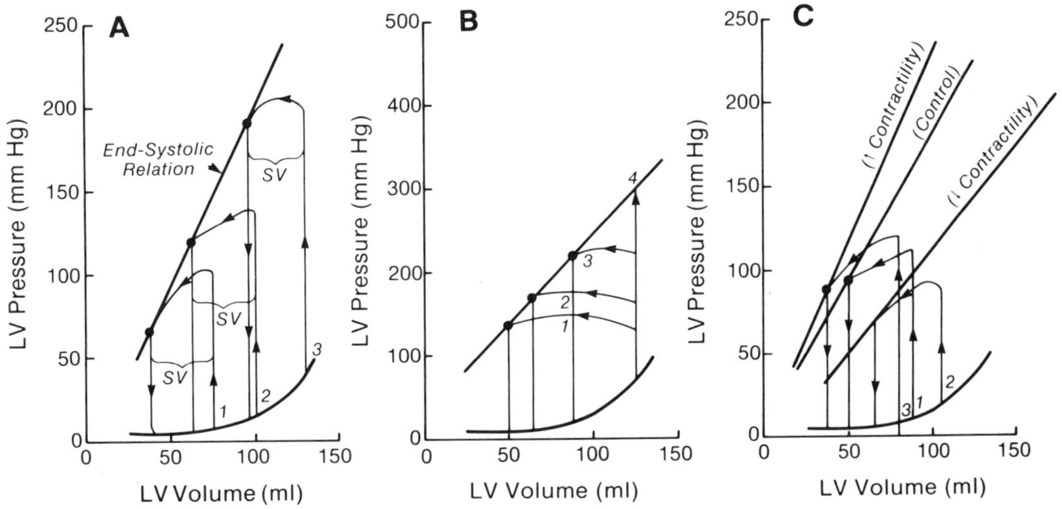

Figure 2-3A Diagrammatic left ventricular pressure–volume loops demonstrating the mechanical response of the chamber to a progressive increase in afterload. Note that end-diastolic volume (preload) increases progressively from beat 1 to beat 3, and the end-systolic pressure–volume coordinates fall along a linear relationship described by its pressure zero intercept (V_o) and its slope (E_{max}).

B Diagrammatic left ventricular pressure–volume loops demonstrating the mechanical response of the chamber when end-diastolic pressure is held constant and the afterload is progressively increased from beat 1 to beat 3. Note that the end-systolic pressure–volume coordinates continue to fall along a linear relationship until the ventricle contracts in an isovolumic fashion (beat 4).

C Diagrammatic left ventricular pressure–volume loops demonstrating the shift in the end-systolic relationship as myocardial contractility is increased from beat 1 to beat 3, and, conversely, is decreased from beat 1 to beat 2. See text for further discussion.

Several investigators have now analyzed the end-systolic pressure–volume relation (ESPVR) and end-systolic stress-volume relation (ESSVR) and their predictive value for determining post-operative myocardial function in patients with volume overload of the left ventricle. Carabello et al[23] applied a measurement of the ratio of end-systolic wall stress (ESWS) to end-systolic volume index (ESVI, normalized to body surface area) in 21 patients with chronic mitral regurgitation as compared to normal subjects. The ESWS/ESVI ratio in normal persons was 5.6 ± 0.9; a smaller ratio indicated progressively worse left ventricular function reflecting an ever larger end-systolic volume for any given afterload. Four of five patients with mitral regurgitation and ESWS/ESVI values less than or equal to 2.2 died postoperatively, and the fifth did not improve his clinical or functional status. Conversely, all those patients with a ratio greater than 2.5 exhibited a favorable outcome to mitral valve surgery. The end-systolic volume index alone did not differ significantly between these subgroups of patients with mitral regurgitation. Thus, it appeared that a reduction in the end-systolic stress measurement was the primary determinant of the reduction in the ESWS/ESVI ratio. While the predictive value of the ESWS/ESVI ratio was apparent in these patients, it should be appreciated that the measured ratio is only one point on a continuum of end-systolic pressure–volume coordinates and is not the same as E_{max} or the slope of the true end-systolic relation as investigated by Suga et al[19] and Sagawa.[20]

We have analyzed the evolution of the left ventricular ESWS/ESV ratio in the chronically instrumented dog (dimensional sonomicrometers, micromanometer gauge, aortic flow probe) over the first 4 weeks after creation of acute mitral regurgitation. While end-systolic stress slowly diminishes, the end-systolic volume progressively increases, and the ratio thus becomes incrementally smaller. In the same animals use of angiotensin II to increase, and nitroprusside to decrease, left ventricular afterload has allowed determination of the slopes of the ESPVR and ESSVR as well as the extrapolated volume at zero force (V_o) (Figure 2-4A). Both the ESPVR and ESSVR showed progressive reduction in slope and an operational shift to

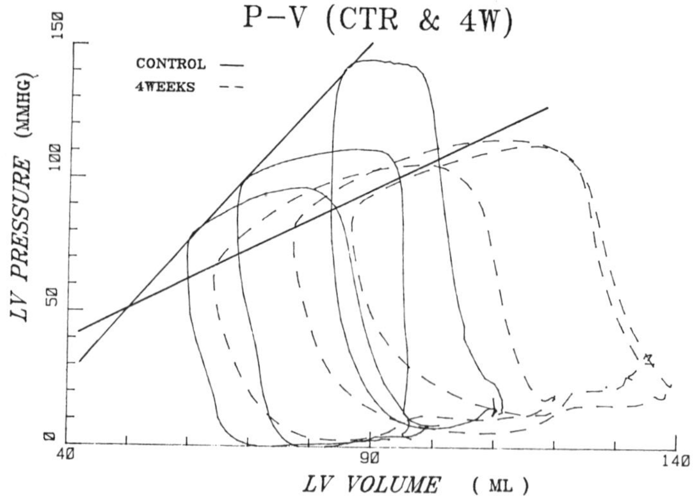

Figure 2-4A Pressure-volume loops at control and 4 weeks after induction of mitral regurgitation in awake, instrumented dogs. To obtain variations in afterload, animal was administered angiotensin II and nitroprusside. End-systolic pressure–volume relation was determined by connecting points of maximal elastance (maximum ratio of pressure to volume).

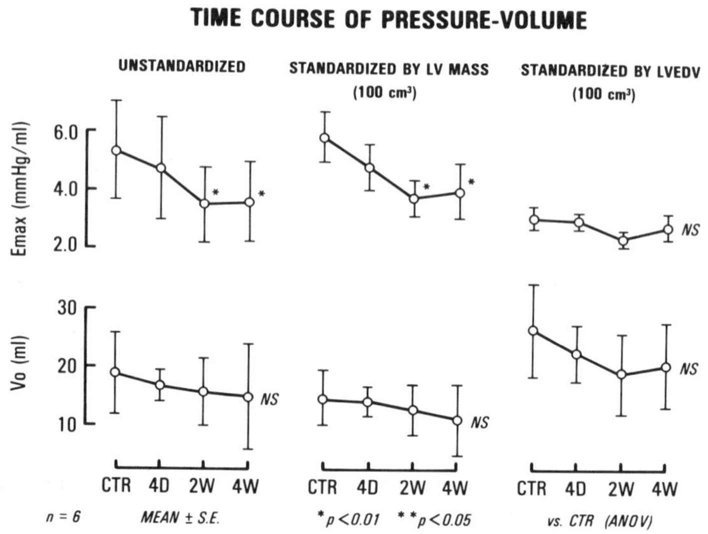

B Analysis of E_{max} (slope of end-systolic pressure–volume relation) and V_o (extrapolated volume at zero pressure) in six dogs before and after induction of mitral regurgitation. CTR = control, ANOV = analysis of variance.

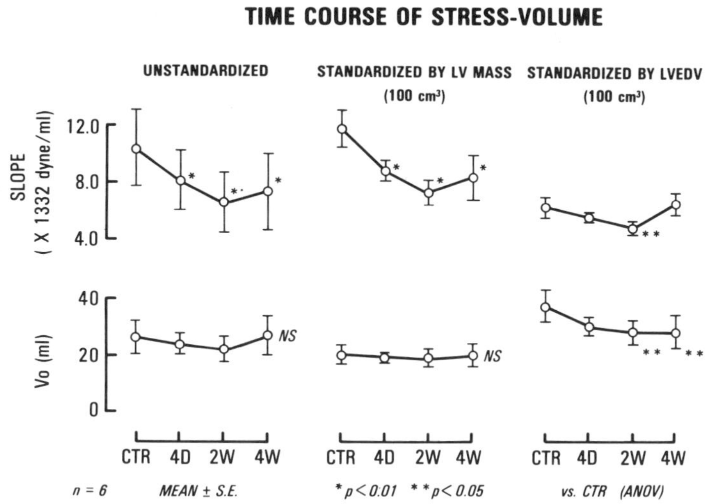

C Analysis of slope of end-systolic stress-volume relation and V_0 (extrapolated volume at zero force) in same six dogs as in Figure 2-4B.

the right while peak dP/dt, ejection fraction, and mean velocity of circumferential shortening remained constant or increased.

The progressive shift to the right of the ESSVR during acute mitral regurgitation in these dogs is explicable both by a diminution in basal end-systolic stress as well as an increase in end-systolic volume. The initial decrease in end-systolic stress (as compared to control) is undoubtedly secondary to low impedance conditions in the left atrium, ie, the left ventricle unloads at a more rapid rate, albeit over an extended period of time, with end-systolic pressure diminishing while end-systolic volume remains constant. However, after 1 week of mitral regurgitation end-systolic stress remains constant and the progressive increase thereafter in end-systolic volume appears to determine the shift of the end-systolic relation to the right.

Thus, the observations in this animal model of left ventricular volume overload indicates that the end-systolic relations are sensitive to the myocardial adaptations occurring in response to acutely imposed mitral regurgitation. To what extent the rightward shift of the relation reflects a reduction in basal contractility (as might be deduced from isolated heart experiments), as opposed to a direct consequence of eccentric hypertrophy, remains conjectural. Serial replication of sarcomeres and fiber slippage could conceivably lead to a larger end-systolic volume for any given stress even though each sarcomere continued to exhibit the same percentage of shortening. In fact, in the above-cited animal experiment, if the slopes of the end-systolic relations are standardized to an index of the number of sarcomeres (eg, end-diastolic volume), a shift to the right in the relation was no longer detected (Figure 2-4B and C).

While providing insight into the effects of acute volume overloading on the left ventricle, animal models, such as the one cited above, will likely never reproduce the pathophysiologic changes occurring over a span of many years in the chronic volume overload states encountered in man. Nevertheless, it seems clear that caution must be exercised in interpreting changes in the end-systolic relation as indicative of depressed myocardial contractility in patients being considered for mitral or aortic valve replacement. That the end-systolic dimensions of well-trained professional athletes are observed to be increased supports the notion that physiologic or adaptive hypertrophy may cause the end-systolic relations to shift rightward.[24] It seems clear that "normal" ranges for the end-systolic pressure–volume and stress-volume relations must be established for the chronically volume-overloaded ventricle with normal contractility.

DIASTOLIC COMPLIANCE AND LEFT VENTRICULAR VOLUME OVERLOAD

Since the early years of use of cardiac catheterization and angiography to study patients with compensated, chronic volume overload states of the left ventricle, it has been noted that the mean pulmonary arterial wedge pressure and the left ventricle end-diastolic pressure often remain within the normal range (< 12 mmHg) despite a two- to threefold increase in end-diastolic volume. It has been inferred from these measurements that the ventricle undergoes "muscle creep" to explain a rightward shift in the passive pressure–volume curve. Similarly, substantial shifts in the diastolic pressure–volume curve of the left ventricle can be demonstrated experimentally during sustained volume loading by means of a large arteriovenous fistula between the aorta and inferior vena cava. In these dogs, a full range of coordinates relating end-diastolic pressure to end-diastolic volume was obtained by acute transfusion and bleeding both before and many weeks after chronic cardiac dilatation had occurred. Although the total curve was shifted along the volume axis to the right, the actual *slope* of the curve was steeper indicating that operational or instantaneous chamber compliance (dV/dP) was decreased[25] (Figure 2-5). Such a comparison of the relative operational range of the left ventricle along its intrinsic pressure–volume curve highlights the importance of normalizing for ventricular size and estimating the pressure at the zero volume intercept.

When studying the distensibility properties of the left ventricle, it is important to recognize the distinction between chamber and muscle compliance. Chamber compliance refers to distensibility properties dictated not only by the intrinsic elasticity of the myocardium but also by its mass (greater force needed to move a thickened wall). Muscle compliance, on the other hand, refers to the intrinsic resistance to stretch of each unit of muscle. In the intact heart, chamber compliance is assessed by the pressure–volume curve: muscle compliance is assessed by modeling a length of myocardium along a given vector, eg, minor axis circumference, and calculating the stress-strain properties of the wall itself. In the relatively few studies published thus far in valvular heart disease, it is apparent that chamber and muscle compliance do not always change proportionately. In fact, in pressure overload secondary to aortic stenosis, chamber compliance can be quite abnormal secondary to the effects of increased muscle mass alone while the intrinsic stiffness of the wall itself remains normal.[26]

Recently Hess et al have published the most comprehensive analysis yet undertaken in man of the diastolic properties of the left ventricle in both pressure and volume overload states related to aortic stenosis and regurgitation.[27] Left ventricular chamber and myocardial stiffness were evaluated with the use of viscoelastic pressure-circumference and viscoelastic stress-strain relationships, respectively, since previous studies (animal models and man) had demonstrated deviations from a monoexponential curve during early diastolic filling and atrial systole. Moreover, Hess et al[27] correlated their mechanical

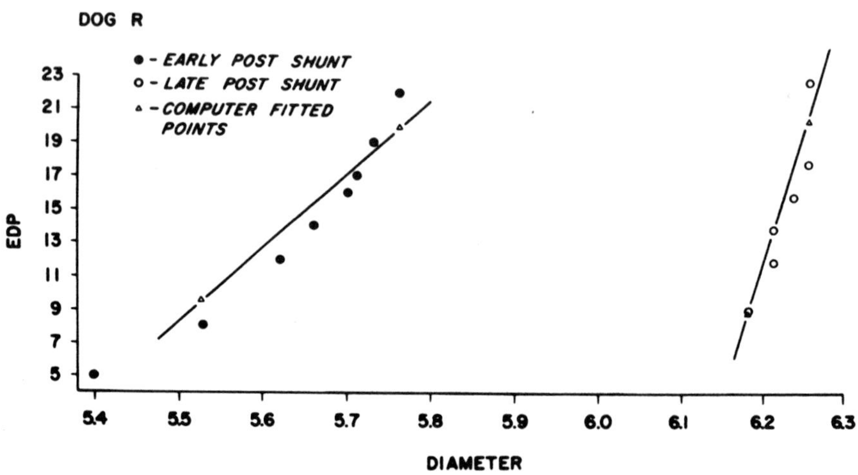

Figure 2-5 Plot of the relation between left ventricular end-diastolic pressure (EDP) and minor axis diameter 1 week after creation of an anteriovenous fistula (closed circles) and later at 12 weeks (open circles). The data points at each time frame are fitted to a linear relation: note the shift to the right of the relation after chronic adaptation as well as the compliance). See text for further discussion. (Reproduced with permission from McCullagh et al and the American Heart Association.[25])

analysis with endomyocardial biopsies taken at the time of cardiac catheterization. They found that the constant of chamber stiffness was slightly although not significantly increased in patients with aortic stenosis, normal in those with combined aortic stenosis and insufficiency, and slightly decreased in those with aortic regurgitation. In the latter group, the end-diastolic volume index averaged 217 mL/m^2, or approximately 2½ times their control patients. Interestingly, the reference midwall circumference at a wall isostress of 1 gm/cm^2 was increased in patients with aortic insufficiency compared to the control group and remained elevated even after correction of the volume overload by aortic valve replacement. These observations would confirm the rightward shift of the pressure–volume and stress-strain relationships for the left ventricle during volume loading. However, they would also suggest that (1) there is no obligatory decrease in either chamber or muscle compliance as a result of this shift, and (2) after correction of the volume overload there is not a complete reversion of the diastolic pressure–volume or stress-strain curves to their original coordinates.

The rightward shift of the diastolic curve during volume overload and eccentric hypertrophy can be explained on the basis of more sarcomeres being laid down in series where each sarcomere unit maintains a normal stiffness (or compliance) constant. However, in some instances, again as shown by the biopsies of Hess et al[26,27], myocardial fibrosis can become prominent in some patients and lead to an increase in both chamber and muscle stiffness in the postoperative state.

REGRESSION OF MYOCARDIAL ADAPTATIONS FOLLOWING RELIEF OF VOLUME OVERLOAD

As operative techniques and mortality statistics for corrective valve surgery have improved, there has been a concomitant interest in improved understanding of the reversibility of the myocardial adaptations and dysfunction which attend mitral or aortic regurgitation. Specifically, a number of investigators have asked: (1) Does left ventricular mass return toward or into the normal range after relief of a volume overload? (2) If myocardial contractility is depressed preoperatively, does this dysfunction persist after surgery? (3) To what extent is the increase in size of the left ventricle reversible after relief of mitral or aortic regurgitation? (4) Are the alterations in diastolic properties of the left ventricle reversible? (5) How do the functional changes noted postoperatively relate to gross and ultrastructural morphology? All of these questions bear importantly on the issue of timing of valve surgery for relief of a long-standing volume

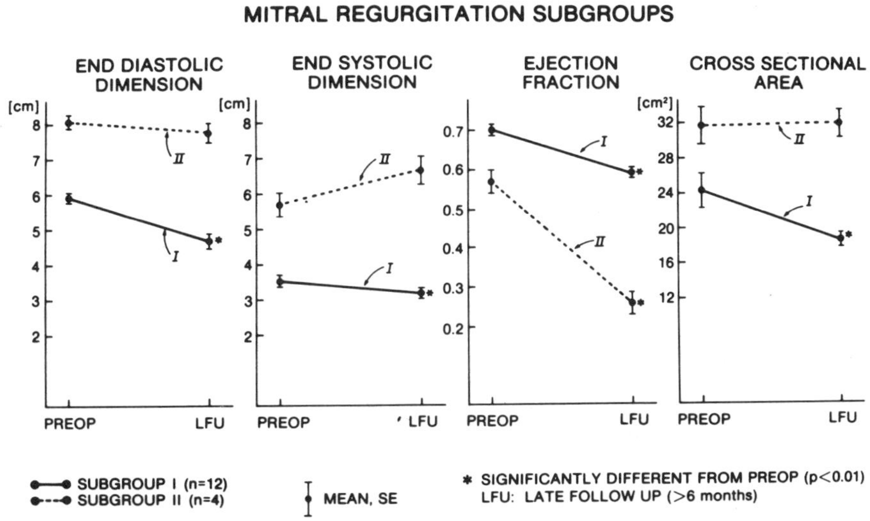

Figure 2-6 Subgroups of patients with chronic mitral regurgitation: comparison of preoperative (PREOP) and late follow-up (LFU) values (> 6 months) for M-mode echocardiographic left ventricular end-diastolic diameter, end-systolic diameter, ejection fraction, and minor axis cross-sectional area of myocardium.[18] (Reproduced with permission from Schuler et al and the American Heart Association.)

overload. Unfortunately, only a limited amount of information is presently available from either experimental or clinical studies.

Experimental pathologic models in either the dog or cat have suggested that myocardial hypertrophy related to either administration of thyroxine or a pressure-overload lesion (aortic obstruction, hypertension) is nearly or totally reversible. In the case of hyperthyroidism, as the stimulus to hypertrophy was removed, papillary muscle function remained mildly depressed suggesting residual ultrastructural or biochemical abnormalities.[28–31] By contrast, after relief of hypertension or obstruction to left ventricular outflow, myocardial mass regresses significantly: analysis of myocardial mechanics in animals with experimental aortic stenosis suggests that myocardial contractility and function remain normal.

A number of experimental and clinical studies have indicated that correction of a volume overload lesion is usually associated with regression of left ventricular hypertrophy.[32–35] For example, as shown in Figure 2-6, we have shown that patients with mitral regurgitation demonstrate progressive reduction in the cross-sectional area of the left ventricle (measured by M-mode echocardiography) over the first 6 months after correction of their leak. However, some patients, particularly those with very large end-diastolic and systolic dimensions, failed to demonstrate this regression and, in fact, showed marked worsening of function as the low impedance leak was eliminated. It is obvious that there is a need for greater understanding of the reversibility of the functional and structural adaptations of the myocardium in volume overload lesions. Unfortunately, there is presently no documentation that there can be complete "normalization" of the ESPVR and ESSVR and a shift of the diastolic pressure–volume curve back toward its original values. A very important area of future research will be the determination of the reversibility of the functional and ultrastructural myocardial adaptations associated with a volume overload. The degree to which these adaptations are reversible will have important bearing on clinical decision-making and the timing of corrective valve surgery.

REFERENCES

1. Vokonas PS, Gorlin R, Cohn PF, et al: Dynamic geometry of the left ventricle in mitral regurgitation. *Circulation* 1973;48:786–796.
2. Fischl SJ, Gorlin R, Herman MV: Cardiac shape and function in aortic valve disease: physiologic and clinical implications. *Am J Cardiol* 1977; 39:170–176.
3. Abdulla AM, Frank MJ, Canedo MI, et al: Limitations of echocardiography in the assessment of left ventricular size and function in aortic regurgitation. *Circulation* 1980;61:148–155.
4. Gould KL, Lipscomb K, Hamilton GW, et al: Relationship of left ventricular shape, function and wall stress in man. *Am J Cardiol* 1974; 34:627–634.
5. Sonnenblick EH, Ross J Jr, Covell JW, et al: Ultrastructure of the heart in systole and diastole. *Circ Res* 1967;21:423.
6. Yoran C, Covell JW, Ross J Jr: Structural basis for the ascending limb of left ventricular function. *Circ Res* 1973;32:297–303.
7. Ross J Jr, Sonnenblick EH, Taylor RR, et al: Diastolic geometry and sarcomere lengths in the chronically dilated canine left ventricle. *Circ Res* 1971;28:49–61.
8. Gabathuler J, Barghava V, Krayenbuehl HP, et al: Left atrial function in aortic valve disease. *J Am Coll Cardiol* 1983;1:640.
9. Payne RM, Stone HL, Engelken FJ: Atrial function during volume loading. *J Appl Physiol* 1971; 31:326–331.
10. Sasayama S, Takahashi M, Osakada G, et al: Dynamic geometry of the left atrium and left ventricle in acute mitral regurgitation. *Circulation* 1979;60:177–186.
11. Spann JF Jr, Buccion RA, Sonnenblick EH, et al: Contractile state of cardiac muscle obtained from cats with experimentally produced ventricular hypertrophy and heart failure. *Circ Res* 1967; 21:341–354.
12. Williams JF Jr, Potter RD: Normal contractile state of hypertrophied myocardium following pulmonary artery constriction in the cat. *J Clin Invest* 1974;54:1266–1272.
13. Turina M, Bussman WD, Krayenbuehl HP: Contractility of hypertrophied canine heart in chronic volume overload. *Cardiovasc Res* 1969;3:486–495.
14. Cooper G, Puga F, Zujko KJ, et al: Normal myocardial function and energetics in volume-overload hypertrophy in the cat. *Circ Res* 1973; 32:140–148.
15. Urschel CW, Covell JW, Sonnenblick EH, et al: Myocardial mechanics in aortic and mitral valvular regurgitation. The concept of instantaneous impedance as a determinant of the performance of the intact heart. *J Clin Invest* 1968;47:867–883.
16. Ross J Jr, McCullagh WH: The nature of enhanced performance of the dilated left ventricle during chronic volume overloading. *Circ Res* 1972; 30:549–556.
17. Gault JH, Covell JW, Braunwald E, et al: Left ventricular performance following correction of free aortic regurgitation. *Circulation* 1970; 42:773–780.
18. Schuler G, Peterson KL, Johnson A, et al: Temporal response of left ventricular performance to mitral valve surgery. *Circulation* 1979; 59:1218–1231.

19. Suga H, Sagawa K, Shoukas AA: Load independence of the instantaneous pressure–volume ratio of the canine left ventricle and effects of epinephrine and heart rate on the ratio. *Circ Res* 1973;32:314–322.
20. Sagawa K: The end-systolic pressure–volume relation of the ventricle: definition, modifications and clinical use. *Circulation* 1981; 63:1223–1227.
21. Mahler F, Covell JW, Ross J Jr: Systolic pressure-diameter relations in the normal conscious dog. *Cardiovasc Res* 1975;9:447–454.
22. Grossman W, Braunwald F, Mann T, et al: Contractile state of the left ventricle in man as evaluated from end-systolic pressure–volume relations. *Circulation* 1977;56:845–852.
23. Carabello BA, Nolan SP, Lockhart BM: Assessment of preoperative left ventricular function in patients with mitral regurgitation: value of the end-systolic wall stress-end-systolic volume ratio. *Circulation* 1981;64:1212–1217.
24. Nishimura T, Yamada Y, Kawai C: Echocardiographic evaluation of long-term effects of exercise on left ventricular hypertrophy and function in professional bicyclists. *Circulation* 1980;61: 832–840.
25. McCullagh WH, Covell JW, Ross J Jr: Left ventricular dilatation and diastolic compliance changes during chronic volume overloading. *Circulation* 1972;45:943–951.
26. Peterson KL, Tsuji J, Johnson A, et al: Diastolic left ventricular pressure–volume and stress-strain relations in patients with valvular aortic stenosis and left ventricular hypertrophy. *Circulation* 1978;58:77–89.
27. Hess OM, Ritter M, Schneider J, et al: Diastolic stiffness and myocardial structure in aortic valve disease before and after valve replacement. *Circulation* 1984;69:855–865.
28. Skelton CL, Prindle KH, Epstein SE: Regression of cardiac hypertrophy induced by chronic hyperthyroidism. *Circulation* 1972;46 (suppl 2):II–46.
29. Sanford CF, Griffin EE, Wildenthal K: Synthesis and degradation of myocardial protein during the development and regression of throxine-induced cardiac hypertrophy in rats. *Circ Res* 1978; 43:688–694.
30. Hall CE, Ogden E: Cardiac hypertrophy in experimental hypertension and its regression following establishment of normal blood pressure. *Am J Physiol* 1953;174:175–178.
31. Cooper G, Harrison CE, Coleman NH: Return to normal myocardial function and energetics after reversal of pressure overload. *Am J Physiol* 1974; 226:1158–1165.
32. Papadimitriou JM, Hopkins BE, Taylor RR: Regression of left ventricular dilatation and hypertrophy after removal of volume overload. *Circ Res* 1974;35:127–135.
33. Schuler G, Peterson KL, Johnson AD, et al: Serial noninvasive assessment of left ventricular hypertrophy and function after surgical correction of aortic regurgitation. *Am J Cardiol* 1979; 44:585–594.
34. Kennedy JW, Stewart D, Douglas K: Left ventricular function before and following aortic valve replacement. *Circulation* 1977;56:944–950.
35. Jamarkani JMM, Graham TP, Canent RV, et al: The effect of corrective surgery on left heart volume and mass in children with ventricular septal defect. *Am J Cardiol* 1971;27:254–258.

CHAPTER 3
Evaluation of the Patient with Valvular Heart Disease

J. David Bristow

Goals for evaluation of the patient with valvular heart disease (VHD) are readily identifiable, and directly influence therapy. Current treatment possibilities are numerous, including digitalis, diuretics, antibiotics, anticoagulants, vasodilators, antiarrhythmic drugs, and cardiac surgery. Intelligent management of VHD depends on systematic, thorough evaluation. This chapter will focus largely on the adult patient, outlining some principles to guide us.

It is important to pose several questions whenever the possibility of VHD is considered:

1. Is VHD actually present?
2. What is the cause of this person's VHD?
3. Has VHD produced hemodynamic abnormalities, and how severe are they?
4. Is the cardiac rhythm normal?
5. Has thromboembolism occurred, or is there reason to expect that it might?
6. Does the patient have infective endocarditis?
7. Are there other health problems which could influence the patient's VHD or its management?

The various procedures considered to investigate suspected VHD should promise to answer these questions. In this chapter, common clinical tools will be discussed broadly in relation to these questions, with the hope that their use will be appropriate and productive. We will start with the four techniques which remain the most important steps in evaluation: the history, physical examination and chest film and ECG. They are universally available and virtually without risk. Thereafter, echocardiography, radionuclide evaluations, and cardiac catheterization will be briefly mentioned.

HISTORY

We need first to determine whether VHD is actually present. The history of a heart murmur that has been consistently heard is helpful, as innocent murmurs may be detected inconstantly or have variable significance attached to them over the years. Murmurs heard from birth or childhood which persist to adolescence or adulthood are less likely to be innocent. A new murmur, especially a diastolic murmur, may have profound diagnostic significance, particularly if the patient or physician is certain that none has been heard previously.

The history may provide clues about the cause of the patient's VHD. For certain valve lesions, this is critical information, whereas the question may have no bearing on management in others. For example, the causes of valvular aortic stenosis are relatively few, and the exact cause may not be absolutely clear in a given, older patient. In that circumstance, the cause is of secondary importance, compared with the hemodynamic severity of the stenosis. On the other hand, causes of regurgitant lesions of the aortic or mitral valves are exceedingly numerous, and some have serious implications for management, eg, dissecting aortic aneurysm, endocarditis, myocardial infarction, etc.[1-3] Although one need not frame questions to explore each conceivable possibility, the history should be detailed enough to uncover familial, general health, social, and other data which might point to the etiology.

Acute rheumatic fever is declining rapidly in the United States, to the extent that many physicians have never encountered it. Nonetheless, its history will heighten suspicion of a rheumatic basis for VHD, especially mitral valve disease, and inquiries should be made.

It is important to be sure that a complete history by systems and past medical history are obtained. Clues about less common causes of VHD will usually come to the fore. For example, venereal disease, arthritis, fever, back pain, skin rash, and trauma, as examples, will each suggest one or more of the etiologic possibilities.

The most frequent concern in evaluating these patients is the accurate assessment of hemodynamic abnormality. Although this may not be done in a quantitative way by the history, it is generally the development of symptoms which leads to other steps. Valvular surgery is rarely performed in patients who have been truly asymptomatic.

Responses of the heart to excessive volume work or obstructions to outflow are limited. Thus, filling pressures may rise on one or both sides of the heart, and the forward cardiac output may be abnormal with rest and/or exercise. The standard cardiorespiratory questions in the history seek evidence that left heart filling pressures are abnormal and are crucial to ask. Questions about dyspnea on exertion, orthopnea, nocturnal dyspnea, and cough explore the possibility of elevated left atrial (and pulmonary capillary) pressure at rest or with exercise. Dependent edema suggests a low cardiac output state and/or elevated right heart filling pressures. Syncope has specific diagnostic connotation for aortic stenosis, but can also occur with an arrhythmia complicating other VHD. Chest pain or pressure, which is characteristic of myocardial ischemia, has a significant bearing on the diagnosis. Low cardiac output translates to exercise intolerance with easy fatigability, exhaustion, and the need for excessive rest. Patients slowly cut back on the level of their physical activity, a change which can be insidious and should be explored. Current limitation of activity may become evident in some patients only when compared with the past.

A history of arrhythmias should be sought. It is also essential to learn in detail about medications the patient has taken in the past or is taking now. This information may have diagnostic utility and may prevent future difficulty if untoward drug responses have already occurred. For example, quinidine could have been prescribed for atrial fibrillation in a patient with mitral valve disease and have been badly tolerated. This type of patient may continue to be a candidate for antiarrhythmic therapy, and it is essential to avoid repetition of past difficulties, such as a ventricular arrhythmia complicating quinidine therapy.

Has there ever been an acute neurologic deficit or other evidence of systemic embolism? Has the patient taken heparin, coumadin, or antiplatelet drugs? Were there difficulties with these drugs? Does the patient have a potential or current problem which could produce undue bleeding if anticoagulants should be otherwise indicated?

Endocarditis would be suggested by fever, malaise, and history of new murmur, pallor, or embolic symptoms. Provocations of endocarditis often are not detected in the history, but should be asked about nonetheless. Any information is helpful in this sometimes difficult diagnosis. Is there a history of antibiotic use recently which might render blood cultures negative?

The list of possibilities for other medical problems which could influence the evaluation of VHD is long and important. For example, is the patient pregnant? Even the first stage of the evaluation is influenced if the answer is "yes," as a chest film may be delayed or avoided entirely during pregnancy. Is there a history of congenital disease in other members of the family with murmurs or premature death? Has endocrinopathy been present in the past? Is there evidence of alcoholism, drug abuse, or addiction? Use of anticoagulant therapy or recommendations about valvular surgery are sometimes radically altered because of such information. Does the patient have symptoms outside the cardiorespiratory system which suggest malignancy or other serious disease which could limit prognosis more than the heart disease?

The foregoing points are illustrative of the medical truism that a complete history is essential when dealing with a potentially serious health problem, which is certainly the case with VHD. From the history, the cause of the VHD may be elucidated, the extent of physiologic derangement first suggested, the need for an operation considered, or the need for prophylaxis of one of several forms recognized. Although the history is routine, its importance is the VHD patient cannot be overstated, and no short cuts should be taken, even if the diagnosis seems evident.

One other essential part of the history in the

patient with symptoms due to VHD should be mentioned. We need to know how well the patient is accepting his/her current situation. The indications for surgery in some regurgitant valvular lesions remain uncertain and are frequently debated. Some forms of VHD have a long asymptomatic phase before irreparable damage is done or operative risks become excessive. The timing of operative will depend to a great extent on the assessment of present disability in comparison with the risks of surgery.

PHYSICAL EXAMINATION

Details of the examination of the various valve lesions are found in the appropriate chapters. Here we will approach the topic briefly from the standpoint of the overall examination, rather than the specific valve lesion.

It hardly requires mention that the physical examination is *the* primary diagnostic test in the evaluation of VHD. From it, the diagnosis follows, and decisions about additional studies depend largely upon the findings. The first, fundamental question about the patient (presence or absence of significant VHD) will usually be answered by this examination.

The general appearance of the patient is exceedingly important. It is striking how often this observation is missing in patients' charts in hospitals. A cachectic appearance with VHD suggests a long-standing, low cardiac output state, eg, the near terminal stage of mitral valve disease. Skin warmth may connote a reasonable cardiac output. Cyanosis may result from a low output with a wide arteriovenous oxygen difference and the resulting low oxygen saturation of venous blood. Further, arterial undersaturation results from elevated pulmonary artery wedge pressure, as in chronic congestive failure and/or mitral valve disease. Profound cyanosis suggests an alternative to a diagnosis of valvular heart disease alone, ie, complex congenital malformation. Petechiae are often absent in endocarditis, but their present in skin and mucous membranes should be sought in all VHD patients. Splinter hemorrhages and funduscopic signs of embolism are also important, although the nail bed signs are far from specific. Head-bob is a sign of a large left ventricular stroke volume with aortic run-off, in severe aortic insufficiency. Osler's nodes and Janeway lesions are uncommon, but certainly ought to be noted.

Accurate evaluation of the jugular venous pulse requires skill which some physicians fail to acquire, but it is of considerable help in many patients. First is the level of the neck veins, read at the top of the internal jugular, preferably on the right side. The height of the waves is roughly indicative of jugular venous pressure but is not the same, as it is the top of a wave in the vein, not identical to the pressure inside the vessel. These two variables, nonetheless, will correspond reasonably well when direct comparisons are made, eg, with the measured right atrial pressure. Loss of the "a" wave is occasionally helpful as a sign of atrial fibrillation, although the irregularlity of the cardiac rhythm is a much more obvious sign. The large systolic "v" wave in tricuspid regurgitation in the jugular veins is a helpful sign, generally in the patient with atrial fibrillation and loss of "a" waves. Most often, it is the level of jugular venous pulse which is helpful diagnostically as an indication of right heart function or abnormal loading. Rarely in VHD, prominent jugular "a" waves could be seen, eg, in tricuspid stenosis or in mitral stenosis with severe pulmonary hypertension, with persistence of sinus rhythm.

Palpation of the arterial pulses is important, first with regard to their presence and equality on the two sides of the body, and between arms and legs. For example, the development of aortic regurgitation with chest pain in a hypertensive patient who has an absent pulse in one brachial artery raises the diagnostic probability of a dissecting aortic aneurysm. Other information potentially available from palpation is the character of the carotid pulse. For generations, the rate of rise of this wave has been described in aortic stenosis. A recent study of "blinded" observers suggests that this sign is not very reliable,[4] excepting perhaps more gross abnormality as in severe aortic stenosis. Notably absent in the study cited above were patients with pure, severe aortic regurgitation.

The very rapidly rising pulse with subsequent collapse is a clear sign in severe aortic regurgitation or other aortic run-off syndromes. The bisferiens pulse of mixed aortic stenosis and regurgitation can be identified. Further, the small, quick pulse of hypertrophic cardiomyopathy is a detectable sign. The author agrees with Spodick et al[4] that more modest degrees of abnormality in the rise of velocity of the carotid pulse, as in many patients with aortic stenosis, is poorly, inconstantly detectable. Although some observers can discern details of the carotid pulse, such as an anacrotic shoulder, this is unlikely to be found by most examiners.

The difficulties in evaluating the carotid pulse should not surprise us, if we consider the variables involved. The total left ventricular stroke volume, the rate of ejection from the ventricle, the ejection time, the stiffness of the arterial tree, the volume at which the arterial tree is operating, and systemic vascular resistance interact to produce the pulse wave. Some of these factors may have influences more potent than, and directly opposite to, changes of the pulse form due to the valve lesion itself.

Palpation of the precordium gives essential information. The location of the cardiac apex is normally to the right of the midclavicular line and in the fifth intercostal space. In the adult it is about 2 cm in diameter, felt as a light tap and not sustained. As the left ventricle becomes volume-loaded as in aortic regurgitation, the impulse expands. In aortic stenosis, the very sustained, forceful apex of left ventricular hypertrophy is an expected sign. A right ventricular lift along the left sternal edge is evidence of pulmonary hypertension, or in mitral valve disease, displacement of the right ventricle anteriorly by the large (posterior) left atrium. A palpable fourth heart sound, ie, double-apex impulse, is a helpful sign, generally reflecting left ventricular hypertrophy. In its most flagrant form it would be found in hypertrophic cardiomyopathy, but it is seen in valvular aortic stenosis as well. It is due to the sudden, exaggerated, late diastolic filling which is found in left ventricular hypertrophy.

The most important maneuver in evaluation of valvular heart disease is auscultation of the heart. Once again, for detail, the reader is referred to the appropriate chapters on the specific valve problems. A very brief overview of some aspects follows below.

The patient must be examined in multiple positions if all important signs are to be found. At the minimum, these are the supine, left lateral position, as well as sitting up, and leaning forward. Faint aortic diastolic murmurs are brought out in the last position, with the breath held in the position of exhalation. The murmur of mitral stenosis and other soft left heart sounds are sometimes heard only when the patient lies on his left side, but not so far turned that the left ventricular apex is buried. Examination of the patient in unusual positions, or during maneuvers such as sustained handgrip, may be helpful in clarifying which valve is diseased.[5]

The intensity of the first heart sound is a useful sign. It is loud and snapping in mitral stenosis with a pliable valve, and soft in acute aortic regurgitation with markedly raised left ventricular diastolic pressure.

The second sound also provides valuable information. Normally both components (aortic and pulmonic) should be separately heard with normal inspiratory splitting. Accentuation of the pulmonic component suggests pulmonary hypertension. A single second sound is consistent with, but not diagnostic of, aortic stenosis or pulmonic stenosis. Paradoxical splitting of the second sound is seen with aortic stenosis, more commonly in the younger patient, but it is also found in left bundle-branch block without valve disease.

A ventricular gallop (third) sound is typically present in volume overload states such as mitral regurgitation and occasionally aortic regurgitation, without necessarily implying left ventricular failure. In aortic stenosis, however, it has that significance. A fourth sound is often a reflection of increased left ventricular diastolic stiffness due to left ventricular hypertrophy, and would be expected in aortic valve disease. The presence of a fourth sound in patients with pure mitral regurgitation suggests a nonrheumatic cause, such as ruptured chordae tendinae.[6]

Broadly speaking, the louder the murmur the more significant the lesion. However, this is only true in a general way. In the older patient with emphysema, aortic stenosis, and a low cardiac output, the murmur may be distant and soft. All experienced cardiologists have seen mitral stenosis with no detectable cardiac murmur. These two examples highlight the need to consider the accompanying physical signs in the overall picture of valvular disease, eg, characteristics of the heart sounds and signs from palpation.

Other Signs

Hepatomegaly is an extremely important sign of VHD, generally indicative of right heart failure with raised systemic venous pressure. Splenomegaly is uncommonly found. Although part of the classical description of subacute bacterial endocarditis, it is not present with most endocarditis, and the diagnostic probability should not be influenced by its absence. Edema can be due to diverse causes, including varicose veins, phlebitis, and hepatic or renal disease. In many patients, there are no pathologic findings. However, substantial edema in the patient with VHD often indicates congestive heart failure, in a fairly advanced stage of the illness.

CHEST FILM AND ELECTROCARDIOGRAM

The standard chest film provides great help in the diagnosis of VHD and evaluation of its severity. The questions that such films may answer include these:

Is cardiac chamber enlargement detectable?
Is valvular calcification present?
Is there evidence of increased pulmonary venous pressure?
Are there signs of pulmonary hypertension?
Is there pleural effusion?
Is the proximal aorta or pulmonary artery enlarged?

Thus, the x-ray films provide clues about the presence or absence of VHD, which valves might be involved, and the severity of the hemodynamic abnormality.

Similarly, the ECG can be of considerable help. For example, there are times when discrimination between aortic and mitral valve disease is difficult, as is the distinction between aortic stenosis and pulmonic stenosis in the occasional younger patient. Given the current level of sophistication of physical diagnosis, this should not often be a problem. When it is, ECG evidence of right ventricular hypertrophy, left ventricular hypertrophy, P-mitrale, etc, is of help. In most patients, a chest film and ECG are basic elements in the initial evaluation.

ECHOCARDIOGRAPHY, DOPPLER ULTRASOUND, RADIONUCLIDE VENTRICULOGRAPHY

Echocardiography, Doppler ultrasound, and radionuclide ventriculography have advanced to the point that almost a complete anatomic and physiologic diagnosis could be established by them in some patients, even without a physical examination. They are relatively expensive procedures, however, and will not supplant the simplicity and accuracy of the physical examination by a well-trained observer. In some circumstances they could even be misleading unless integrated with knowledge from the bedside examination. Their uses at present are to:

1. Confirm the site of VHD
   Abnormal reflectance and motion of a valve (echocardiography)
   Abnormal direction of flow (Doppler ultrasound)
2. Evaluate the severity of VHD
   Maximal velocity of flow through a pathologic valve, notably aortic stenosis (Doppler ultrasound)
   Ventricular dilation in regurgitant VHD (echocardiography, radionuclide ventriculography)
   Comparison of right and left ventricular stroke volumes to estimate aortic or mitral regurgitant flow (radionuclide ventriculography)
   Ventricular hypertrophy (echocardiography)
3. Evaluate ventricular function
   Left ventricular minor axis, fractional shortening (echocardiography)
   Ventricular wall motion and ejection fraction (echocardiography, radionuclide ventriculography)
   Ventricular wall stress calculations (echocardiography, radionuclide ventriculography)
4. Rule out other pathology
   Pericardial effusion (echocardiography)
   Left atrial mass (echocardiography, radionuclide ventriculography)
   Myocardial infarction with segmental ventricular wall motion abnormality (echocardiography, radionuclide ventriculography)
   Aortic root pathology (echocardiography)

How do these studies fit into the evaluation of the patient with VHD? This has become controversial, and the answer depends on the overall approach taken to the original diagnosis and follow-up over time, by the individual physician. For example, the physical examination is the simplest, easiest way to establish the diagnosis of substantial aortic insufficiency. An echocardiographic or Doppler study adds little to establishing that diagnosis. On the other hand, these studies can be useful in determining the presence or absence of mitral stenosis or aortic stenosis when the physical signs are confusing or made less obvious by obstructive pulmonary disease. Thus, the use of Doppler echocardiography in the initial investigation of the patient with VHD will vary with the lesion suspected, the difficulty in identifying it, and other circumstances.

These studies offer much promise for following patients over time, when signs of increased severity of the valve disease or early signs of cardiac dysfunction are important to recognize. This aspect of VHD is discussed next.

EVALUATION AND FOLLOW-UP

Once the initial evaluation has been performed, a clear idea of the lesion present and its significance should have been obtained, ie, the questions posed at the start of this chapter have been addressed. The next problem is to decide how to follow the patient over time. Certainly this is an individual matter from patient to patient, depending on age, severity of the VHD at the time it was first recognized, past problems, the practice situation, and other factors. A few general matters can be discussed.

Patients with VHD certainly ought to be seen on a regularly scheduled basis, one to two times per year for those with milder problems, and more often as the clinical situation indicates. It is important to obtain a history of any new or increased intensity of symptoms. The physical examination will evaluate severity of the disease and detect signs of congestive failure if present. A chest film yearly should be obtained, although in the patient with mild disease and no symptoms a longer interval than a year is satisfactory. An ECG is usually obtained at the same interval. A yearly evaluation in the stable patient by a history, physical examination, chest film, and ECG is not exorhitant in cost and will provide essential information for sequential evaluation.

A few years into the era of the valve replacement, it became evident that some patients did not improve after operation, and others improved initially, only to develop congestive failure later.[7,8] Thus, it was learned that chronic overloading of the left ventricle could lead to permanent left ventricular dysfunction, prior to clinically evident congestive failure and severe symptoms.[9] Concern, therefore, has been directed at finding ways to evaluate cardiac performance, preferably noninvasively, repeatedly, with the hope of identifying the earliest, perhaps reversible, signs of left ventricular dysfunction when valve surgery might be done. Echocardiographic criteria for this purpose have been developed, and been disputed. The problem is a difficult one, perhaps confused by the search, apparently, for a single criterion which can be used in all patients to determine when surgery should be done.

Since many patients with VHD have a protracted course, the present goal in following them is to identify significant change. Such change could be in symptoms, new signs of congestive failure, or in the indices of cardiac function. For the latter purpose, echocardiography, radionuclide ventriculography at rest, and exercise seem promising. Again, the goal may well be *identification of a significant change*, rather than finding an arbitrary abnormality of measurement, eg, a particular end-systolic echocardiographic diameter. Study by echocardiography or radionuclide ventriculography on a yearly basis is surely justified in the patient with significant VHD. In all such measurements, knowledge of the inherent variation of the technique is very important, to avoid overinterpretation of minimal changes.

CARDIAC CATHETERIZATION

One of the great contributions of cardiac catheterization and angiocardiography has been the detailed description of the hemodynamics of VHD. An understanding of its natural history, based on quantitative evaluation, has resulted. Correlations among simple bedside, ECG, and radiographic observations and the information from catheterization have been developed and have reached an advanced level. Thus, it is logical that the question has been raised about the necessity to continue routine catheterization prior to cardiac valve surgery. The issue was discussed recently by St. John-Sutton et al.[10] In an uncontrolled study, a substantial proportion of patients had surgical valve replacement without cardiac catheterization preoperatively. The operative mortality was not different in those who had or did not have cardiac catheterization, and later morbidity and mortality were not different in the first 2 years postoperatively. In discussing these results, the authors entertained several disadvantages to this approach, but failed to consider in detail the most alarming possibility of all, ie, that some uncatheterized, postoperation patients may not have required surgery at the time, had hemodynamic and angiographic findings been known.[10]

St. John-Sutton et al placed remarkable confidence in the M-mode echocardiogram to evaluate the correct diagnosis, the severity of the valve disease, and any resulting ventricular overloading.[10] Support for only limited use of cardiac catheterization preoperatively in selected patients has nonetheless been voiced.[11]

Strong rebuttals to the provocative paper by

St. John-Sutton el al have been published, emphasizing the difference between the correct diagnosis of a particular valve lesion as opposed to evaluation of its pathophysiologic severity.[12,13] Again, the possibility of performing surgery not yet required is a source of concern. A practical issue in the United States, where many VHD patients are middle-aged or older, is the surgeon's requirement for knowing coronary arterial anatomy. Most surgeons will wish to avoid later reoperation for proximal severe coronary disease which was diagnosable before valve replacement, and will also wish to plan intraoperative myocardial protection, based on coronary arteriography.

The major diagnostic challenge in VHD is to define accurately the severity of the valve pathology, the extent of abnormal cardiac loading that is associated, and the resulting cardiac and pulmonary adaptations. A very good approximation can be made by the history, physical examination, chest film and ECG, with occasional use of other noninvasive studies. However, when the time comes to consider valvular surgery, elective cardiac catheterization is advisable for most patients, in the author's opinion. The risk is small, and the appropriate timing and choice of operation are of huge importance to the individual patient. No matter how good the bedside basis for the clinician's decision seems to be, mistakes can be made.

In addition to confirming the correct diagnosis, and defining the pathophysiology, cardiac catheterization data also serve as a baseline for later evaluation if the results of valve surgery are not up to the expected level. If the patient fails to do as well postoperatively as was expected, a reference point for comparison with postoperative hemodynamic data is provided by preoperative cardiac catheterization.

In many patients, the clinical problem is partly due to mechanical valvular disease, and partly to myocardial insufficiency. In order to predict the outcome of valve replacement and to assess surgical prognosis, separation of these two entities is important. Another confounding variable is coronary disease, which can contribute to left ventricular dysfunction, to operative risk, and late prognosis. Despite occasional protestation, most patients with high-grade proximal coronary lesions and operable VHD will have a combined valvular and arterial operation.

The best description of hemodynamic abnormalities in VHD is obtained by cardiac catheterization and angiocardiography. There are occasional times when operation is needed with extreme urgency, and no other procedure should be performed. In my view, however, catheterization should generally be recommended for evaluation before *elective* surgery for VHD.

Despite the above opinion, the day will surely come when the essential information about a patient with VHD will be obtained noninvasively. The emergence of radionuclide and echocardiographic analyses of left ventricular function, and Doppler echo evaluation of transvalvular pressure gradients surely portend such changes in practice, when these and others as yet unforeseen methods will have adequate precision.

CONCLUSIONS

Evaluation of the patient with VHD has been changing, but certain aspects of the process have not. A detailed history is crucial in determining whether a person has a significant problem and in deciding how to attack it. The physical examination is as important as ever in answering several fundamental questions about the diagnosis, and for planning management. Newer techniques frequently provide reassurance about the diagnosis and physiologic severity of VHD, but have not yet replaced the initial evaluation provided by the history, physical examination, chest film and ECG, nor the ultimate quantitation by cardiac catheterization and angiocardiography. The times are changing, however, and noninvasive methods will come to the fore as the definitive studies in VHD.

REFERENCES

1. Braunwald E: Valvular heart disease, in Braunwald E (ed): *Heart Disease*. Philadelphia, WB Saunders Co, 1984, pp 1075, 1106.
2. Fowler NO: *Cardiac Diagnosis and Treatment*. New York, Harper & Row Publishers, 1980, p 565.
3. Silverman ME, Hurst JW: The mitral complex, in Likoff W (ed): *Cardiovascular Clinics*. Philadelphia, FA Davis Co, 1973, pp 37–48.
4. Spodick DH, Sugiura T, Doi Y, et al: Rate of rise of the carotid pulse: An investigation of observer error in a common clinical measurement. *Am J Cardiol* 1982;49:159–161.
5. Rothman A, Goldberger AL: Aids to cardiac auscultation. *Ann Intern Med* 1983;99:346–353.
6. Cohen LS, Mason DT, Braunwald E: Significance of an atrial gallop sound in mitral regurgitation:

A clue to the diagnosis of ruptured chordae tendinae. *Circulation* 1966;35:112–118.

7. Peterson CR, Herr R, Crisera RV, et al: The failure of hemodynamic improvement following valve replacement surgery. *Am Intern Med* 1967; 66:1–24.
8. Bristow JD, Kremkau EL: Hemodynamic changes after valve replacement with Starr-Edwards prostheses. *Am J Cardiol* 1975;35:716–724.
9. Ross J Jr: Left ventricular function and the timing of surgical treatment in valvular heart disease. *Ann Intern Med* 1981;94:498–504.
10. St. John-Sutton MG, St. John-Sutton M, Oldershaw P, et al: Valve replacement without preoperative cardiac catheterization. *N Engl J Med* 1981;305:1233–1238.
11. Brandenberg RO: No more routine catheterization for valvular heart disease? *N Engl J Med* 1981;305:1277–1278.
12. Rahimtoola SH: The need for cardiac catheterization and angiography in valvular heart disease is not disproven. *Ann Intern Med* 1982;97:433–439.
13. Roberts WC: Reasons for cardiac catheterization before cardiac valve replacement. *N Engl J Med* 1982;306:1291–1293.

CHAPTER 4
Congenital Lesions of the Tricuspid Valve

David C. Schwartz

Congenital anomalies of the tricuspid valve are uncommon. Among these lesions only two are of clinical relevance: tricuspid valve atresia and Ebstein's anomaly. Tricuspid incompetence or stenosis due to other types of valve abnormalities are extremely rare pathologic curiosities and generally occur in conjunction with complex forms of congenital heart disease.

TRICUSPID ATRESIA

The absence of right atrial connection to the morphologic right ventricle is the anatomical hallmark of classic tricuspid atresia. Additional cardiac malformations include: a mandatory interatrial communication, hypoplasia of the concordant morphologic right ventricle, interventricular communication, transposition or malposition of the great vessels, and often pulmonary stenosis. Tricuspid atresia is uncommon, accounting for only 1% to 3% of all forms of congenital heart disease, depending on whether one examines autopsy or clinical series.[1] Considerable debate rages with regard to terminology. Bharati and Lev[2] have argued to retain the term tricuspid atresia whereas Anderson et al[3] prefer the term univentricular heart with absence of right atrioventricular (AV) connection. Nonetheless, tricuspid atresia remains in common usage and is desirable for clinicians and surgeons in the context of the pathophysiology of the malformation.

Pathology and Pathophysiology

The pathologic spectrum of tricuspid atresia is wide considering the variation in the anatomical types of atrioventricular orifice atresia as well as

Table 4-1
Classification of Tricuspid Atresia

Type I	Normally related great arteries	
Type II	D-transposition of the great arteries	
Type III	Malposition of the great arteries	
	Subtype 1. L-transposition of the great arteries	
	Subtype 2. Double outlet right ventricle	
	Subtype 3. Double outlet left ventricle	
	Subtype 4. D-malposition of the great arteries (anatomically corrected malposition)	
	Subtype 5. L-malposition of the great arteries (anatomically corrected malposition)	
Type IV	Persistent truncus arteriosus	
		Subgroup a. Pulmonary atresia
		Subgroup b. Pulmonary stenosis or hypoplasia
		Subgroup c. Normal pulmonary arteries (no pulmonary stenosis)

Reproduced with permission from Rao.[8]

ventricular morphology and ventriculoarterial relationships. Various classifications of tricuspid atresia have appeared and depend on the morphology of the atretic orifice,[4,5] radiographic features,[6] and associated cardiac defects.[7] The wide spectrum of tricuspid atresia is due to its association with complex malformations of the heart, where atresia of the right AV orifice is the common denominator among a group of quite different clinical and anatomical entities[8] (Table 4-1). The most common variety is normally related great vessels and situs solitus (type I), where pulmonary blood flow is dependent on a ventricular septal defect, the status of the pulmonary valve, and the development of the pulmonary arteries (Figure 4-1). The size of the ventricular septal defect is variable and may become smaller with increasing age.[9] About 20% of cases are associated with transposition of the great vessels and normal relationship of the left atrium to the mitral valve and left ventricle (type II). In this situation, systemic blood flow is dependent upon the ventricular septal defect and pulmonary blood flow is greatly increased unless there is associated pulmonary stenosis (Figure 4-2). A smaller group of patients have malposition of the great vessels with the aorta anterior and left-sided. This variation is of particular importance to the surgeon, with regard to palliative or physiologically corrective operations. Since in tricuspid atresia the systemic ventricle receives both pulmonary and systemic venous flow, complete mixing is achieved prior to ejection into the great vessels. In this circumstance, pulmonary blood flow is the major determinant of arterial oxygen saturation. In addition, long-term survival is dependent upon the magnitude of pulmonary blood flow and its effect on the pulmonary vascular bed and systemic ventricular function.

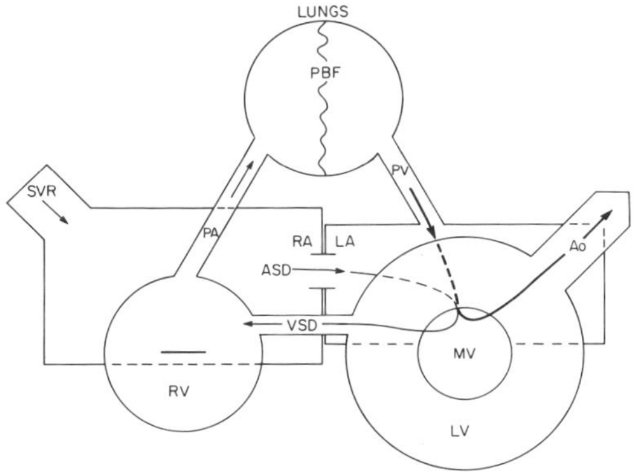

Figure 4-1 Course of the circulation in tricuspid atresia, type I, subgroup b. Pulmonary blood flow is restricted by the interventricular communication and small size of the pulmonary arteries. SVR = systemic venous return, RA = right atrium, RV = right ventricle, PA = pulmonary artery, PBF = pulmonary blood flow, PV = pulmonary veins, LA = left atrium, ASD = atrial septal defect, VSD = ventricular septal defect, MV = mitral valve, LV = left ventricle, Ao = aorta.

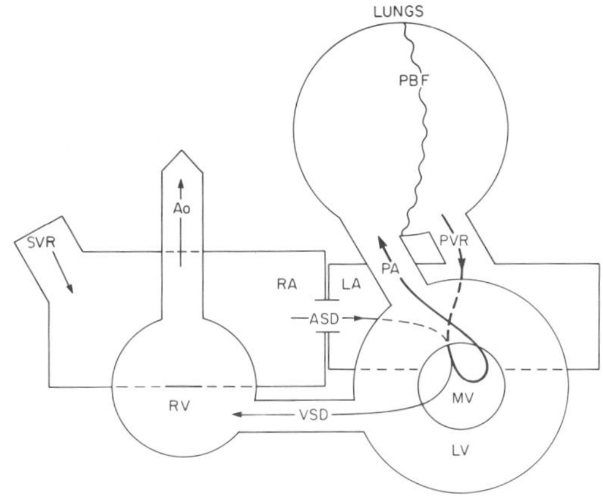

Figure 4-2 Course of the circulation in tricuspid atresia, type II, subgroup c. Ventricular septal defect provides systemic blood flow. Pulmonary blood flow is greatly increased. Abbreviations as in Figure 4-1.

Clinical Features

In general, the clinical picture in tricuspid atresia and diminished pulmonary blood flow is one of cyanosis, clubbing, and polycythemia. In patients with excessive pulmonary blood flow, the cardinal features are severe cardiomegaly and congestive heart failure. The unrestricted pulmonary blood flow in patients with transposition or malposition without pulmonary stenosis (types II and III), leads to pulmonary hypertension, obstructive pulmonary vascular disease, and ultimately to the Eisenmenger syndrome. It is very unusual for pulmonary hypertension to occur in patients with normally related great vessels (type I).[10] If, however, a large aortopulmonary shunt (Pott's or Waterston) was created in infancy or childhood, pulmonary hypertension may develop in these patients as they approach adulthood. Some patients have undergone a previous Glenn shunt (superior vena cava to right pulmonary artery anastomosis) which can result in multiple pulmonary arteriovenous communications leading to increasing cyanosis.[11]

Examination of patients with tricuspid atresia and diminished pulmonary blood flow reveals cyanosis, clubbing, and often delayed growth. The precordium is usually quiet, but there is often left precordial prominence. There is a prominent jugular "a" wave and on auscultation the first sound is loud and single as is the second sound. The pulmonary closure sound is seldom audible except in patients with normally related great vessels and mild pulmonary stenosis, in which case the pulmonary component is delayed and diminished. In most patients, a parasternal systolic murmur is audible, reflecting left-to-right shunt through a restrictive ventricular septal defect or an ejection systolic murmur of pulmonic stenosis, radiating toward the base. Since the pulmonary stenosis is seldom valvar, an ejection click is usually not heard. In patients with increased pulmonary blood flow from a prior shunt and long-standing left ventricular enlargement, there is often a prominent third heart sound at the apex along with a mitral diastolic flow rumble. Some patients in this setting will develop secondary mitral incompetence and have an apical systolic murmur. The Glenn shunt is usually inaudible but the Blalock-Taussig, Pott's, and Waterston shunts are associated with a continuous murmur if they are patent. The Waterston shunt (ascending aorta to right pulmonary artery) is audible over the right chest anteriorly while the Pott's anastomosis (descending aorta to the left pulmonary artery) is heard posteriorly on the left. While the Waterston shunt may become restrictive with increasing age, the Pott's shunt invariably becomes larger resulting in torrential pulmonary blood flow, pulmonary hypertension, and pulmonary vascular obstructive disease.

Electrovectorcardiography

Among patients with cyanotic congenital heart disease, the ECG in tricuspid atresia is virtually diagnostic. The findings include: superiorly oriented QRS axis or left axis deviation, peaked and notched P waves, diminished right ventricular forces, and left ventricular hypertrophy (Figure 4-3). Left ventricular hypertrophy is always present and often with secondary T wave changes, especially in patients with increased pulmonary blood flow or mitral regurgitation. The frontal plane axis varies with the anatomical malformation. In patients with classic tricuspid atresia, normally related great vessels, and an anteriorly positioned but small right ventricle (type I), the frontal plane axis varies between 0° and −90°. Patients with type II or type III malformations have a wide range of frontal plane axis with the major QRS forces oriented leftward and inferiorly, but rarely right-

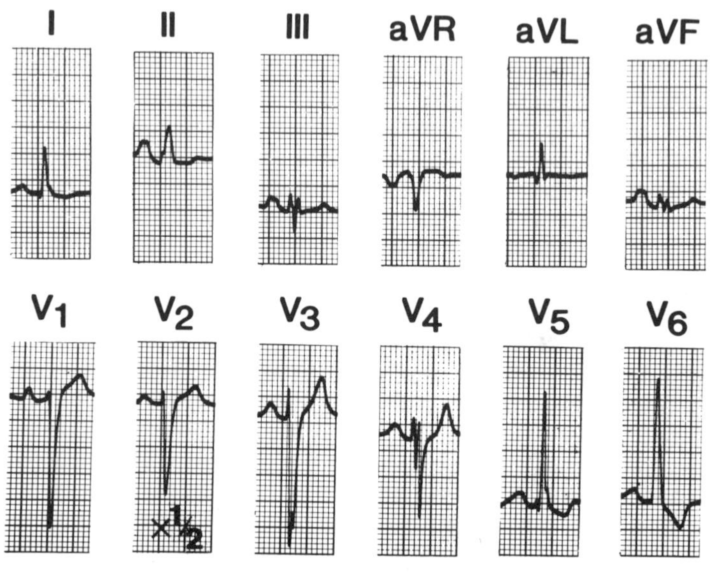

Figure 4-3 Type I tricuspid atresia. The patient is a 30-year-old man who had previously undergone a left Blalock-Taussig shunt in infancy. Wide notched P waves indicate biatrial enlargement. The QRS voltage and T wave changes are consistent with left ventricular hypertrophy.

ward.[12] On the vectorcardiogram, the frontal plane loop is invariably leftward, counterclockwise, and superior. There is virtual absence of anterior and rightward forces in the transverse plane mimicking the findings of an anteroseptal infarction.

Radiographic Features

The radiographic features of tricuspid atresia generally reflect the anatomical alteration and status of pulmonary blood flow. In type I patients, there is an inconspicuous pulmonary artery segment and a prominent right atrium. Pulmonary stenosis is usually present and consequently pulmonary blood flow is greatly diminished. The right atrial contour may be less prominent when left-sided juxtaposition of the atrial appendages is present, which occurs frequently in tricuspid atresia.[13] Pulmonary blood flow is usually increased in type II and type III patients unless surgically restricted by pulmonary artery banding (Figure 4-4). If pulmonary blood flow has been increased surgically, left ventricular enlargement may dominate the radiographic picture (Figure 4-5). In patients in whom a prior Waterston shunt has been performed, the

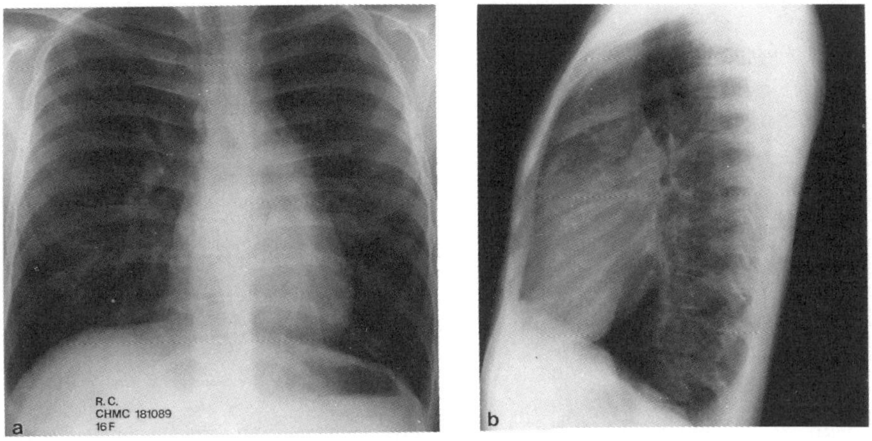

Figure 4-4 Posteroanterior (a) and lateral (b) roentgenograms of a 16-year-old girl with tricuspid atresia, type III, subtype I (malposition of the great vessels with normal pulmonary arteries) who had undergone a pulmonary artery banding in infancy. Pulmonary vascularity is normal. Fullness in the upper left cardiac border is produced by the malpositioned ascending aorta.

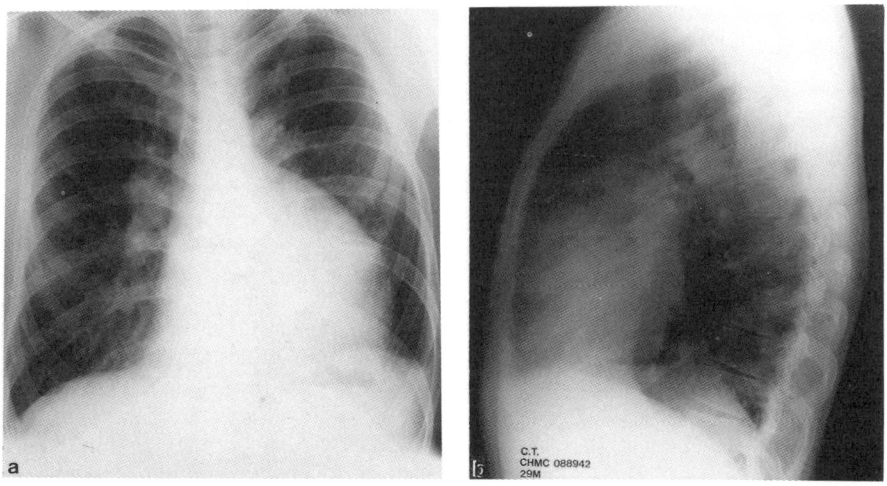

Figure 4-5 Posteroanterior (a) and lateral (b) roentgenograms of a 29-year-old man with tricuspid atresia, type II, subgroup b (D-transposition and pulmonary stenosis) who had undergone a left-Blalock-Taussig shunt in infancy. Shunt vascularity and cardiomegaly reflect the long-standing left-to-right shunt.

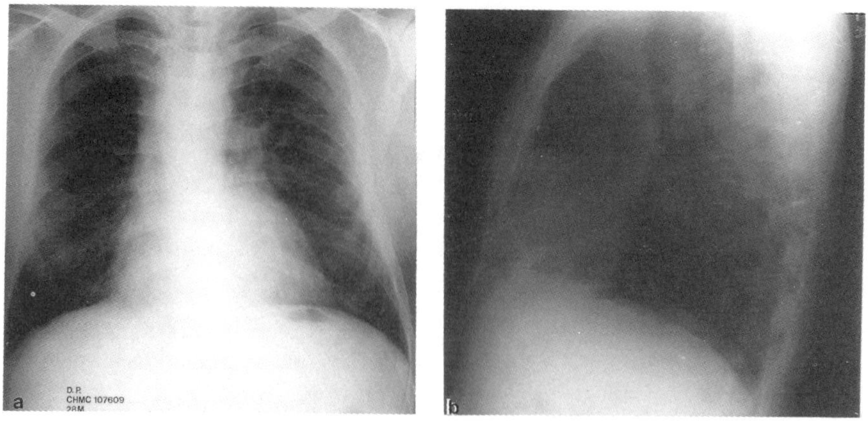

Figure 4-6 Posteroanterior (a) and lateral (b) roentgenograms of a 28-year-old man with type I tricuspid atresia who had undergone a Pott's anatomosis in early childhood. Marked dilatation of the left pulmonary artery and disproportionate shunt vascularity on the left reflect the large aortopulmonary communication.

proximal right pulmonary artery will be greatly dilated. Likewise a Pott's anastomosis will enlarge the left pulmonary artery (Figure 4-6).

Echocardiography

Adequate M-mode echocardiography in infants and children should always reveal some portion of the tricuspid valve. In the adult, especially with severe left ventricular enlargement, the tricuspid valve may not be imaged in spite of exhaustive efforts. Two-dimensional echocardiography is distinctly advantageous over M-mode scanning and permits definitive evaluation of the tricuspid valve, as well as identification of great vessel relationships, the size of the right ventricle, and evaluation of interatrial and interventricular septal defects.[14,15] Echocardiographic contrast studies, especially when imaged in the apical four-chamber view, can identify obligatory right-to-left shunting through the atrial septal defect as well as the failure of contrast to cross the tricuspid valve.[16]

Cardiac catheterization and Angiocardiography

Cardiac catheterization and selective cineangiography clearly establish the diagnosis of tricuspid atresia and are essential in the preoperative assessment when a physiologic corrective procedure is contemplated. Inability to enter the right ventricle directly with a venous catheter and complete admixture of systemic, coronary, and pulmonary venous blood in the left ventricle, are characteristic catheterization findings in tricuspid atresia. The venous catheterization is best performed from the groin to facilitate passage of the catheter across the atrial septum. Although the angiographic anatomy of tricuspid atresia is demonstrated by antegrade venous angiography, selective left ventriculography is necessary to clearly define the origin of the great vessels, source of pulmonary blood flow, and extent of development of the right ventricle.[17] Precise definition of the rudimentary right ventricular chamber and pulmonary arteries may be accomplished by selective angiography in the right ventricle, which can be entered antegrade through the ventricular septal defect. The presence of a pre-existing aortopulmonary shunt permits retrograde catheterization of the pulmonary artery for evaluation of pulmonary artery pressure and pulmonary vascular resistance, as well as performing selective pulmonary angiography.

Natural History and Management

Although virtually all patients with tricuspid atresia have the diagnosis established in infancy or early childhood, increasing numbers of patients have undergone palliative operations permitting prolonged survival. Rarely, a patient will survive into adolescence or adulthood without a prior surgical procedure (Figure 4-7).[18,19] These patients invariably have a ventricular septal defect with pulmonary stenosis perfectly balanced to prevent profound pulmonary congestion, yet not severe enough to result in extreme diminution of pulmonary blood flow and resulting hypoxemia. The majority of adolescents and young adults with tricuspid atresia will have had a

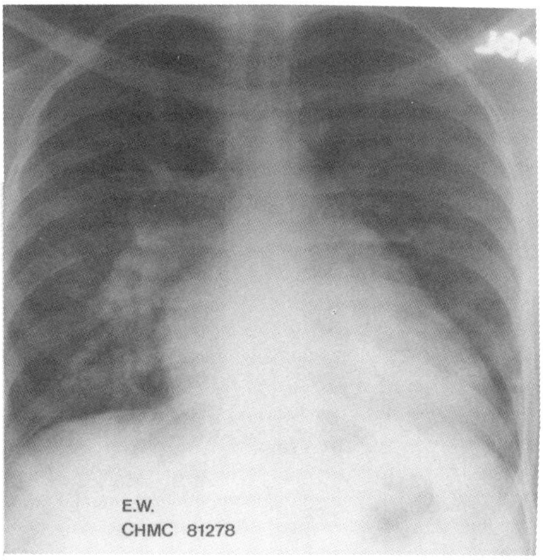

Figure 4-7 Posteroanterior chest roentgenogram of a 32-year-old man with tricuspid atresia, type II, subgroup b (D-transposition with pulmonary stenosis) who is asymptomatic apart from recurrent bouts of supraventricular tachycardia. Poststenotic dilatation of the right pulmonary artery reflects the orientation of the outflow jet through the tranposed pulmonary artery as well as preferential flow to the right lung, characteristic of transposition.

prior shunt procedure. If the shunt has not resulted in chronic left ventricular failure, these patients may be candidates for definitive surgical intervention. Physiologic correction of tricuspid atresia can be accomplished by either direct anastomosis of the right atrium to the main pulmonary artery, or use of a valved conduit which diverts systemic venous blood directly into the lung (Fontan procedure) (Figure 4-8).[20,21] Modifications of this procedure include utilizing a right atrial to right ventricular conduit, with or without an interposed prosthetic valve. Ideal candidates for this type of corrective procedure must have normal pulmonary vascular resistance, a mean pulmonary artery pressure of less than 20 mm Hg, distal pulmonary arteries of adequate size, and good left ventricular function.[22] The procedure is contraindicated in patients with pulmonary vascular obstructive disease or severe left ventricular dysfunction.

Cardiac function after the Fontan repair is often abnormal, particularly during exercise.[23,24] It is common for such patients to have systemic venous congestion, hepatomegaly, pleural effusions, and ascites requiring aggressive diuretic therapy. Nevertheless, most patients who survive the Fontan operation are markedly improved symptomatically and are able to return to active productive lives.

EBSTEIN'S ANOMALY

The most common congenital malformation of the tricuspid valve resulting in stenosis and/or incompetence is Ebstein's anomaly. Published English translations of Ebstein's original description appeared for the first time in 1968[25] and more recently in 1974.[26] Interest in this anomaly as a clinical entity was heightened following a publication in 1950 by Engle et al[27] suggesting for the first time that the diagnosis could be made during life.

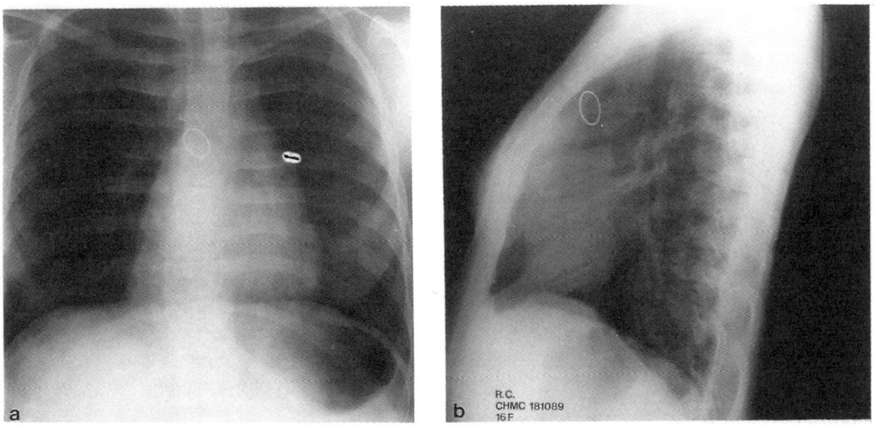

Figure 4-8 Posteroanterior (a) and lateral (b) roentgenograms of a patient with tricuspid atresia, type III (malposition of the great vessels with normal pulmonary arteries) who had undergone a Fontan procedure. Note the position of the porcine xenograft (metal ring) which was interposed between the right atrium and the malpositioned pulmonary artery.

Ebstein's anomaly is among the most unusual of all forms of congenital heart disease, accounting for less than 1% of all cases.[28] The primary anatomical feature is displacement of the proximal attachment of the tricuspid valve leaflets distally into the right ventricle. The displaced valve divides the right ventricle into an inlet portion which is functionally part of the right atrium, the so-called atrialized portion, and the trabecular and outflow portions which become the functional right ventricle.[29] The atrialized portion of the right ventricle is often hypokinetic and contributes very little to right ventricular function. Invariably only the septal and posterior leaflets are displaced while the anterior leaflet retains its normal attachment to the atrioventricular groove.[30] The leaflets are variable in size and usually dysplastic. The severity of the malformation is variable, but the basic pattern of the tricuspid valve displacement is constant. The septal leaflets are often adherent to the right ventricular wall and septum while in some instances, the anterior leaflet is redundant and creates an inflatable curtain or windsock which effectively obstructs the right ventricular outflow (Figure 4-9).[31] Occasionally the tricuspid valve is imperforate, resulting in complete obstruction to pulmonary blood flow, mimicking pulmonary valve atresia.[32,33] In approximately half the cases of Ebstein's anomaly, there is an associated atrial septal defect permitting varying degrees of right-to-left shunting and in the remainder there is usually a patent foramen ovale.

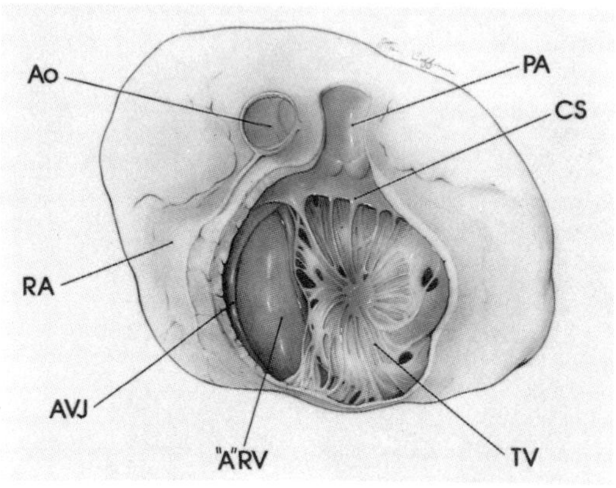

Figure 4-9 · Diagram illustrating abnormal attachment of the anterior leaflet of the tricuspid valve. Fenestrations in the valve leaflet permit limited communication from the inlet portion of the right ventricle to the outflow tract. AO = aorta, RA = right atrium, AVJ = atrioventricular junction, "A"RV = atrialized right ventricle, TV = tricuspid valve, CS = crista supraventricularis, PA = pulmonary artery.

Pathophysiology

The hemodynamic abnormality in Ebstein's anomaly is quite variable and is directly related to the severity of tricuspid incompetence, the impairment of right ventricular function, and the extent of obstruction by the malformed valve. The spectrum of the hemodynamic alteration varies from a severely obstructing tricuspid valve leading to profound reduction in pulmonary blood flow and marked cyanosis in the newborn period (Figure 4-10) to trivial tricuspid regurgitation permiting prolonged and asymptomatic survival into the sixth and seventh decades of life (Figure 4-11).

Clinical features

As the pathology and pathophysiology of Ebstein's anomaly are variable, so too are the clinical features. Cyanosis is the clinical hallmark and occurs at some time during life in 60% to 80% of patients.[34,35] A few patients remain free of symptoms well into adulthood although in the majority, cyanosis and dyspnea appear early and gradually worsen throughout life. Palpitations or sustained tachycardia are common, owing in part to the frequent association of type B Wolff-Parkinson-White pre-excitation.[36] The jugular venous pulse is usually normal despite even moderately severe tricuspid regurgitation. The precordium is surprisingly quiet in most patients. Auscultation in Ebstein's anomaly is often confusing and difficult to evaluate because of wide splitting of the first and second heart sounds, systolic and diastolic murmurs, as well as third and fourth heart sounds.[37] A characteristic superficial scratchy diastolic murmur is often heard and together with the other auscultatory findings, may simulate a pericardial friction rub.[38] The most consistent findings include a widely split first heart sound and a systolic regurgitant murmur of tricuspid incompetence at the low left sternal border characteristically augmented during inspiration.

Electrocardiography

The most striking feature of the ECG in Ebstein's anomaly is the presence of atypical right bundle-branch block in association with low QRS voltage in the right precordium. (Figure 4-12) The right bundle-branch block pattern is often bizarre with polyphasic QRS morphology, especially in the right precordial leads.[39] In

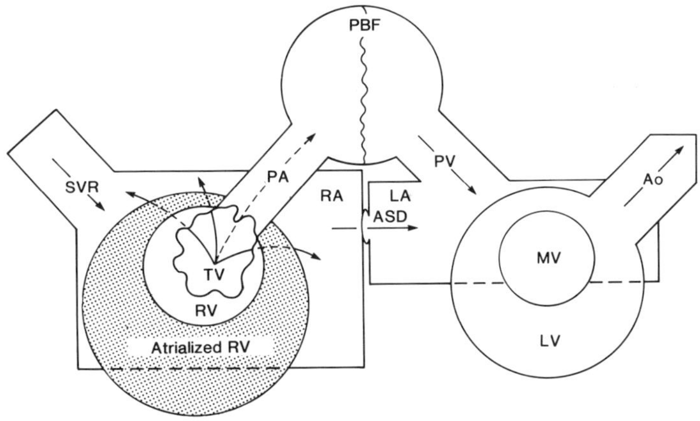

EBSTEIN'S ANOMALY WITH RVOT OBSTRUCTION, TRICUSPID REGURGITATION, R →L ATRIAL SHUNT

Figure 4-10 Pathophysiology of Ebstein's anomaly with predominant tricuspid obstruction. Pulmonary blood flow is reduced (PA, broken line) There is marked tricuspid regurgitation and significant right-to-left atrial shunting (ASD, solid line). TV = tricuspid valve. For other abbreviations, see legend Figure 4-1.

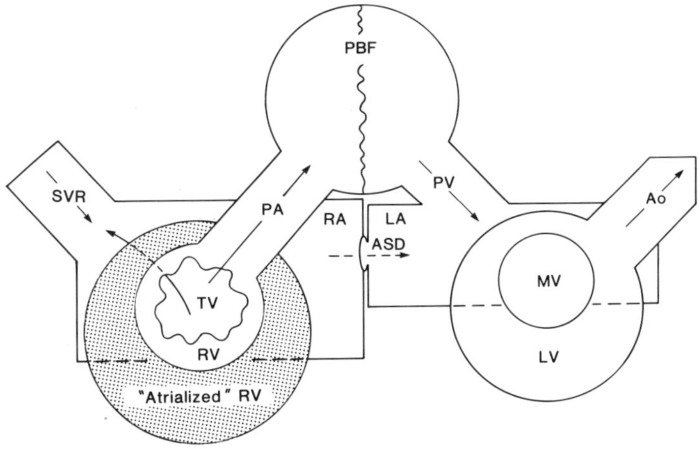

EBSTEIN'S ANOMALY AND TRICUSPID REGURGITATION

Figure 4-11 Hemodynamics in mild Ebstein's anomaly. There is minimal tricuspid regurgitation and intermittent right-to-left atrial shunting (ASD, broken line). Pulmonary flow is normal. For abbreviations, see Figure 4-1 and 4-10.

addition, the P waves are often abnormal both in amplitude and duration. The presence of type B Wolff-Parkinson-White syndrome is quite common, occurring in as many as 25% of cases.[36] Among patients with cyanotic congenital heart disease and type B Wolff-Parkinson-White syndrome, Ebstein's anomaly of the tricuspid valve is by far the most common abnormality. Since preexcitation of the right ventricle tends to counterbalance the effect of right bundle-branch block, Wolff-Parkinson-White syndrome and complete right bundle-branch block are seldom seen together in the same patient.

Radiographic features

In Ebstein's anomaly the radiographic features vary from nearly normal (Figure 4-13) to a relatively distinctive cardiac silhouette charac-

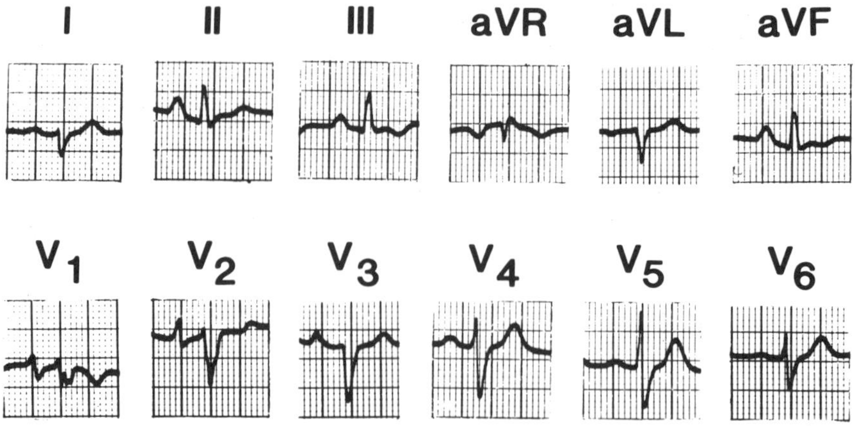

Figure 4-12 The patient is a 27-year-old woman with Ebstein's anomaly and severe tricuspid valve obstruction. Broad peaked P waves with terminal negativity in V_1 indicate biatrial enlargement.

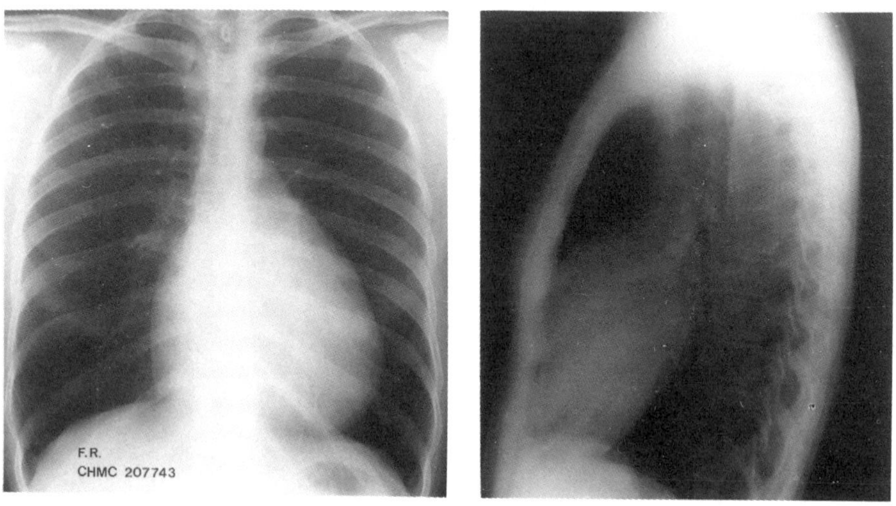

Figure 4-13 Posteroanterior (left) and lateral (right) roentgenograms of a 27-year-old woman with predominant tricuspid obstruction, marked right-to-left atrial shunting and severe cyanosis. Note the absence of right atrial enlargement, diminished pulmonary blood flow, and dilatation of the right ventricular outflow tract.

terized by ballooning of the heart to occupy most of the thorax (Figure 4-14).[36] In most instances the right atrium accounts for the massive enlargement and makes up most of the cardiac silhouette. In the lateral view the enlarged right atrium can project posteriorly and overlap the spine at the level of the diaphragm (Figure 4-15). Characteristically the right ventricular outflow tract is dilated resulting in marked convexity of the left upper cardiac border which, together with the right atrial enlargement, produces the typical boxlike or globular cardiac configuration. The pulmonary vascularity is usually normal or somewhat diminished but almost never increased except in rare instances when there is an associated left-to-right shunt.

Echocardiography

The M-mode echographic features of Ebstein's anomaly include: (1) delayed closure of the tricuspid valve, (2) increased amplitude of the anterior leaflet of the tricuspid valve and the ability to record the tricuspid valve echoes over most of the precordium, (3) abnormal septal

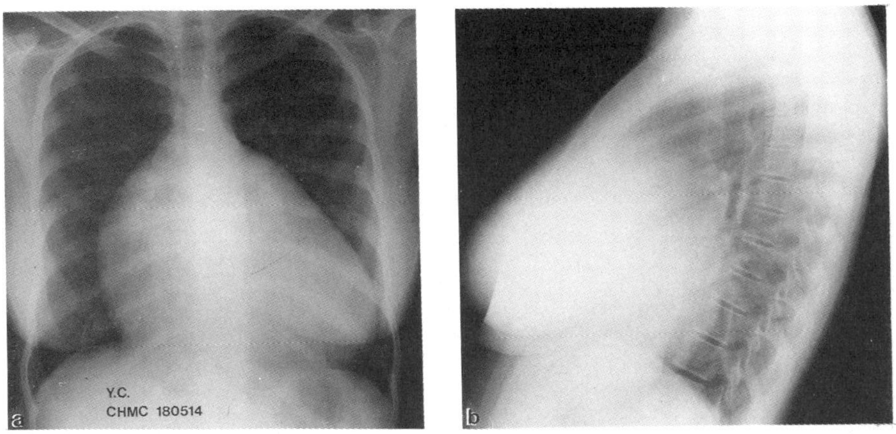

Figure 4-14 Posteroanterior (a) and lateral (b) roentgenograms of a 21-year-old woman with severe tricuspid regurgitation. Marked right atrial enlargement and dilatation of right ventricular outflow tract account for the distinctive cardiac silhouette.

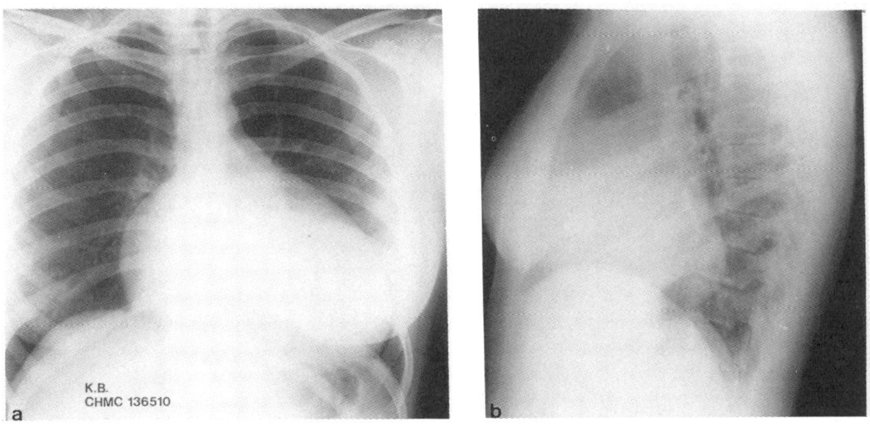

Figure 4-15 Posteroanterior (a) and lateral (b) roentgenograms of a 25-year-old woman with dominant tricuspid incompetence. The greatly enlarged right atrium projects posteriorly and inferiorly to overlap the spine.

motion similar to that seen in patients with right volume overload, (4) decreased diastolic (e-f) slope of the tricuspid valve.[40,41] Among these features the only specific finding in Ebstein's anomaly is the marked delay of tricuspid valve closure.[42] Two-dimensional echocardiography permits a more complete evaluation of the anatomical features. The apical four-chamber view allows excellent visualization of the displaced tricuspid valve, the elongation of the anterior leaflet, and enlargement of the right atrium in conjunction with the atrialized portion of the right ventricle (Figure 4-16).[43] Additional features of Ebstein's anomaly identified by two-dimensional echocardiography include inferior displacement of the septal leaflet, aneurysmal dilatation of the right ventricular outflow tract, and exaggerated tricuspid valve motion. Doppler studies consistently demonstrate tricuspid regurgitation.[44] Angiographic abnormalities of left ventricular contractility have been described by Monibi et al[45] despite the absence of clinical signs of left ventricular dysfunction. In a two-dimensional echocardiographic study of 41 patients by Shiina et al,[46] only two patients were found with abnormalities of left ventricular function. One patient had a previous myocardial infarction and the other was 85 years of age.

Cardiac catheterization and angiocardiography

Despite early admonitions regarding the dan-

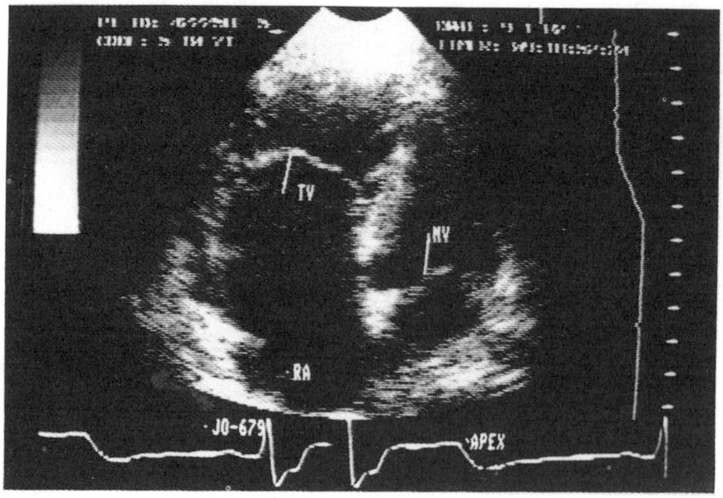

Figure 4-16 Two-dimensional echocardiogram in the apical four-chamber view. Note the marked displacement of the tricuspid valve (TV) into the right ventricle creating the atrialized right ventricle in continuity with the dilated right atrium (RA). MV = mitral valve.

ger of cardiac catheterization in patients with Ebstein's anomaly,[38] extensive invasive studies including electrophysiologic evaluation can be performed with minimal risk.[47] Hemodynamic data typically show modest elevation of right atrial pressure with a dominant "v" wave in those patients with predominant tricuspid regurgitation or a prominent "a" wave in those patients with predominant tricuspid stenosis.[48] The functional right ventricle may be difficult to enter but right ventricular pressure is usually normal. The pulmonary artery may be extremely difficult to catheterize because of displacement of the tricuspid valve into the right ventricular outflow tract. Pulmonary artery pressure is typically normal or slightly decreased especially when there is severe tricuspid regurgitation or partial obstruction of the right ventricular outflow tract by the displaced tricuspid valve. Oximetry frequently demonstrates bidirectional shunting at atrial level with subsequent arterial desaturation. Selective cineangiography in the right ventricle is usually diagnostic of Ebstein's anomaly. The right ventriculogram shows varying degrees of tricuspid regurgitation with subsequent filling of the atrialized right ventricle and native right atrium producing a characteristic three-chambered configuration (Figure 4-17). Cineangiography also demonstrates the abnormal attachment and motion of the tricuspid valve. In the absence of selective angiography, a definitive diagnosis can often be confirmed by intracardiac electrocardiography. Utilizing an electrode-tipped end-hole catheter to record intracavitary pressure, a pullback from the functional right ventricle toward the right atrium demonstrates

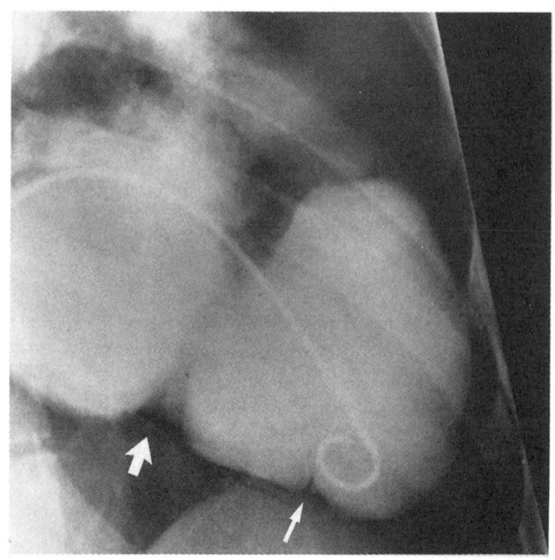

Figure 4-17 Selective right ventriculogram in the right anterior oblique projection showing the angiographic features of Ebstein's anomaly. There is marked tricuspid regurgitation with opacification of the greatly enlarged right atrium. The atrialized portion of the right ventricle is defined by the abnormal attachment of the tricuspid valve distally (thin arrow) and the true tricuspid annulus proximally (thick arrow) creating the typical three-chambered appearance.

continued right ventricular potential after the pressure pulse has changed from a ventricular contour to an atrial contour.[49] The presence of atrial pressure in association with ventricular electrical potentials results from the atrialized portion of the ventricle and is diagnostic of Ebstein's anomaly. In recent years, with improved angiographic techniques and the development of two-dimensional echocardiography, it is seldom necessary to utilize the intracavitary ECG to establish the diagnosis.

Natural history and management

Life expectancy is considerably shortened in the majority of patients with Ebstein's anomaly and death is usually related to hemodynamic alterations leading to congestive heart failure, severe right ventricular outflow tract obstruction, paradoxical embolus and brain abscess or not uncommonly sudden death usually attributed to cardiac arrhythmia.[34,50] Nevertheless, prolonged survival is widely reported[51–53] and it is likely that a number of patients with the mildest form of this anomaly reach adulthood undiagnosed. In a study of 67 patients at the Mayo Clinic with a mean follow-up of 12 years, 26 patients (39%) remained relatively asymptomatic and 41 (61%) progressed to become markedly symptomatic with death occurring in 21% of patients.[35] Factors affecting prognosis included not only progressive symptomatology, but extreme cardiomegaly, profound cyanosis, and symptomatic presentation in early infancy.

The indications for surgical intervention include progressive symptomatology resulting from congestive heart failure, marked cyanosis, and increasing cardiomegaly.[54] Excision of the abnormal valve and replacement with a prosthesis has been widely reported and continues to find a place in the surgical approach to Ebstein's anomaly.[55,–57] Danielson et al have advocated repair of the abnormal valve based on constructing a monocusp valve from the anterior leaflet, plication of the atrialized portion of the free wall of the right ventricle, a posterior tricuspid anuloplasty, and right atrial reduction in those patients with a giant right atrium.[58] Clearly, operative repair is preferred over valve replacement whenever possible since it precludes the problems of prosthetic valve dysfunction and lifetime anticoagulation. The extent to which refractory arrhythmia should influence the decision for surgical repair is uncertain. In patients with recurrent tachycardia, with or without evidence of preexcitation on surface ECGs, detailed electrophysiologic studies to identify the number and location of accessory pathways should be performed if surgical treatment is being considered.[59] In cases where an accessory conduction pathway has been demonstrated in association with refractory arrhythmia, surgical division of the bypass has been successfully performed following intraoperative mapping.[47] In view of the relative ease with which accessory pathways can be isolated and divided surgically, patients with Ebstein's anomaly and preexcitation should undergo operative mapping and division of the accessory pathway at the time of intracardiac repair of the primary lesion, regardless of whether or not they have a history of tachycardia.[60,61]

REFERENCES

1. Rao PS: Demographic features of tricuspid atresia, in Rao PS (ed): *Tricuspid Atresia*. Mt Kisco, NY, Futura Publishing Co, 1982.
2. Bharati S Lev M: The concept of tricuspid atresia complex as distinct from that of single ventricle complex. *Pediatr Cardiol* 1979;1:57–62.
3. Anderson RH, Becker AE, Macartney FJ: Is "tricuspid atresia" a univentricular heart? *Pediatr Cardiol* 1979;1:51–56.
4. Van Praagh R, Ando M, Dungan WT: Anatomic types of tricuspid atresia; Clinical and developmental implications. *Circulation*, 1971;43–44 (suppl 2):11–115.
5. Weinberg PM: Anatomy of tricuspid atresia and its relevance to current forms of surgical therapy. *Ann Thorac Surg* 1980;29:306.
6. Gasul BM, Arcilla RH, Lev, M: *Heart Disease in Children: Diagnosis and Treatment*. Philadelphia, JB Lippincott Co, 1966, pp 656–685.
7. Rao PS: A unified classification of tricuspid atresia. *Am Heart* J, 1980;99:799–804.
8. Rao PS: Classification of tricuspid atresia, in Rao PS (ed): *Tricuspid Atresia*. Mt Kisco, NY, Futura Publishing Co, 1982.
9. Rao PS: Natural history of the ventricular septal defect in tricuspid atresia and its surgical implications. *Bri Heart J* 1977;39:276.
10. Dick M, Flyer DC, Nadas AS: Tricuspid atresia; Clinical course in 101 patients. *A J Cardiol* 1975; 36:327–337.
11. McFaul RC, Tajik AJ, Mair DD, et al: Development of pulmonary arteriovenous shunt after superior vena cava–right pulmonary artery (Glenn) anastomosis. *Circulation* 1977;55:212.
12. Kulanjara RJ, Boineau JP, Moore HV, et al: Electrovectorcardiographic features of tricuspid atresia, in Rao PS (edi): *Tricuspid Atresia*. Mt Kisco, Futura Publishing Co, NY, 1982.
13. Deutsch V, Shem-Tov A, Yahini J, et al: Juxtaposition of atrial appendages; angiographic observations. *Am J Cardiol* 1974;34:240.
14. Beppu S, Nemura Y, Tamai M, et al: Two-

dimensional echocardiography in diagnosing tricuspid atresia. *Br Heart J* 1978;40:1174.
15. Silverman NH, Schiller NB: Apex echocardiography: A two-dimensional technique for evaluating congenital heart disease. *Circulation* 1978; 57:503.
16. Koiwaya Y, Watanabe K, Orita Y, et al: Contrast two-dimensional echocardiography in diagnosis of tricuspid atresia. *Am Heart J* 1981;101:507.
17. Schwartz D: Angiography in tricuspid atresia, in Rao PS (ed): *Tricuspid Atresia* Mt Kisco, NY, Futura Publishing Co, 1982.
18. Jordan JC, Sanders CA: Tricuspid atresia with prolonged survival. *Am J Cardiol* 1966;18:112.
19. Bohm R, Schmidt KH, Gunther KA et al: Tricuspid atresia with ventricular septal defect in a 31 year old woman. *Cardiologia* 1968;53:11–18.
20. Fontan F, Bandet E: Surgical repair of tricuspid atresia. *Thorax* 1971;26:240.
21. Kreutzer G: Recent surgical approaches to tricuspid atresia, in *The Child with Congenital Heart Disease After Surgery*. Kidd BSL, Rowe RD (eds): Mt Kisco, NY, Futura Publishing Co, Inc. 1976.
22. Graham TP Jr: Tricuspid atresia in adolescents and adults, in Rao PS (ed): *Tricuspid Atresia*, Mt Kisco, NY, Futura Publishing Co, 1982.
23. Shackar GB, Fuhrman BP, Wang Y, et al: Rest and exercise hemodynamics after Fontan procedure. *Circulation* 1982;65:1043–1048.
24. Graham TP Jr: Ventricular performance in adults after operation for congenital heart disease, in Engle MA, Perloff J (eds): *Congenital Heart Disease after Surgery*. Yorke Medical Books, 1983.
25. Schiebler GL, Gravenstein JS, Van Mierop LH: Ebstein's anomaly of the tricuspid valve, translation of original description and comments. *Am J Cardiol* 1968;22:867.
26. Sekelj P, Benfey BG: Historical landmarks: Ebstein's anomaly of the tricuspid valve. *Am Heart J* 1974;88:108–114.
27. Engle MA, Payne TPB, Bruins C, et al: Ebstein's anomaly of the tricuspid valve. Report of 3 cases and analysis of clinical syndrome. *Circulation* 1950;1:1246.
28. Rowe RD, Freedom RM, Mehrizi, A, et al: The neonate with congenital heart disease. Philadelphia, WB Saunders Co, 1981, p 517.
29. Zuberbuhler JR, Allwork SP, Anderson RH: The spectrum of Ebstein's anomaly of the tricuspid valve. *J Thorac Cardiovasc Surg* 1979;77:202–211.
30. Lev M, Lieberthson RR, Joseph RH et al: The pathologic anatomy of Ebstein's disease. *Arch Path*, 1970;90:334–344.
31. Anderson KR, Zuberbuhler JR, Anderson RH, et al: Morphologic spectrum of Ebstein's anomaly of the heart. *Mayo Clin Proc* 1979;54:174–180.
32. Newfeld EA, Cole RB, Pave MH: Ebstein's malformation of the tricuspid valve in the neonate. Functional & anatomic pulmonary outflow tract obstruction. *Am J Cardiol* 1967;19:727.
33. Rao PS, Jue KL, Isabel-Jones J, et al: Ebstein's malformation of the tricuspid valve with atresia. *Am J Cardiol* 1973;32:1004–1009.
34. Genton E, Blount SG: The spectrum of Ebstein's anomaly. *Am Heart J* 1967; 73:395–425.
35. Giuliani ER, Fuster V, Brandenburg RO, et al: The clinical features and natural history of Ebstein's anomaly of the tricuspid valve. *Mayo Clin Proc* 1979;54:163–173.
36. Bialostozky D, Horwitz S, Espino-Vela J: Ebstein's malformation of the tricuspid valve. A review of 65 cases *Am J Cardiol* 1972; 29:826–836.
37. Perloff J: Ebstein's anomaly of the tricuspid valve, in *Clinical Recognition of Congenital Heart Disease*, ed 2. Philadelphia, WB Saunders Co, 1978, pp 246–249.
38. Wood P: *Diseases of the Heart and Circulation* ed Philadelphia, 3, JB Lippincott Co, 1968, pp 411–418.
39. Chou T-C: *Electrocardiography in Clinical Practice*. New York, Grune & Stratton, Inc, 1979, pp 320–321.
40. Meyer RA: Echocardiography in congenital heart disease. *Am J Med* 1977; 63:41–49.
41. Farooki ZQ, Henry JG, Green EW: Echocardiographic spectrum of Ebstein's anomaly of the tricuspid valve. *Circulation* 1976;53:63–68.
42. Milner S, Meyer RA, Venables AW et al: Mitral and tricuspid valve closure in congenital heart disease. *Circulation* 1976;53:513–518.
43. Ports TA, Silverman NH, Schiller, NB: Two-dimensional echocardiographic assessment of Ebstein's anomaly. *Circulation* 1978;58:336–343.
44. Waggoner AD, Quinnones MH, Young JB, et al: Pulsed Doppler echocardiographic detection of right-sided valve regurgitation. *Am J Cardiol* 1981;47:279.
45. Monibi AA, Neches WH, Lenox CC et al: Left ventricular anomalies associated with Ebstein's malformation of the tricuspid valve. *Circulation* 1978;57:303–306.
46. Shiina A, Seward JB, Edwards WD, et al: Two-dimensional echocardiographic spectrum of Ebstein's anomaly: Detailed anatomic assessment. *J Am Coll Cardiol* 1984;3:356–370.
47. Smith WM, Gallagher JJ, Kerr CR, et al: The electrophysiologic basis and management of symptomatic recurrent tachycardia in patients with Ebstein's anomaly of the tricuspid valve. *Am J Cardiol* 1982;49:1223–1234.
48. Takayasu S, Obunai Y, Konno S: Clinical classification of Ebstein's anomaly. *Am Heart J* 1978; 95:154–162.
49. Watson H: Electrode catheters and the diagnosis of Ebstein's anomaly of the tricuspid valve. *Br Heart J* 1966;28:161–171.
50. Watson H: Natural history of Ebstein's anomaly of the tricuspid valve in childhood and adolescence. *Br Heart J* 1974;36:417–427.
51. Seward JB, Tajik AJ, Feist DJ et al: Ebstein's anomaly in an 85 year old man. *Mayo Clinic Proc* 1979;54:193–196.
52. Cabin HS Wood TP, Smith JO, et al: Ebstein's anomaly in the elderly. *Chest* 1980; 80:212–214.
53. Makous N, Vander Veer JB: Ebstein's anomaly and life expectancy: Report of survival to over age 79. *Am J Cardiol* 1966;18:100–104.
54. Danielson GK, Fuster V: Surgical repair of Ebstein's anomaly. *Ann Surg* 1982;196:499.
55. Bove EL, Kirsh MM: Valve replacement for Ebstein's anomaly of the tricupid valve. *J Thorac Cardiovasc Surg* 1979;78:229.
56. Shigenobu M, Mendez MA, Zubiate P, et al:

Thirteen years experience with the Kay-Shiley disc valve for tricuspid replacement in Ebstein's anomaly. *Ann Thorac Surg* 1980;29:423.

57. Barbero-Marcial M, Verginelli G, Awad M, et al: Surgical treatment of Ebstein's anomaly: Early and late results in twenty patients subjected to valve replacement. *J Thorac Cardiovasc Surg* 1979;78:416.
58. Danielson GK, Maloney JD, Devloo RAE: Surgical repair of Ebstein's anomaly. *Mayo Clin Proc* 1979;54:185–192.
59. Kugler JD, Gillette PC, Duff DF, et al: Elective mapping and surgical division of the bundle of Kent in a patient with Ebstein's anomaly who required tricuspid valve replacement. *Am J Cardiol* 1978;41:602–605.
60. Ott DA, Cooley DA, Reul, GJ, Jr. et al: Surgical treatment of patients with tachydysrhythmia, in *Pediatric Cardiac Dysrhythmias*, Gillette C, Garson Jr, A (eds): New York, Grune & Stratton, Inc 1981, pp 437–449.
61. Gallagher JJ, Sealy WC, Cox JL, et al: Results of surgery for preexcitation caused by accessory atrioventricular pathways in 267 consecutive cases, in *Tachycardias: Mechanism, Diagnosis, Treatment*. Josephson ME Wellens HJ (eds): Philadelphia, Lea & Febigu G, 1984, pp 259–269.

CHAPTER 5
Acquired Tricuspid Valve Disease

Bruce H. Brundage
Stuart Rich
Sidney Levitsky
Jeffrey G. Shanes

The evaluation of patients with acquired valve disease often gives little consideration to the valves of the right ventricle. This situation is particularly common in the United States where the incidence of rheumatic fever and subsequent rheumatic heart disease has decreased markedly in the last three decades. The annual incidence of acute rheumatic fever in 1935 was 40 per 100,000 population and recently was reported to be 0.64 per 100,000 in Memphis.[1,2]

However, some diseases of the tricuspid valve such as infective endocarditis in drug addicts have increased in frequency.[3] As unfortunate as this disease is, the clinician must be aware of its presenting symptoms, characteristic physical findings, and some of the unique epidemiologic manifestations, such as regional differences in infecting organism.[4]

Tricuspid valve disease is often not detected during the physical examination and yet it frequently produces visible abnormalities of the jugular venous pulse.

New diagnostic methods such as echocardiography have increased the physician's awareness of tricuspid valve abnormalities such as tricuspid valve prolapse. Recognition of this abnormality may be the first clue to the presence of Marfan's syndrome.

Treatment of tricuspid valve disease still poses some difficult problems. While valve replacement has proved to be successful treatment for aortic, pulmonic, and mitral valve disease, tricuspid valve replacement is less satisfactory because of the greater propensity for tricuspid prosthetic valves to develop thrombus or pannus. Tilting disc valves develop obstructive thrombosis in 20% of cases.[5] Although the incidence is lower with ball valve and heterograft prostheses, it remains higher than for aortic and mitral valves.

This chapter will review the more common etiologies of tricuspid valve disease, with emphasis on the changing patterns, compare the pathophysiology of stenosis and regurgitation, describe the pertinent features of the history and physical examination, detail the traditional diagnostic modalities, and describe several new methods of diagnosis. Finally, the principles of the medical and surgical treatment of the disease will be discussed.

ETIOLOGY

Tricuspid Regurgitation

Throughout the world, rheumatic valvulitis is the most common cause of tricuspid valve disease. However its incidence has dropped dramatically in economically well-developed areas like the United States, Europe and Japan. The incidence is also beginning to fall in rapidly developing Third World countries such as Taiwan.

The rheumatic process may cause valve leaflet fusion producing stenosis as seen with mitral valvulitis. However, retraction of the tricuspid leaflets with loss of valve substance is more common making tricuspid regurgitation the more common clinical form of rheumatic tricuspid valve disease. Isolated rheumatic involvement of the tricuspid valve almost never, if ever, occurs but is usually associated with significant rheumatic involvement of the mitral valve. Pulmonary hypertension is a common sequela of rheumatic mitral valve disease and often produces chronic right-sided heart failure which may result in a secondary form of tricuspid regurgitation. Indeed, the most common cause of tricuspid regurgitation in patients with rheumatic heart disease is mitral valve disease. In some economically underdeveloped countries primary rheumatic tricuspid valve disease is quite frequent, but even in these countries tricuspid regurgitation secondary to pulmonary hypertension is probably more frequent than primary regurgitation.

The development of right heart failure is often heralded by the appearance of tricuspid valve regurgitation when pulmonary hypertension is present. Initially the volume of regurgitant blood is often small but with chronic heart failure the amount may become substantial. If compensation of the right ventricular function can be accomplished with treatment, the regurgitation will often diminish or disappear. With long-standing right heart failure the regurgitation may be irreversible and when open heart surgery is performed for the mitral valve, the tricuspid valve may have so much loss of valvular substance that it too requires replacement or repair. This appearance of the tricuspid valve at surgery often raises questions as to whether the etiology of the tricuspid regurgitation is primary or secondary.

In the United States, the development of tricuspid endocarditis is nearly always associated with intravenous (IV) drug abuse. A review of infective endocarditis in addicts collated the reported incidence of isolated tricuspid valve involvement and found it occurred in an average of 52% of all cases.[6] The range, however, was highly variable. The incidence of tricuspid involvement in nonaddicts is between 1% and 6%. Infective endocarditis of the tricuspid valve always results in some regurgitation. The regurgitation, even when substantial, is well tolerated as long as pulmonary vascular resistance is normal (Figure 5-1). However, the tricuspid vegetations are often bulky and friable and sometimes embolize to the pulmonary arteries. Extensive embolization may result in pulmonary hypertension. With the development of pulmonary hypertension, the tricuspid regurgitation is worsened and morbidity and mortality are increased.

Staphlococcus aureus is the cause of tricuspid endocarditis in more then 50% of addicts and apparently is introduced into the bloods stream during the self-administration of drugs. However, the staphlococcus organism usually cannot be cultured from the street drugs used or from the drug paraphenalia. Therefore it is presumed

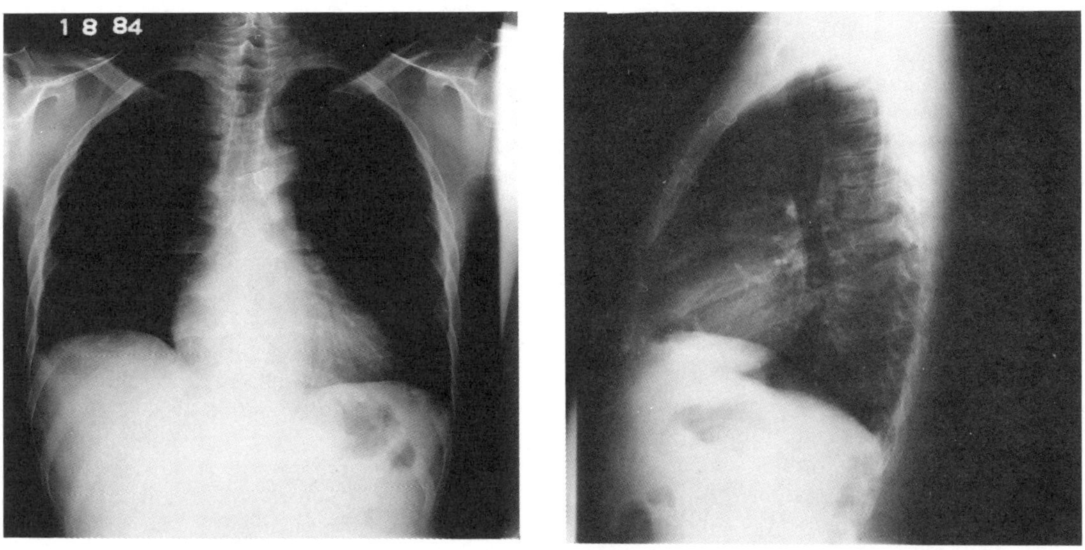

Figure 5-1 These posteroanterior (left) and lateral (right) chest films of an addict 4 years after tricuspid valvectomy show evidence of mild to moderate right atrial enlargement. The films are remarkable for the relatively mild changes despite an absent tricuspid valve.

to come from the addict's skin or nasopharynx.[6] In large midwestern cities such as Chicago, *Pseudomonas aeruginosa* is a frequent Gram-negative cause of tricuspid endocarditis in addicts. In San Francisco, *Serratia marcescens* is reported to be a frequent Gram-negative cause.[4] Other Gram-negative organisms and fungi also cause endocarditis in addicts.[6,7]

Carcinoid tumors of the gastrointestional (GI) tract, when they metastasize to the liver, may produce a unique type of endocardial fibrosis of the right ventricle that often involves the tricuspid valve and may cause regurgitation and occasionally stenosis.[8] On occasion the cardiac manifestations of the disease may be so severe that the symptoms of systemic venous hypertension predominate in the clinical picture. The fibrotic process is believed to be caused by vasoactive substances released by the tumor into the hepatic veins.

Myxomatous degeneration of the tricuspid valve is much less common than of the mitral valve, but is said to be present in one third of patients with mitral valve prolapse.[9] Myxomatous involvement of the tricuspid valve is most often present in Marfan's syndrome. Whenever the tricuspid valve is affected, the mitral valve is almost always involved too. Clinical sequelae from myxomatous degeneration of tricuspid valve are uncommon but nonejection clicks and tricuspid regurgitation murmurs may be present.

Tricuspid regurgitation has been observed infrequently after right ventricular infarction,[10] in thyrotoxicosis,[11] in association with aneurysm of the ventricular septum,[12] and with Löffler's endocarditis.[13] Both penetrating and nonpenetrating chest trauma may also cause tricuspid regurgitation.[14]

Tricuspid Stenosis

Tricuspid stenosis is clinically much less frequent than tricuspid regurgitation. In the United States, where the incidence of rheumatic fever and rheumatic heart disease have declined dramatically, clinically significant tricuspid stenosis is uncommon.

Tricuspid stenosis may result from surgical annuloplasty for tricuspid regurgitation. Occasionally this iatrogenic form of stenosis is severe enough to require reoperation.

Tumors which involve the right side of the heart may cause obstruction of the tricuspid orfice. This obstruction may be intermittent as occurs with right atrial myxoma or it may be unrelenting as observed with sessile metastatic tumors of the right atrium and right ventricle (Figure 5-2). The carcinoid syndrome, Löffler's endocarditis, and constrictive pericarditis are rare reported causes of tricuspid stenosis.[8,15,16]

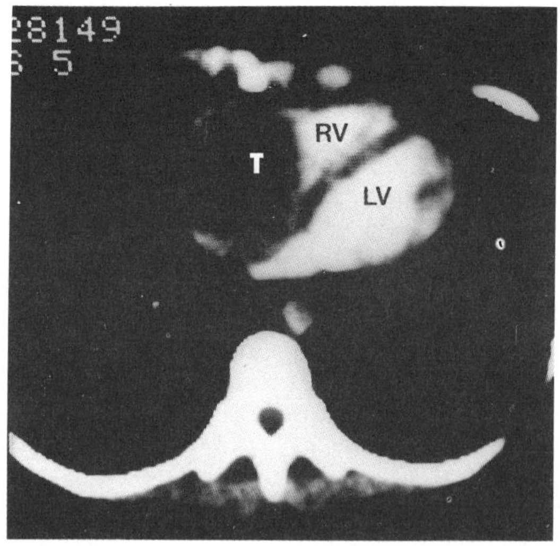

Figure 5-2 This contrast-enhanced computed tomographic (CT) scan of the heart shows a large thymoma metastasis (T) occupying the right atrium. LV = left ventricle, RV = right ventricle.

PATHOPHYSIOLOGY

Tricuspid Regurgitation

Tricuspid regurgitation, when severe, produces two hemodynamic effects. It causes a pulsatile systemic venous hypertension which may result in hepatic congestion, ascites, and peripheral edema. The regurgitation may also limit the ability of the right ventricle to increase stroke volume when necessary as during exercise. This limitation can cause symptoms of malaise and easy fatiguability.

The regurgitant volume in primary causes of tricuspid regurgitation as seen with infective endocarditis in addicts or with trauma can be large without producing systemic venous hypertension or low cardiac output because the resistance in pulmonary circulation is usually normal. When pulmonary pressure is normal, tricuspid regurgitation is well tolerated and the patients are usually asymptomatic.

Contrarily, secondary tricuspid regurgitation often leads to systemic venous hypertension and reduced cardiac output. Secondary tricuspid regurgitation occurs as a result of chronic right ventricular systolic hypertension. Initially the tricuspid valve is anatomically normal but after long periods (usually years) there may be retraction of the leaflet edges, loss of valve substance, and annular dilatation. The amount of regurgitation is linked directly to the level of right ventricular systolic pressure; the greater the pressure the greater the regurgitation. Usually the right ventricular systolic overload is caused by pulmonary hypertension and this is most frequently related to elevation of pulmonary capillary and venous pressures caused by left heart problems such as mitral stenosis. Recently, the role of annular dilatation and malalignment of the tricuspid leaflets has been emphasized as a pathogenetic mechanism in secondary or functional tricuspid regurgitation.[17] However, in annular dilatation, lack of leaflet coaptation or loss of valve substance play a role in secondary tricuspid regurgitation; the usual final common pathway is pulmonary hypertension and the severity of regurgitation and symptoms are directly correlated with the severity of pulmonary hypertension. In fact the best means of determining whether tricuspid regurgitation is primary or secondary is to determine whether significant pulmonary hypertension is present. Even in rheumatic heart disease where both primary and secondary causes of tricuspid regurgitation can coexist, the predominant mechanism is likely to correlate with pulmonary pressure.

Tricuspid Stenosis

Like tricuspid regurgitation, tricuspid stenosis produces the same two hemodynamic abnormalities: systemic venous hypertension and restriction of the heart's ability to increase cardiac output in response to increased demand. The major signs and symptoms produced by tricuspid stenosis are likewise related to increased systemic venous pressure. Tricuspid stenosis is usually of rheumatic etiology and in this case is nearly always accompanied by disease of the mitral valve and the disturbed physiology is often dominated by the effects of the mitral valve disease. The pulmonary hypertension that often accompanies mitral valve disease may reduce cardiac output so much that the presence of organic tricuspid stenosis is masked.

Alteration of the diastolic filling pattern of the right ventricle caused by tricuspid stenosis is another important feature of the pathophysiology and it provides important diagnostic clues which can be observed in the jugular venous pulse wave. Rarely the venous congestion produced by the valve obstruction may be so severe that the clinical presentation is a malabsorption or nephrotic syndrome. Occasionally tricuspid stenosis may be confused with constrictive pericarditis.

CLINICAL FEATURES

History

Patients with tricuspid stenosis or regurgitation usually complain of symptoms related to systemic venous hypertension with peripheral edema being most common. In more severe forms of the disease, ascites and periorbital edema may also occur. Fatigue is another frequent symptom in advanced tricuspid disease, because of the limited cardiac output response to physical exertion. However, because many patients with tricuspid valve disease have rheumatic involvement of other cardiac valves, the symptoms related to these associated abnormalities may dominate the clinical picture.

The history is important in providing clues to the presence of tricuspid valve disease, but its greatest value is in uncovering the etiology of the tricuspid disease. Because the etiologies are so varied, from tumor to infection, and the treatments so different, from surgery to observation, the need to identify the underlying cause of the tricuspid valve disease is obvious.

Physical Examination

The clinician is afforded a unique opportunity when evaluating tricuspid valve disease compared to bedside assessment of other forms of valvular heart disease. Noninvasive hemodynamic assessment of the disease is possible at the bedside because the neck veins reflect right atrial pressure events (Figure 5-3). Measurement of the height of the venous column above the angle of Louis provides accurate determination of right atrial pressure. Inspection of the venous pulsations gives important clues to the presence of tricuspid regurgitation and tricuspid stenosis. The characteristic regurgitant wave of tricuspid regurgitation (Figure 5-3) may be the only clue to insufficiency of the tricuspid valve because the murmur may be very faint or absent. With severe degrees of regurgitation the "v" wave may cause outward movement of the ear lobes, pulsation of the eyeballs, and commonly pulsation of the liver. Tricuspid stenosis also modifies the jugular venous pulse but in a more subtle way. The slope of the downward limb of the "v" wave, known as

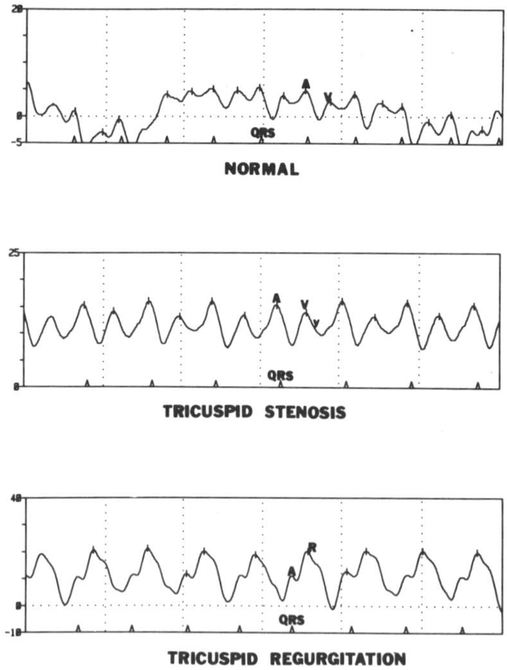

Figure 5-3 Right atrial phasic pressure measurements obtained during cardiac catheterization are shown from a patient with a normal heart, a patient with tricuspid stenosis, and a patient with tricuspid regurgitation. A = "a" wave, V = "v" wave, y = y-descent, ORS = onset of systole.

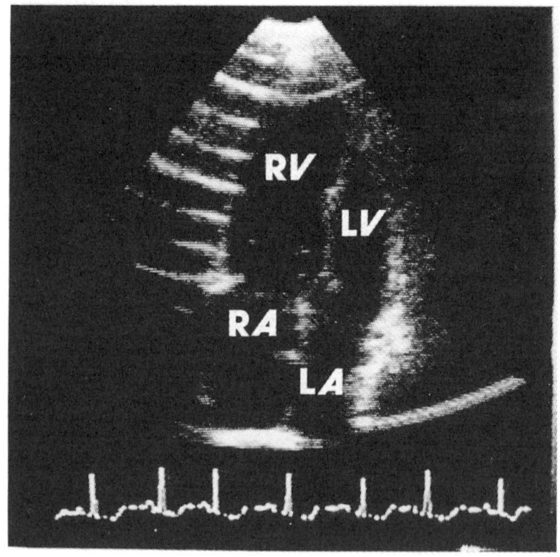

Figure 5-4 Apical four chamber, freeze-frame two-dimensional echocardiographic image of a patient with right ventricular enlargement secondary to tricuspid regurgitation. This view illustrates how the enlarged right ventricle is now the predominating structure over the apex of the heart. LA = left atrium, LV = left ventricle, RA = right atrium, RV = right ventricle.

the y-descent, is reduced and when the stenosis is severe this slow emptying of the jugular vein may be detected at the bedside (Figure 5-3). Also the amplitude of the "a" wave is increased.

The volume overload of the right ventricle in moderate to severe tricuspid regurgitation causes a palpable right ventricular lift. The more severe degrees of tricuspid regurgitation may produce so much right ventricular dilatation that the cardiac apex is formed by the right ventricle rather than the left (Figure 5-4). Failure to recognize this development may result in the misinterpretation of right ventricular enlargement as left ventricular enlargement.

Auscultation provides important clues of tricuspid valve disease. Tricuspid regurgitation usually produces a holosystolic murmur at the lower left sternal border. Sometimes inspiratory augementation of the murmur confirms its right-sided origin (Carvallo's sign). However, lack of an inspiratory increase in the murmur's intensity does not exclude the diagnosis of tricuspid regurgitation. When the murmur is suspected to be tricuspid in origin it has been reported that firm pressure applied to the liver during auscultation brings out respiratory augmentation.[18] In some cases of regurgitation, even severe ones, no systolic murmur may be audible if right ventricular systolic pressure is normal. Most likely this absence of sound is due to the lack of a significant systolic pressure gradient between the right ventricle and atrium. When the amount of regurgitation is large, a third heart sound or diastolic flow rumble may be audible at the lower left sternal border. In the presence of marked right ventricular dilation (Figure 5-4) the murmur of tricuspid regurgitation is well heard at the apex and this finding may result in the misinterpretation of the murmur as mitral regurgitation. When tricuspid prolapse is present, single or multiple nonejection clicks may be heard with or without an accompanying systolic murmur.

Rheumatic tricuspid stenosis produces a murmur similiar to mitral stenosis: an opening snap followed by a diastolic rumble. The rumble is often less intense than with mitral stenosis because of the smaller transvalvular gradient and often will demonstrate inspiratory augmentation. However, in rheumatic valve disease, the murmur of tricuspid stenosis may be masked by the louder accompanying mitral stenosis murmur.

Postannuloplasty tricuspid stenosis may produce a short diastolic rumble but it is more commonly recognized by elevation of the jugular venous pressure accompanied by a slow y-descent in the pulse.

Pedunculated right atrial tumors, which are usually myxomas, may produce a tumor "plop," diastolic rumble, or systolic murmur. However, these tumors are rare and physical findings may be occult or absent.

LABORATORY EVALUATION

The noninvasive laboratory evaluation of right heart disease is usually more difficult than assessment of left heart disease. The chest film, ECG, and echocardiogram are all more sensitive for detecting left-sided heart disease. However, all of the traditional and some of the new cardiac diagnostic tests can provide some useful information about patients with tricuspid valve disease.

CHEST ROENTGENOGRAM

The chest film may not detect mild forms of right ventricular and right atrial enlargement but usually right ventricular dilatation of a moderate to severe degree is noted on the lateral chest film as crowding of the retrosternal space (Figure 5-1). However, when pulmonary pressure is normal, severe tricuspid regurgitation may produce suprisingly little alteration in the cardiac contour. Right atrial enlargement is recognized on the posteroanterior chest film as more heart shadow to the right of the sternum than usual and increased convexity to the right heart border (Figure 5-1). Tricuspid valve calcification may be identified on the lateral chest film but it usually is difficult to differentiate from concomitant mitral valve calcification. Fluroscopy performed in the left anterior oblique projection separates the two valves.

ELECTROCARDIOGRAM

The ECG may show right atrial enlargement in tricuspid valve disease, particularly in tricuspid stenosis (Figure 5-5), but these patients are often in atrial fibrillation so this diagnostic clue is lost. Right ventricular and right atrial enlargement may cause clockwise "rotation" of the heart in the horizontal plane so there is reduced R wave height in the anterior V leads. Electrocardiographic signs of right ventricular hypertrophy indicate pulmonary hypertension is present and do not result from the primary effects of tricuspid regurgitation (Figure 5-5).

ECHOCARDIOGRAM

Although the tricuspid valve has been characteristically difficult to visualize in the normal

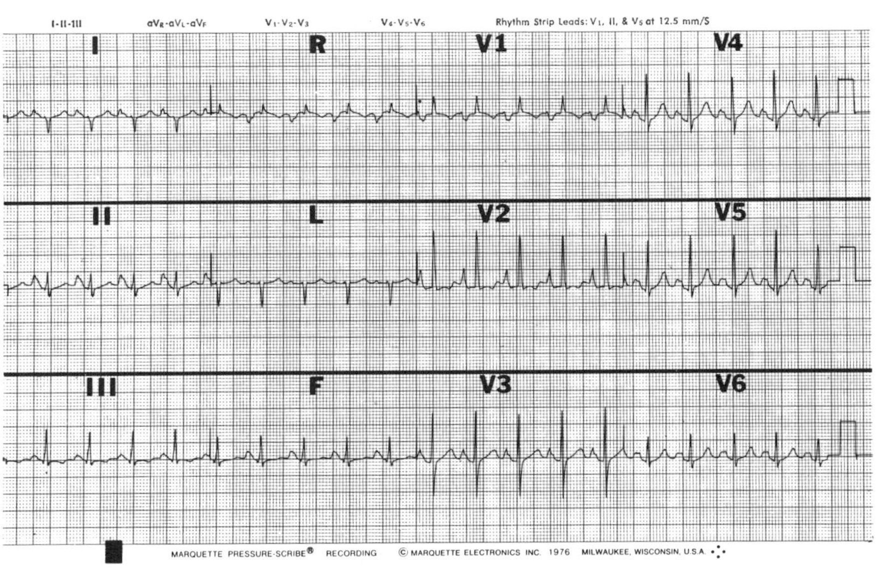

Figure 5-5 Marked right atrial and right ventricular hypertrophy is seen in the ECG of a patient with severe tricuspid and mitral stenosis.

patient with M-mode echocardiography, two-dimensional echocardiography usually provides adequate assessment of its structure and motion. The anterior leaflet is easier to visualize than the posterior and septal leaflets. The triscupid valve has motions similar to the mitral valve on the echocardiogram. The tricuspid valve opens earlier because the peak systolic pressure of the right ventricle is much lower than the left and thus less time is required for right ventricular pressure to fall below right atrial pressure. Tricuspid valve closure, however, occurs after mitral valve closure because electrical activation of the left ventricle precedes that of the right ventricle. Right atrial activation and contraction occurs before that of the left atrium; therefore the tricuspid's "a" wave occurs first.

The M-mode echocardiographic findings of rheumatic tricuspid stenosis are a thickened valve, reduced valve excursion, and diminished E–F slope. Doming of the valve leaflets in diastole can be seen with two-dimensional echocardiography and is characteristic of rheumatic tricuspid stenosis.[19]

Tricuspid regurgitation is diagnosed with echocardiography by indirect findings. Tricuspid regurgitation produces right ventricular volume overload, which is often associated with paradoxical septal motion. Many patients will also have dilation of the tricuspid annulus detected.

Other indirect echocardiographic signs of tricuspid regurgitation are: (*a*) the right ventricular volume overload contraction pattern of an increase in right ventricular size with accompanying increase in fractional shortening, (*b*) right atrial enlargement, and (*c*) increase in the size and pulsations of the inferior vena cava. These secondary findings can be corroborated by the infusion of agitated saline which will produce "bubbles" that can be seen to move to and fro across the insufficient tricuspid valve with two-dimensional echocardiography. The appearance of the saline microcavitations, after injection into an upper extremity vein, in the inferior vena cava and hepatic veins synchronous with the "V" wave, is diagnostic of tricuspid regurgitation.[20] The diagnosis of tricuspid regurgitation by these criteria is largely qualitative. One recent study, however, suggested that the severity of the regurgitation could be quantitated by measuring right atrial volumes in systole and diastole using a computerized light-pen system and thus determining the regurgitant volume.[21]

The increasing application of two-dimensional echocardiography to evaluate the right heart has led to the recognition of tricuspid valve prolapse as a clinical entity. The diagnosis is made by visualizing the closure of the tricuspid valve leaflets behind the tricuspid valve ring in systole. However, like mitral valve prolapse, tricuspid valve prolapse suffers from lack of an adequate standard for comparison and the true sensitivity and specificity of echocardiography for detecting tricuspid valve prolapse is unknown. Tricuspid valve prolapse is rarely seen alone and has been associated with mitral valve prolapse in 6% to 49% of cases.[22,23]

Although endocarditis of the tricuspid valve is relatively uncommon except in drug addicts, echocardiography has significantly improved our ability to detect this infection. The echocardiographic diagnosis of tricuspid valve endocarditis is based on the visualization of vegetations which are often large, very echo-reflective, and shaggy in appearance.[24] Tricuspid vegetations are usually seen on the atrial side of the valve.

DOPPLER ULTRASOUND

At the present time, Doppler ultrasonic techniques are primarily being used in tricuspid disease for the qualitative assessment of valve flow and regurgitation. Normal tricuspid valve flow can usually be distinguished from mitral flow by a lower peak velocity and respiratory variation in the velocity. Recordings from the tricuspid valve are usually easily made because of the anterior location of the right ventricle.

Tricuspid regurgitation is diagnosed with Doppler ultrasound by noting a reverse velocity of systolic flow at the tricuspid orfice which projects back into the right atrium (Figure 5-6). The regurgitation is usually noted to begin with tricuspid valve closure and continues after the second heart sound until the tricuspid valve opens. Doppler studies can provide a qualitative and semiquantitative assessment of the amount of regurgitation. Significant regurgitation is recorded further from the tricuspid orfice into the right atrium and the intensity of the Doppler signal is usually higher.[25] In addition, the forward flow velocity of blood across the tricuspid valve is also increased. When a very large regurgitant lesion is present, the increased forward velocity signal can be recorded in the right ventricle. Early studies have shown that vena cava flow is also abnormal in the presence of tricuspid regurgitation, with forward flow into the right heart greatest during ventricular diastole, opposite to the pattern that occurs normally.[26]

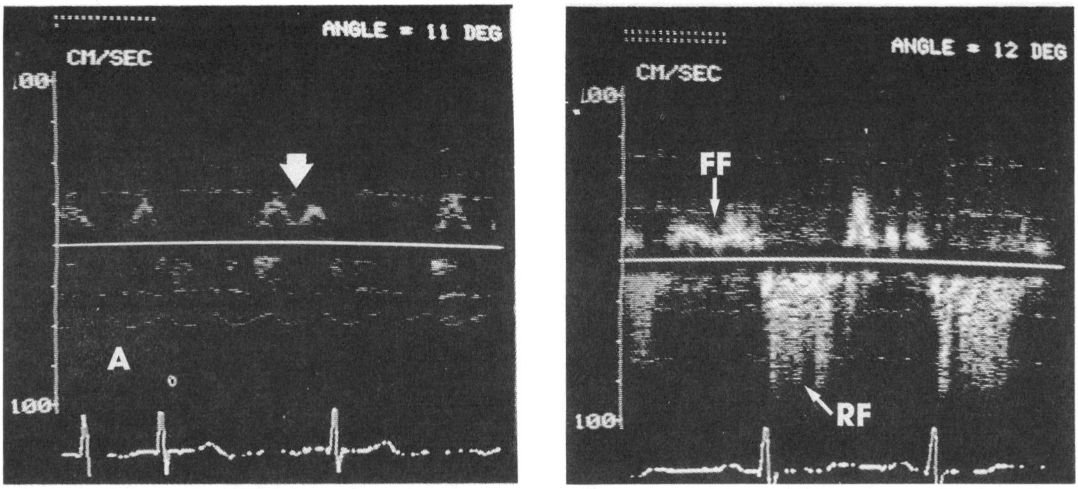

Figure 5-6 A Pulsed Doppler recording sampled in the right atrium, just behind the tricuspid valve, in a normal patient. Note, the characteristic low velocity M-shaped laminar (arrow) flow pattern of the velocity curves seen in diastole. The timing of the Doppler waveforms can be correlated with the ECG that appears below the tracing.
B Pulsed Doppler sample taken from the right atrium, just behind the tricuspid valve, in a patient with tricuspid regurgitation. Note, as compared to the normal tracing, the following typical features: (*a*) slight turbulence in the forward flow (FF) pattern and (*b*) a high velocity regurgitant jet (RF) going backwards in the right atrium. The timing of the regurgitation coincides with the QRS complex of the ECG.

Validation studies suggest that Doppler ultrasound may be the most sensitive method for diagnosing mild tricuspid regurgitation. Experience seems to suggest that mild regurgitation may be detected across the tricuspid valve in some patients who lack overt clinical findings. The true specificity and sensitivity of Doppler ultrasound for tricuspid regurgitation is still unknown. One study compared pulsed Doppler ultrasound with right ventriculography in 62 patients with suspected tricuspid regurgitation on clinical grounds, and detected regurgitant flow in 58 (94%)[27] In addition, there was a good correspondence in the severity of tricuspid regurgitation as graded by ventriculography *v*. Doppler studies. Quantitative studies on the amount of regurgitation detected may provide a particularly useful means of assessing the severity of the lesion in mild cases.

Doppler ultrasound can also be used to detect and grade tricuspid stenosis. When an obstruction to flow exists, the velocity of flow across the obstruction increases, while the pressure distal to the obstruction falls (modified Bernoulli equation). The pressure drop, or in this case the valve gradient, will be directly proportional to the increase in velocity that occurs.

Like mitral stenosis, tricuspid stenosis is characterized by high velocity diastolic turblent flow into the right ventricle with a diminished or absent "a" wave. The severity of the stenosis is assessed by the relative increase in flow velocity between samples from the right atrium and right ventricle. Moderately increased velocities decrease slowly during diastole and the respiratory variation is more pronounced than noted in normal subjects. Tight tricuspid stenosis may result in flow velocities that exceed the ability of pulsed Doppler systems to measure them accurately. Validation studies using Doppler ultrasound to quantify tricuspid stenosis have not yet been reported,but should be possible.

CARDIAC CATHETERIZATION

Cardiac catheterization provides the most definitive hemodynamic assessment of tricuspid valve disease. Measurement of cardiac output and the transvalvular gradient is still the most accurate method of determining the severity of tricuspid stenosis. The valve gradient is often small so great care must be taken to be sure the pressure measurements are very accurate. Indeed it is best to use two catheters or a double lumen catheter in order to measure right atrial

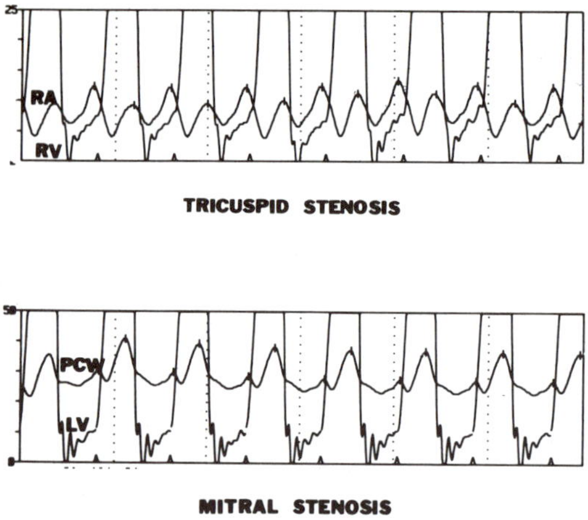

Figure 5-7 The relatively small tricuspid valve gradient associated with clinically significant stenosis is contrasted with the much larger gradient observed in the same patient with significant mitral stenosis.
RA = right atrial pressure, RV = right ventricular pressure, PCW = pulmonary capillary wedge pressure, LV = left ventricular pressure.

and right ventricular pressure simultaneously (Figure 5-7). Pressure manometers must be carefully balanced and the catheter connection should be reversed and the pressures remeasured to exclude artifactual differences between right atrial and right ventricular pressure. In the absence of moderate to large amounts of regurgitation, a gradient of 2 to 3 mmHg indicates that significant tricuspid stenosis may be present. We do not find the calculation of a valve area particularly helpful in making therapeutic decisions but cardiac output and heart rate must be considered when evaluating the significance of a valvular gradient. The greater the output and heart rate, the less important the gradient.

Right ventricular angiography is the best method for assessing the severity of tricuspid regurgitation. Even though a catheter lays across the valve in this procedure, artifactual regurgitation is minimal permitting reliable assessment of the functional significance of the leak.[28] Although the value of right ventricular angiography for evaluating tricuspid regurgitation has been questioned in the past, many cardiologist feel, as we do, that angiography should be performed during cardiac catheterization if there is any evidence that suggests significant valvular insufficiency.

Phasic pressure measurements from the right atrium will demonstrate the same changes in wave form as observed in the neck veins — a large systolic regurgitant wave in tricuspid regurgitation and a reduced y-descent in tricuspid stenosis. Patients in sinus rhythm may also have a large "a" wave in tricuspid stenosis (Figure 5-3).

Cardiac catheterization is indicated for the evaluation of tricuspid valve disease whenever symptoms are not adequately controlled with medical therapy. The functional status of the tricuspid valve should be carefully assessed in any patient undergoing cardiac catheterization for rheumatic heart disease as the signs and symptoms of significant disease are often masked by the effects of mitral and aortic valve disease.

RADIOISOTOPES

Recently a radioisotope method has been devised for comparing right and left ventricular stroke volume.[29] The difference in end-systolic and end-diastolic counts for each ventricle provides an index of the stroke volume ratio. Comparison of the two indices provides a semiquantitative means of determining the severity of the regurgitation. When the left ventricular/right ventricular stroke volume index ratio exceeds 1.0, it indicates mitral or aortic valve regurgitation; when less than 1.0, tricuspid or pulmonary valve regurgitation. The further the ratio from 1.0 the greater the regurgitation. Assessment of the radioactivity of the liver during a nuclear angiogram may also provide clues to the presence of tricuspid regurgitation.[29] When multiple valve regurgitation is present this method cannot determine the amount contributed by each valve. For example, in balanced tricuspid and mitral regurgitation the ratio would be normal. Furthermore, it is sometimes difficult to separate right ventricle radioactivity from that of the left ventricle or right atrium, making the results of this test inaccurate. The clinical utility of this method is still unproven.

COMPUTED TOMOGRAPHY

X-ray transmission–computed tomography (CT) is a new diagnostic technology only recently applied to the evaluation of cardiac disease.[30] The method is still under development and its clinical value has not yet been determined. However, CT offers real promise as a method that can accurately measure cardiac chamber volumes and such measurements would be of value in tricuspid regurgitation (Figure 5-8). A new ultrafast CT scanner, with a 50-ms scan time,

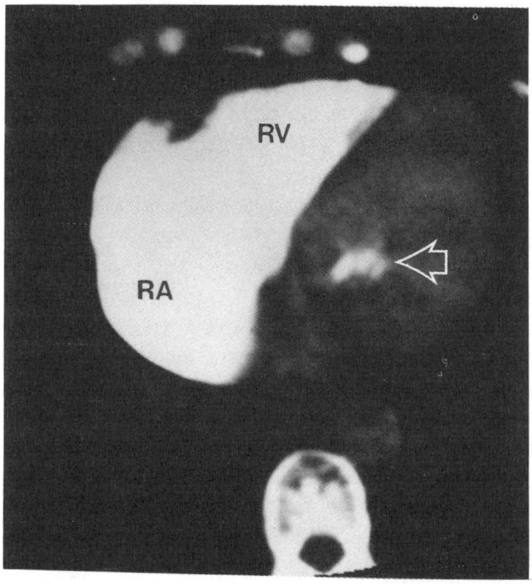

Figure 5-8 This CT scan of a patient with calcific mitral stenosis (arrow), pulmonary hypertension, and secondary tricuspid regurgitation shows a dilated right atrium (RA) and right ventricle (RV) during an IV bolus of contrast medium.

will permit accurate simultaneous measurement of right ventricular and left ventricular stroke volume providing an absolute regurgitation index similar to the radioisotope method.[31]

Cardiac output can be determined by CT from the analysis of contrast medium indicator dilution curves.[32] By comparing this measurement of forward stroke volume to CT geometric measurements of right ventricular stroke volume, an accurate measurement of tricuspid regurgitant volume should be possible. At this time it is unknown whether ultrafast CT will be a useful imaging method for evaluating tricuspid valve stenosis but valve motion has been detected in initial studies with the ultrafast scanner.[33]

MANAGEMENT

Medical Treatment

The medical treatment of tricuspid valve disease, whether regurgitation, stenosis, or both, is directed primarily at reducing systemic venous hypertension. In most cases this is achieved by administering diuretics which decrease circulating blood volume. Restriction of dietary salt is also quite effective and often underemphasized. As previously outlined, tricuspid regurgitation is often secondary to pulmonary hypertension. Therefore, any therapy that will lower pulmonary pressure will very likely decrease the amount of regurgitation and related symptoms. Vasodilators that lower systemic vascular resistance may be particularly helpful in aortic and mitral insufficiency by increasing forward cardiac output and thereby indirectly lowering left atrial pressure.[34,35] Reduction of left atrial and consequently pulmonary capillary wedge pressure will lower pulmonary artery pressure and diminish tricuspid valve regurgitation. In a similar manner, vasodilators may improve myopathic left ventricular function and thereby reduce tricuspid regurgitation. Pulmonary hypertension secondary to parenchymal lung disease, such as emphysema, may be improved with vasodilator therapy.[36] Secondary tricuspid regurgitation in these patients may be reduced if this therapy lowers pulmonary pressure.

Atrial fibrillation frequently accompanies tricuspid and mitral valve disease; therefore digitalis is useful in slowing heart rate and thereby prolonging the diastolic filling period. This therapy is particularly important in tricuspid stenosis and may contribute to reducing systemic venous hypertension. Indirectly, digitalis therapy may reduce secondary tricuspid regurgitation in patients with mitral stenosis by lowering left atrial pressure and effecting a reduction in pulmonary artery pressure.

Surgery

Surgical treatment of acquired tricuspid valve disease continues to remain controversial for a variety of reasons including problems in understanding anatomy and function of the valve apparatus,[37] difficulty in documenting severity of the disease process especially in the insufficiency state, and the poor long-term results associated with prosthetic valve replacement.

Tricuspid insufficiency under consideration for surgical repair often occurs as a consequence of rheumatic heart disease involving stenosis of the mitral valve and is secondary to dilatation of the right heart. Other than documenting the presence of tricuspid insufficiency preoperatively, quantification of the degree of insufficiency is sometimes difficult, given present diagnostic aids. At the present time, the surgeon is often still required to assess the severity of the tricuspid insufficiency in the operating room by closed digital palpation of the valve through the atrial appendage before initiating cardiopulmonary bypass. Even in 1986, the estimate of the degree of insufficiency remains empirical and dependent on the experience of the surgeon. One of the authors (S.L.) estimates severity on the basis of annular diameter, velocity of the insufficient valve jet, and the distance from the valve annulus that the jet can be appreciated. The decision to replace the tricuspid valve rather than perform an annuloplasty is made only after the valve is visualized. Because tricuspid valve replacement carries a higher mortality, annuloplasty is initially attempted in all insufficiency cases. After the mitral valve is repaired or replaced, attention is turned to the tricuspid valve. It is difficult to distinguish primary from secondary tricuspid regurgitation and repair is similar despite differences in etiology. Rarely is the subvalvular apparatus, eg, chordae or papillary muscles, involved. Dilatation of the tricuspid annulus occurs along the anterior and posterior leaflets; the septal leaflet, which is part of the fibrous skeleton of the heart, does not dilate and is used as a landmark for quantitating the optimum diameter of the valve annulus. Tricuspid annuloplasty is accomplished by plicating the anterior and posterior leaflets together by use of either a purse-string suture by the method of DeVega[38,39] or by implanting a ring device as described by Carpentier et al [40] and Duran and Vbago.[41] Operative mortality (30 days) is approximately 5% and significant residual regurgitation is present in less than 15% of cases studied postoperatively.[39]

Tricuspid stenosis occurs in 3% to 15% of patients with rheumatic heart disease[42] and is always associated with either mitral or aortic valvular disease. Commissurotomy is usually performed between the anterior and septal leaflet and occasionally through the anteroseptal and posteroseptal commissures. If subvalvular stenosis is present, it may be necessary to sharply slit the fused chordae and papillary muscles. Residual insufficiency is treated by use of one of the annuloplasty techniques previously described.

Tricuspid valve replacement with mechanical devices has been associated with an unusually high operative mortality in the range of 10% to 58%.[43] Much of this high mortality can be attributed to a mismatch in geometric configuration between the right ventricle and either the ball valve or disc valve mechanical prosthesis. Operative mortality has significantly decreased to the 7% to 12% range since the porcine heterograft prosthesis has been used. Late mortality over 5 years reflects the status of the ventricle before the original operative procedure and varies from 7% to 28%.[44]

Acute drug-resistant endocarditis of the tricuspid valve, usually present in drug addicts, represents a unique surgical problem. Total valvectomy without prosthetic valve replacement results in complete cure of the infection and is well tolerated on a long-term basis.[45]

SUMMARY

Tricuspid valve disease has not received the same attention as mitral and aortic disease but clearly there is an increased awareness among clinicians about its changing etiology. There are new promising diagnostic tools for assessing tricuspid valve disease and they are likely to further our understanding of its pathophysiology. Newer surgical techniques introduced in the past decade have improved survival and hemodynamic outcome.

REFERENCES

1. DiSerarcio G, Taranta A: Rheumatic fever in children. *Am Heart J* 1980;99:635–658.
2. Land MA, Bisno AL: Acute rheumatic fever, a vanishing disease in suburbia. *JAMA* 1983;249: 895–898.
3. Lang M, Salaki JS, Middleton JR, et al: Infective endocarditis in heroin addicts: epidemiological observations and some unusual cases. *Am Heart J* 1978;96:144–152.
4. Mills J, Drew D: *Serratia marcescens* endocarditis: a regional illness associated with intravenous drug abuse. *Ann Intern Med* 1976;84:29–35.
5. Thorburn CW, Morgan JJ, Shanahan MX, et al: Long-term results of tricuspid valve replacement and the problem of prosthetic valve thrombosis. *Am J Cardiol* 1983;51:1128–1132.
6. Reisberg B: Infective endocarditis in the narcotic addict. *Prog Cardiovas Dis* 1979;22:193–203.
7. Corne P: Infective endocarditis: current perspectives. *Compr Ther* 1982;8:57–70.
8. Roberts WC, Sjoerdsma A: The cardiac disease associated with the carcinoid syndrome (carcinoid heart disease). *Am J Med* 1964;36:5–34.
9. Wooley CF: Rediscovery of the tricuspid valve. *Curr Probl Cardiol* 1981;6:1–41.
10. Silverman BD, Carabajal NR, Chorches MA, et al: Tricuspid regurgitation and acute myocardial infarction. *Arch Intern Med* 1982;142:1394–1395.
11. Dougherty MJ, Craige E: Apathetic hyperthyroidism presenting as tricuspid regurgitation. *Chest* 1973;63:767–778.
12. Esaghpour E, Kawai N, Linhart JW: Tricuspid insufficiency associated with aneurysm of the ventricular septum. *Pediatrics* 1978;61:586–592.
13. Chusid MJ, Dale DC, West BC et al: The hypereosenophilic syndrome: analysis of fourteen cases with review of the literature. *Medicine* 1975;54: 1–27.

14. Fracasso A, Pothen P. Gallucci V: Tricuspid regurgitation caused by blunt chest trauma in association with pericardial agenesis: surgical correction after eight years. *Thorax* 1982;37:75–76.
15. Weyman AE, Rankin R, King H: Loeffler's endocarditis presenting as mitral and tricuspid stenosis. *Am J Cardiol* 1977;40:438–444.
16. McGuinn JB, Zipes DP: Constrictive pericarditis producing tricuspid stenosis. *Arch Intern Med* 1972;129:487–490.
17. Mikami T, Kudo T, Nobuko S, et al: Mechanisms for development of functional tricuspid regurgitation determined by pulsed doppler and two-dimensional echocardiography. *Am J Cardiol* 1984;53:160–163.
18. Cha SD, Gooch AS: Diagnosis of tricuspid regurgitation, current status. *Arch Intern Med* 1983; 143:1763–1768.
19. Joyner CR, Hey BE, Jr, Johnson J, et al: Reflected ultrasound in the diagnosis of tricuspid stenosis. *Am J Cardiol* 1967;19:66–73.
20. Meltzer RS, Hoogenhuyze D, Serruys PW, et al: Diagnosis of tricuspid regurgitation by contrast echocardiography. *Circulation* 1981;63:1093–1099.
21. DePace NL, Jian-Fang R, Kotler MN, et al: Two-dimensional echocardiographic determination of right atrial emptying volume: a non-invasive index of quantifying the degree of tricuspid regurgitation. *Am J Cardiol* 1983;52:525–529.
22. DeMaria A, Bommer W, Neuman A, et al: Evaluation of tricuspid valve prolapse by two-dimensional echocardiography. *Circulation* 1978; 58 (suppl 2):43.
23. Mardelli TJ, Morganroth J, Chen CC, et al: Enhanced diagnosis of tricuspid valve prolapse by cross-sectional echocardiography. *Chest* 1981; 79:201–205.
24. Kisslo J, Von Ramm OT, Haney R, et al: Echocardiographic evaluation of tricuspid valve endocarditis, an M-mode and two-dimensional study. *Am J Cardiol* 1976;38:502–507.
25. Curtis JM, Thyssen M, Brewer HWM, et al: Doppler versus contrast echocardiography for diagnosis of tricuspid regurgitation. *Am J Cardiol* 1985;56:333–336.
26. Benchimol A, Barreto EC, Tio S: Phasic right atrium and superior vena caval flow velocity in patients with tricuspid insufficiency. *Am Heart J* 1970;79:603–612.
27. Miyatake K, Okamato M, Kinoshita N, et al: Evaluation of tricuspid regurgitation by pulsed doppler and two-dimensional echocardiography. *Circulation* 1982;66:777–784.
28. Ubego JL, Figueroa A, Colman T, et al: Right ventriculography as a valid method for the diagnosis of tricuspid regurgitation. *Cathet Cardiovasc Diagn* 1981;7:433–441.
29. Handler B, Pavel DG, Pietras R, et al: Equilibrium radionuclide gated angiography in patients with tricuspid regurgitation. *Am J Cardiol* 1983; 51:305–310.
30. Brundage BH: Computed tomography: a new view of cardiovascular disease. *Primary Cardiol* 1983;9:57–72.
31. Boyd DP, Gould RG, Quinn JR, et al: A proposed dynamic cardiac 3-D densitometer for early detection and evaluation of heart disease. *IEEE Trans Nucl Sci* 1979;26:2724.
32. Herfkens RJ, Axel L, Lipton MJ, et al: Measurement of cardiac output by computed transmission tomography. *Invest Radiol* 1982;17:550–553.
33. Brundage BH, Herfkens RJ, Kramer PH, et al: Evaluation of infarct size by contrast enhanced computed tomography in humans. *Circulation* 1983;68(III):137.
34. Greenberg BH, DeMots H, Murphy E, et al: Mechanism for improved cardiac performance with anteriolar dilators in aortic insufficiency. *Circulation* 1981;63:263–268.
35. Greenberg BH, Massie BM, Brundage BH, et al: Beneficial effects of hydralazine in severe mitral regurgitation. *Circulation* 1978;58:273–279.
36. Rubin LJ, Peter RH: Hemodynamics at rest and during exercise after hydralazine in patients with cor pulmonale. *Am J Cardiol* 1981;47:116–122.
37. Silver MD, Lam JH, Ranganthan N, et al: Morphology of the human tricuspid valve. *Circulation* 1971;43:333–348.
38. DeVega NG: La anuloplastia selectiva reguable y permanente. *Rev Esp Cardiol* 1972;25:6.
39. Grondin P, Meere C, Limet R, et al: Carpentier's annulus and DeVega's annuloplasty. *J Thorac Cardiovasc Surg* 1975;70:852–861.
40. Carpentier A, Deloche A, Dauptain J, et al: A new reconstructive operation for correction of mitral and tricuspid insufficiency. *J Thorac Cardiovasc Surg* 1971;61:1–13.
41. Duran CMG, Vbago JL: Clinical and hemodynamic performance of a totally flexible prosthetic ring for atrioventricular valve reconstruction. *Ann Thorac Surg* 1976;22:458–463.
42. Kitchin A, Turner R: Diagnosis and treatment of tricuspid stenosis. *Br Heart J* 1964;26:354–379.
43. Sanfelippo PM, Giuliani ER, Danielson GK, et al: Tricuspid valve prosthetic replacement. Early and late results with the Starr-Edwards prosthesis. *J Thorac Cardiovasc Surg* 1976;71:441–445.
44. Jugdutt BI, Fraser RS, Less SJ, et al: Long-term survival after tricuspid valve replacement. Results with several different prostheses. *J Thorac Cardiovasc Surg* 1977;74:20–27.
45. Levitsky S, Mammana RB, Silverman NA, et al: Acute endocarditis in drug addicts: Surgical treatment for gram-negative sepsis. *Circulation* 1982;66 (suppl 1):I135–I138.

CHAPTER 6
Pulmonic Valve Disease

Henry J. Issenberg

The most frequent anomaly of the pulmonic valve is congenital stenosis. Acquired lesions are rare and may present later in life with regurgitation rather than stenosis. Pulmonic stenosis as a sole lesion affects the sexes equally and accounts for approximately 10% of all types of congenital heart disease, being the third or fourth most common in large series.[1,2] It may also occur as an associated lesion with other cardiac defects in up to 30% of those with congenital heart disease. Some of these associated lesions may include ventricular septal defect, hypoplastic right ventricle, Ebstein's anomaly of the tricuspid valve, or transposition of the great vessels. Pulmonic stenosis with or without an atrial septal defect has been reported to make up 15% of adult cardiac catheterization cases.[3]

Over the last four decades there has been a dramatic evolution in the recognition, diagnosis, and therapy of valvar pulmonic stenosis and other forms of right ventricular outflow tract obstruction. The initial pathologic description is credited variously to de Senac (1749) or Morgagni (1761). In 1888 Fallot described the "trilogy" as those with severe pulmonary stenosis and right-to-left atrial shunting to be separated from those with tetralogy who have right-to-left ventricular shunting. Pulmonic stenosis was considered rare with occasional sporadic case reports appearing in the literature. In 1936 Abbott described 1000 cases of congenital cardiac malformations, including nine cases with "simple pulmonic stenosis."[5] In 1947 Taussig stated that she had "not had the opportunity to study a proven case of pure pulmonary stenosis" and "ordinarily the condition is only compatible with life for six to eight months."[6] Three years later Wood correlated the physical findings and catheterization data of 28 patients with right ventricular outflow tract obstruction of varying severity, after having remarked that "No form of congenital heart disease has caused so much confusion and muddled thinking as pulmonary stenosis."[7] From this morass of confusion developed a generally accepted classification system based on the anatomical and physiologic findings and an effective, nearly curative, surgical repair.

In the majority of cases, outflow obstruction from the right ventricle occurs at the pulmonary valvar level. There may also be congenital or acquired obstruction either above or below this level (Figure 6-1). Below the valve, anomalous muscle bundles may obstruct flow within the body of the right ventricle, or at the entrance to the infundibulum, from enlargement of the parietal band (also called the crista supraventricularis or conal septum) creating a subvalvar chamber inferior to the pulmonary valve. Narrowing distal to the valve may be discrete, at the superior margin of the valve cusps, forming a ring, or diffuse, narrowing the entire main pulmonary artery along with the right and left branch pulmonary arteries. Peripheral pulmonary arterial narrowing can be discrete, circumferential, membranous, or diffuse long-segment hypoplasia. Any combination of these anatomical abnormalities may coexist simultaneously. The physiologic outcome will be the same — elevation of the systolic pressure in some portion of the system proximal to the obstruction with the development of a systolic pressure gradient across the area of obstruction. Right ventricular myocardial hypertrophy will be the direct result of this pressure overload.

The description of the disease includes both the exact anatomical location of the obstruction,

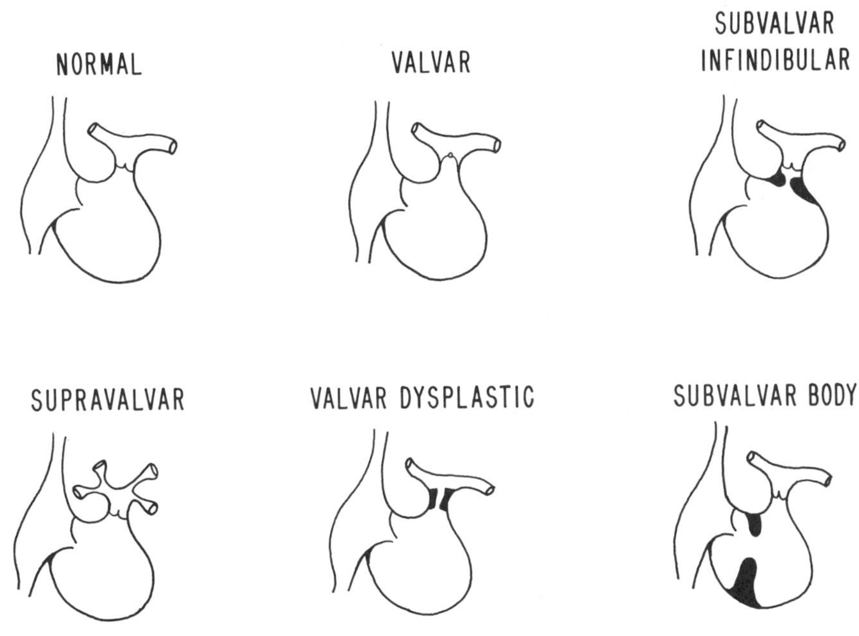

Figure 6-1 Schematic representation of different levels of right ventricular and outflow tract obstruction.

the severity of the obstruction as judged by the systolic pressure gradient and peak right ventricular pressure, and the presence or absence of right-to-left atrial shunting secondary to decreased right ventricular diastolic compliance and patency of the foramen ovale. Large natural history studies[8,9] have arbitrarily used gradients to divide severity into four groups: (1) trivial — peak systolic ejection gradient <25 mmHg; (2) mild — peak systolic ejection gradient 25 to 50 mmHg; (3) moderate — peak systolic ejection gradient 50 to 75 mmHg; and (4) severe — peak systolic ejection gradient > 75 mmHg. Another classification system uses the ratio of peak right ventricular systolic pressure to left ventricular or systemic pressure[10,11]: if moderate, the pressure in the right ventricle is one half to two thirds the pressure in the aorta; if severe, the pressure in the right ventricle equals or exceeds the systemic pressure. Elevations in right atrial pressure, secondary to an increased right ventricular end-diastolic pressure, which produces right-to-left atrial shunting and systemic desaturation, is usually considered severe, since the diastolic compliance problems of the right ventricle imply a degree of congestive heart failure.

PATHOLOGY

The most frequently encountered form of obstruction lies at the valvar level. The pulmonary valve may be poorly differentiated histologically with three thickened dysplastic myxoid leaflets, or poorly developed with a small annulus and indistinct raphae and leaflets.[12] In the most common presentation of moderate to severe disease, the annulus is normal to mildly hypoplastic in diameter.[4] The leaflets are well developed and differentiated with three distinct raphae that represent the commissural fusion line, between the cusps.[13] Occasionally, the valve may be bicuspid or quadracuspid.[12,14] The central valvar orifice may be circular or ovoid, with its diameter being as small as 1 to 2 mm^2 in the severest of cases. The commissural fusion prevents leaflet retraction into the sinuses of Valsalva during ventricular systole, and instead the valve "domes" as a parabolic billowing membrane into the main pulmonary artery. Depending on the length of each fused commissure, the central orifice may be eccentric and direct the jet of blood laterally into the wall of the main pulmonary artery, or posteriorly toward the left pulmonary artery. The turbulence and eddies created by the stenosis are one reason given for the aneurysmal dilation of the proximal main pulmonary artery segment, along with the possibility of a primary elastic defect in the arterial wall that may also be associated with valvar pulmonic stenosis.[15] With time, the valve undergoes secondary degenerative changes. The leaflets become thickened, irregular, and less pliable. Small fibrous nodules form along the arterial side of the orifice and the leaflets may undergo focal calcification in older patients,[16–18] which results in further rigidity, orifice narrowing, and increased obstruction[19]

With increasing severity, the conal septum, along with other right ventricular muscle bands and myocardium, will thicken. As the conal septum hypertrophies, the infundibulum will narrow. This subvalvar narrowing may become another site of hemodynamic obstruction. The myocardial hypertrophy will be most prominent in the papillary muscles and the trabeculum and may seem to encroach on the cavity of the right ventricle. The endocardium becomes fibrotic, glistening, and thickened as a result of subendocardial ischemia from the increased myocardial oxygen demand from the pressure overload and wall stress.[20] True transmural ischemia or myocardial infarction is rarely seen outside of infancy and childhood.[21]

With hypertrophy the ventricular compliance decreases, and the right atrium may undergo enlargement and hypertrophy. Also, as an end-stage phenomenon associated with heart failure, the tricuspid valve becomes regurgitant, placing an additional volume overload on the right atrium and right ventricle. As the pressure in the right atrium rises and the atrium dilates, right-to-left shunting may occur through the stretched foramen ovale which is patent in the majority of patients.[22] Systemic cyanosis may precede the findings of right-sided congestive heart failure as the right atrium decompresses.

Hepatic congestion from severe right ventricular outflow tract obstruction that leads to cirrhosis[23] has been described in the presurgical era, but now is infrequently encountered.

After the onset of a right-to-left atrial shunt, the left ventricle may dilate in response to the volume overload. The aortic arch is left-sided; if it is right-sided, infundibular obstruction with a closing ventricular septal defect should be suspected.[22,25] Aortic to pulmonary collateralization may occur in cases with long-standing cyanosis.

Lung hypoplasia is seen in congenital pulmonary stenosis. This has been determined with pulmonary vascular morphometrics performed on laboratory animals,[26] along with pulmonary function studies of the vascular bed in adults.[27] The investigators concluded that alterations in hemodynamics may play a significant factor in lung growth and development.

Acquired valvar disease is rare (Table 6-1).

Table 6-1
Acquired Pulmonic Valve Disease

1. Infectious
   a. Endocarditis
   b. Tuberculous
   c. Syphylitic
2. Inflammatory
   a. Rheumatic
   b. Collagen-vascular
3. Carcinoid
4. Atheromatous
5. Primary tumor
   a. Sarcoma
   b. Myxoma
   c. Blood cyst
6. Connective tissue disorders (Marfan's syndrome)
7. Pulmonary hypertension
8. Surgical/iatrogenic
   a. Catheter-induced
   b. Surgical

Bacterial endocarditis has been reported to both increase obstruction because of secondary scarring and healing changes, and also to decrease the outflow tract obstruction or cause regurgitation with perforation or dissolution of the leaflet tissue. Rheumatic heart disease, blood cysts,[28,29] carcinoid syndrome,[30] and atheroma have all been described as a source of valvar obstruction, along with tumors and aortic aneurysms[30–33] as a source of subvalvar obstruction.

In pulmonary hypertension, either primary or secondary, as the pulmonary arterial diastolic pressure rises, the valve may become regurgitant. Valvar damage leading to regurgitation has also been seen with prolonged use of monitoring catheters crossing the outflow tract.[34]

NATURAL HISTORY

The majority of those with pulmonic stenosis will be discovered at birth or in early infancy because of the presence of a murmur,[35] most often thought to be hemodynamically significant. Some will have symptoms of congestive heart failure or cyanosis. Data from the New England Regional Infant Cardiac Program[36] included all infants born in New England from 1968 to 1977 with congenital heart disease who within the first year of life required cardiac catheterization or surgery, or who were discovered at autopsy. Pulmonic stenosis had an incidence of 0.073/1000 live births, making it the ninth most common lesion detected, and forming 3.3% of all types of congenital heart disease in this selected series. Of these 79 infants, 17 (22%) died within 1 year. Mild cases may come to the physician's attention beyond infancy when it becomes the third or fourth most commonly encountered lesion, forming 7.5% to 11% of all congenital heart disease.[1,9,22]

A large proportion of the infants will be followed clinically for signs of progressive obstruction or symptoms. Generally, those with hemodynamically moderate to severe disease, even if free of symptoms, will be surgically corrected in childhood if detected. The mild to moderate group may be asymptomatic and stable for long periods, as the valve orifice area may grow along with the child.[37,38]

In the multicentered natural history study[8] 261 patients from birth to 21 years of age, mostly with mild to moderate stenosis, were followed medically, along with a group of 304 patients treated surgically. Of the 181 who were treated medically and had a second cardiac catheterization within 4 or 8 years, the gradient remained unchanged in 72%, decreased in 14%, and increased in 14%. Of those in whom the gradient increased, it was most common in the group under 4 years of age, when the initial gradient was greater than 40 mmHg. Through the follow-up period, there were no cardiac deaths or cases of endocarditis in the medically followed group.

Periods of rapid somatic growth, as may occur during infancy or puberty, will require vigilant observation for dramatic increases in obstruction or the development of the symptoms.[38] After these periods of rapid growth, there are data to support the nonprogression of stenosis in the asymptomatic adult with mild to moderate obstruction. Johnson et al followed a group of 21 adults an average of 15 years after initial evaluation by cardiac catheterization.[3] The group was weighted toward those with mild to moderate disease, with only two having a right ventricular pressure greater than 100 or a peak systolic ejection gradient greater than 75. There was no evidence of clinical deterioration based on physical examination, chest x-ray films, or ECG and there were no cardiac deaths or cases of endocarditis.

Though there are numerous case reports of survival into the seventh decade,[39,40] there is an attrition that occurs in the first three decades, when viewed through an analysis of postmortem studies. Of the 77 postmortem reports, Fabricius[41] reported that only 22 (29%) were over 40 years of age. Fontana et al[22] reviewed 123 cases of pulmonic stenosis, with a median age of death of 20 years. Twelve percent were over 40 years old. The leading cause of death was cardiac failure (28%), with a median of 22 years, followed by sudden death (9%), endocarditis (7%), and acute cyanosis with dyspnea (7%).

CLINICAL FEATURES

History

Symptoms are rarely seen in those people with mild to moderate right ventricular outflow tract obstruction.[42] Those with severe obstruction may complain of dyspnea on exertion, fatigue, or decreased exercise capacity. These will be manifestations of limitations in cardiac output from the obstructive valve orifice or congestive heart failure from the long-standing pressure overload. Tricuspid regurgitation or a supraventricular tachyarrhythmia may further embarrass forward cardiac output and lead to right-sided congestion, often as a terminal event.

If right-to-left atrial shunting through the foramen ovale occurs as the right-sided filling pressures rise, systemic cyanosis will be seen. The degree of systemic desaturation at rest and with exercise will determine the patient's subjective well-being, along with his/her exercise capacity. Hypercyanotic spells as seen in tetralogy of Fallot are not seen. Other complications from right-to-left shunting such as brain abscess or cerebrovascular accident may occur.[22]

Chest pain, anginal in quality,[43] is only seen in severe right ventricular outflow tract obstruction and reflects the unmet myocardial oxygen demand from increased wall stress. This may be aggravated by exercise when the right ventricular pressure climbs further, to suprasystemic levels.

Fainting and syncope are indications of a severely limited cardiac output.[43] As with other paroxysmal events, cardiac dysrhythmias, either supraventricular or ventricular, may be the cause. These are potentially fatal, and require immediate relief of obstruction. Sudden death has been seen.[44,45] Though the final series of events has not been elucidated, myocardial infarction and dysrhythmias can be implicated.[46]

Genetics

The family and maternal history is rarely contributory. Maternal rubella infection in the first trimester was a frequent etiology of right ventricular outflow tract obstruction, especially peripheral pulmonary stenosis, but with the advent of an effective vaccine in 1969 it has subsequently become rare.[47]

If a single parent without a syndrome transmitted through clear mendelian genetics has pulmonic stenosis, there is a 3.5% risk of it occurring in an offspring. Should a sibling have pulmonic stenosis, then the risk of recurrence in a subsequent sibling is 2.7%.[48] These percentages are based on a multifactorial mode of inheritance, and are numerically quite similar for all forms of congenital heart disease. Frequently, different forms of congenital heart disease may be observed in probands, such as pulmonic stenosis in one and an atrial septal defect in another. Therefore, concordancy in the inherited anomaly is not the rule.

Many syndromes are associated with pulmonic stenosis (Table 6-2). Noonan's syndrome[49] is autosomal dominant with normal chromosomes. It is associated with short stature, webbed neck, hypertelorism, delayed puberty, and pectus excavatum. It is frequently termed the Turner phenotype. It may occur in either male or female, and contrary to Turner's syndrome (45 XO), the affected are fertile. Though pulmonic stenosis is the most frequent form of heart disease in this syndrome (62.1%), other anomalies including atrial septal defect (25.2%) and hypertrophic cardiomyopathy (17.0%) may be found, along with smaller percentages of others.[50] The pulmonic valve is frequently dysplastic; the leaflets are poorly differentiated with myxomatous thickening, rigid cusps, and no evidence of commissural fusion. This is best demonstrated with right ventricular angiography with the thickened cusps seen most clearly during diastole.[51,52]

Physical examination

On physical examination (Table 6-3) the vast majority of patients are acyanotic. The presence of cyanosis, indicating right-to-left atrial shunting, is a hallmark of severe disease. If not present, it does not rule out severe obstruction. It may be mild, and only detectable with oximetry,

Table 6-2
Etiologic Basis of Pulmonic Valve Disease and Right Ventricular Outflow Tract Obstruction

Chromosomal	Mendelian		Infectious
	Dominant	Recessive	
Turner's syndrome (45 XO)	Holt-Oram syndrome	Cutis laxa	Rubella
Trisomy 18	Leopard syndrome	Laurence-Moon-Bardet-Biedl syndrome	
Trisomy 13–15	Hypertrophic cardiomyopathy		
Trisomy 21	Neurofibromatosis		
	Noonan's syndrome		
	Williams syndrome		
	Marfan's syndrome		
	Ehlers-Danlos syndrome		

Table 6-3
Physical Findings in Pulmonic Valve Disease

	Mild (PSEG < 50 mmHg)	Moderate (PSEG 50–75 mmHg)	Severe (PSEG > 75 mmHg)
Cyanosis	–	–	+/–
Jugular venous "a" wave	+/–	+	++
Precordial systolic thrill	+	+++	+++
Systolic ejection click	+++	++	+/–
Pulmonic closure (P_2)	nl	nl to ↓	inaudible
Murmur grade	2–5/6; ends before A_2	3–5/6	4–6/6; late peaking, lasting to P_2

PSEG = peak systolic ejection gradient.

or may be quite obvious, centrally and peripherally. If long-standing, digital clubbing will be observed.

The jugular venous pulse demonstrates a prominent "a" wave, indicating a forceful atrial contraction into a right ventricle with decreased compliance. Unless right ventricular failure has occurred, or tricuspid regurgitation is coexistent, the "v" wave will not be elevated.

The chest is normally formed without deformity or bulge. Often a right ventricular heave can be palpated below the midsternum or xyphoid. A systolic thrill is invariably felt at the left upper sternal border or suprasternal notch, in hemodynamically significant disease. Because the pulmonary arterial pressure is normal, the pulmonic component of the second sound is not felt. An early systolic ejection click may be palpable at the left upper sternal border; its intermittency as it varies with respiration defines its origin as pulmonic.

During auscultation, by analyzing the pulmonic component of the second sound (P_2), the presence or absence of the systolic ejection click and the characteristics of the murmur, the examiner can easily and accurately diagnose pulmonic stenosis, assess its severity by predicting gradient, and determine its level in the right ventricular outflow tract. The data to support this had been developed by independent observers, and confirmed by large multicenter studies with multiple clinical participants.[8,11] Phonocardiography has allowed refinement and graphic reproduction of the acoustic impressions, so that clinical parameters could be correlated to specific measurements.[53]

The first sound is always of normal intensity and is closely followed (within 0.15 second) by an often loud variable pulmonary ejection click best heard at the left upper sternal border (Figure 6-2). Through phonocardiographic and echocardiographic timing correlations, the click occurs as the leaflets have reached their maximal opening excursion.[54] As ventricular ejection begins, the systolic ejection murmur also starts, and continues until the leaflets close, as represented by the second component of the second sound, P_2. A third heart sound is heard only if the ventricle is failing. A fourth heart sound is correlated with the right atrial contraction and may be of variable intensity, as it changes during the respiratory cycle, as does the systolic ejection click.

The distinguishing characteristic of the pulmonary ejection click is its variability with respiration.[55] Because of changes in diastolic filling of the right ventricle, the click becomes less audible during inspiration and returns in intensity at end expiration. Since the click represents valve movement during systole, one can infer something about the leaflet texture and pliability, depending on whether the sound is heard or, if in longitudinal follow-up, the sound is lost. The ejection click is not heard if the valve is myxomatous[51,56] or if the obstruction is either subvalvar or supravalvar.[57]

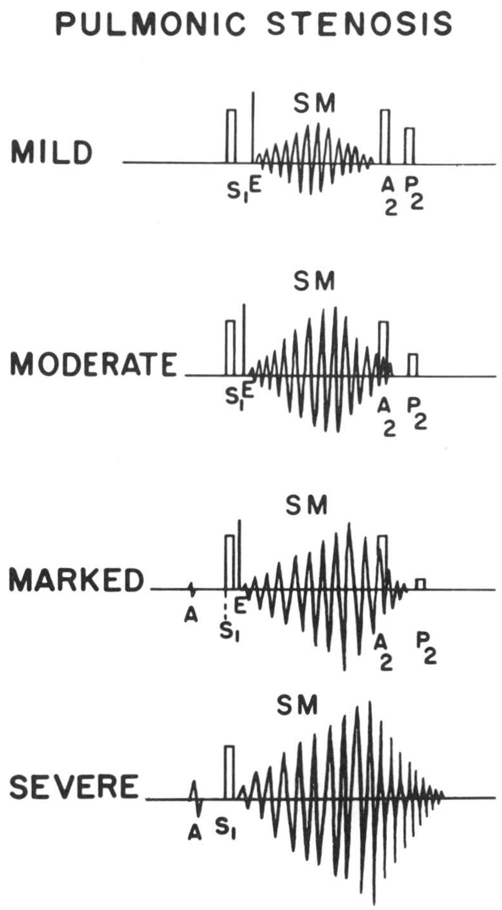

Figure 6-2 Schematic representation of heart sounds and murmur with increasing levels of severity in valvar pulmonic stenosis. S_1 = first heart sound, E = ejection click, SM = systolic murmur, A_2 = aortic closure sound, R = pulmonic closure sound, S_4 = fourth heart sound. Reproduced with permission from Perloff.[57]

The interval between the first sound and the ejection click is also related to the severity of obstruction. As obstruction increases, the interval shortens, to where the ejection click may be superimposed and indistinguishable from the first sound.[58] At this point, in severe obstruction, often the click does not occur since the valve leaflets are immobile, and the murmur begins with the first sound. The interval between A_2 and P_2 also lengthens with increasing severity, and reflects a prolonged right ventricular ejection time.[58] The intensity of P_2, pulmonary valve closure, decreases relative to the leaflet pliability, as does the ejection click. Therefore, in severe disease it is often inaudible.

The systolic murmur of valvar pulmonic stenosis begins with the opening of the valve and increases, peaks, and decreases in loudness, ending at valve closure. There is no diastolic murmur, as pulmonary insufficiency is rarely associated. Generally, as the severity increases, so does the intensity of the murmur, along with the interval from the first sound (or the ECG Q wave) to the peak of the crescendo.[58]

Electrocardiogram

The ECG is an easily obtainable noninvasive method to document and estimate the amount of right ventricular hypertrophy, and therefore approximate the degree of pressure overload from the stenosis. In the past, various elaborate regression formulas have been derived from single and multiple measurements of the scalar and vector ECG.[59] Since these formulas are complicated, difficult to remember, and frequently inaccurate, their application in clinical practice has not gained widespread utility. The trends based on certain criteria are generally correct, and allow the separation into the three hemodynamic classifications of mild, moderate, or severe, as the degree of right ventricular hypertrophy, and other signs of right heart pressure overload increase.

In mild stenosis the ECG is most frequently normal.[10,59,60] Since the right ventricular dominance of childhood regresses during the adolescent years, a comparison of serial studies should be made in the young to avoid any confusion in overdiagnosing the presence of right ventricular hypertrophy. The earliest ECG sign may be a rightward shift in the QRS axis. This would be followed by increasing right precordial-anterior forces, as the increased right ventricular mass from hypertrophied muscle dominates the depolarization vector.

In moderate pulmonic stenosis, a normal ECG is seen infrequently, less than 10% of the time.[61] The QRS axis is rightward (90° to 130°), and the right precordial-anterior forces are increased, as evidenced by increased voltages, and a conduction delay of right ventricular depolarization (incomplete right bundle-branch block). The normal peripubertal change of the T wave in V_1 becoming upright may not occur, as the increased right ventricular forces persist into adulthood. At this stage, the degree of right ventricular hypertrophy may be marginally abnormal for age, and can also be confused with the pattern seen in an atrial septal defect with a right ventricular volume overload and increased right ventricular mass, along with a normal right ventricular pressure.

In severe stenosis the ECG shows signs of right ventricular hypertrophy in nearly all cases[10] (Figure 6-3). If the degree is questionable, a vector cardiogram may be more sensitive in determining the initial anterior voltage/time inscription.[62] Rarely, a normal ECG will be seen in severe disease.[60] One can infer that this (1) represents a methodologic error in determining right ventricular hypertrophy electrocardiographically, or (2) biologic variability in the amount of hypertrophy needed to generate elevated right ventricular pressures.

If the ECG is in conflict with other physical findings and appears to be underestimating the stenosis, the gradient may be proximal to the pulmonary valve, such as in the body of the right ventricle.[63] In this case the proximal high pressure area and the hypertrophied portion may be relatively small,[64] and not be as obvious on the scalar ECG where a summation of forces are seen.

Arrhythmias are rarely seen, and with the exception of end-stage disease, cannot be correlated with severity. Right atrial enlargement is frequently seen as the severity increases, and often implies hemodynamic significance with decreased right ventricular compliance from hypertrophy and increased right atrial mass and enlargement.[2,10]

The QRS axis will continue moving rightward with increasing severity and the QRS interval may continue to widen. The right-anterior forces may become so great that the left-sided posterior ventricular forces are not seen in V_1, yielding a pure R wave, and S greater than R in V_6. Ventricular "strain" is defined as associated repolarization changes, noticeably in the T wave, or the development of a QR pattern in V_1.

With severe stenosis the T wave axis may become discordant from the QRS; it may move leftward, and superiorly and posteriorly. Therefore, the T wave in leads II, III, av_F, and V_1 may be inverted. If accompanied by ST-T wave depression in V_1 to V_4,[60] one can assume the

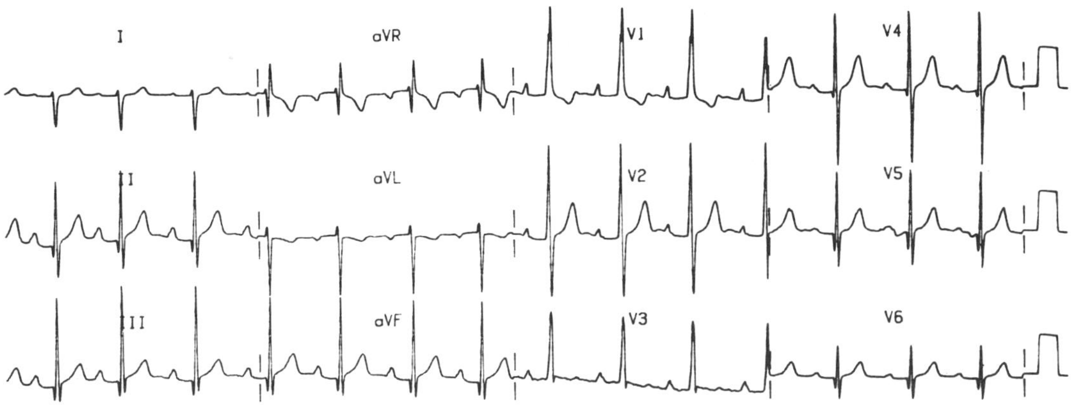

Figure 6-3 Scalar ECG in severe valvar pulmonic stenosis with right atrial enlargement. First-degree atrioventricuar block, right axis deviation (QRS 135), and right ventricular hypertrophy with ST-T wave abnormality, from an 18-year-old with a peak systolic ejection gradient of 76 mmHg and a peak right ventricular pressure of 90 mmHg.

myocardium is suffering ischemic changes from the detrimental pressure overload.[45] After adequate relief of the gradient, the ST-T wave abnormality may not normalize, as the other changes resolve.

Chest Roentgenogram

The cardiothymic silhouette is usually normal in size except in severe cases where right ventricular failure has occurred, producing an enlarged right atrium, and ventricle.[65] Occasionally, the right atrial border on the anteroposterior projection may become abnormally convex.[66] Some prominence of the right ventricle may be seen, especially in the retrosternal area on the lateral projection. The left ventricle is of normal size and contour, though the left atrium frequently shows mild enlargement in less than 50% of cases.[66] Intracardiac calcification in the region of the valve is rare, and only seen in adults.[19]

Pulmonary blood flow and the pulmonary venous pattern are normal. Some have described an asymmetry of perfusion with the left lung appearing greater than the right, thought to be from preferential streaming into the left pulmonary artery, across a narrowed eccentric valvar orifice.[67]

The main and left pulmonary arteries, because of poststenotic dilation, are unusually prominent on the anteroposterior projection (Figure 6-4), forming a convexity along the left upper heart border. The right pulmonary artery is of normal caliber. The degree of dilation may vary, but this cannot be correlated with the severity of the obstruction. In fact, mild disease is often seen with the most prominent poststenotic dilation. This finding can be seen without right ventricular outflow tract obstruction, especially in adolescence as "idiopathic dilation of the pulmonary trunk," in which case no murmur is present [40] (Figure 6-5). In adults, the left main pulmonary

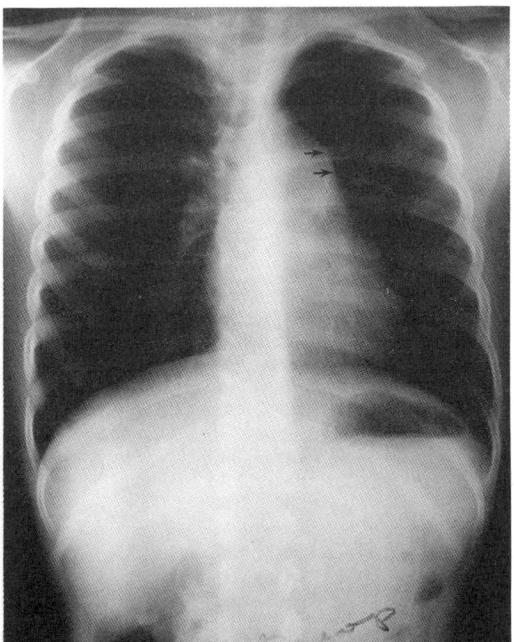

Figure 6-4 Posteroanterior chest film preoperation in a 12-year-old girl with moderate valvar pulmonic stenosis demonstrating a normal heart size, contour and pulmonary blood flow, with marked main pulmonary arterial poststenotic dilation (arrows).

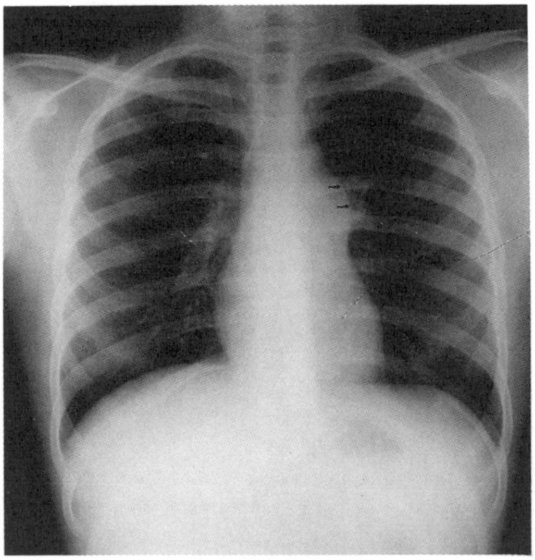

Figure 6-5 Posteroanterior chest film showing idiopathic dilation of main pulmonary artery (arrows) in a 13-year-old girl without evidence of right ventricular outflow tract obstruction.

artery may become enlarged and radiodense; it has been confused with a perihilar tumor.[66] Fluorscopy may help to further define the mass as vascular. Poststenotic dilation is not frequently seen if the valve is dysplastic[51] or the obstruction is below the valvar level.

The aortic arch is on the left.[57] Though a right aortic arch has been described with an intact ventricular septum, it is rare, and its presence should arouse the suspicion of a concomitant ventricular septal defect or subvalvar obstruction.[24]

Echocardiography

Noninvasive imaging techniques, along with Doppler interrogation, have offered a new opportunity to evaluate the anatomy of the right ventricular outflow tract and estimate the severity.

There are no definitive diagnostic features on the M-mode echocardiogram.[68] The supportive features attempt to separate a right ventricular volume overload pattern with a dilated right ventricle and reversed interventricular septal motion, from the pressure overload pattern. This would show a thickened right ventricular free wall and a deep pulmonary valve "a" wave excursion, reflecting a forceful atrial contraction, into a "stiffened" ventricle with decreased myocardial compliance.[69] This may also be found in other situations of elevated right ventricular end-diastolic pressure with a low pulmonary arterial pressure and is therefore nonspecific.[70] False-negatives are also frequently found.[71]

Pulmonary valve leaflet motion can be visualized, but rarely is more than one cusp seen. Because of ultrasonic beam angulation, along with cardiac motion, often, only the posterior leaflet is seen.[68] Since a severely obstructive valve may be a pliable domed structure anatomically, its motion during the cardiac cycle on M-mode echocardiography may appear normal. The actual size of the orifice cannot be accurately determined.

Systolic leaflet flutter is not diagnostic of severity or location of obstruction, though it is often seen with isolated subvalvar narrowing.[72] Fine harmonic leaflet flutter may be consistent with insignificant low-intensity systolic murmurs.

Subvalvar narrowing may cause violent leaflet flutter with early systolic closure, indicating a dynamic obstructive component similar to that

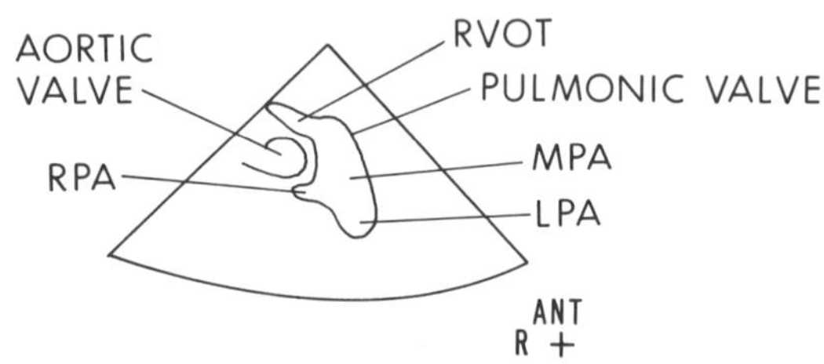

Figure 6-6A

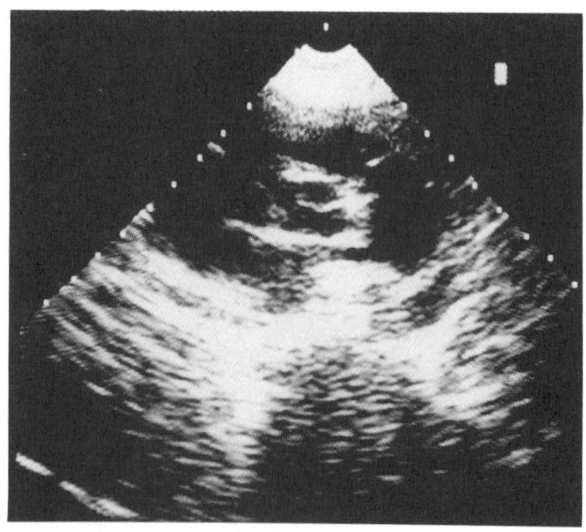

Figure 6-6B

Figure 6-6A&B Two-dimensional echocardiogram of an 11-year-old with mild valvar pulmonic stenosis. Systolic frame shows doming of anterior cusp with poststenotic main pulmonary arterial (MPA) dilation. RVOT = right ventricular outflow tract, LPA = left pulmonary artery, RPA = right pulmonary artery.

seen on the aortic valve with idiopathic hypertrophic subaortic stenosis.[72]

Systolic time intervals can be generated from a simultaneous M-mode echocardiogram of the pulmonary valve, along with an ECG tracing. They have not demonstrated any clinical utility in determining the severity of pulmonic stenosis.[54]

Two-dimensional echocardiography With adequate equipment, the right ventricular outflow tract can be visualized from a number of standard views, and the level of obstruction, along with an estimation of severity, can be determined. Similar findings to angiography may be visualized: annular narrowing, leaflet thickening with doming, and decreased mobility.[73] The proximal main pulmonary artery will be dilated[74] (Figure 6-6 A and B).

Recently, pulsed-gated Doppler ultrasound has been used to more accurately define the level and severity of obstruction. The area of Doppler interrogation may be maneuvered through the right ventricular outflow tract into the main

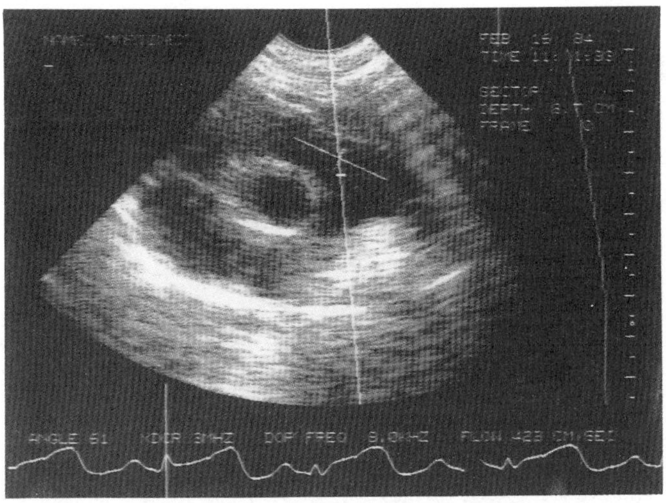

Figure 6-7A Two-dimensional echocardiogram with Doppler sample in main pulmonary artery, and incident angle of 40° to flow.

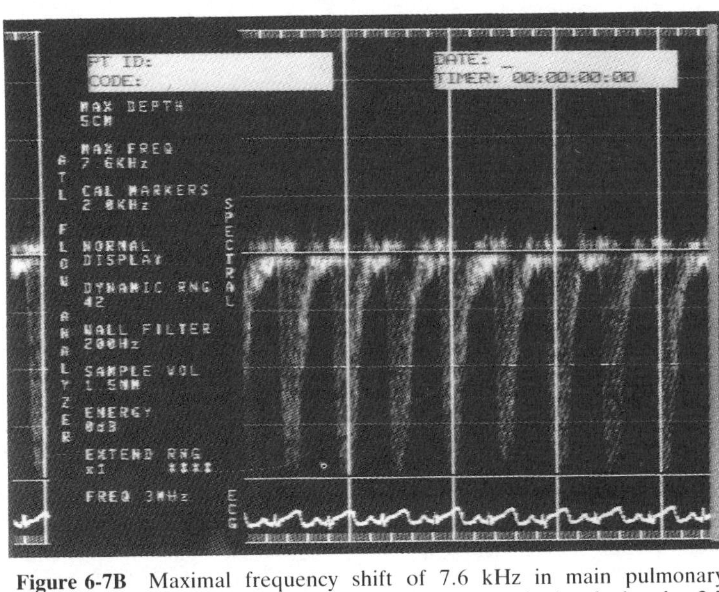

Figure 6-7B Maximal frequency shift of 7.6 kHz in main pulmonary artery distal to stenotic valve. The maximal flow velocity is calculated at 2.7 m/sc, and when placed in the modified Bernoulli equation yields a peak systolic ejection gradient of 28 mmHg. This correlated to a catheterization-derived gradient.

pulmonary artery, and by measuring the Doppler frequency shift, along with the incident angle of the Doppler beam, the peak blood flow velocity (V) can be determined (Figure 6-7 A and B). When placed into the simplified Bernoulli equation, as modified by Hatle et al[75], a peak systolic ejection gradient (PSEG) may be calculated:

$$PSEG = 4 \times V^2$$

This has an excellent correlation to hemodynamically derived measurements.[76] Multiple levels of obstruction, or other causes of chaotic turbulence, such as pulmonary insufficiency or a subpulmonary ventricular septal defect, may result in an error due to the inability to record a clear Doppler signal.[77]

CARDIAC CATHETERIZATION

By the time the sequence of clinical and noninvasive studies are performed, the anatomical location and severity of right ventricular outflow tract obstruction have already been established with a high degree of accuracy. Therefore, the purpose of cardiac catheterization has changed from being a primary diagnostic tool that supplied all of the imaging and physiologic data, to a more selective methodology for answering questions left unresolved, and to further elucidate the anatomy with angiography. With further advances in noninvasive imaging along with Doppler evaluation of cardiac flow and gradient, cardiac catheterization may be further supplanted, or even become superfluous for the preoperative evaluation in pulmonic valve disease.

The physiologic determinations are separated into saturation measurements, pressure measurements, and hemodynamic calculations, such as flow and valve area.

The catheter course is unremarkable, with a high frequency of patency of the foramen ovale, allowing entry into the left atrium, left ventricle, and aorta, antegrade. In severe disease, with a decreased cardiac output or tricuspid regurgitation, manipulating a balloon-tipped catheter from the right atrium into the right ventricle may be difficult. The same difficulty may be encountered in crossing the right ventricular outflow tract. In cases of severe stenosis with a tiny valve orifice, the catheter diameter or flow-directed balloon tip may totally obstruct the right ventricular output and create an additional afterload strain on an already precarious ventricle. Bradycardia, cyanosis (from right-to-left atrial shunting), or ventricular ectopy may ensue. Therefore, prior to attempting to cross the right ventricular outflow tract when the right ventricular pressure is systemic or greater, or if systemic cyanosis exists, an arterial (peripheral systemic or aortic) line should be in place for saturation sampling and systemic pressure monitoring (Figure 6-8).

Unless the atrial septum is deficient, there will be no significant saturation step-up seen from the superior vena cava to the right atrium, or a step-

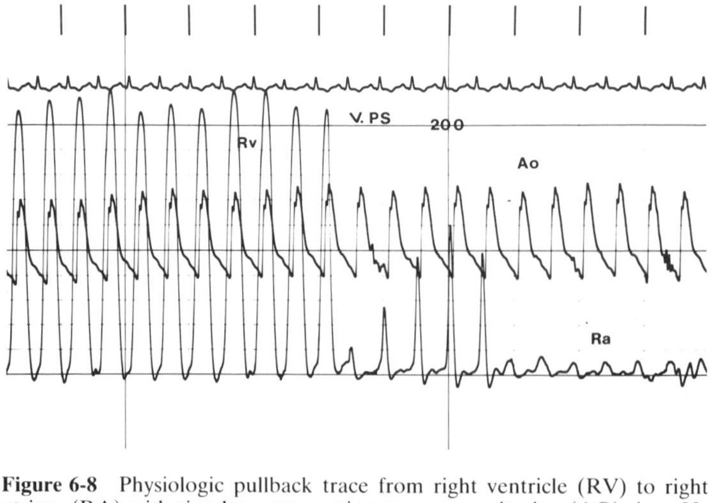

Figure 6-8 Physiologic pullback trace from right ventricle (RV) to right atrium (RA) with simultaneous aortic pressure monitoring (AO), in a 22-year-old with severe valvar pulmonic stenosis and suprasystemic right ventricular pressure (226 mmHg). Entry into the main pulmonary artery across the pulmonary valve was not attempted.

down (from right-to-left shunting) seen between a pulmonary vein and the left atrium. A left-to-right atrial shunt implies an atrial septal defect (primum, secondum, sinus venosus) or an anomalous pulmonary vein draining into the right atrium, as opposed to a "stretched" foramen ovale. The corollary is not true; a right-to-left shunt may be seen with a stretched foramen ovale that would be competent if the pressure in the right atrium were less. Further pressure or angiographic data are needed to define truly the anatomical site of the shunt. If right-to-left atrial shunting is occurring and systemic cyanosis exists, the right ventricular outflow tract obstruction is by definition severe.

The systolic pressure in the right ventricle will always be elevated, with a peak pressure greater than that seen in the main pulmonary artery. The difference in these two peak pressures, if measured simultaneously, is termed the peak systolic ejection gradient. Since simultaneous pressure monitoring is rarely performed, a pullback from the main pulmonary artery across the outflow tract into the body of the right ventricle usually suffices as a "gradient" measurement (Figure 6-9). An end-hole or single side-hole physiologic catheter should be used for the slow pullback from the main pulmonary artery, through the right ventricle to the right atrium with careful observation for any further pressure changes at either the infundibulum or within the right ventricular body.[76] If confusion as to the location of multiple gradients exists, the catheter should be positioned at the right ventricular apex, and then slowly withdrawn to the right atrium, thereby specifically searching for a gradient between inflow and apex.

The right atrial pressure may be normal or show an accentuation of the usually prominent "a" wave. If a "v" wave predominates, tricuspid regurgitation from severe pulmonic stenosis or right ventricular failure should be inferred. The left atrial and right atrial mean pressures should be unequal on pullback, if the atrial septum is intact, or if the foramen ovale is stretched. If the foramen ovale has become physiologically unrestrictive, and allows equalization of mean pressures, an atrial septal defect (anatomical location unknown) is diagnosed.

There is no diastolic gradient from the right atrial "a" wave to the right ventricular end-diastolic pressure, which like the "a" wave may be elevated if the right ventricle has become less compliant from hypertrophy.

The left atrial and left ventricular pressures are within the normal range. Occasionally, in severe, long-standing disease, often associated with systemic cyanosis and right ventricular failure, the left ventricular end-diastolic pressure may also be elevated. The left ventricular dysfunction is partially from the shared contribution that the interventricular septum makes to both ventricles.

Using the Gorlin formula,[79] the valve orifice area can be calculated:

$$\text{Area (cm}^2) = \frac{\text{flow (systolic)/}}{44.5\ \sqrt{\text{mean systolic pressure different across pulmonary valve}}}$$

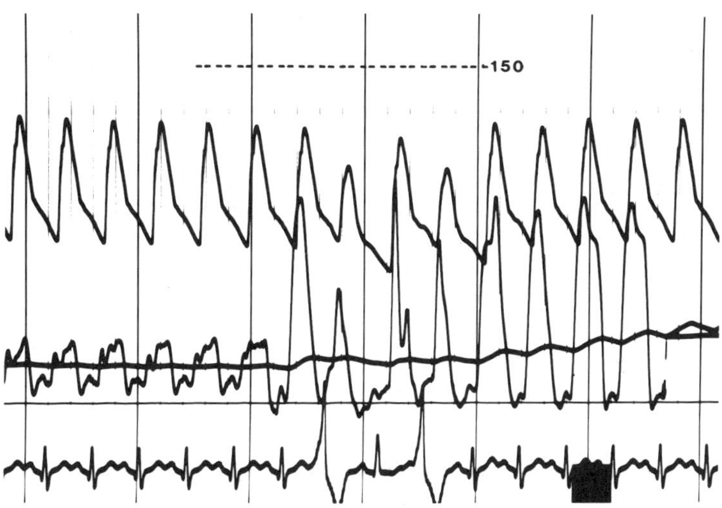

Figure 6-9 Physiologic pullback trace from main pulmonary artery to right ventricle demonstrating a peak systolic ejection gradient of 66 mmHg, and a right ventricle at three-fourths systemic pressure (aortic trace).

This has been simplified by Moller and Adams,[80] so as to utilize the peak right ventricular pressure and mean pulmonary arterial pressure, thereby eliminating the tedium of measuring the mean gradient. This formula is only accurate in pure valvar disease, since it was derived for flow across an orifice and therefore cannot be used if an infundibular gradient or pulmonary insufficiency coexist.[78] The normal calculated valve area is approximately 2.0 cm^2/m^2. Mild to moderate stenosis will yield an area of 1.0 to 2.0 cm^2/m^2, and in severe stenosis the valve area will be less than 0.50 cm^2/m^2.[78] The measured gradient will vary directly with the cardiac output, given a fixed stenotic valve orifice. Therefore, the hemodynamic measurements and valve area can be redetermined after manipulations are made in cardiac output, with either exercise or inotropic drugs,[81,82] if the degree of severity is in question. The ratio of peak right ventricular pressure/systemic pressure, along with gradient, should be used, rather than the peak right ventricular pressure alone. Also, an inappropriate increase in cardiac output with work or oxygen consumption (an abnormal exercise factor) can be used as an additional determinant of severity in borderline cases, along with the development of right-to-left atrial shunting, or an increase in the right ventricular end-diastolic pressure.[83–85] Exercise will often unmask abnormalities in the right ventricular diastolic properties from myocardial hypertrophy, fibrosis, or ischemia.[86] These abnormalities at a given right ventricular pressure are more frequently seen with increasing age,[87] along with the inability to increase the cardiac output appropriately with exercise.

Angiocardiography

In cases where surgical intervention is anticipated, angiocardiography is essential to accurately define the anatomy of the right ventricular outflow tract, and to observe right ventricular and tricuspid valve function. It should be performed with biplane projection to allow a spatial appreciation of asymmetric structures. Cineangiocardiography with rapid sequence filming allows precise analysis of the pulmonary valve motion during the cardiac cycle, along with the differentiation of dynamic *v* fixed infundibular stenosis.

The catheter should be placed with the injecting ports near the right ventricular apex, while free in the cavity and not entrapped. Unless there is a right ventricular volume overload from an atrial septal defect, tricuspid regurgitation, or pulmonary insufficiency, the contrast load per injection does not have to exceed 1.0 mL/kg, or have to be injected at rapid rates. In biplane projection, the right ventricle should be imaged anteroposteriorly (AP) or laterally, or preferably in the right anterior oblique (RAO)/left anterior oblique (LAO) projection, which will allow a better visualization of the infundibular area, especially the RAO view, along with a view en face of the pulmonary valve. If pulmonary artery branch stenosis is suspected by pullback pressure gradients, cranial angulation of the RAO or AP camera will facilitate visualization, especially of the right branch takeoff, as it arises from the main pulmonary artery.

The right ventricular cavity volume is normal,[88,89] but may seem crowded because of hypertrophied trabeculae and papillary muscles. The right ventricular wall thickness is increased, in proportion to the severity, and is especially obvious in the right ventricular free wall. If the right ventricular pressure is suprasystemic, the interventricular septum may bow toward the left ventricular cavity.[78]

The pulmonary valve leaflets will have various amounts of thickening that may be asymmetric. The cusps can be counted and often an estimation of orifice size can be made either by the positive contrast jet coming through the valve, or by the later negative jet of unopacified blood. The known catheter size can be used as a "relative" standard for estimation of the orifice diameter. The leaflets dome toward the main pulmonary artery with ventricular systole (Figure 6-10). As they lose their pliability, the leaflets tend to "rock" to and fro during the cardiac cycle. If the leaflets are very thickened and the cusps not well defined, a myxomatous, dysplastic valve should be suspected. In this case systolic doming and leaflet motion is not seen and the pulmonary valve annulus is small.

The infundibular area should be examined closely for both fixed and dynamic narrowing. When the conal septum hypertrophies, a subvalvar chamber may form above the obstructing muscle band. During diastole, differentiation of dynamic obstruction is possible, as the area in the biplane projection opens to a diameter approximating the annulus. Other large muscle bands in the body of the ventricle should also be sought.

The main pulmonary artery and proximal left pulmonary artery show dilation, often maximal at the point where struck by the angiographic jet. The right and left branch pulmonary arteries

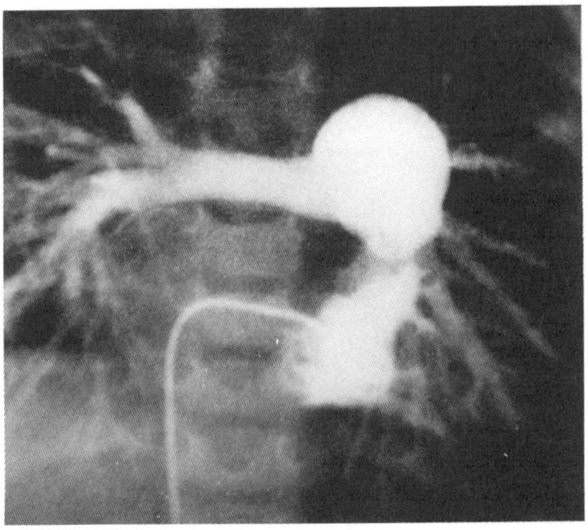

Figure 6-10A

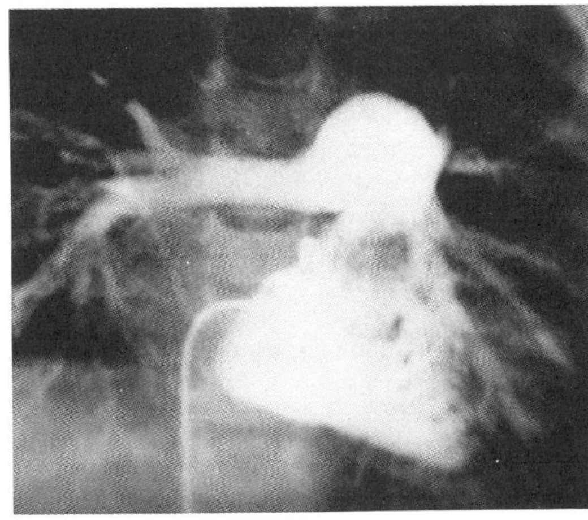

Figure 6-10C

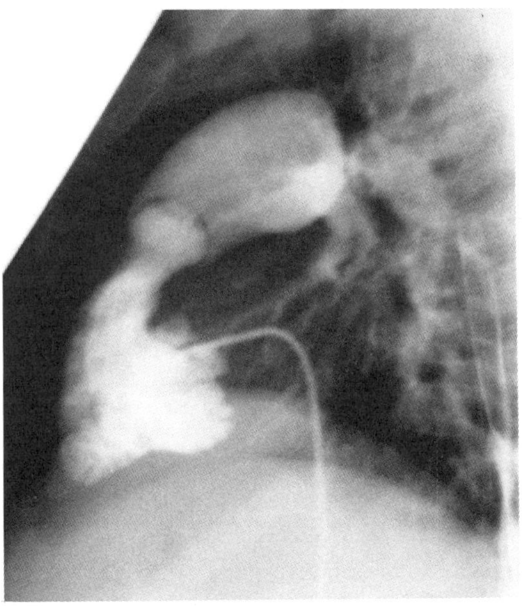

Figure 6-10B

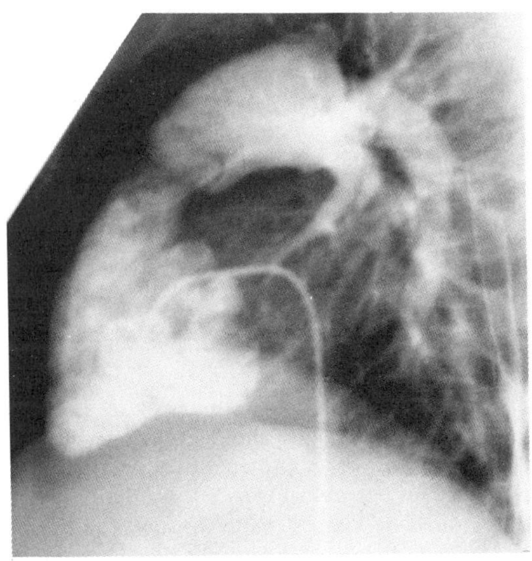

Figure 6-10D

Figure 6-10 Anteroposterior and lateral right ventricular cineangiogram. A and B Systolic cavity encroachment by hypertrophy with dynamic infundibular narrowing. The pulmonary valve domes superiorly during systole (lateral) as the poststenotic main pulmonary arterial dilation is maximal. C & D. Diastolic enlargement of right ventricular cavity and infundibulum. Thickened pulmonary valve leaflets continue to be visible, with normal annular diameter.

should be inspected for obstruction from either narrowing or intraluminal membranes.

On levophase, contrast will return via the pulmonary veins to the left atrium, and left-to-right atrial shunting can be detected and evaluated both for location and magnitude. A separate left ventricular angiogram is often performed to further rule out any associated lesions such as ventricular septal defect, aortic stenosis, or large systemic to pulmonary arterial collateral vessels.

TREATMENT

The treatment of pulmonary stenosis is obviously based on removal of the area of obstruction. This procedure was first performed by

Doyen in 1913, using a small tenotomy knife through the right ventricle. The patient died soon after surgery.[90] In 1948 Brock[90] and Sellors,[91] each working independently, resurrected and successfully modified the procedure. The operation was performed without extracorporeal circulation, via a transventricular approach using a specially constructed apparatus passed through a purse-string stitch in the right ventricular free wall, extending through the stenotic valve and into the main pulmonary artery. This procedure was widely used for all forms of right ventricular outflow tract obstruction, including that associated with tetralogy of Fallot.

Inflow occlusion and the development of extracorporeal circulation allowed the surgeon to open the main pulmonary artery and visualize the valve from above, prior to performing the valvotomy.[92] Depending on the anatomy, the commissures can be opened and the subpulmonic area can be explored. Various operating room evaluations of adequacy have been used, including sizing the annulus with dilators and also measuring the residual gradients directly from right ventricular and pulmonary arterial pressure monitoring.

Open pulmonary valvotomy is easily and safely performed with a 2% to 4% mortality in large series.[93–96] The determinants of a poor outcome are cyanosis, congestive heart failure, and associated anomalies.[93,95]

If the annulus is small, the valve leaflets dysplastic (myxomatous), or the infundibular obstruction nondynamic, simple valvotomy will not adequately decrease the degree of right ventricular outflow tract obstruction. Therefore, a more extensive surgical repair is warranted.[93] A longitudinal incision is made through the infundibulum and carried through the pulmonary valve annulus. A patch is sewn over the outflow tract annulus and main pulmonary artery. This patch forms a new elevated "roof" to the outflow tract, thereby creating a larger channel from the right ventricle to the main pulmonary artery. This patch can be constructed from autologous pericardium, or prosthetic material such as Dacron mesh or PTFE (Gortex). Any intracavitary obstructing muscle bundles can also be excised through the ventriculotomy.

In the group that undergoes valvotomy alone, subvalvar obstruction from a dynamic hypertrophied infundibulum may develop despite returning the pulmonary valve orifice to a near-normal diameter. This dynamic obstruction may be severe, but if given time, it usually regresses.[97,98]

The surgical relief of obstruction is excellent, both in the short term and long term. This was seen in the multicentered natural history study which followed the clinical course of 245 patients aged 2 to 21 years who were treated surgically and had pre- and postoperative catheterization measurements of gradient.[8] There was one surgical mortality. On postoperative recatheterization only four out of 245 patients had a residual peak systolic ejection gradient greater than 50, thereby implying a 98% success rate for surgery. Twenty-nine patients had two postoperative catheterizations at a median interval of 5.7 years. The gradients did not increase; therefore, restenosis did not occur. This indicates that the postoperative decrease in gradient is long-lasting.

Specially constructed balloon dilation catheters have been used successfully to relieve obstruction in selected cases of valvar disease.[99–103] The approach and equipment have been a refinement of the techniques developed for systemic and coronary arterial angioplasty.[104]

At the time of cardiac catheterization, the balloon catheter is passed over a wire and positioned across the annulus of the pulmonary valve. The balloon is distended with fluid under high pressure. It becomes rigid, and tears the membranous fused leaflets. The short-term results have been encouraging, with a drop in the systolic pressure gradient.[100,103] The long-term effects, including the incidence of re-stenosis or the subsequent need for surgical intervention, have not been evaluated.

An associated atrial septal defect can be closed surgically with the patient on cardiopulmonary bypass. If there is right-to-left atrial shunting because of elevated right ventricular filling pressures, the advisability of the procedure is controversial. By eliminating the site of the shunt, the patient will not have persistent cyanosis, the potential cost being manifestations of right ventricular failure and decreased cardiac output. Often, if the defect is left open and the right ventricular outflow tract obstruction is adequately relieved, the diastolic properties of the right ventricle will improve, and the right-to-left atrial shunt may reverse, or the septum primum may spontaneously close the defect.

A dysplastic pulmonary valve frequently is not amenable to a simple commissurotomy. Upon visualization, the surgeon may elect to remove one of the cusps, or if the annulus is also narrowed, to incise across it, for placement of a patch.[98] Even if the pulmonary arterial pressure is normal, the physical findings of pulmonary insufficiency will be noted. The small right ventricular volume overload is much better tolerated than the severe pressure overload.

COURSE AND PROGNOSIS

The course and prognosis of pulmonic valve disease are directly related to the severity of the right ventricular outflow tract obstruction. The most accurate measurement of severity is the cardiac catheterization–derived gradient, along with the ratio of right ventricular to systemic pressure, since this may reveal additional information on the hemodynamic state. Included in the decision-making process are the presence of symptoms or decreased exercise capacity, if the hemodynamic criteria are borderline.

Mild stenosis is rarely progressive, and therefore the hemodynamic burden can easily be tolerated for a "normal" life.[105] It should not be a source of symptoms or decreased exercise capacity. Pregnancy and delivery carry no greater risk than in the general population. Bacterial endocarditis remains a small but real risk, and lifetime prophylaxis is recommended. Though the incidence of bacterial endocarditis is difficult to determine, Keith et al[2] found it to be less than 2% while Engle et al [10] noted it in 7% of patients. After an initial evaluation, the patient can be followed infrequently with noninvasive procedures, and if the patient's state remains consistent with mild disease, cardiac catheterization may never be warranted.

The asymptomatic patient with moderate stenosis generally has a well-tolerated pressure overload, that may or may not progress in severity or cause deterioration of right ventricular function. The group with moderate stenosis, therefore, creates a terrible dilemma for the clinician. By hemodynamics alone, there may not be adequate criteria for surgical intervention, but the presence of mild symptoms or ECG evidence of right ventricular strain may coerce the clinician to recommend surgery. Otherwise, regular clinical and noninvasive follow-up is warranted with repeat cardiac catheterization predicated on changing symptoms or noninvasive studies. Often an exercise tolerance test may be of value in objectifying exercise capacity,[106] often reported subjectively as "normal," along with detecting any exercise-induced arrhythmias or repolarization phenomena from the right ventricular hypertension.

Since surgical therapy provides nearly a "cure", with a drop in gradient, little chance of restenosis, and low mortality and morbidity, it is often favored over subjecting the right ventricle to the long-term effects of the moderate pressure overload. This pressure overload may either progress and require operation later under less favorable conditions, or cause possibly irreversible myocardial fibrosis and right heart damage.[107]

Severe stenosis, defined as a gradient greater than 75 mmHg and/or a right ventricular pressure equal to or greater than the systemic pressure, with or without cyanosis from right-to-left atrial shunting, has to be alleviated to prevent further development of right ventricular myocardial fibrosis and failure, both of which would increase the surgical risk and lessen the opportunity for a good outcome. Prior to the advent of right ventricular failure, the procedure can be performed safely with minimal morbidity.[93] Very few severe cases will be seen after the second decade, either because of attrition in the natural history or the more liberal and early use of surgery.

Fortunately, a patient with severe disease is rarely seen de novo. Most often those with moderate disease may have progression in signs and symptoms that will push the balance in favor of surgical relief of the obstruction, even though the gradient may or may not have increased when measured at cardiac catheterization.

After surgical intervention, the physical examination should reflect the decreased right ventricular outflow tract obstruction that has now been replaced by mild pulmonary insufficiency in 60% of patients.[8] Invariably, the systolic murmur will decrease in intensity by several grades. If it has not, one should suspect inadequate relief of obstruction, either at the valvar or infundibular level. Dynamic infundibular obstruction may decrease slowly with time as the hypertrophy regresses. The findings of right ventricular failure and tricuspid regurgitation may or may not improve. The ECG often shows a slow decrease in right ventricular hypertrophy. The chest film remains unchanged. Since physical and laboratory findings are rarely "normal" after surgery,[95] there is a tendency toward recatheterization. Because of the near universal achievement of a good surgical result with a drop in gradient, this is unwarranted on a routine basis on statistical grounds, but the evaluation should be individualized.

After surgery, symptoms will be relieved and exercise capacity should be improved.[108,109]

Though there has not been a long-range natural history study on surgical outcome, it is considered that if an adequate valvotomy is performed prior to the advent of right ventricular failure, and the residual pulmonary insufficiency is mild, a normal longevity without any physical limitations can be expected. A large right ventricular volume overload from pulmonary insufficiency may have a detrimental long-term effect on right ventricular performance and limit exercise capacity.[110,111] Routine endocarditis prophylaxis is necessary postoperatively for the patient's lifetime.

REFERENCES

1. Nadas AS, Fyler DC: *Pediatric Cardiology*, ed 3, Philadelphia, WB Saunders Co, 1972.
2. Keith JD, Rowe RD, Vlad P: *Heart Disease In Infancy And Childhood*. New York, Macmillan Publishing Co, Inc, 1958.
3. Johnson LW, Grossman W, Dalen JE, et al: Pulmonic stenosis in the adult. Long-term follow-up results. *N Engl J Med* 1972;287:1159–1163.
4. Bankl H: *Congenital Malformations of the Heart and Great Vessels*. Munich, Urban & Schwarzenberg, 1977.
5. Abbott ME: *Atlas of Congenital Cardiac Disease*. New York, American Heart Association, 1936.
6. Taussig HB: *Congenital Malformations of the Heart*. New York, The Commonwealth Fund, 1947.
7. Wood P; Congenital heart disease: A review of its clinical aspects in the light of experience gained by means of modern techniques. *Br Med J* 1950;2:693–698.
8. Nugent EW, Freedom RM, Nora JJ, et al: Clinical course in pulmonic stenosis. *Circulation* 1977;56:(suppl 1)38–47.
9. Wood, P: *Diseases of the Heart and Circulation*, ed 2, London, Eyre & Spotteswoode, 1956.
10. Engle, MA, Ito T, Goldberg HP: The fate of the patient with pulmonic stenosis. *Circulation* 1964; 30:554–561.
11. Levine OR, Blumenthal S: Pulmonic stenosis. *Circulation* 1965;31,32:(suppl 3)33–41.
12. Becker AE, Anderson RE: *Pathology of Congenital Heart Disease*. London, Butterworths & Co Ltd, 1981.
13. Brock RC: *The Anatomy of Congenital Pulmonary Stenosis*. London, Cassell & Co Ltd, 1957.
14. Moore, GW, Hutchins GM, Brito JC, et al: Congenital malformations of the semilunar valves. *Hum Pathol* 1980;11:367–372.
15. Holman E: On circumscribed dilation of an artery immediately distal to a partially occluding band: Poststenotic dilatation. *Surgery* 1954; 36:3–24.
16. Hardy WE, Gnoj J, Ayres SM, et al: Pulmonic stenosis and associated atrial septal defects in older patients. *Am J Cardiol* 1969;24:130–134.
17. Alday LE, Moreyra E: Calcific pulmonary stenosis. *Br Heart J* 1973;35:887–889.
18. Gabriele OF, Scatliff JH: Pulmonary valve calcificiation. *Am Heart J* 1970;80:299–302.
19. Roberts WC, Mason DT, Morrow AG, et al: Calcific pulmonic stenosis. *Circulation* 1968;37: 973–978.
20. Hoffman JIE: The natural history of congenital isolated pulmonic and aortic stenosis. *Annu Rev Med* 1969;20:15–28.
21. Franciosi RA, Blanc WA: Myocardial infarcts in infants and children. I. A necropsy study in congenital heart disease. *J Pediatr* 1968;73: 309–319.
22. Fontana RS, Edwards JE: *Congenital Cardiac Disease*. Philadelphia, WB Saunders Co, 1962.
23. Campbell M: Simple pulmonary stenosis. Pulmonary valvular stenosis with a closed ventricular septum. *Br Heart J* 1954;16:273, 1954.
24. Gamble WJ, Nadas AS: Severe pulmonary stenosis with intact ventricular septum and right aortic arch. *Circulation* 1965;32:114–119.
25. Hastreiter AR, D'Cruz IA, Cantez T: Right-sided aorta. *Br Heart J* 1966;28:722–739.
26. Levin DL, Heyman MA, Rudolph AM: Morphological development of the pulmonary vascular bed in experimental pulmonic stenosis. *Circulation* 1979;59:179–182.
27. DeTroyer A, Yernault JC: Lung hypoplasia in congenital pulmonary valve stenosis. *Circulation* 1977;56:647–651.
28. Liese GJ, Brainard, SC, Goto U: Giant blood cyst of the pulmonary valve. *N Engl J Med* 1963; 269:465–467.
29. Jiminez-Martinez M, Franco-Vazquez S, Angulo-Hernandez O, et al: Blood cysts of the pulmonary valve producing pulmonic stenosis. *J Thorac Cardiovasc Surg* 1968;56:165–169.
30. Davies MJ: *Pathology of Cardiac Valves*. London, Butterworths & Co Ltd, 1980.
31. Bulkley BH, Hutchins GM, Ross RS: Aortic sinus of valsalva aneurysms simulating primary right-sided valvular heart disease. *Circulation* 1975;52:696–699.
32. Drachler DH, Willis PW: Acquired right ventricular outflow tract obstruction. *Am Heart J* 1971;82:536–540.
33. Griffith DNW, Myers A: Obtruction of right ventricular outflow tract solitary ovarian metastasis. *Br Heart J* 1978;40:700–702.
34. O'Toole JD, Wurtzbacher JJ, Wearner NE, et al: Pulmonary valve injury and insufficiency during pulmonary artery catheterization. *N Engl J Med* 1979;301:1167–1168.
35. Hoffman JIE, Christianson R: Congenital heart disease in a cohort of 19,502 births with long-term follow-up. *Am J Cardiol* 1978;42:641–647.
36. Flyer DC: Report of the New England Regional Infant Cardiac Program. *Pediatrics* 1980;65: 375–461.
37. Moller JH, Adams P: The natural history of pulmonary valvular stenosis. Serial cardiac catheterizations in 21 children. *Am J Cardiol* 1965;16: 654–664.
38. Danielowicz D, Hoffman JIE, Rudolph AM: Serial studies of pulmonary stenosis in infancy and childhood. *Br Heart J* 1975;37:808–818.
39. Genovese PD, Rosenbaum D: Pulmonary steno-

sis with survival to the age of 78 years. *Am Heart J* 1951;41:755–761.

40. Greene DG, Baldwin ED, Baldwin JS, et al: Pure congenital pulmonary stenosis and idiopathic congenital dilatation of the pulmonary artery. *Am J Med* 1949;6:24–40.
41. Fabricius J: *Isolated Pulmonary Stenosis*. Copenhagen, Munksgard, 1959.
42. Abrahams DG, Wood P: Pulmonary stenosis with normal aortic root. *Br Heart J* 1951;13: 519–548.
43. Wood P: Congenital heart disease. A review of its clinical aspects in the light of experience gained by means of modern techniques. *Br Med J* 1950;2:639–645.
44. Lambert EC, Menon VA, Wagner HR, et al: Sudden unexpected death from cardiovascular disease in children. *Am J Cardiol* 1974;34:89–96.
45. Marquis RM: Unipolar electrocardiography in pulmonary stenosis. *Br Heart J* 1951;13:89–101.
46. Dimond EG, Lin TK: The clinical picture of pulmonary stenosis (without ventricular septal defect). *Ann Intern Med* 1954;40:1108–1124.
47. Noonan JA: Association of congenital heart disease with syndromes or other defects. *Pediatr Clin North Am* 1978;25:797–816.
48. Lamy M, DeGrouchy J, Schweisguth O: Genetic and non-genetic factors in the etiology of congential heart disease: a study of 1188 cases. *Am J Hum Genet* 1957;9:17–41.
49. Noonan JA: Hypertelorism with Turner phenotype. A new syndrome with associated congenital heart disease. *Am J Dis Child* 1968;116:373–380.
50. Pearl W: Cardiovascular anomalies in Noonan's syndrome. *Chest* 1977;71:677–679.
51. Koretzky ED, Moller JH, Korns ME, et al: Congenital pulmonary stenosis resulting from dysplasia of valve. *Circulation* 1969;40:43–53.
52. Jeffery RF, Moller JH, Amplatz K: The dysplastic pulmonary valve: A new roentgenographic entity. *Am J Roentgenol Ther Radium Nucl Med* 1972;114:322–339.
53. Vogelpoel L, Schrire V: Auscultatory and phonocardiographic assessment of pulmonary stenosis with intact ventricular septum. *Circulation* 1960;22:55–72.
54. Tavel ME: *Clinical Phonocardiography and External Pulse Recording*, ed 3, Chicago, Year Book Medical Publishers, Inc, 1978.
55. Hultgren HN, Reeve R, Cohn K, et al: The ejection click of valvular pulmonic stenosis. *Circulation* 1969;40:631–639.
56. Linde LM, Turner SW, Sparkes RS: Pulmonary valvular dysplasia. A cardiofacial syndrome. *Br Heart J* 1973;35:301–304.
57. Perloff J: *The Clinical Recognition of Congenital Heart Disease*, ed 2, Philadelphia, WB Saunders Co, 1978.
58. Gamboa R, Hugenholtz PG, Nadas AS: Accuracy of the phonocardiogram in assessing severity of aortic and pulmonic stenosis. *Circulation* 1964;30:35–46.
59. Ellison RC, Freedom, RM, Keane JF, et al: Indirect assessment of severity in pulmoary stenosis. *Circulation* 1977;56(suppl I)14–20.
60. Boyle D. McC, Pantridge JF: The electrocardiogram in pulmonary valve stenosis with intact ventricular septum. *Br Heart J* 1964;26:477–480.
61. Emmanouilides GC, Baylen BG: Pulmonary Stenosis, in Adams FH, Emmanoulides GC (eds): *Moss' Heart Disease/In Infants, Children and Adolescents*, ed 3. Baltimore, Williams & Wilkins 1983, pp 234–262.
62. Gamboa R, Hugenholtz PG, Nadas AS: Corrected (Frank), uncorrected (Cube), and standard electrocardiographic lead systems in recording augmented right ventricular forces in right ventricular hypertension. *Br Heart J* 1966; 28:62–74.
63. Rowland TW, Rosenthal A, Castaneda AR: Double-chamber right ventricle: experience with 17 cases. *Am Heart J* 1975;89:455–462.
64. Danielowicz D, Ishmael R: Anomalous right ventricular muscle bundle: Clinical pitfalls and extracardiac anomalies. *Clin Cardiol* 1981;4: 146–150.
65. Swischuk LE: *Plain Film Interpretation in Congenital Heart Disease*, ed 2. Baltimore, Williams & Wilkins Co, 1979, pp 159–168.
66. Elliott LP, Schiebler GL: *The X-ray Diagnosis of Congenital Heart Disease in Infants, Children, and Adults*, ed 2. Springfield, Ill, Charles C Thomas Publisher, 1979.
67. Chen JTT, Robinson AE, Goodrich JK, et al: Uneven distribution of pulmonary blood flow between left and right lungs in isolated valvular pulmonary stenosis. *Am J Roentgenol* 1969;107: 343–350.
68. Williams RG, Tucker CR: *Echocardiographic Diagnosis of Congenital Heart Disease*. Boston, Little Brown & Co, 1977.
69. Weyman AE, Dillon JC, Feigenbaum H, et al: Echocardiographic patterns of pulmonary valve motion in valvular pulmonary stenosis. *Am J Cardiol* 1974;34:644–651.
70. Feigenbaum H: *Echocardiography*, ed 3. Philadelphia, Lea & Febiger, 1981.
71. Goldberg SJ, Areias JC, Spitaels SEC, et al: Echo Doppler detection of pulmonary stenosis by time-interval histogram analysis. *J Clin Ultrasound* 1979;7:183–189.
72. Weyman AE, Dillon JC, Feigenbaum H, et al: Echocardiographic differentiation of infundibular from valvular pulmonary stenosis. *Am J Cardiol* 1975;36:21–26.
73. Weyman AE, Hurwitz RA, Girod DA, et al: Cross-sectional echocardiographic visualization of the stenotic pulmonary valve. *Circulation* 1977;56:769–774.
74. Gussenhoven EJ, Becker AE: *Congenital Heart Disease*. London, Churchill Livingstone Inc, 1983.
75. Hatle L, Angelsen BA, Tromsdal A: Non-invasive assessment of aortic stenosis by Doppler ultrasound. *Br Heart J* 1980;43:284–292.
76. Lima CO, Sahn DJ, Valdes-Cruz LM, et al: Noninvasive prediction of transvalvular pressure gradient in patients with pulmonary stenosis by quantitative two-dimensional echocardiographic Doppler studies. *Circulation* 1983;67:866–871.
77. Hatle L, Angelsen B: *Doppler Ultrasound in Cardiology*. Philadelphia, Lea & Febiger, 1982.
78. Rudolph AM: *Congenital Diseases of the Heart*. Chicago, Year Book Medical Publishers, 1974.

79. Gorlin R, Gorlin SG: Hydraulic formula for calculation of the area of the stenotic mitral valve, other cardiac valves, and central circulatory shunts. *Am Heart J* 1951;41:1–29.
80. Moller JH, Adams P: A simplified method for calculating the pulmonary valvular area. *Am Heart J* 1966;72:463–465.
81. Truccone NJ, Steeg CN, Dell R, et al: Comparison of the cardiocirculatory effects of exercise and isoproterenol in children with pulmonary or aortic valve stenosis. *Circulation* 1977;56:79–82.
82. Rao PS, Awa S, Linde LM: Role of kinetic energy in pulmonary valvar pressure gradients. *Circulation* 1973;48:65–73.
83. Lewis JM, Montero AC, Kinard SA, et al: Hemodynamic response to exercise in isolated pulmonic stenosis. *Circulation* 1964:29: 854–861.
84. Moller JH, Rao S, Lucas RV: Exercise hemodynamics of pulmonary valvular stenosis: Study of 64 children. *Circulation* 1972;46:1018–1026.
85. Ikkos D, Jonsson B, Linderholm H: Effect of exercise in pulmonary stenosis with intact ventricular septum. *Br Heart J* 1966;28:316–330.
86. Hugenholtz PG, Nadas AS: Exercise studies in patients with congenital heart disease. *Pediatrics* 1983;2:769–775.
87. Howitt G: Haemodynamic effects of exercise in pulmonary stenosis. *Br Heart J* 1966;28:152–160.
88. Nakazawa M, Marks RA, Isabel-Jones J, et al: Right and left ventricular volume characteristics in children with pulmonary stenosis and intact ventricular septum. *Circulation* 1976;53:884–890.
89. Graham TP, Jarmakani JM, Atwood GF, et al: Right ventricular volume determinations in children. Normal values and observations with volume or pressure overload. *Circulation* 1973;47: 144–153.
90. Brock RC: Pulmonary valvulotomy for the relief of congenital pulmonary stenosis. *Br Med J* 1948;1:1121–1126.
91. Sellors TH: Surgery of pulmonary stenosis. *Lancet* 1948;1:988–989.
92. Varco RL: in discussion Muller WH, Longmire WP: The surgical treatment of cardiac valvular stenosis. *Surgery* 1951;30:41–42.
93. Danielson GK, Exarhos ND, Weidman WH, et al: Pulmonic stenosis with intact ventricular septum. *J Thorac Cardiovasc Surg*. 1971;61: 228–234.
94. Silverman BK, Nadas AS, Wittenborg MH, et al: Pulmonary stenosis with intact ventricular septum. *Am J Med* 1956;20:53–64.
95. Tandon R, Nadas AS, Gross RE: Results of open-heart surgery in patients with pulmonic stenosis and intact ventricular septum. *Circulation* 1965;31:190–201.
96. McIntosh HD, Cohen AL: Pulmonary stenosis: The importance of the myocardial factor in determining the clinical course and surgical results. *Am Heart J* 1963;65:715–716.
97. Engle MA, Holswade GR, Goldberg HP, et al: Regression after open valvotomy of infundibular stenosis accompanying severe valvular pulmonic stenosis. *Circulation* 1958;17:862–873.
98. Brock RC: The surgical treatment of pulmonary stenosis. *Br Heart J* 1961;23:337–356.
99. Kan JS, White RI, Mitchell SE, et al: Percutaneous balloon valvuloplasty: A new method for treating congenital pulmonary-valve stenosis. *N Engl J Med* 1982;307:540–542.
100. Kan JS, White RI, Mitchell SE, et al: Percutaneous transluminal balloon valvuloplasty for pulmonary valve stenosis. *Circulation* 1984;69: 554–560.
101. Lababidi Z, Wu J-R: Percutaneous balloon pulmonary valvuloplasty. *Am J Cardiol* 1983;52: 560–562.
102. Pepine CJ, Gessner IH, Feldman RI: Percutaneous balloon valvuloplasty for pulmonic valve stenosis in the adult. *Am J Cardiol* 1982;50: 1442–1445.
103. Rocchini AP, Kveselis DA, Crowley D, et al: Percutaneous balloon valvuloplasty for treatment of congenital pulmonary valvular stenosis in children. *J Am Coll Cardiol* 1984;3:1005–1012.
104. Dotter CT, Judkins MP: Transluminal treatment of arterosclerotic obstruction: description of a new technique and a pulmonary report of its application. *Circulation* 1964;30:654–670.
105. Nadas AS: Pulmonic stenosis. Indications for surgery in children and adults, editorial. *N Engl J Med* 1972;287:1196–1197.
106. Cumming GR: Maximal exercise capacity of children with heart disease. *Am J Cardiol* 1978; 42:613–619.
107. Campbell M: Natural history of congenital pulmonary stenosis. *Br Heart J* 1969;31:394.
108. Finnegan P, Ihenacho HNC, Singh SP, et al: Haemodynamic studies at rest and during exercise in pulmonary stenosis after surgery. *Br Heart J* 1974;36:913–918.
109. Stone FM, Bessinger FB, Lucas RV, et al: Pre- and postoperative rest and exercise hemodynamics in children with pulmonary stenosis. *Cirulation* 1974;49:1102–1106.
110. Wessel HU, Cunningham WJ, Paul MH, et al: Exercise performance in tetralogy of Fallot after intracardiac repair. *J Thorac Cardiovasc Surg* 1980;80:582–593.
111. Rocchini AP: Hemodynamic abnormalities in response to supine exercise in patients after operative correction of tetrad of Fallot after early childhood. *Am J Cardiol* 1981;48:325–330.

CHAPTER 7
Congenital Mitral Valve Disease

Gerald R. Marx

Recognition of congenital mitral valve disease is important because of its association with significant morbidity and mortality. However, diagnosis is obscured by its coexistence with other congenital heart defects, such as in Shone's syndrome, a complex consisting of supravalvar mitral ring, parachute mitral valve, subaortic stenosis, and coarctation of the aorta.[1] Congenital mitral valve disease can also occur with cyanotic heart defects,[2] single ventricle,[2] and hypoplasia of the left ventricle.[3]

Diagnosis of congenital mitral valve disease is further complicated by its nonspecific findings on physical examination, chest films, and ECG. However, recent advances in technology have enhanced the clinician's capability to diagnose this disease. Improvements in cineangiography provide better recognition of mitral valve defects at cardiac catheterization. Real-time two-dimensional echocardiography allows more precise visualization of the mitral valve orifice, leaflets, and tensor apparatus. With recent advances in Doppler echocardiography, the degree of mitral valve regurgitation, mitral valve stenosis, and orifice area can be determined.

In this chapter, not all aspects of congenital mitral valve are presented. Specifically, mitral atresia, overriding or straddling mitral valve, hypoplastic left heart syndrome, and mitral valve prolapse are excluded. Mitral valve disease associated with endocardial cushion defects is included to emphasize associated abnormalities of the papillary muscles.

The purpose of this chapter is to aid the clinician in recognizing congenital mitral valve disease by presenting (1) the anatomy of this disease, (2) findings on history, physical examination, chest film, and ECG, and (3) the use of cineangiography, and two-dimensional and Doppler echocardiography in the diagnosis of this disease.

ANATOMY OF CONGENITAL MITRAL VALVE DISEASE

Davachi et al[4] provide a useful classification of congenital mitral valve disease by categorizing the defects according to the anatomical location. These abnormalities can occur at the (1) leaflets, (2) commissures, (3) chordae tendineae, and (4) papillary muscles. More than one abnormality can exist simultaneously.

Leaflet abnormalities include clefts in either the anterior or posterior leaflets, accessory orifice of the mitral valve, and accessory mitral leaflet tissue (the latter can create left ventricular outflow tract obstruction). Cleft mitral valve leaflets usually occur with primum atrial septal defects.[5,6] In embryonic development, the endocardial tissues coalesce to form a portion of the atrial and ventricular septae, anterior leaflet of the mitral valve, and septal leaflet of the tricuspid valve.[5,6] Therefore, disruptions at this stage of development usually result in atrial (primum) and/or ventricular endocardial cushion defects with or without abnormalities of the mitral and/or tricuspid valves. However, cleft mitral valve leaflets are reported with secundum atrial septal defects[7–10] and in isolation.[11–12]

In the second category, the most common congenital abnormality of the commissures is fusion. This can occur as an isolated event, but can also be associated with a supravalvar mitral ring, a circumferential ridge of connective tissue within the left atrium. When a supravalvar mitral ring is attached to the atrial surface of the mitral valve, it can prevent normal diastolic excursion of the leaflets causing inflow obstruction.

Mitral valve disease at the level of the chordae tendineae can exist when the chordae are excessively foreshortened or long. When the chordae tendineae are foreshortened, inadequate coaptation of the leaflets during ventricular systole can occur, causing mitral regurgitation. Excessively long chordae tendineae can result in prolapse of the mitral valve leaflets into the left atrium, also resulting in mitral regurgitation.

The fourth anatomical substrate associated with congenital mitral valve disease is abnormality of the papillary muscles. Mitral valve arcade is an abnormality in which the anterolateral and posteromedial papillary muscles are fused, forming a bridge of fibrous tissue that is continuous with the free aspect of the anterior mitral leaflet. The mitral commissures are not fully developed, and the chordae tendineae are thickened and foreshortened. Mitral valve arcade can be associated with either severe mitral stenosis and/or regurgitation.

Another type of mitral valve disease caused by abnormalities at the level of the papillary muscles is that of parachute mitral valve. In this abnormality, the chordae tendineae from both mitral valve leaflets insert into a single papillary muscle, the chordae tendineae are foreshortened, and the mitral valve orifice is reduced. This can also occur when two papillary muscles exist, but they are either fused or closely opposed. (More detail and specific clinical examples of these defects are presented later in the chapter.)

ACQUIRED DISEASE

Acquired mitral valve disease in the pediatric age group requires mention in order to differentiate it from congenital defects. Probably the most prevalent form of acquired disease is rheumatic heart disease. Other causes of inflammation of the mitral valve can occur secondary to viral, bacterial, or fungal infection.[13] Metabolic disorders of Hurler's syndrome (a defect in mucopolysaccharide metabolism), and homycystinuria (a defect in amino acid metabolism), and connective tissue diseases of rheumatoid arthritis and Marfan's syndrome can involve the mitral valve.[13] Infarction of the papillary muscles resulting in mitral regurgitation can occur with severe aortic stenosis, aortic coarctation, endocardial fibroelastosis, and anomalous left coronary artery.[13]

INCIDENCE

Congenital mitral valve disease is reported to be rare. Most studies consist of collaborative autopsy series or isolated case reports. In one autopsy review of pediatric patients with congenital heart disease, mitral stenosis occurred in 1.2% of cases.[2] During the same time period, the ratio of patients with mitral stenosis admitted was 0.17 per 1000 hospital cases. In a 7-year period from 1968 to 1975, six (0.2%) of 2178 infants admitted to the New England Regional Infant Care Program had congenital mitral stenosis.[2] From 1950 to 1973, 30 (0.2%) of 15,104 patients cared for at the Hospital for Sick Children in Toronto had congenital mitral valve disease.[14]

SYMPTOMS

The symptoms of congenital mitral valve disease are attributable to the severity of pulmonary venous congestion and decrease in cardiac output. However, because mitral valve disease is often associated with other cardiac abnormalities, precise etiology for the symptoms can be difficult to determine. In mitral stenosis and/or insufficiency, neonates and infants present with recurrent respiratory infections, irritability, decreased feeding, and poor growth.[2,15–17] These infants have difficulty with breathing, especially during feeding. Cyanosis may be present if significant pulmonary venous congestion exists.[2,17] Older children and young adolescents may complain of shortness of breath, dyspnea on exertion, and poor exercise tolerance.[15,17] In cases of severe mitral stenosis, syncope may occur.[17] Difficulty arises when mitral valve stenosis is associated with left ventricular outflow tract obstruction. The latter alone can be associated with chest pain, syncope, and even sudden death.

The symptoms of mitral valve disease may not be apparent until after surgical intervention. For example, preoperatively in a patient with mitral stenosis, ventricular septal defect, and pulmonary artery band, there will be decreased pulmonary blood flow. After removal of the pulmonary artery band, even with closure of the ventricular septal defect, pulmonary blood flow may be significantly increased. This can result in increased transmitral flow across a stenotic mitral valve causing left atrial hypertension, pulmonary venous congestion, and symptoms of dyspnea.[18] Another example is a patient with an atrial septal defect and mitral valve disease. Preoperatively, the atrial septal defect will decompress the left atrium. Once the defect is closed, if there is significant mitral valve disease, left atrial hypertension and pulmonary venous congestion may develop.[18]

PHYSICAL EXAMINATION

Mitral Stenosis

Infants and children with moderate to severe mitral valve stenosis will fail to thrive, with weight disproportionately less than height.[2] The patients may be tachycardic and tachypneic.[2,16,19] Cyanosis may be present secondary to either pulmonary edema or decreased cardiac output and increased oxygen extraction.[2,17] When pulmonary hypertension exists, a prominent lift along the left sternal border will be evident.[20] Because of decreased left ventricular filling, the precordial impulse is inconspicuous or absent.[15,20] Rales may be present secondary to pulmonary congestion.[16] In almost all cases of congenital mitral stenosis, the first heart sound is of increased intensity.[2,15,17,20] Left atrial pressure is high with moderate to severe mitral stenosis; leaflet closure is delayed, causing it to occur at a time when left ventricular pressure is rapidly rising. Hence, coaptation of the leaflets is abrupt and the closure sound is increased.[20] The second heart sound is usually split, but the splitting may be narrowed and the pulmonic component increased in intensity, depending on the degree of pulmonary artery hypertension.[20] An opening snap is usually absent,[15,17,20] as opposed to rheumatic mitral stenosis. However, when an opening snap is present,[2] the interval between aortic closure and the opening snap tends to be short when stenosis is severe, since high left atrial pressure opens the mitral valve earlier in diastole.[20]

The most common murmur of congenital mitral stenosis is a low-pitched apical diastolic murmur, with presystolic accentuation.[2,16,17,20] However, patients with normal mitral valves can have a middiastolic rumble caused by increased transmitral flow, such as occurs with a ventricular septal defect, patent ductus arteriosus, or severe mitral regurgitation.

Mitral Regurgitation

Mitral regurgitation is also associated with tachycardia, tachypnea,[21,22] and failure to thrive. Rales are present when there is pulmonary edema. If both left and right ventricular dilation exist, hepatomegaly will be present.[21] An increased precordial impulse will be palpable secondary to left ventricular enlargement.[21] If pulmonary artery hypertension coexists, a parasternal lift may also be present.[7–9] Mitral regurgitation produces an apical, pansystolic, blowing murmur which is maximal at the apex.[11,19–22] This murmur can radiate to the apex and to the back.[21] In cases of papillary muscle dysfunction, the murmur may occur either in mid- or late systole.[20] With significant mitral regurgitation, a prominent third heart sound followed directly by middiastolic rumble is audible.[20,21] As opposed to mitral stenosis, the first heart sound is decreased or of normal intensity.[20] The second heart sound is usually normally split, but if pulmonary artery hypertension exists, the splitting will be narrowed and the pulmonic component will be increased in intensity.[20]

CHEST ROENTGENOGRAM

The cardiac silhouette on the chest film in patients with mitral stenosis will show left atrial enlargement.[2,15–17] With significant pulmonary artery hypertension, the right ventricle may also be enlarged. In significant mitral stenosis, signs of pulmonary edema may be present.[2,15–17]

Left atrial and left ventricular enlargement are seen on chest film with significant mitral regurgitation.[11,19,21] With severe mitral regurgitation, left atrial enlargement may compress either the left or right main stem bronchus, causing atelectasis.[19,21]

ELECTROCARDIOGRAPHY

The ECG findings of congenital mitral stenosis are left atrial enlargement.[2,16] Right ventricular hypertrophy[2,16] will be present in severe cases with pulmonary artery hypertension. Patients with congenital mitral insufficiency will also have ECG findings of left atrial enlargement.[11,19] In contrast to mitral stenosis, findings of left ventricular enlargement will also be present.[11,21] Again, if pulmonary artery hypertension exists, there will be signs of right ventricular hypertrophy.[22]

CARDIAC CATHETERIZATION

The usual physiologic parameters of congenital mitral stenosis and/or insufficiency[23] may not be present in pediatric patients who have associated defects. Patients with a large atrial septal defect may not have an increased atrial "a" wave, or elevated left atrial or pulmonary capillary wedge pressure with simultaneous decreased left ventricular end-diastolic pressure, even in the presence of severe mitral stenosis. Similarly, elevated "v" or filling waves in the left atrium may not be present in patients with severe mitral insufficiency with an atrial septal defect. The gradients across stenotic mitral valves may be reduced in situations of decreased pulmonary blood flow, which may occur with associated pulmonary outflow tract obstruction. Therefore, emphasis at catheterization has also been placed on the angiographic diagnosis of congenital mitral disease. Although significant advances in the angiographic diagnosis of all congenital heart defects has occurred with improvements in technology and introduction of axial cineangiography,[24,25] only an "indirect" visualization of the mitral valve apparatus is possible.

Although contrast injections in the pulmonary artery or left atrium may provide information about the size of the left atrium and mitral valve annulus, a left ventricular injection better demonstrates the valve leaflets and anatomy of the chordae tendineae and papillary muscles.[26] With right and left oblique projections, abnormal filling defects can be visualized if the papillary muscles are abnormally enlarged and/or fused, as would occur with a parachute mitral valve. In this disease, McCartney et al have described a typical "egg-timer" appearance on the left ventricular angiogram.[26] During diastole, the posterior superior portion of the filling defect results from the coned mitral leaflets and chordae tendineae, and the anterior inferior filling defect results from the single enlarged papillary muscle. However, a specific note of caution about determination of the anatomy of the papillary muscles on angiography is warranted. In one study which evaluated left ventricular angiograms in 50 patients with no mitral valve disease, no papillary muscles were seen in 10%, and only one papillary muscle could be visualized in 36% of patients.[17] In another report of patients with congenital mitral stenosis, the number and position of the papillary muscles could be visualized on the left ventricular angiogram in only 20% of patients.[2]

TWO-DIMENSIONAL ECHOCARDIOGRAPHY

Two-dimensional echocardiography can provide the clinician with a direct visualization of the entire mitral valve apparatus.[27–31] Because the abnormalities in congenital mitral disease can occur at several anatomical levels, a step-by-step progression of examination is advised.

First, the mitral valve annulus should be inspected for size and orientation. Second, the mitral valve leaflets should be visualized for thickness, mobility, and position during systole and diastole. Third, the insertion of the leaflets onto the chordae tendineae, and the position, length, and interchordal distance should be examined. Fourth, the insertion of the chordae tendineae onto the papillary muscles, and the size, number, and position of the papillary muscles relative to each other and to the ventricular wall, must be carefully inspected. Although "standard" echocardiographic views may provide better visualization for certain aspects of mitral valve disease, all views should be employed. The apical four-chamber and subcostal long axis views provide good visualization of the mitral valve annulus, leaflets, and chordae tendineae. However, the number, size, and position of the papillary muscles are best visualized on short axis views, either in a parasternal or subcostal position.[27–31] Depending on the orientation of the left ventricle on a short axis plane, the papillary muscles can occur in a variety of positions. In general, the interpapillary distance is approximately 80° on a 360° circle.[31] (Figure 7-1 shows a short axis view with the papillary muscles in their normal position. Figure 7-2 is the same view in a patient with a parachute mitral valve deformity; note the large fused papillary muscle group on the anterolateral wall of the left ventricle.) To determine the anatomical relation of the mitral valve annulus to the leaflets, chordae tendineae, and papillary muscles, a complete progressive sweep of the left ventricle in the short axis plane is recommended.

Diseases that may mimic congenital mitral valve disease can also be differentiated by two-dimensional echocardiography. Supravalvar mitral ring on two-dimensional echocardiography appears as a distinct membrane superior to the valve that moves through the annulus in diastole and away from the valve in systole.[27] However, even on echocardiography the supravalvar mitral ring may not be diagnosed if it is so close to the mitral valve that it adheres to the leaflets causing them to appear thickened.[27,29]

When a membrane is suspected in the left atrium, cor triatriatum must also be considered. Cor triatriatum is as an embryonic failure of the common pulmonary veins to become incorpor-

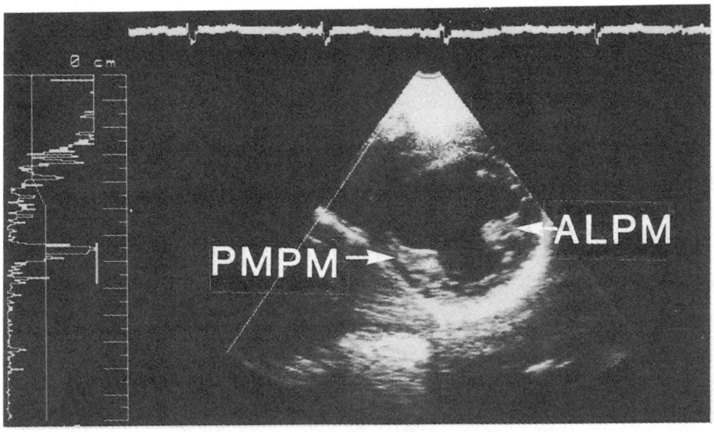

Figure 7-1 Short axis view of the left ventricle. ALPM = anterior lateral papillary muscle, PMPM = posterior medial papillary muscle.

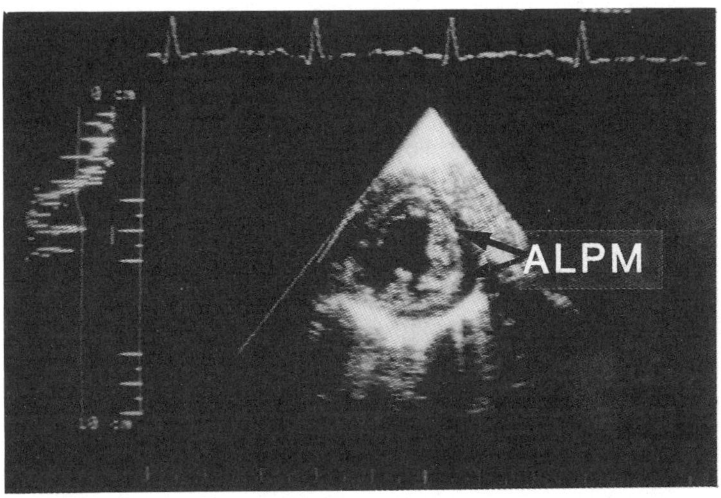

Figure 7-2 Short axis view of the left ventricle in a patient with parachute mitral valve deformity. ALPM = anterior lateral papillary muscle.

ated into the left ventricle, with a membrane causing left ventricular inflow obstruction.[22] On two-dimensional echocardiography, cor triatriatum appears as an oblique echo-dense line that bisects the left atrium into two components with the superior dorsal component receiving the pulmonary veins and the lower, more anterior chamber communicating with the left ventricle via the mitral valve.[18,27,29]

DOPPLER ECHOCARDIOGRAPHY

Doppler echocardiography can determine noninvasively the presence and estimate the severity of both mitral stenosis and mitral regurgitation.

The diagnosis of mitral regurgitation is dependent upon finding systolic flow in the left atrium opposite to the usual antegrade diastolic flow[32,33] (Figure 7-3). Since mitral regurgitation begins at mitral valve closure, and continues until mitral valve opening, the systolic flow of regurgitation is continuous with the normal diastolic flow. This timing can help to differentiate the systolic flow of mitral regurgitation from aortic stenosis.[33] With increasing severity of mitral regurgitation, the spectral analysis will be of higher intensity.[33] The distance the jet disturbance can be imaged posteriorly into the left atrium also relates to the severity of regurgitation.[33] An estimate of regurgitant fraction can also be obtained by Doppler flow determination.[32] First, total flow across the

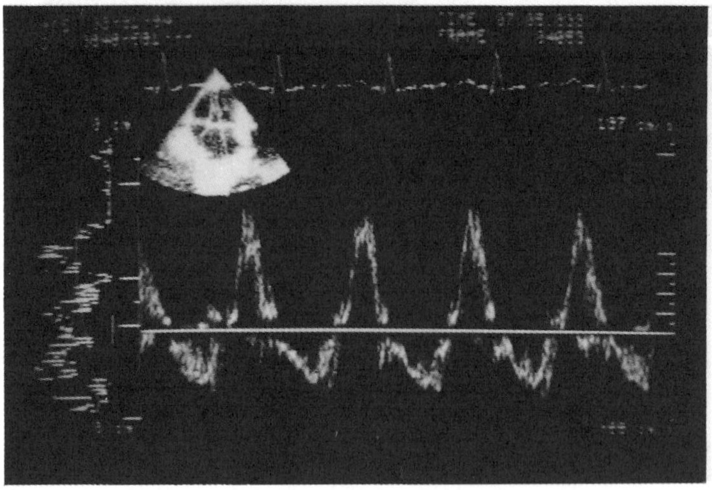

Figure 7-3 Range-gated Doppler interrogation in the left atrium in a patient with mitral insufficiency. Normal positive (above baseline) diastolic flow is continuous with abnormal systolic negative flow (below baseline) of mitral regurgitation.

mitral valve is calculated. Next, net forward flow across the aortic valve is obtained. The regurgitant flow is then the total forward flow across the mitral valve minus the net forward flow across the aorta.[32]

Doppler echocardiography can also determine the severity of mitral stenosis.[33] The procedure allows measurement of increased velocities across a stenotic orifice; this increase in velocity is a result of a pressure drop. Using the modified Bernoulli equation, both the mean and maximal pressure drop across stenotic orifices can be calculated.[33] Excellent correlation has been reported by Hatle and Angelsen who compared Doppler measurements across stenotic mitral valves to pressure measurements at catheterization.[33]

Since the pressure drop is dependent upon flow, Hatle and Angelsen demonstrated that the Doppler-measured mitral valve pressure half-time can differentiate between an increased pressure drop secondary to increased flow and/or stenosis.[33] The pressure half-time is the time for the peak transmitral pressure drop to decrease by one half. In mitral stenosis, the pressure half-time is prolonged, whereas in patients with normal mitral valves with a flow-related gradient, the pressure half-time is normal. Hatle and Angelsen have shown that pressure half-time also provides a good estimation of mitral valve area, with excellent correlation to values obtained at catheterization. (For details of pressure half-time calculation, see Hatle and Angelsen.[33])

DIAGNOSIS AND MANAGEMENT

Difficulty of Recognition

In a 7-year period at a large children's medical center, 38 patients were admitted with the diagnosis of mitral valve disease.[2] Twenty of the 38 patients had associated cardiovascular defects. Although the diagnosis of heart disease was made at an average of 1.5 years of age, and the mean age at first hospitalization was 2.1 years, the diagnosis of congenital mitral valve disease was not established until 4.5 years of age. In nine of the 38 patients, the diagnosis of mitral valve disease was not made until surgery or autopsy. (This study was reported before many of the advances in cineangiography and Doppler echocardiography had taken place. This may in part explain difficulties in diagnosis. Equally important was that 50% of the patients in the above study had other significant cardiovascular defects.)

The remainder of this chapter provides specific cases to illustrate the diagnosis, medical and surgical treatment of patients with congenital mitral valve disease.

CASE REPORTS

Mitral stenosis

This patient was admitted at 20 months of age with failure to thrive. His height was at the 25th percentile and weight at the fifth percentile for his age. He was tachycardic and tachypneic and had a hyperdynamic precordial impulse with no palpable thrills. There was an increased first heart sound and a normal second heart sound. A grade 3/6 harsh systolic ejection murmur at the left sternal border and an apical middiastolic rumble with presystolic accentuation was present. The pulses in the upper extremities were mildly decreased and the pulses in the lower extremities were barely palpable. Blood pressure in the right arm was 90 mmHg and in the leg 70 mmHg. Chest films demonstrated pulmonary venous congestion and left atrial enlargement. Findings of left atrial enlargement with right ventricular hypertrophy were present on the ECG.

A two-dimensional echocardiogram demonstrated a subaortic membrane. The aortic valve was normal. On the short axis parasternal views, interrogation from the base to the apex of the left ventricle demonstrated chordae tendineae attached to a single papillary muscle.

At cardiac catheterization, hemodynamic measurements confirmed mitral stenosis, subaortic stenosis, and coarctation of the aorta. Angiography demonstrated subaortic stenosis. The aortic valve appeared normal. A large filling defect in the anterolateral portion of the left ventricle and only one set of papillary muscles was visualized, implicating the diagnosis of parachute mitral valve. The aortic root angiogram showed a distinct coarctation, distal to the left subclavian artery.

The patient had subclavian artery flap angioplasty repair of the coarctation of the aorta. One week later, he had a mitral valve annuloplasty with resection of portions of the papillary muscle, and fenestration of the restrictive components of the mitral valve leaflets and chordae tendineae. In addition, the subaortic stenosis was resected.

Cardiac catheterization 8 months later demonstrated persistent significant mitral stenosis with no regurgitation. However, the decision of the medical/surgical team was not to intervene surgically since further mitral valve annuloplasty would not significantly alleviate mitral stenosis without creating mitral insufficiency. Prosthetic valve replacement was not yet warranted, considering the decreased longevity of heterograft valves, and problems inherent with anticoagulation for metallic valves in this age group.

This case illustrates the coexistence of congenital mitral valve disease with other congenital heart defects. This association was first reported by Swan et al in 1949.[34] They described an 18-year-old female who had congenital mitral stenosis associated with a patent ductus arteriosus and coarctation of the aorta. In 1963, Shone et al[1] reported the syndrome of parachute mitral valve, supravalvar mitral ring, subaortic stenosis, and coarctation of the aorta. Even in this early report, variations of this complex occurred, ie not all aspects was present. The case reported here represents a variation of Shone's syndrome in which three of four of the abnormalities are present.

The original description by Swan et al[34] of a parachute mitral valve was one "in which the chordae tendineae were shortened and fused to form a funnel-shaped, firmly fixed, almost solid sheet of tissue that obstructed the orifice of the valve. The blended chordae were inserted into the apex of the solitary, double-bellied papillary muscle which arose from the posterior wall of the left ventricle near the margin of the intact interventricular septum. Viewed from above, the mitral valve resembled the inverted top of a salt shaker."[34] In addition to this excellent description, in parachute mitral valve, the chordae tendineae are short and thickened causing the interchordal space to be reduced as the chordae converge into a single papillary muscle. Thus, left ventricular inflow obstruction occurs not only at the annulus and leaflets, but also at the convergent chordae tendineae.[3,4,15] Because of decreased leaflet mobility, parachute mitral valve can also be associated with insufficiency.[15,22]

In general, surgery for congenital mitral valve disease has been moderately successful. One surgical series reported a 38% intraoperative mortality for valvotomy, and 29% for mitral valve replacement.[2] In three patients, only an atrial septectomy was attempted, but all three died intraoperatively. The overall survival rate was 53% at 10 years, and 18% after 18 years. (It again should be emphasized that many of these patients had significant associated malformations.)

Other surgical series have reported improved success with valvuloplasty repair for congenital mitral valve disease.[35] In a report of 47 patients with an assortment of congenital mitral valve defects, 38 had valve reconstruction and nine valve replacement. In the patients undergoing valve reconstruction, three died at operation; no late deaths occurred. In the valve replacement group, three patients died intraoperatively, and three died later. Eighty-six percent of the patients who had valve annuloplasty improved clinically. Postoperative cardiac catheterization was performed in 50% of these, and in all but one, both pulmonary artery and pulmonary capillary wedge pressure had decreased significantly.[35]

Surgical reports of operation for isolated parachute mitral valve disease are rare. In one review of the literature, 28 patients were operated on, and 13 of the 28 survived.[18] Mitral commissurotomy was ineffective in the majority of cases, and the authors concluded that the appropriate operation for parachute mitral valve, regardless of age, should be valve replacement. In one case report of mitral valve arcade creating severe stenosis, valvuloplasty was also not considered feasible, and the infant had successful placement of a prosthetic valve.[16]

Although surgical placement of prosthetic valves in children can be performed with low morbidity and mortality,[36] use of prosthetic valves in the pediatric age group is fraught with significant complications. Use of metallic valves carries the risk of thromboembolic phenomenon. Anticoagulation therapy in children and adolescents is hazardous, since restriction of activities to prevent hemorrhagic episodes is difficult. Anticoagulation with warfarin sodium is further complicated by children's constant rate of growth, changing nutritional status, and the requirements of antibiotic therapy for recurrent infections. All three parameters will alter prothrombin activation. Third, because of increasing size, pediatric patients may require serial valve replacement, metallic or otherwise, despite a normally functioning valve.

Accelerated fibrocalcific disease of porcine heterograft valves in children has required their early replacement.[37,38] In one series of Hancock porcine heterograft valve placements in children, three of the nine children developed severe fibrocalcific obstruction requiring replacement after 3.5, 3.6, and 4.0 years.[37] During the same time span, in 561 adult patients, only two had developed similar changes. In a different series,[38] 44 pediatric patients had placement of 47 porcine xenograft valves. In 25 patients followed 20 months or longer, eight required valve replacement. Only 50% had intact valves after 45 months. In this series, of the eight patients who required valve replacements, all were 10.3 years or less at initial operation. In those patients with normally functioning valves, the mean age at initial valve placement was 15.0 years.

Mitral insufficiency

A 1.2-kg premature baby presented in the first day of life with respiratory distress and low cardiac output, which was presumed secondary to perinatal asphyxia. No murmur was audible except for an S_3 and S_4 gallop. The PO_2 from the right radial artery was 300 torr and from the descending aorta 40 torr, confirming a significant right-to-left shunt across a patent ductus arteriosus. The chest films showed marked cardiac enlargement, pulmonary venous congestion, and a dilated left atrium compressing the left main stem bronchus. The two-dimensional echocardiogram showed severe left atrial and left ventricular enlargement with a decreased percent fractional shortening of 18% (Figure 7-4) (normal in this age group is 32% to 36%). Althoug there was poor coaptation of the leaflets, the mitral valve appeared normal. Interrogation at the root of the ascending aorta on short axis parasternal views confirmed normal anatomy of the right and left coronary arteries. Pulsed Doppler interrogation from an apical four-chamber view with the sample volume in the left atrium demonstrated a systolic jet of mitral regurgitation (Figure 7-5). Doppler aortic flow from the suprasternal notch was obtained, and the calculated cardiac output was markedly decreased at 1.8 L/min/m^2.[32] Doppler-derived mitral valve regurgitant fraction was

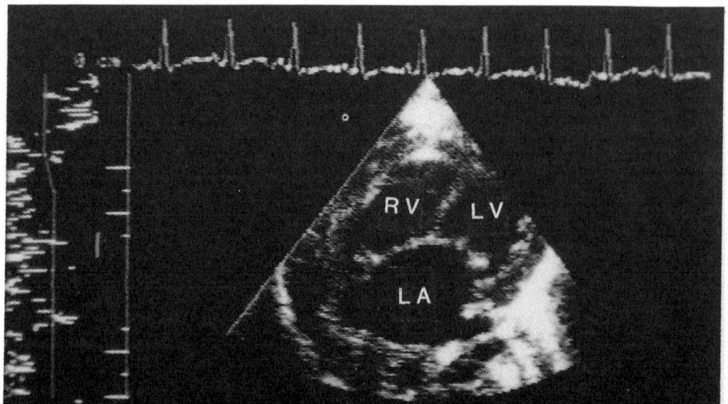

Figure 7-4 Apical four-chamber view in a premature infant with massive left atrial dilation. LV = left ventricle, LA = left atrium, RV = right ventricle.

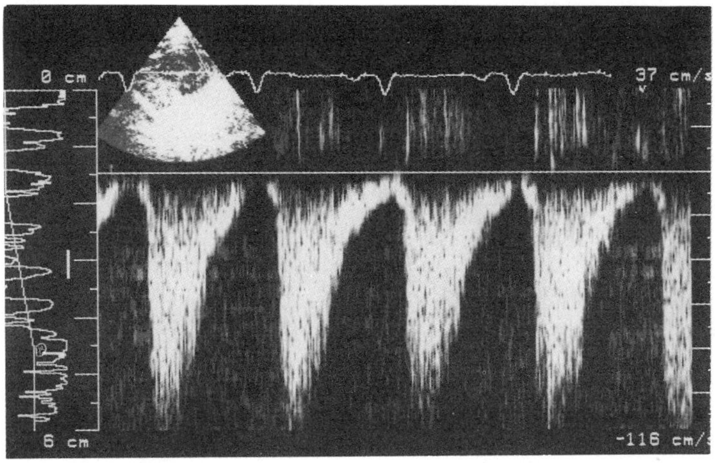

Figure 7-5 Doppler interrogation in the left atrium demonstrates severe mitral regurgitation in a 1.2-kg premature infant.

70%.[32] The patient was started on dobutamine to increase cardiac output, and nitroprusside to further increase cardiac output and decrease the regurgitant fraction. Unfortunately, several weeks later, the baby deteriorated and died. No postmortem examination was obtained.

Congenital mitral valve insufficiency is extremely rare. Primary abnormalities of the mitral valve, ie, parachute mitral valve, mitral valve arcade, clefts in the leaflets, and redundant chordae tendineae can all be associated with mitral regurgitation. The etiology of this neonate's mitral disease may have been severe perinatal stress resulting in left ventricular dysfunction, left atrial dilation, and mitral regurgitation. Another possible etiology was that this infant may have had an intrauterine viral illness causing myocarditis. However, viral confirmation was not obtained. Since this patient was premature and weighed only 1.2 kg, mitral valve replacement was not possible. Echocardiographic examination did not reveal anatomical abnormalities amenable to mitral valve annuloplasty.

Mitral regurgitation associated with coarctation of the aorta

This infant presented at 7 months of age with a history of irritability, difficulty feeding, and failure to thrive. She was pale, tachycardiac and tachypneic, with weight below the third percentile for her age. She had significant hepatomegaly and diffuse rales were heard over the chest. A heaving precordial impulse was palpable, but there were no thrills. The first heart sound was normal, and the second was narrowly split with an increased pulmonic component. A grade 3/6 blowing holosystolic murmur, 2/4 diastolic rumble, and an S_3 and S_4 gallop were easily heard. She had excellent pulses in the upper and barely perceptible pulses in the lower extremities. Doppler blood pressure in the right arm was 130 mmHg and in the right leg 85 mmHg. A dilated left atrium and left ventricle with diminished left ventricular function was seen on two-dimensional echocardiography. The mitral valve apparatus appeared normal. Suprasternal notch echocardiographic interrogation demonstrated a severe coarctation of the aorta beyond the left subclavian artery. By Doppler interrogation, a significant regurgitant systolic jet of mitral insufficiency was interrogated in the left atrium.

At cardiac catheterization, the pulmonary capillary wedge, left atrial, and left ventricular end-diastolic pressures were all elevated at 20 mmHg. The catheter could not be advanced across the coarctation segment site. Left ventricular angiography showed severe mitral regurgitation and aortic coarctation (Figure 7-6). The only flow to the descending thoracic aorta was via collaterals distal to the left subclavian artery. The next day, the patient successfully underwent subclavian flap angioplasty repair of the coarctation. Four months later, the patient had significant weight gain. No gradient from the ascending to descending thoracic aorta could be obtained by cuff sphygmomanometry, and the murmur of mitral regurgitation was less intense. On the chest film, the cardiac enlargement and pulmonary venous congestion had significantly decreased.

This case illustrates the important association of congenital mitral valve disease and coarctation of the aorta. Autopsy series report that 60% of patients with coarctation have mitral valve de-

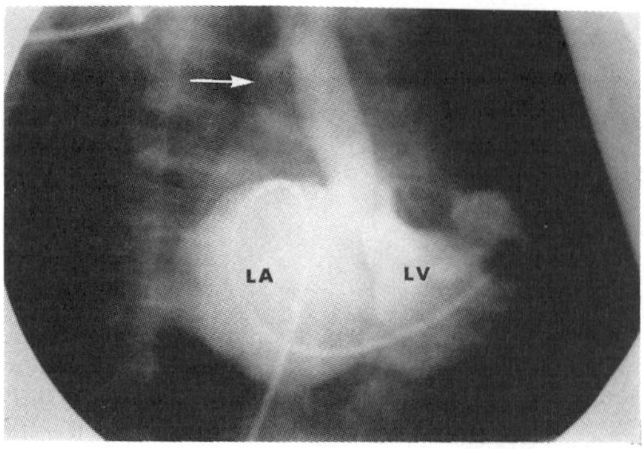

Figure 7-6 Left ventricular angiogram in a right anterior oblique projection demonstrating severe mitral regurgitation in an infant with critical aortic coarctation (arrow). LA = left atrium, LV = left ventricle.

fects;[39] 7% are parachute mitral valve. Two-dimensional echocardiographic studies report a similar incidence of associated mitral valve disease, 59%,[30] with 37% being severe defects consisting of either supravalvar mitral ring, congenital mitral stenosis, prolapse, or parachute mitral valve.

In a large series of infants with aortic coarctation, 18 (2%) of 861 patients, had mitral regurgitation.[40] In three patients who died intraoperatively, and in two who required mitral valve replacement, the valve was severely deformed. One patient had a mitral valve arcade, the second had ruptured chordae tendineae, the third had a commissural gap, and there was a perforation in the posterior leaflet in the fourth patient. In the 13 patients who did not have mitral valve replacement (including two patients who did not have the coarctation repaired), mitral regurgitation became worse in four (27%) patients, did not change in six (46%) patients, and improved in four (27%) patients.

Parachute mitral valve association with endocardial cushion defect

An infant presented at 6 weeks of age with a history of severe failure to thrive and difficulty in feeding. On physical examination, she was tachypneic, tachycardiac, and pale. She had normal pulses in the upper and lower extremities. A bulging precordial impulse could be easily palpated. An increased first and single second heart sound, S_3 and S_4 gallop, and a 2/6 systolic ejection murmur with a diastolic rumble were heard. On abdominal examination, the liver was palpable 3 cm below the right costal margin. Chest films showed marked cardiac enlargement, pulmonary venous congestion, and increased pulmonary blood flow. There was a superior axis, counterclockwise loop, and right ventricular hypertrophy on the ECG. Two-dimensional echocardiography demonstrated a primum atrial septal defect. The patient was treated with digoxin and diuretic therapy, but returned at 3 months of age with persistent congestive heart failure. Cardiac catheterization confirmed an ostium primum endocardial cushion defect, pulmonary artery hypertension, and a significant coarctation of the aorta. The left ventricular angiogram showed the typical gooseneck deformity of an endocardial cushion defect with minimal mitral regurgitation. The pulmonary artery angiogram showed a significant left-to-right shunt across a primum atrial septal defect. The patient subsequently underwent a successful subclavian flap angioplasty repair of the coarctation. Severe congestive heart failure persisted despite optimal medical therapy. At 4 months of age, the primum atrial septal defect was closed. Postoperatively, the patient was in low cardiac output, from which she eventually died.

A parachute mitral valve deformity was recognized post mortem. The chordae tendineae coalesced predominantly into a single large papillary muscle on the anterolateral wall of the left ventricle (Figure 7-7A). The left atrium was enlarged and the atrial septal defect patch was in place. The left ventricle was smaller than normal. On review of the echocardiogram, the long axis parasternal view showed the mitral valve chordae tendineae attached to a single large papillary muscle group on the anterolateral wall of the ventricle (Figure 7-7B). A large filling defect in the same position could be visualized on the right anterior oblique projection of the left ventricular angiogram (Figure 7-7C).

Left ventricular papillary muscle abnormalities have recently been reported in patients with complete atrioventricular canal. In an autopsy series of 164 patients with complete atrioventricular canal, 7% had either a single papillary muscle or papillary muscles closely opposed.[41] The authors concluded that when the anterior leaflet of the atrioventricular valve is sutured, the mitral valve orifice and the interchordal spaces are restricted, creating mitral stenosis. In a two-dimensional echocardiographic study of 31 infants with complete atrioventricular canal, three (10%) had three papillary muscles, and three (10%) a single papillary muscle.[31] All patients with a single papillary muscle, and two of the three with three papillary muscles died postoperatively. The authors also conclude that suturing of the cleft between the superior and inferior components of the anterior mitral leaflet may result in either severe stenosis, or increased tension on the leaflet tissue, causing dehiscence of the mitral valve reconstruction and sudden onset of mitral regurgitation.

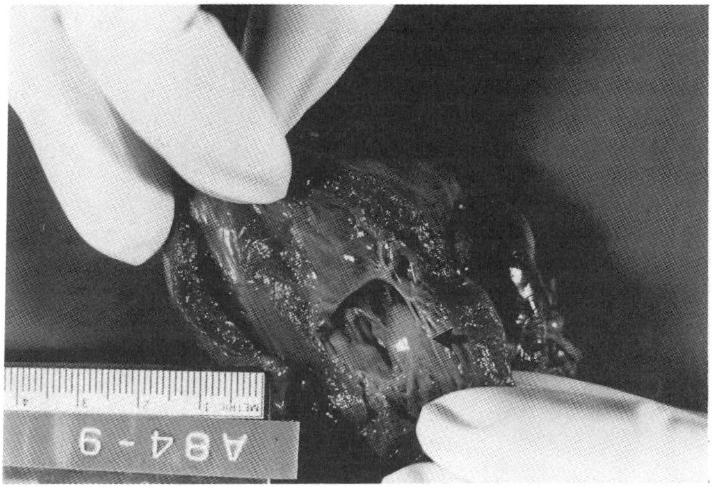

Figure 7-7A Left ventricle held open with black arrow pointing to single large papillary muscle on the anterior lateral wall.

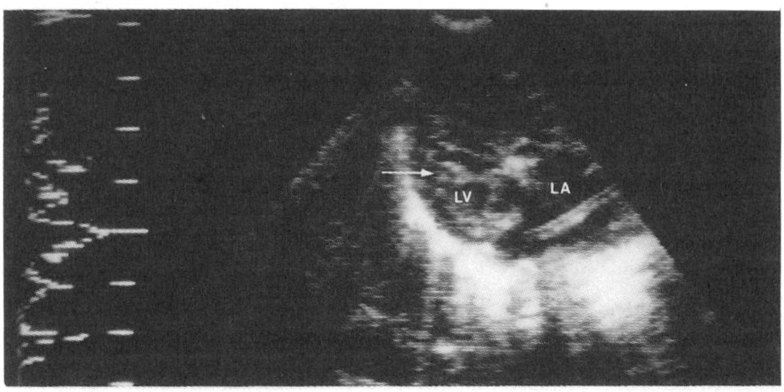

7B Long axis parasternal view showing a dilated left atrium, small left ventricle, and chordal attachments to single large papillary muscle (arrow) on the lateral wall of the left ventricle. LA = left atrium, LV = left ventricle.

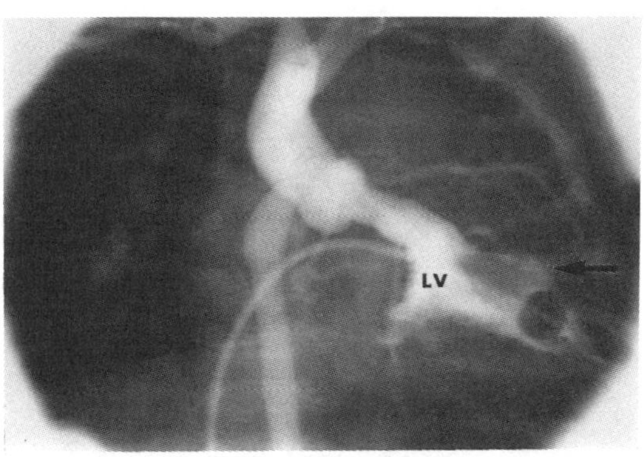

7C Left ventricular angiogram in right anterior oblique projection in an infant with parachute mitral valve deformity (large filling defect demonstrated by black arrow). LV = left ventricle.

Cleft mitral leaflet

A child who had closure of an atrial septal defect at 7 years of age presented at 21 years of age with gradual onset of dyspnea on exertion, orthopnea, and paroxysmal nocturnal dyspnea. On physical examination, a bulging precordial impulse was present. The first and second heart sounds were normal and a pansystolic blowing murmur with a diastolic rumble was heard at the apex. The ECG showed left atrial and left ventricular enlargement with a superior axis and counterclockwise loop (the latter associated with endocardial cushion defects). Chest films also showed significant left atrial and left ventricular enlargement, with pulmonary congestion. On a short axis parasternal view, the two-dimensional echocardiogram demonstrated a cleft anterior mitral valve leaflet with a perforation (Figure 7-8). At cardiac catheterization, there was con-

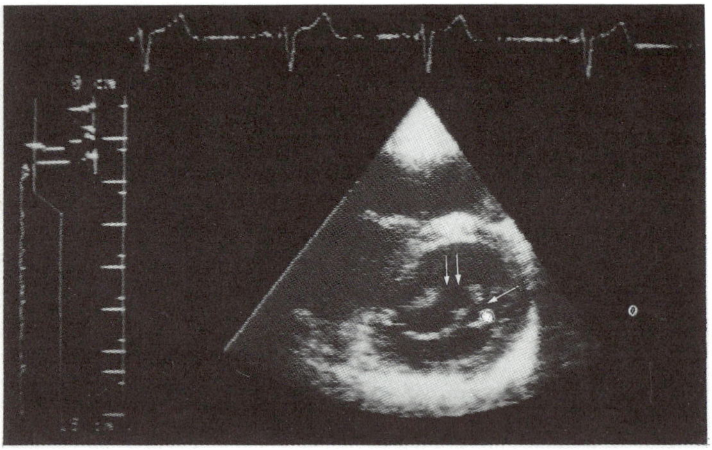

Figure 7-8 Short axis parasternal view of left ventricle. Cleft in the anterior mitral valve leaflet (double arrows) and perforation (single arrow) are seen.

firmation on left ventricular angiography of severe mitral regurgitation with dye refluxing into the pulmonary veins. The patient subsequently had successful annuloplasty repair of the mitral valve. The cleft in the anterior leaflet was sutured, and the perforation in the leaflet repaired. Postoperative Doppler echocardiography revealed no mitral stenosis or insufficiency.

Diagnosis of cleft mitral valve by angiography[5,24,25] and two-dimensional echocardiography[11,42,43] is not difficult. Problems arise in deciding whether at the time of surgical closure of the atrial septal defect to repair the cleft. When significant mitral regurgitation exists, most cardiologists and surgeons would concur that suturing of the cleft is warranted. The decision to suture the cleft is more problematic when the preoperative evaluation demonstrates only mild to moderate regurgitation. Increased left atrial hypertension and pulmonary venous congestion can develop postoperatively if the cleft is not sutured, and the atrial septal defect closed. However, it has been reported that mitral insufficiency can be worsened by closure of the mitral valve cleft.[6] Suturing of the cleft may result in further decreased excursion of mitral valve leaflets causing abnormal coaptation and increased insufficiency.[6]

Accessory endocardial cushion tissue creating left ventricular outflow tract obstruction

A 2-month-old infant was referred for evaluation of a grade 2/6 systolic ejection murmur. Left ventricular hypertrophy was noted on the ECG. On two-dimensional echocardiography a moderately sized mass was seen in the subaortic outflow tract attached to the anterior leaflet of the mitral valve. The mass protruded through the aortic valve during systole and back into the left ventricular outflow tract during diastole. Suprasternal notch interrogation with Doppler echocardiography demonstrated a gradient of 36 mmHg. Cardiac catheterization was performed which confirmed the gradient. The measurements and angiograms were obtained by placing the catheter across a patent foramen ovale, the mitral valve, and into the left ventricle. Because the patient was active and well, no intervention was undertaken.

Two months later, the patient had a thrill and an increased grade 4/6 systolic ejection murmur. Repeat two-dimensional echocardiography showed that the mass was significantly larger (Figure 7-9A). Doppler interrogation by continuous wave in the suprasternal notch predicted a gradient of 57 mmHg (Figure 7-9B). Because this mass seemed to severely occlude the outflow tract, surgery was performed, and a gelatinous subaortic pedunculated mass attached to the mitral valve annulus and membranous interventricular septum was excised. Postoperatively, Doppler echocardiography measured peak velocities across the aortic outflow tract that calculated an aortic gradient of 20 mmHg. No aortic insufficiency was seen.

Previous case reports have described left ventricular outflow tract obstruction caused by accessory mitral valve tissue.[44,45] As in our patient, the tissue was attached to the anterior leaflet of the mitral valve and membranous portion of the interventricular septum.

This last case illustrates the use of two-dimensional Doppler echocardiography in the diagnosis

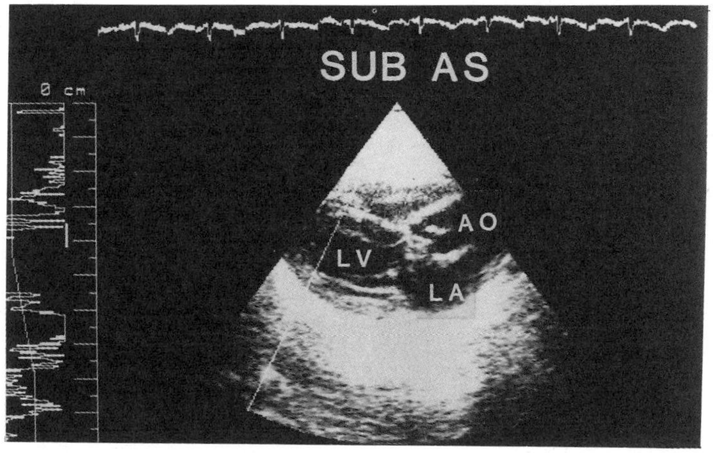

Figure 7-9A Long axis parasternal view showing large mass in the left ventricular outflow tract attached to the mitral valve apparatus. LA = left atrium, LV = left ventricle, AO = aorta.

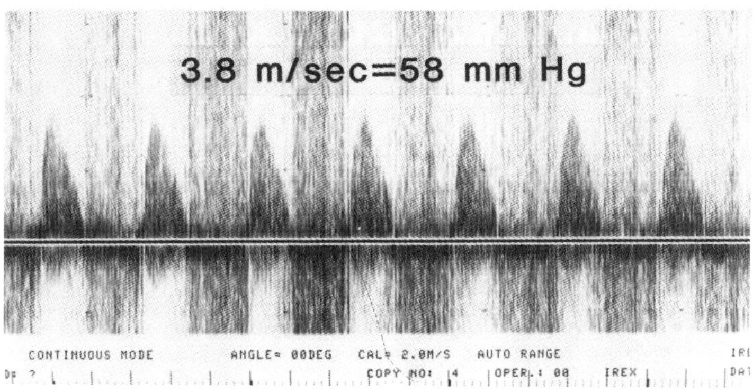

9B Suprasternal notch continuous wave Doppler interrogation in a two-month-old infant with subaortic stenosis.

and treatment of congenital mitral valve disease. Repeat cardiac catheterization would have provided little additional information and could have caused significant morbidity if the catheter had dislodged the tissue mass, potentially causing it to embolize to other vital organs.

SUMMARY

The accurate diagnosis of congenital mitral valve disease has been obscured by its nonspecific findings on clinical examination, ECG, and chest roentgenogram, and by its association with other cardiovascular abnormalities. Improvements in cineangiography and two-dimensional echocardiography have enhanced the recognition of congenital mitral valve disease. Combined Doppler echocardiography has aided in the noninvasive demonstration and quantitation of mitral regurgitation and stenosis.

In the past 10 years, there has been significant improvement in the surgical treatment of congenital heart disease. This, along with earlier and more accurate diagnosis, should improve the outlook for patients with congenital mitral valve disease. With increased experience, mitral valve annuloplasty repair will continue to improve. In addition, with newer research and development, the use of metallic valves should result in decreased morbidity and mortality. It is hoped that the cause(s) of accelerated fibrocalcification of xenograft valves in children will be explained, so that bioprosthetic valves will experience greater longevity in these patients. With these advances, the prognosis for infants and children with congenital mitral valve disease will continue to improve.

REFERENCES

1. Shone JD, Sellers RD, Anderson RC, et al: The developmental complex of "parachute mitral valve," supravalvular ring of left atrium, subaortic stenosis, and coarctation of the aorta. *Am J Cardiol* 1963;11:714–725.
2. Collins-Nakai RL, Rosenthal A, Castaneda AR, et al: Congenital mitral stenosis: A review of 20 years' experience. *Circulation* 1977;56:1039–1047.
3. Ruckman RN, Van Praagh R: Anatomic types of congenital mitral stenosis: Report of 49 autopsy cases with consideration of diagnosis and surgical implications. *Am J Cardiol* 1978;42:592–601.
4. Davachi F, Moller JH, Edwards JE: Diseases of the mitral valve in infancy. An anatomic analysis of 55 cases. *Circulation* 1971;43:565–79.
5. Baron MG: Abnormalities of the mitral valve in endocardial cushion defects. *Circulation* 1972;45:672–680.
6. Van Mierop LHS, Alley RD: The management of the cleft mitral valve in endocardial cushion defects. *Ann Thorac Surg* 1966;2:416–423.
7. Hara M, Char F: Partial cleft of septal mitral leaflet associated with atrial septal defect of the secundum type. *Am J Cardiol* 1966;17:282–285.
8. Goodman DJ, Hancock EW: Secundum atrial septal defect associated with a cleft mitral valve. *Br Heart J* 1973;35:1315–1320.
9. Snow NJ, Ankeney JL: Congenitally cleft atrioventricular valves associated with secundum atrial septal defects. *Thorac Cardiovasc Surg* 1976; 72:925–928.
10. Davies RS, Green DC, Brott WH: Secundum atrial septal defect and cleft mitral valve. *Ann Thorac Surg* 1977;24:28–33.
11. Di Segni E, Bass JL, Lucas RV Jr, et al: Isolated cleft mitral valve: A variety of congenital mitral regurgitation identified by 2-dimensional echocardiography. *Am J Cardiol* 1983;51:927–931.
12. Di Segni E, Edwards JE: Cleft anterior leaflet of the mitral valve with intact septa; A study of 20 cases. *Am J Cardiol* 1983;51:919–926.
13. Vlad P: Mitral valve anomalies in children, editorial. *Circulation* 1971;43:465–466.
14. Keith J, Rowe R, Vlad P: *Heart Disease in Infancy and Childhood*, ed 3. New York, MacMillan Publishing Co, 1978.
15. Zamalloa O, De Franceschi A, Leachman RD: Clinical and angiographic diagnosis of the parachute mitral valve. *Acta Cardiol* 1969;24:101–111.
16. Castaneda AR, Anderson RG, Edwards JE: Congenital mitral stenosis resulting from anomalous arcade and obstructing papillary muscles. *Am J Cardiol* 1969;24:237–240.
17. Macartney FJ, Scott O, Ionescu MI, et al: Diagnosis and management of parachute mitral valve and supravalvar mitral ring. *Br Heart J* 1974; 36:641–652.
18. Jacobstein MD, Hirschfeld SS: Concealed left atrial membrane: Pitfalls in the diagnosis of cor triatriatum and supravalve mitral ring. *Am J Cardiol* 1982;49:780–786.
19. Schachner A, Varsano I, Levy MJ: The parachute mitral valve complex. Case report and review of the literature. *J Thorac Cardiovasc Surg* 1975; 70:451–457.
20. Zuberbuhler JR: *Clinical Diagnosis in Pediatric Cardiology*. New York, Churchill Livingstone Inc, 1981.
21. Schieken RM, Friedman S, Waldhausen J, et al: Isolated congenital mitral insufficiency: Pathologic and surgical variations in five children. *J Pediatr Surg* 1971;6:49–55.
22. Nojek C, Agosti J, Castro A, et al: Surgical treatment of the "parachute mitral valve" complex in infancy. *J Cardiovasc Surg* 1978;19:401–406.
23. Grossman W: *Cardiac Catheterization and Angiography*, ed 2. Philadelphia, Lea & Febiger, 1980.
24. Bargeron LM, Elliott LP, Soto B, et al: Axial cineangiography in congenital heart disease. Section I. Concept, technical and anatomic considerations. *Circulation* 1977;56:1075–1083.
25. Elliott LP, Bargeron LM Jr, Bream PR, et al: Axial cineangiography in congenital heart disease. Section II. Specific lesions. *Circulation* 1977;56: 1084–93.
26. Macartney FJ, Bain HH, Ionescu MI, et al: Angiocardiographic/pathologic correlations in congenital mitral valve anomalies. *Eur J Cardiol* 1976;4:191–211.
27. Snider AR, Roge CL, Schiller NB, et al: Congenital left ventricular inflow obstruction evaluated by two-dimensional echocardiography. *Circulation* 1980;61:848–855.
28. Smallhorn J, Tommasini G, Deanfield J, et al: Congenital mitral stenosis; anatomy and functional assessment by echocardiography. *Br Heart J* 1981;45:527–534.
29. Silverman N, Snider R: Two-dimensional echocardiography in congenital heart disease. Norwalk, Conn, Appleton-Century-Crofts, 1982.
30. Celano V, Pieroni D, Morera JA, et al: Two-dimensional echocardiographic examination of mitral valve abnormalities associated with coarctation of the aorta. *Circulation* 1984;69:924–932.
31. Chin AJ, Bierman FZ, Sanders SP, et al: Subxiphoid 2-dimensional echocardiographic identification of left ventricular papillary muscle anomalies in complete common atrioventricular canal. *Am J Cardiol* 1983;51:1695–1699.
32. Goldberg SJ, Allen HD, Marx GR, et al: *Doppler Echocardiography*. Philadelphia, Lea & Febiger, 1984.
33. Hatle L, Angelsen B: *Doppler Ultrasound in Cardiology. Physical Principles and Clinical Applications*, ed 2. Philadelphia, Lea & Febiger, 1985.
34. Swan H, Trapnell JM, Denst J: Congenital mitral stenosis and systemic right ventricle with associated pulmonary vascular changes frustrating surgical repair of patent ductus arteriosus and coarctation of the aorta. *Am Heart J* 1949;38: 914–923.
35. Carpentier A, Branchini B, Cour JC, et al: Congenital malformations of the mitral valve in children. *J Thorac Cardiovasc Surg* 1976;72: 854–866.
36. Bloodwell RD, Hallman GL, McNamara DG, et

al: Cardiac valve replacement for congenital mitral valvular disease in children. *J Pediatr Surg* 1969; 4:9–16.

37. Kutsche LM, Oyer R, Shumway N, et al: An important complication of Hancock mitral valve replacement in children. *Circulation* 1979;60(I): 98–103.
38. Sanders SP, Levy RJ, Freed MD, et al: Use of Hancock porcine xenografts in children and adolescents. *Am J Cardiol* 1980;46:429–438.
39. Rosenquist GC: Congenital mitral valve disease associated with coarctation of the aorta. *Circulation* 1974;49:985–993.
40. Freed MD, Keane JF, Van Praagh R, et al: Coarctation of the aorta with congenital mitral regurgitation. *Circulation* 1974;49:1175–1184.
41. David I, Castaneda AR, Van Praagh R: Potentially parachute mitral valve in common atrioventricular canal. *J Thorac Cardiovasc Surg* 1982;84: 178–186.
42. Hagler DJ, Tajik AJ, Seward JB, et al: Real-time wide angle sector echocardiography: Atrioventricular canal defects. *Circulation* 1979;59:140–150.
43. LaCorte JA, Cooper RS, Kauffman SL, et al: Atrioventricular canal ventricular septal defect with cleft mitral valve. Angiographic and echocardiographic features. *Pediatr Cardiol* 1982;2: 289–295.
44. Furuta N, Luhmer I, Hetzer R, et al: Abnormal accessory mitral leaflet simulating left ventricular outflow tract tumor. *Thorac Cardiovasc Surg* 1983; 31:249–253.
45. Mathewson JW, Riemenschneider TA, McGough EC, et al: Left ventricular outflow tract obstruction produced by redundant mitral valve tissue in a neonate. Clinical, angiographic, and operative findings. *Circulation* 1975;53:196–199.

CHAPTER 8
Mitral Valve Disease

Melvin D. Cheitlin
Randolph C. Byrd

The mitral valve is the guardian of the lungs. During diastole when it is open, the mitral valve has a functional area of about 6 cm^2 and thus presents no obstruction to the flow of blood from the lungs into the left ventricle. The left atrium normally acts as a conduit rather than a chamber during this time. During systole, proper closure of the mitral valve allows systemic pressure development in the left ventricle without significantly affecting the pressure in the left atrium. Since the hydrostatic pressure in the pulmonary capillary bed is the same as the left atrial pressure, a properly functioning mitral valve which is mobile, flexible, and opens completely is responsible for maintaining a normal low pressure in the left atrium.

ANATOMY AND FUNCTION OF THE MITRAL VALVE

The mitral valve apparatus from proximal to distal consists of the mitral annulus, the leaflets, the chordae tendineae, the papillary muscles and the left ventricular wall. Since the mural leaflet is continuous with the endocardium of the left atrial wall, some authors include the left atrium also as a structure involved in the mitral valve apparatus.[1] The mitral valve is a thin, flexible structure with two major leaflets, an anterior or aortic leaflet which is semicircular in shape, and a larger narrower quadrangular leaflet, the posterior or mural leaflet.[2] The area of the mitral leaflets is about 2.5 times the area of the orifice at the annular level. The mural leaflets' fibrous structure arises from the thin fibrous mitral annulus in the atrioventricular groove. The mitral annulus is not complete but is open at the portion of the aortic leaflet extending up to the aortic annulus and becoming continuous with the left coronary cusp and the anterior portion of the noncoronary cusp.[3]. The portion of the anterior leaflet that extends up to the aortic valve is known as the intervalvular membrane. The intervalvular membrane valve moves less than the free portion of the anterior leaflet during diastole, thus forming the "hinge" portion of the anterior leaflet. If this part of the mitral valve calcifies, the anterior leaflet will not open completely under normal pressure.

The major commissures are located anterolaterally and posteromedially. Under these two commissures are the two papillary muscles which give rise to chordae supporting both leaflets. The mural leaflet has two minor commissures which divide the leaflet into three functional "scallops": an anteromedial, a middle, and a posteromedial scallop.[4]

The chordae tendineae branch once or twice before reaching the leaflets and have been named first, second, and third order chordae. The chordae arise from the papillary muscles and attach to the leading edge of the valve and to the ventricular surface of the leaflets up to 1 cm back from the edge, termed the "rough zone." From the mural leaflet only, chordae arise from the ventricular wall and attach to the rough zone. The rough zone is thicker than the rest of the valve, deepest in the center of the leaflet, thinning toward the commissures. The chordae at each major and lesser commissure are characterized by a fanlike branching.[5] The function of the chordae is to keep the edges of the leaflet in the left ventricle during systole. After passing through the mitral orifice, the blood passes through the multiple chordae into the body of the left ventricle. Thickening and fusion of the chordae can result in subvalvular obstruction to flow.

The histologic structure of the leaflet itself is of importance. The leaflet is composed of three layers: a thin fibrous layer facing the atrium, the atrialis; a tough collagen fibrous layer facing the ventricle, the ventricularis; and a thin, loose myxomatous layer sandwiched in between, the spongiosa. An intact, tough ventricularis is essential to the integrity of the valve. In prolapsing mitral valve, the weaker spongiosa is much thicker than normal, invading and replacing the fibrosa and frequently undermining the attachments of the chordae.[6] This allows the valve leaflet under left ventricular systolic pressure to stretch, thus increasing the surface area of the valve which prolapses back into the atrium. Weakened chordal attachments make them more susceptible to rupture under the force of the left ventricular systolic pressure.

The competence of the mitral valve during systole depends on the anatomical and functional integrity of the entire valve apparatus.[1,3] Examples of diseases affecting primarily each of the structures of the mitral valve apparatus and resulting in mitral insufficiency are: mitral annular and subannular calcification affecting the mitral annulus; rheumatic fever, infective endocarditis, and prolapse of the mitral valve affecting leaflets; idiopathic rupture of the chordae tendineae; acute myocardial infarction with rupture of a papillary muscle; and left ventricular muscle disease such as coronary artery disease and cardiomyopathy affecting the left ventricular wall.

The left ventricle is a muscular structure forming a cuplike structure with a proximal opening called the ostium of the left ventricle. Within the ostium anteromedially is the aortic annulus with the aortic valve, and posterolaterally the mitral annulus with the mitral valve. During systole, the circumferential muscles of the left ventricle surrounding the ostium of the left ventricle contract, decreasing the area which will be closed off by the billowing mitral valve leaflets. During diastole the leaflets hang like a curtain into the left ventricle with a 6-cm^2 opening connecting the left atrium and the left ventricle making them a common chamber. with essentially no pressure gradient across the mitral valve. As the left ventricle fills from the atrium, the left ventricular pressure rises and the valve floats toward the closed position. With a properly timed atrial contraction the velocity of the blood from the left atrium is increased and turbulence is created which forces the atrial surface of the leaflets together via the Venturi effect. The coaptation of the atrial contact surface of the leaflets involves the distal 1 cm of the valves, the part of the leaflet supported by the chordal attachments or the rough zone. The valve is now normally functionally closed at the end of diastole. In ventricular systole, the closed valve is tensed toward the left atrium with the edges held into the left ventricle by the chordae.

Competence of the mitral valve depends on proper functioning of the entire mitral valve apparatus. With decreased left ventricular contractility and dilatation of the left ventricle, the ostium of the left ventricle and the mitral annulus dilate, enlarging the orifice which the valve must cover. The area of coaptation of the leaflets is consequently decreased, thus diminishing the forces pressing the leaflets together and favoring mitral insufficiency. Normally, the papillary muscles and the chordae are oriented along the long axis of the left ventricle. Therefore the force exerted along the chordae is parallel to the axis that keeps the edges of the valve in the ventricle. With left ventricular dilatation, the papillary muscles are moved apart and the force along the chordae is directed at an angle to the long axis of the left ventricle, thus decreasing the effective force keeping the leaflet edges in the left ventricle.[3] Finally, with left ventricular ejection the kinetic energy of the blood is directed out the aortic valve and parallel to the anterior leaflet of the mitral valve, therefore exerting no force on the anterior leaflet. With dilatation of the left ventricle, the aortic leaftet during systole is oriented more horizontally and perpendicularly to the kinetic vector. This exerts a force on the anterior leaflet pushing the leaflet back toward the left atrium.

Because the mitral valve is difficult to obstruct, there are few diseases causing mitral stenosis. However, because competence of the complex mitral apparatus requires all parts of the mitral apparatus to function properly, there are multiple diseases that result in mitral insufficiency.[2]

MITRAL STENOSIS

Etiology

For practical purposes, rheumatic fever is the etiology of mitral stenosis in the vast majority of cases. There are two other diseases which are recognized etiologies of mitral stenosis: congenital mitral stenosis and calcification of the mitral annulus and subannular areas.[7,8] Recently, with the older population increasing it has been recognized that mitral annular and subannular calcification results not only in mitral insufficiency, which has been known for many years, but also that the exuberant atheromatous calcification under the mural leaflet can cause sufficient decrease in the valve area as to result in mitral stenosis. Other diseases which occasionally cause mitral stenosis are Whipple's disease[9,10] and malignant carcinoid.[11] For practical purposes, when mitral stenosis is diagnosed, rheumatic heart disease is the etiology.

In the differential diagnosis of mitral stenosis any disease which obstructs flow into the left ventricle and causes elevation of pressure in the left atrium can result in the pathophysiologic changes seen in mitral stenosis. Such diseases as left atrial myxoma, supravalvular mitral ring, and cor triatriatum all cause obstruction to flow above the mitral valve. Obstruction can occur under the mitral valve from intraventricular tumors, hypertrophic cardiomyopathy, and the parachute mitral valve where all chordae come from a single papillary muscle.[7]

Pathophysiology

Rheumatic heart disease involves the contact edges of the leaflets as well as the chordae resulting in synechiae of the commissures, fibrosis and thickening of the leaflets, and fusion and shortening of the chordae[2] (Figures 8-1 and 8-2). At times, thick fused chordae form a mass of tissue below the valve, causing subvalvular obstruction. Later calcification of the valve occurs involving contact surfaces of the leaflets as well as the hinge point of the anterior leaflet. All these changes result in narrowing of the orifice and obstruction of blood flow across the mitral valve in diastole. When the valve orifice narrows to below 2 cm^2, there is a breaking up of laminer flow across the valve and turbulence of flow results in a minimal gradient and diastolic murmur especially at times of peak flow early in diastole. On further narrowing of the valve, the left atrium and left ventricle are no longer a common chamber in diastole. In order to keep the stroke volume normal a pressure gradient develops across the mitral valve in diastole. When the valve area is reduced to the level of about 1 cm^2, severe stenosis of the mitral valve exists.

As the area of the mitral valve orifice decreases, resistance to flow across the valve increases, thereby raising the pressure in the left atrium. This results in elevation in the pressure in the pulmonary veins and pulmonary capillaries and an increase in total pulmonary resistance faced by the right ventricle during systole.

The consequences of the obstruction therefore are an increase in left atrial pressure and pulmonary capillary hydrostatic pressure as well as "passive" pulmonary hypertension. The net movement of fluid out of the capillary bed is caused by the hydrostatic intravascular pressure

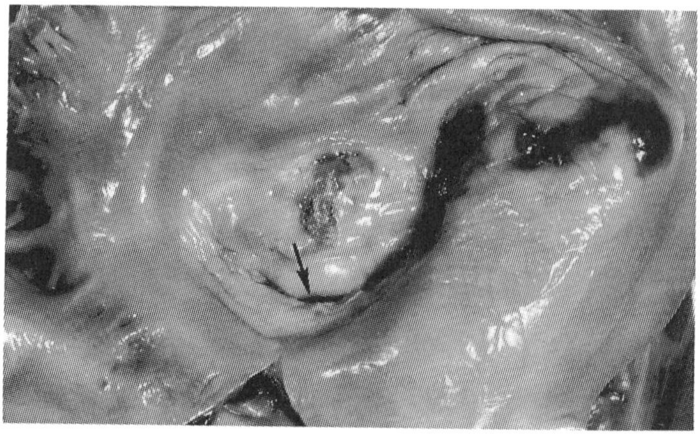

Figure 8-1 Patient with rheumatic mitral stenosis. Left atrium opened. Pectinate muscles of opened atrial appendage seen on left. Arrow indicates "fish mouth" orifice of mitral valve. Anterolateral and posteromedial commissure fused. Endocardial lesion on atrial surface of aortic leaflet of mitral valve above arrow.

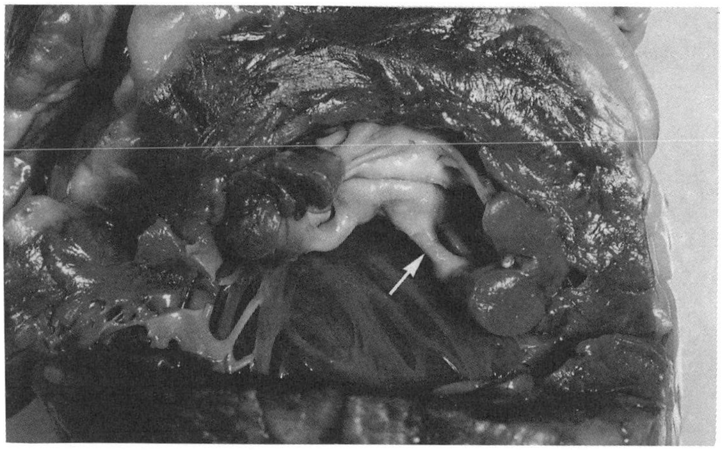

Figure 8-2 Patient with rheumatic mitral stenosis. Ventricular surface of mitral valve seen from left ventricle. Note thickened, shortened, and fused chordae tendineae.

and balanced by the colloid osmotic pressure, exerted mostly by serum albumin in the intravascular blood. Although there are opposing forces in the interstitial space, these forces under normal circumstances are minimal.

Once in the interstitial space the fluid is removed by the lymphatic system and prevented from moving into the alveoli.[12] The increase in lung water results in stiffening and reduced dynamic compliance of the lung, increasing work of the respiratory muscles in expanding the lung during inspiration, as well as stimulation of intrapulmonary and thoracic cage receptors.[13] These pulmonary changes and the increase in inspiratory work result in the sensation of dyspnea.[14] If the increase in hydrostatic pressure occurs acutely, as it does in acute myocardial infarction, when the hydrostatic intravascular pressure rises to 25 mmHg the increasing net flow of fluid out of the capillaries into the interstitial space can no longer be compensated for by the protective mechanism of the normal lung lymphatics, the proteinaceous fluid spills into the alveoli, and pulmonary edema occurs. With a gradual increase in obstruction and hydrostatic pressure over a period of months, the resulting increase in interstitial fluid flow is balanced by an increased capacity of the pulmonary lymphatic system to drain the interstitial space. For this reason, and because there is an adaptation to the chronic increase in lung water, a much higher left atrial and pulmonary capillary pressure can be maintained without the sensation of dyspnea. It is therefore not unusual to see patients with mitral stenosis who have resting wedge pressures of 30 to 35 mmHg without very much in the way of symptoms at rest or with mild exertion.

As the left atrial pressure and pulmonary capillary pressure increase, there is an increased resistance to right ventricular systole and systolic pressure rises in the pulmonary artery and right ventricle. In mitral stenosis, in about one third of the cases, there is an active increase in pulmonary artery pressure as a result of the marked increase in pulmonary vascular resistance. This comes about because of the increase in interstitial water. Since the interstitium is a common interconnecting space, in the upright position the interstitial water gravitates to the dependent portion of the lung, increasing the extramural pressure on small vessels and small airways of the lower lung. The extramural pressure on the small vessels results in an increase in pulmonary vascular resistance which is compounded by the vasoconstriction effects of an increase in local hypoxia and acidosis due to pressure on small airways.[14,15] Together with an increase in the thickness of the smooth muscle of the media of the small pulmonary vessels, the increase in vascular resistance to flow in the lower lung results in a redistribution of blood flow to the upper lungs[16–18] as well as an "active" increase in pulmonary artery pressure. Since the increased interstitial water is primarily responsible for the increase in pulmonary vascular resistance, the decrease in lung water brought about by lowering the left atrial pressure by relieving mitral stenosis results in decrease in pulmonary vascular resistance.

Pulmonary hypertension causes an afterload burden on the right ventricle. Even with only passive increases in pulmonary artery pressure, the right ventricle may hypertrophy and dilate and right ventricular ejection fraction decrease.[19] With active increases in pulmonary vascular resistance, the pulmonary artery pressure can rise to systemic levels, and cause severe right ventricular hypertrophy. Finally right ventricular dilatation and tricuspid and pulmonary valve insufficiency occur and signs of right ventricular failure appear.

The relationships of pressure gradient to diastolic flow across the mitral valve are expressed in the Gorlin equation[20] which is derived from the steady flow relationship:

$$Q \; \alpha \; A \times \sqrt{P1 - P2}.$$

where Q = flow, A = area of obstruction, and P1 − P2 = the pressure drop across the obstruction A. Gorlin and Gorlin rearranged the formula to estimate mitral valve area. Since the flow across the mitral valve occurs only in diastole, Q in the formula becomes cardiac output divided by the number of seconds/minute occupied by diastole — the diastolic filling period. The new relationship is therefore:

$$MVA \; \alpha \; \frac{CO}{DFP \times \sqrt{LAd - LVd}}.$$

where MVA = mitral valve area, CO = cardiac output, DFP = diastolic filling period, LAd = left atrial pressure in diastole, and LVd = left ventricular pressure in diastole.

For the clinician it is useful to rearrange the formula to look at the determinants of left atrial pressure and the gradient.

$$LAd - LVd \; \alpha \; \left(\frac{CO}{(DFP \times MVA)}\right)^2$$

From this relationship it can be seen that when cardiac output drops, the pressure in the left atrium must also drop. In this way pulmonary hypertension, by causing right ventricular failure and dropping cardiac output, will "protect" the capillary bed by decreasing the left atrial pressure.

Since the loudness of the murmur of mitral stenosis is related to the gradient, with a decrease in cardiac output the gradient will drop and therefore the loudness of the murmur will decrease. Conversely, if the cardiac output is increased or the heart rate is increased, thereby decreasing diastolic filling period, the left atrial pressure and the gradient will rise and the murmur will increase.

The time period over which mitral valve stenosis increases is not known. It is not known whether continued rheumatic activity causes further fibrosis or whether, as is more likely, the turbulence caused by commisural fusion over the years promotes further fibrosis and later calcification. It is also not known whether the stenosis progresses steadily or, as is more likely, is episodic and periodic.[21] Because of the exponential relationship of the mitral valve area to the gradient it is apparent that with gradual decreases of mitral valve area at some point there is a rapid rise in the gradient so that slightly more obstruction results in a sharply increased left atrial pressure.

Mitral Stenosis with Mitral Insufficiency

When significant mitral stenosis and insufficiency coexist, the pathophysiologic consequences are similar to those of mitral stenosis. The regurgitant volume results in a larger volume flow with each diastole thus increasing the left atrial pressure and the diastolic gradient. The natural history is similar to that of mitral stenosis and the major difference is that if surgery is necessary, mitral valve replacement is required since at present valvuloplasty in these cases is usually not possible.

The Clinical Picture of Mitral Stenosis

Rheumatic fever is rare before the age of 3 years and unusual before the age of 5. The peak incidence of acute rheumatic fever is between the ages of 5 and 25 years. Over the age of 20, if rheumatic fever occurs for the first time, it usually does not involve the heart but only the joints. The younger the patient is with the first episode, the more likely the patient is to have cardiac involvement.[22] The only significant chronic residuum of acute rheumatic fever is valvular disease. In the past and presently in some parts of the world, the patient may have repeated episodes of rheumatic fever yearly, each time having another episode of rheumatic carditis with further valvular involvement. For this reason, in countries such as India, it is not unusual to see young people under the age of 20 and even at the end of the first decade with severe multivalvular involvement or severe mitral stenosis.[23] Acute rheumatic fever is a mimetic disease when it recurs and if carditis were not present with the first episode it is unlikely to occur with a second episode.[24]

With acute rheumatic carditis, mitral and/or aortic insufficiency can be seen immediately. Mitral stenosis on the other hand is the most frequent chronic sequela of rheumatic fever. Because commissural fusion and fibrosis is required, mitral stenosis does not occur until 2 or more years after the acute episode of rheumatic fever. The gradual development of the obstruction allows for the compensations described above to develop and therefore it is not unusual to find the murmur of mitral stenosis even with severe obstruction in patients who are asymptomatic.[25]

Physical Findings

The sounds of mitral stenosis are: (1) the loud first heart sound; (2) the opening snap; (3) the diastolic murmur of mitral stenosis heard best at the apex in the left lateral postion; (4) the increased pulmonary component of S_2; (5) the findings of pulmonary hypertension: right ventricular S_4, tricuspid insufficiency, and pulmonary insufficiency.

Reference to the left-sided pressure curves from the patient with mitral stenosis will help to understand the physical findings created by obstruction to flow across the mitral valve. Since the left atrium and the left ventricle are connected by a small opening during diastole and are no longer a common chamber, at the end of diastole the pressure in the left atrium remains higher than that in the left ventricle and the mitral valve is pressed into its position of maximum opening. With ventricular systole, the pressure relationships are reversed and the valve with its fused commissures is moved suddenly through its maximum range of motion to a tensed closed position. If the valve is flexible this sudden rapid displacement of blood and sudden checking of motion results in a loud first heart sound. The loudness is dependent on the flexibility of the leaflets. In the presence of a stiff fibrotic or calcific valve, the leaflets move less freely, and the first sound will be softer.

For similar reasons, at the beginning of diastole, when the pressure in the left ventricle drops below the left atrial pressure, the valve suddenly moves from a tensed closed position to a tensed open position, its movement suddenly checked by the lack of mobility caused by the fused commissures. This results in a high pitched sound 0.04 to 0.12 second after the A_2 — the mitral opening snap.

In general, there is an inverse relationship between the A_2–opening snap interval and the height of the left atrial pressure. Therefore the tighter the mitral stenosis, the higher the left atrial pressure and the shorter the A_2–opening snap interval. The height of the left atrial pressure, the timing of closure of the aortic valve, and the opening of the mitral valve depend on the cardiac output, compliance of the aorta, and the systemic vascular resistance as well as the stiffness of the mitral valve, where the interval from the actual mitral valve opening to opening snap is prolonged.[26] Therefore the A_2–opening snap interval must be interpreted with care when estimating the severity of the mitral stenosis.

Because of the small mitral valve orifice, the stroke volume crosses the mitral valve during diastole impelled by a relatively low gradient. This results in a diastolic low-frequency murmur starting after the opening snap and going to the first heart sound, frequently with enough energy to be loud enough to result in a palpable apical thrill. Since the murmur is generated in the left ventricle below the mitral valve, it is transmitted to the chest wall best where the left ventricle contacts the chest wall: at the point of maximal impulse (PMI). Because the low frequency murmur is transmitted poorly through other structures, the murmur may not be heard away from the PMI. For this reason the murmur is best heard with the bell of the stethoscope lightly applied at the PMI.

Occasionally, even in the presence of severe mitral stenosis, the murmur is difficult or impossible to hear. There are several possible reasons for this: low cardiac output and right ventricular dilatation. If the cardiac output is low the gradient may be very small and the murmur inaudible; with liberal use of diuretics it is becoming more frequent to cause hypovolemia and to drop the cardiac output precipitously. With pulmonary hypotension and dilatation of the right ventricle, the left ventricular apex is moved away from the chest wall and the murmur may be inaudible at the body surface. The increase in the pulmonary artery pressure, whether passive or active, results in the signs of pulmonary hypertension: increase in pulmonic component of S_2, right ventricular hypertrophy, and finally dilatation of the right ventricle with tricuspid and even pulmonary valve insufficiency.

Pulmonary valvular insufficiency results in a high-pitched, decrescendo blowing diastolic murmur along the left sternal border indistinguishable from aortic insufficiency and called the Graham-Steele murmur. With right ventricular failure, the signs of right heart failure occur with an elevated venous pressure, edema, hepatomegaly, and finally ascites.

Symptoms

Since mitral stenosis results in an increase in left atrial and pulmonary capillary pressure, it is understandable that dyspnea should be an early symptom. Anything that increases cardiac output and decreases the diastolic filling period should increase the left atrial pressure and therefore cause dyspnea. Dyspnea on exertion is therefore frequently the earliest symptom developing in a patient with mitral stenosis. Other more infrequent causes of increased heart rate and cardiac output such as infection, anemia, and thyrotoxicosis also result in dyspnea, orthopnea, or even pulmonary edema. Since mitral stenosis is four times as common in women as in men, it is not unusual for the murmur of mitral stenosis to be first discovered during pregnancy.[27] Since cardiac output increases by 30% to 50% by the 20th to 24th week of pregnancy, it is common for the patient suddenly to have acute dyspnea, paroxysmal nocturnal dyspnea, or even an episode of pulmonary edema for the first time. In fact the commonest cardiac cause of death in pregnancy before the era of diuretics was mitral stenosis.

In mitral stenosis, since the elevation in left atrial pressure is not determined by left ventricular failure, but by obstructed flow past a stenotic valve, marked elevations and decreases in left atrial pressure can occur rapidly. For this reason, the patient can suddenly have orthopnea, paroxysmal nocturnal dyspnea, or even pulmonary edema and after treatment within minutes to hours have marked improvement. After diuresis it is possible for patients to return to entirely normal activity, even athletic activity, without symptoms.

Since the left atrial pressure is elevated, the left atrium enlarged, and possibly also since the rheumatic disease has damaged atrial muscle, atrial fibrillation is a common relatively early complication. With atrial fibrillation, the patient becomes more symptomatic because of the irregular rapid heart rate, and decrease in the diastolic filling period, but also because of the loss of atrial contraction which especially in moderate mitral stenosis has an important role in increasing left ventricular filling and maintaining the stroke volume.[28,29] Thompson et al demonstrated in mitral stenosis that the loss of atrial contraction decreased cardiac output by 20%.[30] The onset of atrial fibrillation frequently marks the beginning of the reduction in the patient's exercise tolerance and a marked change in physical activity.

With the development of pulmonary hypertension and right ventricular failure, there is a decrease in the ability to increase cardiac output or even a decrease in resting cardiac output. This in part is beneficial because the left atrial pressure may decrease with the decrease in cardiac output and may not rise as much with activity. Therefore there is less orthopnea, paroxysmal nocturnal dyspnea, and dyspnea on exertion may not be as prominent. The trade-off, however, is that there is an inability to increase cardiac output, resulting in easy fatigability and marked decrease in exercise capacity.

With right heart failure, the final stages are characterized by extremely poor cardiac output with stasis cyanosis due to marked extraction of oxygen from the blood and venous desaturation, increasing peripheral edema, hepatic engorgement and dysfunction, and finally ascites. The final picture is that of a patient with severe cachexia, jaundice, and ascites who appears to have end-stage cirrhosis.

Two symptoms that occur in patients with mitral stenosis deserve special mention: hemoptysis and hoarseness. The onset of hemoptysis is often sudden; it occurs after a coughing spell and consists of bright red blood, from small amounts to larger frightening amounts of a half cup or more. Rarely, large volumes of blood are coughed up occasionally requiring emergency mitral commissurotomy.[31] The basis for the hemoptysis is the dual drainage of the bronchial veins through the azygous veins into the systemic venous system as well as through collaterals into the pulmonary venous system. With increase in the pulmonary venous pressure, these collaterals are enlarged and a left-to-right shunt occurs increasing the flow of fully saturated blood in the bronchial veins. The enlarged bronchial veins are submucosal in the airways and with coughing can rupture, resulting in hemoptysis.[32] Hemoptysis is always a sign of severe mitral stenosis but occassionally can be the first sign even in a patient with good exercise tolerance.

Another classic symptom in mitral stenosis is the development of hoarseness due to paralysis of the left recurrent laryngeal nerve (Ortner's syndrome). This is the result of the peculiar anatomical course of the left recurrent laryngeal nerve looping around the ligamentum arteriosum which connects the proximal descending aorta and the pulmonary artery. With tight mitral stenosis and pulmonary hypertension, left atrial and pulmonary artery enlargement together crowd the "aortic window" and put pressure on the left recurrent laryngeal nerve causing paralysis.[33]

With left atrial enlargement, especially with atrial fibrillation, abetted by a decrease in cardiac output, formation of a left atrial thrombus is common and systemic embolization is a complication, at times tragic in consequence.

Course

In the classic descriptions of mitral stenosis of Olesen,[34] Wood,[35] and Rowe et al,[25] the usual time course was the development of symptomatology toward the end of the third decade after 10 to 20 years of minimal problems, increasing symptoms by the fourth decade, and death by the end of the fifth decade. There are many studies of patients' survival after the discovery of mitral stenosis.[34–36] All studies have shown that survival is related to the functional capacity of the patient at the time of discovery: the more symptomatic the patient, the shorter the survival. Average survival for the entire group is about 60% at 5 years, and 40% at 20 years. In Olesen's series[34] seen during the presurgical era, functional class III patients had a 5-year survival of 62% compared to a 15% 5-year survival in class IV patients. At 10 years survival was 38% in functional class III patients with no class IV patients surviving after 8 years. The latest series from the time the diagnosis was made to death in a random series of patients with mitral stenosis was Rapaport's,[37] published in 1975, which showed an 80% survival at 5 years and 60% alive at 10 years.

Since most of the series were published in the 1950s and since oral diuretics were first introduced in the mid-1950s, it is highly probable that this natural history is no longer the natural history of mitral stenosis and that improved medical management will mean a less symptomatic and longer life even for the unoperated patient.

Chest Roentgenogram

The chest film classically shows left atrial enlargement expanding posteriorally and rightward.[38] The left atrial appendage appears under the main pulmonary artery segment on the frontal projection and results in a convexity just under the pulmonary artery. With pulmonary artery enlargement, this straightens or makes convex the left border of the heart (Figure 8-3) which has been referred to as "mitralization" of the heart. The left atrium enlarging rightward forms a double density behind the right atrium and finally bulges beyond the right border of the heart. As the left atrium enlarges posteriorly, it displaces the left mainstem bronchus posteriorly and superiorly and the barium-filled esophagus posteriorly and rightward. Right ventricular hypertrophy may distort the cardiac silhouette by tipping up the apex of the heart off the diaphragm, and right ventricular dilatation enlarges the transverse diameter of the heart.

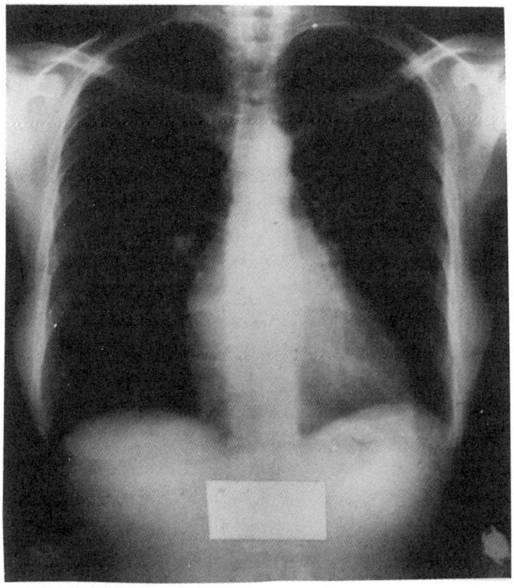

Figure 8-3 Posteroanterior chest film of 40-year-old woman with mitral stenosis. Left atrium seen enlarging on the right. Note double density in right upper portion of cardiac silhouette and straightening of left border of heart.

Enlargement of the right ventricle in the frontal plane can be difficult to differentiate from left ventricular enlargement. In the lateral film, the right ventricle may fill more than one third of the retrosternal space (Figure 8-4) and the left mainstem bronchus may be displaced posteriorly by the enlarged left atrium. Occasionally, calcification of the mitral valve can be seen in the lateral or oblique views but it is better seen on fluroscopy. Calcification of portions of the left atrial wall occasionally can be seen, usually best on lateral films, and in our experience only with

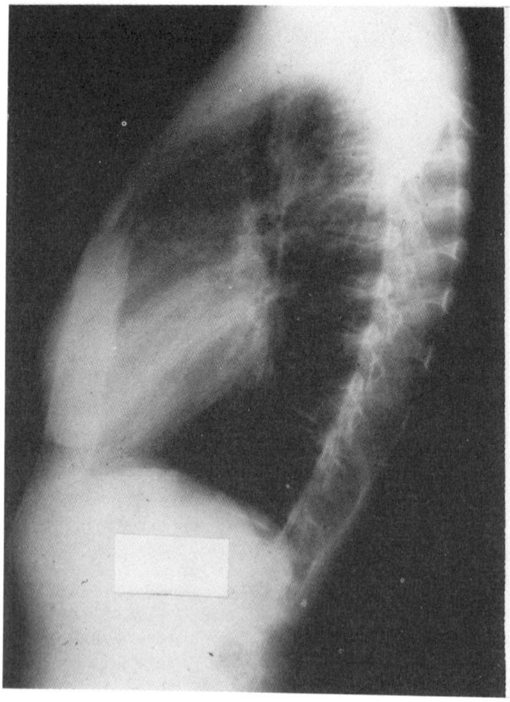

Figure 8-4 Left lateral chest film of same patient as in Figure 8-3. Note posterior bulge of left atrium in superior posterior portion of the cardiac silhouette. Note filling of retrosternal space secondary to right ventricular hypertrophy.

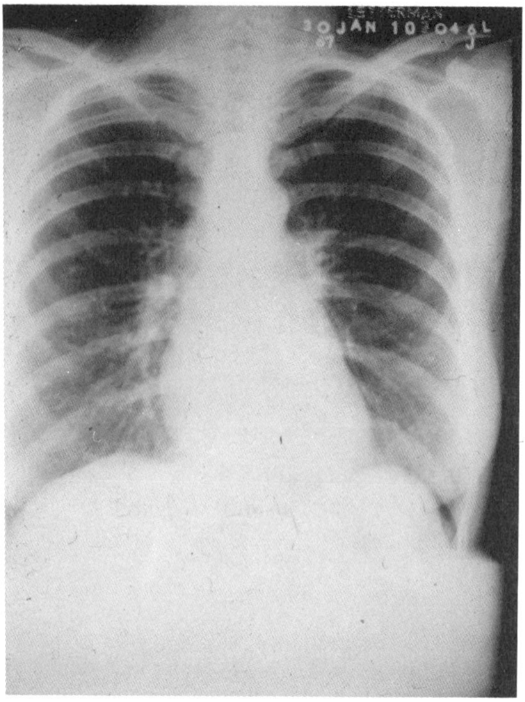

Figure 8-5 Posteroanterior chest film of 35-year-old woman with mitral stenosis. Note vascular redistribution with prominent vascularity, especially in left upper lobe. Note also convexity of left atrial appendage under main pulmonary artery segment along left cardiac border.

mitral stenosis and invariably a predictor of thrombus in the left atrium.

As left atrial pressure rises, the pulmonary blood flow redistributes and the upper lobe pulmonary vessels appear more prominent than the lower vessels (Figure 8-5). Signs of increased interstitial fluid become apparent consisting of haziness of the outlines of vessels; cuffing around the airways; Kerley B lines, which are straight 1 cm or longer lines which are best seen in the costophrenic angles in the lateral lung fields; Kerley A lines, long curving lines arising from the hilum; and finally pulmonary edema. Attempts have been made to predict the hemodynamic severity of mitral stenosis from the chest x-ray film appearance, especially using the size of the pulmonary arteries, the presence of signs of vascular redistribution, pulmonary congestion, and interstitial edema.[39–41] In general there is good correlation of these findings with the severity of the mitral stenosis but since left atrial pressure and therefore pulmonary capillary and pulmonary artery pressures are dependent on not only mitral valve area but also on cardiac output and heart rate, the correlation is not perfect.[42] Mitral stenosis is one cause of pulmonary edema with a relatively small heart on chest film. With right heart failure pleural effusion occurs with fluid in the minor and major fissures and finally free pleural effusion.

Electrocardiogram

With mild mitral stenosis the ECG can be within normal limits. As mitral stenosis becomes more severe, the ECG usually shows left atrial abnormality with broadening and notching of the P wave and the increased terminal posterior vector of the P wave causing an abnormal negative terminal P wave in V_1. Eventually atrial fibrillation occurs. With pulmonary hypertension, there are signs of right ventricular hypertrophy — right axis deviation, and a terminal QRS vector which is directed anteriorly and rightward. This results in an rSR′ in V_1, an R/S ratio in V_1 greater than 1, and large R waves in V_1 and terminal S waves in V_5 and V_6.[42,43]

Echocardiography

With M-mode echocardiography, the most

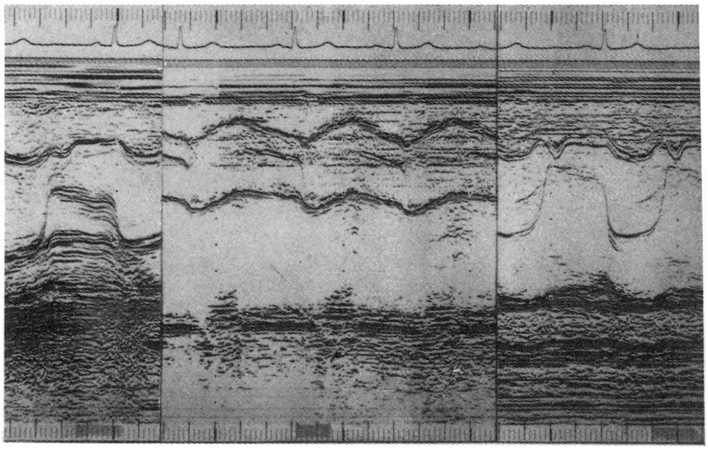

Figure 8-6 M-mode echocardiogram of patient with mitral stenosis. Left panel: Note anterior leaflet with flat e-f slope. Anterior and posterior leaflet in diastole move in the same anterior direction. There are increased echoes from both leaflets. Note loss of anterior motion of anterior leaflet ("a" wave) with atrial contraction. Middle panel: Large left atrium posterior to aortic root echo. Note that closure of aortic valve is asymmetric due to bicuspid aortic valve. Right panel: Maximum excursion of anterior leaflet 2.8 cm consistent with flexible mitral leaflets.

important findings are the abnormal movements of the mitral leaflets.[44] The increased pressure in the left atrium compared to left ventricle during diastole prevents the anterior leaflet from rapidly moving away from the septum. The e-f slope is decreased and with severe mitral stenosis may become less than 10 mm/s (Figure 8-6), although there is no reliable relationship allowing the prediction of severity of mitral stenosis from this measurement.[45] The valve leaflets can be thickened if fibrosis is severe or calcification occurs. With severe mitral stenosis the anterior motion of the anterior mitral leaflet with systole (the "a" wave) is decreased and disappears. In a study of 35 catheterization-proven mitral stenosis patients in normal sinus rhythm, Dabestani et al reported that no patient with an "a" wave had a mitral valve area less than 1.2 cm^2.[46] The usually opposite movement of the mural leaflet disappears with commissural fusion and both leaflets in mid- and late diastole move in the same direction. In early diastole the mural leaflet can move posteriorly, even in severe mitral stenosis. Left atrial enlargement occurs and finally right ventricular hypertrophy and enlargement.

With two-dimensional echocardiography, it is possible to visualize the mitral orifice during diastole[48] (Figure 8-7). In addition to seeing a restricted orifice, the diaphragmlike restricted motion of the leaflets is apparent. The thickening of the mitral valves can be seen as well as the subvalvular fused, shortened chordae.[49,50] Left atrial and right ventricular enlargement are easily appreciated especially in the apical four-chamber view. Since the mitral orifice can be visualized, it can also be planimetered and, in general, measurement of the mitral orifice correlates well with the severity of the mitral stenosis and the valve area by catheterization.[48,51,52,53] As is often the case, mild and severe mitral stenosis can easily be separated. The problem in differentiating degrees of severity comes when moderate mitral stenosis is present.

Left atrial thrombus is very difficult to identify in M-mode echocardiography and especially difficult to rule out. It is also a problem with two-dimensional echocardiography. Since most often the thrombus is in the atrial appendage, it is impossible to rule out thrombus with the latter technique.

Doppler Ultrasound

Until recently, there was no noninvasive technique that accurately assessed intracardiac pressures or gradients. With the development of Doppler ultrasound techniques this is no longer true. Using the principle of the Doppler frequency shift, the difference between the frequency of sound projected into the heart and that reflected from moving blood cells is proportional to the velocity of the blood cells. With present technology, it is possible to measure with

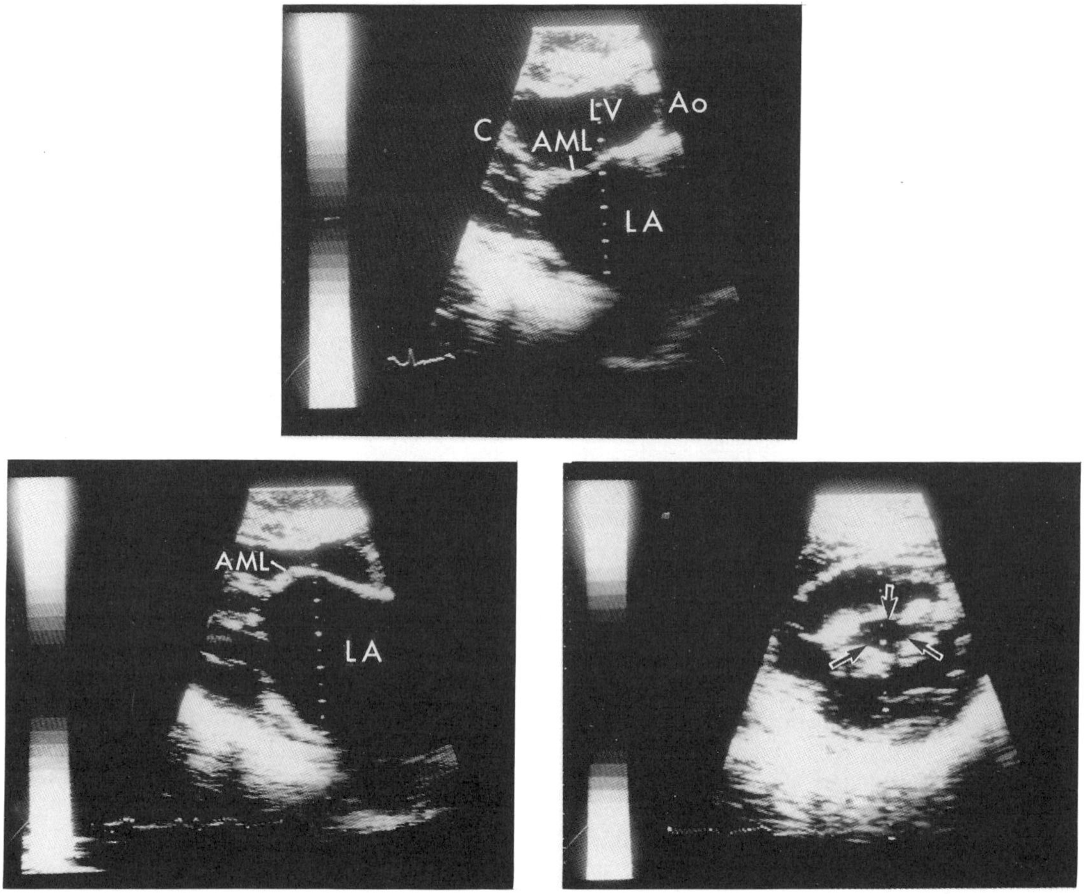

Figure 8-7 Two-dimensional echocardiogram of a 21-year-old asymptomatic woman, 22 weeks pregnant, with mitral stenosis.
A. Long axis view in systole. Mitral valve is closed. Left atrium is enlarged. Chordae are thickened. LA = left atrium, Ao = aortic valve, C = chordal structures, LV = left ventricular outflow tract, AML = anterior mitral leaflet.
B Long axis view in diastole. Anterior leaflet (AML, pointer) edge is tethered and anterior leaflet is bowed anteriorly. Left atrium is enlarged.
C Short axis view in diastole at level of smallest orifice of the mitral valve. Orifice (arrows) planimetered opening at 0.6 cm^2. Mitral valve is abnormally reflectant.

a pulsed Doppler ultrasound technique the velocity of blood moving in a sample volume from a specific location of the heart chosen by two-dimensional echocardiography recorded simultaneously. With the continuous Doppler technique the maximum velocity of the jet can be measured. High velocities are not recorded accurately by the pulsed Doppler technique.

The principle used in relating velocity of blood to pressure gradient is that when blood passes through a restricted orifice, velocity of blood flow increases and a high velocity jet is formed downstream from the stenosis. The relation between the pressure drop and the velocity is given by the Bernoulli equation.[54] With simplification, dropping terms of small magnitude, the pressure drop can be calculated from the maximal velocity of the jet:

$$\text{Gradient (mmHg)} = 4 \times V^2$$

where V = maximal velocity of jet (m/s)

Holen et al[55] showed that the pressure drop across a stenotic mitral valve can be calculated from transcutaneous Doppler ultrasonic measurements of blood velocity.

Holen et al,[56] Hatle et al,[54] and others[57] have since validated the accuracy with which Doppler ultrasound can predict the diastolic gradient obtained at catheterization. The sources of error are the inability to find the maximum jet velocity below the valve either because of anatomical position or lung attenuation of the signal. The angle of the ultrasonic beam to the direction of maximum velocity is important. The larger the angle, the greater the underestimation of the gradient. Also this technique estimates gradient, not absolute pressures in the left atrium or left ventricle. The gradient is dependent on diastolic flow across the valve and diastolic filling period as well as effective mitral valve area in diastole. For instance, a higher jet velocity can be accounted for by an increase in cardiac output, or an increase in diastolic flow due to severe mitral insufficiency in the face of a lesser degree of mitral stenosis. Similarly, a lower velocity jet can occur either because of a lesser degree of obstruction or because the cardiac output is markedly diminished. With recognition of the problems in interpretation, if the patient's clinical picture is taken into account, two-dimensional echocardiography and Doppler ultrasonography are able to predict accurately the severity of mitral stenosis.

Catheterization

During catheterization, the pressure gradient across the mitral valve must be measured. This is usually done by simultaneously measuring the pulmonary artery wedge pressure, which reflects left atrial pressure, and the left ventricular pressure. With tight mitral stenosis and a normal diastolic filling period there is always a pressure gradient throughout diastole with the left atrial pressure and the left ventricular pressure never equilibrating. If with a normal diastolic filling period equilibration occurs (Figure 8-8), this is strong evidence against tight mitral stenosis and can be seen in a patient who has predominant mitral insufficiency with mild mitral stenosis. The left atrial mean pressure is elevated and because the cardiac output and stroke volume are not increased, the "a" and "v" waves in the left atrial pressure curve are equally elevated. The "v" wave is not markedly elevated compared to the mean left atrial pressure, as is the case in severe dominant mitral insufficiency.

Pulmonary artery pressures are often elevated in proportion to the elevation of left atrial pressure. However, pulmonary artery pressures can be increased at times to systemic levels. The right ventricular diastolic pressure and right atrial pressure can be normal or elevated with right ventricular failure. With tricuspid insufficiency, the right atrial pressure can be elevated with a prominent "v" wave.

The left ventricular diastolic pressure is usually normal. Although there is great controversy in the literature concerning possible left ventricular dysfunction in mitral stenosis,[58,59] the evidence is quite convincing that in pure mitral stenosis left ventricular function is normal if the diastolic volume of the left ventricle is normal,[60] although

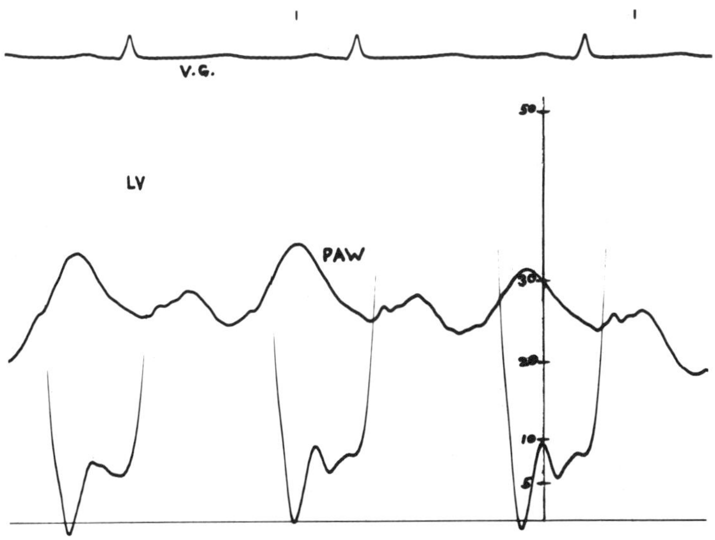

Figure 8-8 Simultaneous pulmonary artery wedge (PAW) and left ventricular (LV) pressures in a patient with severe mitral stenosis (mitral valve area 0.65 cm^2). Paper speed 100 mm/s. Mean PAW pressure is 30 mmHg. Note pressure gradient (mean 24 mmHg) between PAW and LV pressure in diastole.

in some patients reduced stroke volume and ejection fraction may be related to abnormally increased afterload without adequate preload compensation.[61] With angiocardiography and echocardiography there is frequently some regional localized left ventricular wall motion dysfunction in the area of the left ventricular ostium, especially if there is heavy fibrosis and calcification of the mitral valve. If the right ventricle is markedly dilated, especially with severe tricuspid insufficiency, there can be interference with left ventricular filling on the basis of the dilated right ventricle distorting the interventricular septum and interaction with left ventricular filling through the pericardium.

During catheterization, it is important to measure cardiac output, diastolic filling period, and pressure gradient as closely together as possible in order to calculate the mitral valve area. The smaller the gradient the less accurate the calculated mitral valve area. If the cardiac output is diminished with a relatively small gradient, it is imperative that the cardiac output be raised by exercise. The valve area calculation is more accurate when the gradient is higher. A special problem is the patient who has received large doses of diuretics, especially furosemide. Excessive diuresis can markedly decrease cardiac output and almost eliminate the gradient at rest. Under these conditions the left atrial pressure may be markedly decreased so that it can be within normal limits even with severe mitral stenosis. It is our practice to stop diuretics 24 to 48 hours before catheterization, when appropriate, to reduce the incidence of this problem.

Another problem in estimating the severity of mitral stenosis occurs in the presence of severe aortic insufficiency. With rapid filling of the left ventricle from retrograde flow from the aorta, the left ventricular diastolic pressure is elevated and the mitral valve is moved earlier in diastole into a closed position, so that even with severe mitral stenosis in a patient with a normal or slow heart rate, the mean diastolic gradient across the mitral valve may be small. In this case the majority of the mitral diastolic flow occurs early and the valve is in the closed position with flow minimal at the end of diastole. In this situation if the heart rate is increased with exercise, this source of error is minimized and the mean diastolic gradient will reflect the severity of the mitral stenosis.

Since surgery is usually recommended in mitral stenosis to alleviate symptoms, the question arises as to whether cardiac catheterization is necessary in all patients with mitral stenosis prior to surgery. Effron et al[62] reviewed 82 patients undergoing catheterization for isolated mitral stenosis. Of 47 patients with New York Heart Association functional class III or IV disease, 46 had hemodynamic confirmation of severity of stenosis sufficient to warrant surgery. In 35 patients who were in class II, surgery was not recommended as a result of catheterization in nine (26%) with normal or only moderately elevated pulmonary artery wedge pressures. Coronary arteriography was done in 44 patients (54%) and identified four patients with significant luminal narrowing in one or two arteries. Their conclusion was that catheterization was not needed in class III and IV patients with classic mitral stenosis and no clinical evidence of aortic valve or coronary artery disease.[62] In less symptomatic patients catheterization should be done to confirm the presence of severe mitral stenosis before surgery.

Our experience with 82 patients with mitral stenosis who had coronary arteriography confirmed the fact that classic angina pectoris was literally always related to the presence of coronary artery disease.[63] Of 16 patients with significant coronary artery disease we also found four (25%) patients who did not have angina but whose coronary disease was in one or two vessels and in no case was coronary bypass surgery indicated or performed. Therefore, it is probably not necessary to do coronary arteriography in patients with mitral stenosis without angina pectoris or prior myocardial infarction.

We have also seen functional class III patients in atrial fibrillation who had an elevated left atrial pressure with minimal exercise on the basis of a rapid increase in ventricular rate and decrease in diastolic filling period in response to exercise. These patients did well with β-blocking drugs decreasing the ventricular response.[64] Our recommendation is that whenever the patient has atypical features or any question arises as to the cause of the symptoms, the patient should be catheterized prior to surgery.

Treatment

The asymptomatic patient needs careful observation, but may need no treatment other than prophylaxis for rheumatic fever,[65] and prophylactic antibiotics at the time of bacterimia to prevent infective endocarditis.[66] In adults over the age of 30 years the need for prophylaxis for rheumatic fever is controversial. Some authorities recommend penicillin or sulfa prophylaxis for life. We feel that the incidence of recurrent rheumatic fever after age 30 at present is so unusual that it is safe not to give prophylaxis against rheumatic fever in these patients. Certainly sore throats in these patients and infection with group A streptococcus should be promptly evaluated and treated. Even though it is reported that infective endocarditis with pure mitral stenosis is unusual, it is our practice to recommend antibiotics to prevent infective endocarditis at the time of bacteremias, especially with dental procedures.

With the development of dyspnea on exertion, orthopnea, or paroxysmal nocturnal dyspnea, diuretics are the first therapy that should be employed. If atrial fibrillation develops, digitalis is effective in controlling the ventricular rate and together with diuretics frequently returns the patient toward normal activity. Consideration to cardiovert the patient to normal sinus rhythm should be given, especially if the left atrium is not markedly enlarged, since in normal sinus rhythm the incidence of embolization is low and the presence of a good atrial contraction may be important in maintaining normal stroke volume.

With atrial fibrillation, the possibility of systemic emboli raises the question of chronic anticoagulation.[67,68] The incidence of systemic embolization over the patient's lifetime is quite high in this situation, estimated to be about 20%,[69] and if the patient is a reliable candidate for long-term anticoagulation, we recommend warfarin sodium anticoagulation to minimize this possibility. The incidence of embolization is four to five times higher in mitral stenosis and mitral stenosis associated with mitral insufficiency, than in mitral insufficiency alone.[69] The question of chronic anticoagulation in mitral stenosis patients without prior embolism in normal sinus rhythm is even more controversial. We feel that the dangers of anticoagulation do not justify their use in this group of patients. Any patient with prior embolism should be anticoagulated chronically regardless of rhythm.

With pregnancy and other problems that increase heart rate and/or cardiac output, special care must be taken to decrease physical activity and to minimize salt and fluid retention to prevent sudden pulmonary edema.

At times, patients with only moderate mitral stenosis and valve areas between 1.2 and 1.8 cm^2 will develop dyspnea on normal or less than normal exertion. These patients are frequently in atrial fibrillation and the symptomatology may occur in spite of the fact that ventricular response at rest is well controlled with digitalis. In these patients the ventricular rate with mild to moderate exercise frequently rapidly increases, thereby markedly decreasing the diastolic filling period and increasing left atrial pressure. In these patients, low-dose β-blocking agents frequently will adequately control ventricular response to exercise and increase the patient's exercise tolerance.[64]

Surgery

In 1925, Souttar performed a closed mitral commissurotomy in a patient with mitral stenosis.[70] The operation was not performed again until the late 1940s when Bailey in Philadelphia[71] and Harkin in Boston,[72] reintroduced closed mitral commissurotomy. Since then, surgery has become an option for the patient with symptomatic mitral stenosis. There are three surgical procedures possible for the patient with mitral stenosis: the closed mitral commissurotomy, the open mitral commissurotomy on cardiopulmonary bypass, and mitral valve replacement.

Whenever surgical intervention is considered, it is necessary to balance the dangers and benefits of surgical intervention against those of nonintertervention, in this case, the natural history of the medically treated patient.

The problems and dangers faced by the patient with mitral stenosis are: (1) symptomatology limiting physical activity, (2) pulmonary edema, (3) pulmonary hypertension and right heart failure, (4) embolization, (5) infective endocarditis, and (6) decreased survival. The problems with surgery vary depending on the surgical procedure. With closed and open commissurotomy the mortality at the present time is quite low, from 1% to 3%,[73,74] the morbidity at the time of surgery is low, and the clinical results are excellent.[75,76] The incidence of re-stenosis with open commissurotomy is low, with Housman et al[73] reporting in 100 patients followed an average of 46 months an incidence of reoperation of 9% at 5 years. In a study reported by Smith et al[77] the reoperation rate was 10% at 4 years follow-up. After 10 years the incidence of reoperation will probably be higher. The incidence of complications after surgery such as embolization is decreased.[76,78] There are furthermore few late problems resulting from commissurotomy itself, with the exception of the development of severe mitral insufficiency caused by the surgery, which at present is uncommon.[75,78] With these benefits and the relatively low incidence of complications it is possible to offer the functional class II patient who is becoming symptomatic with mitral stenosis a commissurotomy.[79] This is also true for patients who are asymptomatic on treatment who are unhappy taking daily drugs. The symptomatic relief after surgery is good and the long-term benefits excellent,[80,81] even in those patients whose only complication is an embolus. There is some evidence that successful surgery will reduce the incidence of embolization by approximately one half. By reducing the pressure in the left atrium, it is possible to return the patient to normal sinus rhythm and avoid the problems of long-term anticoagulants.

It is possible with a high probability to predict who can benefit from commissurotomy by recognizing that the patient with a mobile, flexible nonleaking valve is amenable to commissurotomy. The signs predicting flexibility and competency of the valve are (1) a loud mitral first heart sound, (2) loud opening snap, (3) absence of more than minimal mitral insufficiency by physical examination and by catheterization, (4) minimal or no calcification of the valve on fluroscopy, and (5) good mobility of mitral apparatus by echocardiography. These signs are seen most often in young patients under the age of 55 years.

With mitral valve replacement a different magnitude of problems and risks are present. A detailed description of prothestic valve problems is presented in chapter 17, but to summarize: (1) Perioperative mortality is from 3% to 10%.[79,82] (2) Surgical morbidity is higher than in commissurotomy. (3) Late mortality in the patient with a prosthetic valve is in the range of 2% to 3%/yr, mostly from problems associated with the prosthetic valve. In a 20 year follow-up study on patients operated on by Starr from 1960 to 1980, the long-term survival for mitral valve replacement was 56% at 10 years and 44% at 15 years.[83] (4) Late morbidity is significant consisting of (*a*) thromboembolic problems even with anticoagulation of 3% to 4%/yr, (*b*) anticoagulant complications, (*c*) paraprosthetic leaks and dihiscence, (*d*) prosthetic valve dysfunction which is uncommon with mechanical valves but more a problem with tissue valves, especially after 5 to 10 years, (*e*) a higher incidence of late infective endocarditis in the range of 0.5% to 1%/year, (*f*) mildly obstructed valve orifice with the prosthetic valves of less than 2.5 cm^2, the so-called valve prosthesis–patient mismatch,[84] and (*g*) other less common problems such as hemolysis, later left ventricular dysfunction, and sudden death.[83,85,86]

The benefits of valve replacement, on the other hand, are marked improvement in physical capacity with a return of the patient to functional class I or II. Although it is difficult to prove that life is prolonged in patients who are in class III or IV, there is some evidence to indicate that it is.[36,87] Certainly, since the patient is either asymptomatic or markedly improved, whether life is prolonged or not is a moot question. Life, if not prolonged, is certainly markedly improved in quality.

For these reasons we do not recommend valve replacement for patients unless they are in functional class III, ie, symptomatic on ordinary activity, after full medical management. Since anticoagulation is necessary it is obvious that mitral valve replacement unlike commissurotomy is not indicated for patients whose only problem has been embolization. In these patients anticoagulation is the treatment, not valve replacement. In those patients with severe pulmonary hypertension, especially those with a dilating right ventricle, we believe that surgery is indicated even if it requires valve replacement and even if the patient is less symptomatic, ie, in class II on treatment. The reason for this opinion is that once the right ventricle has failed and the tricuspid valve has become incompetent, the results of surgery are not as good and frequently the patient never returns to completely normal function and activity.

CHRONIC MITRAL INSUFFICIENCY

Etiology

Unlike mitral stenosis, mitral insufficiency has many etiologies.[1,2], The common causes of mitral insufficiency commonly seen in clinical practice are:

1. Rheumatic heart disease which is presently becoming less frequent in the United States.
2. Mitral valve prolapse, the commonest cause of mitral insufficiency. The pathologic basis for prolapse is found in about 5% of the population and there is a similar incidence by echocardiography.[88,89] Even with a small fraction of the patients developing severe incompetence, mitral valve prolapse is being recognized as a common cause of isolated severe mitral insufficiency at present.
3. Arteriosclerotic heart disease; papillary muscle and left ventricular wall dysfunction

commonly cause mitral insufficiency. Balu et al[90] reported on 1530 patients catheterized with coronary artery disease, of whom 104 (6.8%) had associated mitral insufficiency. Gahl et al[91] reported a series of 127 patients with coronary artery disease catheterized because of symptoms prior to going to surgery. Thirty-nine patients (31%) had mitral insufficiency.[91] Severe transient mitral insufficiency can result from ischemia of the papillary muscle and the left ventricular wall, and severe, rapidly fatal mitral insufficiency can occur during acute myocardial infarction from rupture of the tip of the papillary muscle.[92]

4. Idiopathic rupture of the chordae tendineae with or without mitral valve prolapse.[93,94]
5. Calcification of the mitral annulus and subannular area.[95] Savage et al[96] reported a prevalence in the population of 2.8% mitral annular calcification in the Framingham population. Over 90% of the patients with calcification were over age 59 years.[96]
6. Infective endocarditis.
7. Cardiomyopathy with left ventricular dilatation.[2]

There are many other causes of mitral insufficiency which are less common.[97]

1. Congential defects such as clefting of the mitral valve with or without other lesions resulting from endocardial cushion defect such as ostium primum atrial septal defect or atrioventricular canal, and parachute mitral valve[98]
2. Other collagen diseases such as disseminated lupus erythematosus and rheumatoid arthritis
3. Other connective tissue diseases such as Marfan's syndrome, Ehlers-Danlos syndrome
4. Trauma, both penetrating and nonpenetrating
5. Hypertrophic cardiomyopathy
6. Left atrial and left ventricular myxoma
7. Fibroelastosis (endocardial fibroelastosis)

The usual causes of acute mitral insufficiency, which have a specific clinical picture that is different from chronic mitral insufficiency, are: (1) rupture of the chordae tendineae; (2) infective endocarditis; (3) rupture of the papillary muscle tip in acute myocardial infarction; (4) trauma; (5) prosthetic valve dehiscence.

Pathology

The pathologic findings depend on the etiology of the mitral insufficiency.[2] With rheumatic disease there is fibrosis and retraction of the contact surfaces of the mitral valve with decreased valve area and failure of coaptation. This is complicated and made worse by fibrosis, fusion, and shortening of the chordae tendineae.

With mitral valve prolapse, there is thickening of the spongiosa of the valve with weakening of the fibrosis, ventricular and atrial, and bulging and redundancy of the leaflet.[99,100] The chordae also can be stretched and elongated. Rupture of the chordae is a common cause for the development of sudden and severe mitral insufficiency. The patient by history has had a nonejection click and/or late systolic murmur and therefore has mitral valve prolapse.

With infective endocarditis, vegetations cause weakening of the connective tissue of the valve and tearing of the leaflet edge, the chordae, or perforation of the valve leaflet. With left ventricular failure and dilatation, there is a dilatation of the left ventricular ostium and mitral annular dilatation. A decrease in the contact area of the opposing leaflets during systole, displacement of the papillary muscles, and changes in the geometry of the left ventricle result in mitral insufficiency. With calcification of the mitral annulus and subannular areas, there is splinting of the left ventricular ostium so that narrowing cannot take place during systole, and entrapment of the mural leaflet of the mitral valve, both of which can result in mitral insufficiency.

In coronary disease a portion of the myocardial wall supporting a papillary muscle may fail to contract normally as compared to other parts of the myocardium, causing lack of support of a portion of the mitral valve during systole. A regurgitant orifice may form during systole resulting in a murmur which may be pansystolic or only present in early, mid- or late systole.[101,102] With cardiomyopathy and dilatation of the left ventricle the regurgitant orifice and therefore mitral insufficiency may be present. As ventricular compensation improves with diuretics and the left ventricular volume becomes smaller, the area of the regurgitant orifice may decrease and the murmur may become softer or disappear.

Pathophysiology

Mitral insufficiency is the classic diastolic volume overload lesion of the left ventricle.[103] With gradually increasing mitral insufficiency, with each systole there is regurgitation of blood back into the left atrium which returns with each subsequent diastole. This regurgitating blood joins the blood coming from the lungs and the volume of blood in the next diastole is increased by the amount of the regurgitant volume. The increased diastolic left ventricular volume stimulates synthesis of new sarcomeres and growth of the left ventricle. The larger left ventricle allows continued filling at the same normal low diastolic pressure. Total left ventricular stroke volume increases in order to maintain normal effective forward stroke volume despite the blood regurgitating into the left atrium, known as the regurgitant volume.

The left atrial pressure and therefore the pulmonary capillary pressure depends on: (1) the volume of blood filling the left atrium and pulmonary venous bed; this is composed of the forward stroke volume coming through the lungs plus the regurgitant volume leaking back from the left ventricle; (2) the compliance of the left atrium–pulmonary venous "chamber"; (3) the left ventricular filling pressure.[104]

If the mitral insufficiency develops gradually, the volume of the left atrium–pulmonary venous chamber is also increased, thus accomodating the larger volume in systole. Since the left atrium–pulmonary venous complex is relatively noncompliant, the increased volume during systole causes an earlier rise of systolic pressure in the left atrium, the "v" wave. The height of the "v" wave depends on the regurgitant volume and the left atrium–pulmonary venous compliance. If the left atrium stretches and becomes very large, the rise in the "v" wave will be dampened. If the left atrium remains relatively small in the face of large regurgitant volume, the "v" wave will be large. Since the "v" wave is of short duration, as long as the left ventricular filling pressure remains normal the mean left atrial pressure and therefore the mean pulmonary capillary pressure will remain relatively low. As long as the forward stroke volume and the pulmonary capillary pressure remain normal, the patient will have little symptomatology.[105]

The volume-loaded left ventricle has an advantage in mitral insufficiency in that when the left ventricle contracts, the blood is unloaded under low pressure directly into the left atrium. In other words, there is no isovolumic period of contraction where the left ventricular pressure rises at the maximum left diastolic volume. Since the ventricular radius becomes smaller as the pressure rises, the rise in left ventricular wall tension is minimized.[104,106] Eckberg et al [107] estimated that in severe mitral insufficiency half the regurgitant volume enters the left atrium before the aortic valve opens.

The left ventricular stroke volume is increased in proportion to the increase in left ventricular diastolic volume. For this reason, the ejection fraction remains normal or is elevated as long as left ventricular contractility remains normal. Eventually, when left ventricular contractility begins to decrease, left ventricular stroke volume decreases at the expense of forward stroke volume, end-systolic volume increases, and end-diastolic volume increases returning left ventricular stroke volume toward normal by the Frank-Starling mechanism. Eventually this increase in left ventricular end-diastolic volume cannot keep up with the large left ventricular stroke volume and the forward stroke volume begins to fall. End-systolic volume increases out of proportion to the left ventricular end-diastolic volume and the ejection fraction decreases.[108] As the left ventricular end-diastolic volume increases, the left ventricular filling pressure increases, thus increasing the mean left atrial pressure and the pulmonary capillary pressure. Now the patient is unable to increase cardiac output to meet the physiologic demands of exercise and develops fatigue. The elevated left atrial pressure and pulmonary capillary pressure cause dyspnea. With increasing left atrial pressure, there is the development of pulmonary hypertension and eventually, very late in the course, right heart failure.

Clinical Course

Chronic mitral insufficiency developing slowly can become very severe with regurgitant fractions of 50% to 80%, and with a very large dilated left ventricle and left atrium, but without the patient having any limitation of activity at all. Eventually, the left ventricle cannot maintain the large left ventricular stroke volume, and the left ventricular end-systolic and end-diastolic volume increase results in elevation of the left ventricular filling pressure. The patient begins to experience easy fatigability and dyspnea on exertion. Finally, orthopnea, paroxysmal nocturnal dyspnea, and pulmonary edema develop with pulmonary hypertension, and, ultimately, right ventricular failure.

The course of gradually developing mitral insufficiency can be very long indeed with the patient remaining asymptomatic for 10 to 20 years. In Rapaport's study,[37] survival at 5 years from the discovery of the lesion was 80% and at 10 years 60%, values similar to those of the patients with mitral stenosis. In patients with combined mitral stenosis and insufficiency survival was worse with 67% surviving 5 years and 30% surviving 10 years. Hammermeister et al,[87] in a study with patients characterized hemodynamically as having moderately severe mitral insufficiency, reported a survival of 55% at 5 years. There was a higher mortality with increased arteriovenous oxygen difference reflecting decreased forward effective cardiac output and increasing end-diastolic volume.[87]

The clinical picture may differ depending on the etiology of the mitral insufficiency. For instance, with infective endocarditis the patient usually has a febrile course and there may be embolic events or problems such as glomerulonephritis and petechiae related to immune complex injury to capillaries in the kidneys and skin.

Most patients with mitral valve prolapse are asymptomatic and the degree of mitral insufficiency remains minimal.[99,100,109] The course is usually benign although infective endocarditis is still a feared complication.[110] There is in many cases a familial tendency with a high incidence of mitral valve prolapse found in relatives such that the evidence suggests inheritance as a dominant characteristic.[111] Frequently, thoracic skeletal abnormalities are present such as a narrow anterior-posterior chest diameter, kyphoscoliosius, or pectus excavatum.[112] A variety of symptoms have been attributed to mitral valve prolapse including chest pain, usually atypical but occasionally typical for angina, palpitations, faintness, weakness, and shortness of breath in the absence of severe mitral insufficiency. Frequently there are ST-T wave changes in the diaphragmatic-lateral leads of the ECG. This clinical picture has been called the billowing mitral leaflet syndrome by Barlow[99] and Barlow's syndrome by everyone else. Whether these symptoms are related to abnormal sensitivity to catecholamines,[113] a dysautonomia, to an abnormal responsiveness to sympathetic stimulation,[114] or whether they are simply common problems seen in the population and for the most part unrelated to mitral valve prolapse is at present controversial.

What *is* seen in a very small proportion of patients who, after all, constitute 5% of the population, are certain complications.

1. Progression to severe mitral insufficiency with and without chordal rupture[110]
2. Infective endocarditis[115]
3. Arrhythmias, both ventricular and atrial; tachyarrhythmias, sinus node dysfunction, and atrioventricular block[116]
4. Sudden death[117]
5. Thromboembolic phenomena[118]

Since so many people have the underlying abnormality, even with a small proportion of the population progressing to severe mitral insufficiency, mitral valve prolapse represents one of the commonest etiologies for isolated severe mitral insufficiency. Infective endocarditis is again very unusual but it does constitute a danger requiring the physician to advise prophylactic antibiotics at the time of possible bacteremia. Arrhythmias of all varieties are described and are probably common in these persons. Most worrisome are the ventricular ectopic rhythms, especially in the unusual patient who has runs of ventricular tachycardia. Very rarely sudden death is seen in these patients. The last complication to be described has been that of thromboembolic phenomena, usually manifested as transient ischemic episodes or a cerebral vascular accident. The basis for emboli is probably the disruption of the endothelial lining of the atrial surface of the redundant valve with deposition of platelet aggregates and occasionally thrombi which can serve as a source of emboli.[119]

Physical Findings

With a small abnormal opening of the mitral valve during systole forming the regurgitant orifice, a jet of blood regurgitates into the left atrium creating a murmur, which begins with the high frequency component of the first heart sound and ends with the second heart sound. The regurgitant volume is small and propelled by a large gradient. Therefore the murmur is high-pitched and of similar intensity throughout systole, the so-called pansystolic or holosystolic murmur. The murmur is best heard at the apex. If the regurgitant volume is small, no abnormality in the left atrial pressure curve is seen.

With a larger regurgitant orifice and a large regurgitant volume the murmur is louder with lower frequency sounds. With a very large regurgitant volume there may be a short diastolic rumbling murmur just after A_2, the aortic component of the second heart sound, consistent with a large flow of blood into the left ventricle in early diastole. A third heart sound at the apex is also not unusual.

The duration of the murmur in systole depends on the time during systole when the regurgitant orifice is present. With rheumatic heart disease and leaflet retraction, the regurgitant orifice is present throughout systole and so there is a murmur throughout systole — a pansystolic murmur. With a prolapsed mitral valve, the regurgitant orifice may not develop until the ventricle has emptied significiantly and systole is well under way. In this case, the murmur starts after the first heart sound in mid- or late systole and may continue up to the second sound. In arteriosclerotic heart disease, the regurgitant orifice may be present only early in systole or in mid- or late systole. The murmur will therefore not be pansystolic in these cases.

With small amounts of mitral insufficiency the rhythm usually remains a sinus rhythm. Frequently, by the time mitral insufficiency becomes severe, because of the increase in left atrial pressure and dilatation of the left atrium, the patient develops atrial fibrillation.

The radiation of the murmur depends on the direction of the jet. If the jet into the left atrium is directed anteromedially, as it is with rupture of the chordae to the middle scallop of the posterior leaflet, the jet will impinge on the anterior interatrial septum which is just posterolateral to the aortic root. The murmur will then radiate well to the base and possibly be confused with the murmur of aortic stenosis.[120] If the jet is directed posterolaterally as it is with mitral insufficiency due to prolapse of the anterior leaflet, the murmur will be loudest at the apex and will radiate well to the axilla and left lung base. If the anterolateral commissure is insufficient, the jet will be directed posteromedially. With the left atrium against the spine, the murmur will radiate well to the left lung base and widely up and down the spine posteriorly.

With severe chronic mitral insufficiency, the left ventricular apex will be enlarged and displaced to the left and inferiorally. With palpation, there will be hyperactivity of the apex. With systole there can also be a forceful late systolic anterior movement of the precordium caused by the left atrium expanding against the spine and pushing the heart forward.

With pulmonary hypertension, there is an increase in the pulmonic component of the second heart sound and with right heart failure there is elevation of systemic venous pressure and signs of right heart failure.

Certain findings are common with specific etiologies of mitral insufficiency. For instance, the nonejection click–late systolic murmur is frequently seen in prolapsed mitral valve. Mitral insufficiency in the presence of fever should suggest infective endocarditis. A tall person with pectus excavatum or carinatum, wearing glasses with thick lenses, with long arms and legs, thin long fingers, and a high arched palate, possibly with a murmur of aortic insufficiency, suggests Marfan's syndrome.

Chest Roentgenogram

With mild mitral insufficiency the chest film is normal. As the regurgitant volume increases, the left ventricle and left atrium increase in size. The left ventricle as it enlarges dilates leftward and inferiorally with the left ventricular apex dipping below the diaphragm. The left atrium in severe mitral insufficiency is larger than in severe mitral stenosis. In fact, the largest left atria seen, where the cardiac silhouette touches the right chest wall, the so-called giant left atrium, is almost exclusively seen in severe mitral insufficiency. When left ventricular failure occurs the findings of pulmonary vascular redistribution, interstitial edema, and pulmonary edema are seen.

Calcification of the mitral valve, especially with rheumatic heart disease, is more commonly seen in mitral stenosis than in mitral insufficiency. Specific etiologies of mitral insufficiency can be suggested by radiologic findings. For instance, calcification of the mitral annulus and subannular areas can be seen in the chest film, especially the lateral view.[121] In Marfan's syndrome, a long chest, with long, thin bones and thoracic skeletal abnormalities such as pectus excavatum, may be seen.

Electrocardiogram

The ECG in minimal mitral insufficiency is usually within normal limits. With severe mitral insufficiency, the ECG shows voltage and ST-T wave changes consistent with left ventricular hypertrophy. Left atrial abnormality also occurs and eventually atrial fibrillation. With prolapsed mitral valve, isolated inferior-lateral ST-T wave changes have been described.

Echocardiography

Unlike mitral stenosis, echocardiography only inferentially suggests the presence of mitral insufficiency. Although it has been suggested that in rheumatic mitral regurgitation two-dimensional echocardiography can identify the presence of mitral insufficiency by showing failure of the leaflets to close completely, echocardiography has been most helpful in identifying the effects of severe mitral insufficiency on ventricular function and the size of the left ventricle and left atrium.[122] Since there is a large amount of blood returning to the left ventricle from the left atrium in diastole, there is frequently a wide excursion of the mitral leaflets. As long as contractility is normal there will be large excursions of the left ventricle in systole with a enlarged left ventricular diastolic diameter, a relatively normal end-systolic diameter, and an excellent ejection fraction. With ventricular failure, the end-systolic volume diameter increases and the ejection fraction decreases.

Echocardiography provides clues to the etiology of mitral insufficiency. For instance, with prolapsed mitral valve there is an abnormal posterior movement of the posterior and/or anterior leaflets during systole. This abnormal posterior motion can be pansystolic or late systolic.[123] There are also multiple echoes from the redundant leaflets seen on M-mode echocardiography. With rheumatic heart disease, the leaflets tend to be thickened and have increased echo density with perhaps some degree of mitral stenosis manifested by decrease of the e-f slope and similar anterior motion of the anterior and posterior leaflet during systole. With infective endocarditis the echo-dense, mobile vegetations on the mitral valve can at times be seen. With left atrial myxoma, the echo-dense myxoma can be seen to fall behind the anterior leaflet of the mitral valve during diastole. In Marfan's syndrome there are large mitral leaflets with large excursion, a wide left ventricular ostium, and a large aortic root, at times with diastolic vibrations of the mitral valve seen due to aortic insufficiency.

With mitral annular calcification there is an echo-dense mass behind the mural leaflet of the mitral valve which disappears abruptly as the echo beam sweeps from the left ventricle at the level of the mitral leaflets to the level of the aorta–left atrium.[121] With rupture of a chorda tendineae, there are marked excursions of the left ventricular cavity with coarse vibrations on one or both leaflets in diastole[124]; at times, echoes appear above the valve plane in the left atrium in systole.

Doppler ultrasound

Because the regurgitant flow occurs as a jet, Doppler ultrasound can detect abnormal regurgitant flow in the left atrium and therefore predict the presence of mitral insufficiency with a high degree of sensitivity[125,126] The only false-negative studies have occurred in mild mitral insufficiency with highly discrete jets. Unlike mitral stenosis, the gradient does not predict the severity of mitral insufficiency and therefore quantitation is poor with the Doppler technique.[127] Efforts have been made to judge how far posterior to the mitral valve the jet can be detected and to relate the distance to the severity of the mitral insufficiency.[128] Of importance is the fact that Doppler echocardiography can detect the presence of mitral regurgitation in the patient with a paraprosthetic valvular leak where the murmur may be unimpressive or even absent. Quinones et al[125] reported on 17 paraprosthetic leaks; 16 (94%) were correctly identified by the pulsed Doppler technique.

Radioisotope Evaluation

Determination of ejection fraction and left ventricular volumes in diastole and systole are all possible with the relatively noninvasive technique of radioactive labeling of the blood and blood-pool imaging. Ventricular volumes can be obtained either by geometric assumptions similar to those used to calculate volumes in angiocardiography, or more reliably, by using the principle that the counts within the total area of the left ventricle are proportional to the volume of blood in the ventricle. The ratio of the counts leaving the ventricle with each systole (stroke volume) to the number of counts in the ventricle at end diastole, with correction for background, is the ejection fraction. With correction for the concentration of counts per milliliter of blood, the ventricular volumes can be calculated.[129]

Taking care to eliminate as much as possible overlap with counts from the right and left atria, the right and left ventricles can be imaged in the left anterior oblique position and the right and left ventricular stroke volume ratios obtained. With mitral insufficiency the left ventricular stroke volume is greater than the right ventricular stroke volume, proportional to the magnitude of the regurgitant volume.[130] Ideally, in the normal person, the ratio of left ventricular to right ventricular stroke volume should be 1.0. In practice, because of some overlap with atrial counts, the ratio is 0.9 to 1.3 in normal controls.[131] Patients with mitral insufficiency have ratios significantly greater than 1.5. By this method, the severity of mitral insufficiency can be roughly quantitated. The degree of mitral regurgitation has been estimated by these radioisotope techniques and compared to regurgitant fractions obtained by standard angiocardiographic techniques. There was moderately good correlation between the two methods (r value = .70 to .86).[131,132]

Since these measurements are important in assessing left ventricular function, and are relatively noninvasive and can be repeated over the years, radioisotope studies have become useful in following some patients with mitral insufficiency in order to decide when catheterization should be performed.

Acute Mitral Insufficiency

What has been said so far refers to chronic mitral insufficiency. With acutely developing severe mitral insufficiency such as that seen with ruptured mitral valve with infective endocarditis and with a ruptured chord, a very different pathophysiology and therefore clinical picture occurs.[133] With sudden severe mitral insufficiency the regurgitant volume is suddenly added to the forward stroke volume and in the next diastole increases the left ventricular volume within a fibrous noncomplaint pericardium. The sudden increase in volume is resisted by the left ventricular myocardium and pericardium and so the left ventricular filling pressure rises suddenly and markedly. The regurgitant volume in systole suddenly increases the volume of the left atrium–pulmonary venous chamber, a structure which is relatively noncomplaint.[134] The "v" wave in systole is very high in severe acute mitral insufficiency, on the order of 40 to 70 mmHg. This approaches the pressure of the left ventricle in end systole and "ventricularizes" the left atrial pressure. Both systolic and diastolic left atrial pressures are increased and the mean left atrial–pulmonary capillary pressure is suddenly increased markedly. Pulmonary congestion and edema is early and frequent.

With sudden increases in left atrial pressure, there is a sudden increase in pulmonary artery pressure and consequently there is frequently right ventricular failure due to the marked increase in resistance to the right ventricular ejection. Another possible reason for right ventricular failure is the sudden increase in left ventricular volume in a tight pericardial sac. With increase in left ventricular volume, there is an increase in pericardial pressure and distortion of the interventricular septum, both of which change the filling characteristics of the right ventricle in diastole which raises right ventricular filling pressure.[135] Therefore, some of the increase in systemic venous pressure seen in acute mitral insufficiency may be the result of interference of diastolic filling of the right ventricle.

The clinical picture is also changed in acute mitral insufficiency. Because the left atrial pressure is suddenly increased in systole and approaches left ventricular pressure, the gradient

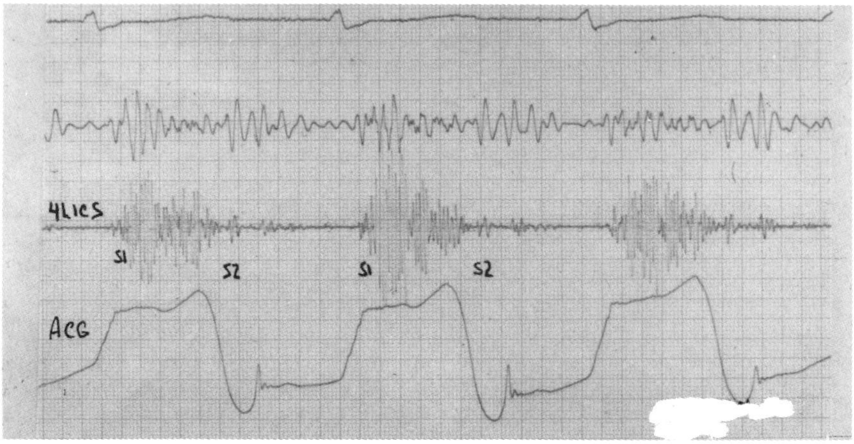

Figure 8-9 Phonocardiogram and apex cardiogram of a patient with perforated valve and acute mitral insufficiency with infective endocarditis. From top to bottom: ECG, phonocardiogram in fourth left intercostal space (4LICS) with low and medium frequency bands; and bottom, apex cardiogram (ACG). Note systolic murmur beginning with the first heart sound (S1) and decreasing, almost disappearing before the aortic component of the second heart sound (S2). Note the S3 gallop (unmarked) at the time of the sharp spike on the ACG marking the transition from the rapid to the slow filling phase. Note absence of P wave on ECG and "a" wave on ACG. There is also a short low frequency diastolic rumble after the S3.

between the left ventricle and left atrium decreases and the murmur frequently decreases toward the end of systole (Figure 8-9).[136] The murmur remains pansystolic and is usually loud — frequently loud enough to cause a systolic apical thrill. If left ventricular function is decreased or the regurgitant orifice large enough so that little turbulence results from the regurgitant flow, the murmur may be soft or even absent.[137]

The left ventricle and left atrium are increased in size only by the amount of the regurgitant volume. The left ventricle therefore is not markedly dilated but the point of maximum impulse (PMI) is frequently very forceful and hyperactive due to the large left ventricular stroke volume. At the same time, the effective stroke volume is often decreased because of the large regurgitant volume. Thus, in the face of a hyperkinetic apex, there is a rapidly rising but small-volume carotid arterial pulse.

Since the left atrium is not severely dilated, the rhythm is usually a normal sinus rhythm. Since the left ventricular end-diastolic pressure is high, with atrial systole a fourth heart sound is frequent,[138] as is a short early diastolic rumble and a third heart sound, both of which are related to the increased flow across the mitral valve during early diastole. Signs of pulmonary hypertension including a palpable P_2, a right ventricular precordial thrust, and murmurs of pulmonary valve insufficiency and tricuspid valve insufficiency are not uncommon.

The chest film may not show obvious left ventricular and left atrial enlargement. Enlargement, however, can be seen if the heart is compared to the preacute mitral insufficiency film if one is available. (See Figure 8-10) With a relatively normal size heart, pulmonary congestion and even pulmonary edema is seen.

The ECG is frequently not abnormal, left ventricular hypertrophy is not common early, and frequently only ST-T wave changes are seen. Left atrial abnormality may or may not be present and the patient, as previously stated, is usually in normal sinus rhythm.

The echocardiogram shows a mildly dilated left ventricle and left atrium usually with a large excursion of the left ventricle in systole. With chordal rupture, echoes in the left atrium above the valve plane in systole can frequently be seen, with vibration of the unsupported portion of the anterior or mural leaflet in diastole or at times in systole. With infective endocarditis, vegetations causing echo densities moving with mitral leaflets

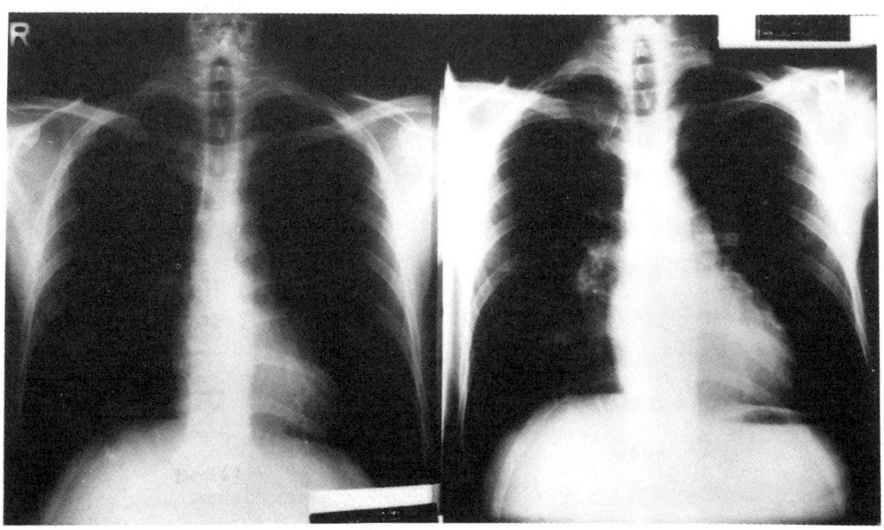

Figure 8-10 A 32-year-old man with perforation of the anterior leaflet of the mitral valve from *Staphylococcus aureus* endocarditis.
Right: Posteroanterior chest film after treatment for pulmonary congestion. Note prominent main pulmonary artery segment and prominent left ventricle. The overall heart size does not appear to be markedly enlarged.
Left: Posteroanterior chest film of same patient almost 3 years before endocarditis and mitral valve perforation. Heart size is considerably smaller than after valve perforation. Comparing the two films it is now obvious that the left ventricle and main pulmonary artery segment are markedly enlarged compared to the film before perforation.

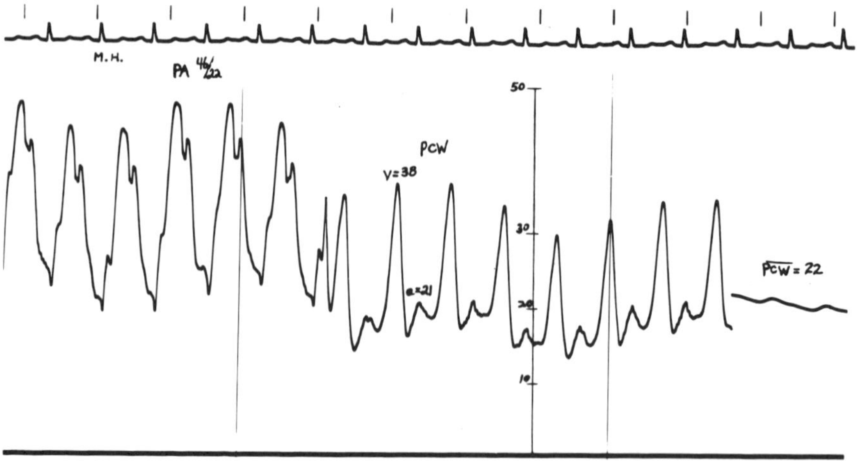

Figure 8-11 Pressure curves from a patient with severe chronic mitral insufficiency. Left portion of the pressure curve shows pulmonary artery pressure (PA) of 46/22 mmHg. The right portion of the curve shows the catheter wedged and the pressure curve changing subtly to a pulmonary artery wedge (PAW) with a "V" wave of 38 mmHg and an "a" wave of 21 mmHg. Mean pulmonary capillary pressure (PCW) is 22 mmHg. Although the two curves look similar and can be confused, note the difference in the sharp upstroke at the time of the QRS in the PA curve and the late upstroke after the QRS of the "v" wave.

but frequently more mobile with greater excursion can be seen.[124]

Catheterization and Angiocardiography

Cardiac catheterization is at present the gold standard for assessing the severity of mitral insufficiency and its effect on cardiac function. Left atrial pressures can be obtained by entering the left atrium through a patent foramen ovale, from the right atrium, or by puncture of the atrial septum by a long needle, the transseptal or Brockenbrough technique. More often, reflected left atrial pressure is obtained by pulmonary capillary wedge pressures. In mitral insufficiency with a normally functioning left ventricle, the x-descent is decreased since the "v" wave begins earlier than it does normally (Figure 8-11) The "v" wave is abnormally high. The height of the "v" wave depends not only on the magnitude of regurgitation but also on the compliance of the left atrium–pulmonary venous chamber. With sudden acute mitral insufficiency and a relatively small left atrium, the "v" wave may be 40 to 70 mmHg and with chronic mitral insufficiency and a dilated left atrium, the "v" wave may be 15 to 40 mmHg or even normal in the face of severe mitral insufficiency.[133]

With a competent left ventricle the left atrial mean pressure may not be markedly elevated, even with a 30-mmHg "v" wave since diastolic pressures are still low. With left ventricular failure, the diastolic left atrial pressure rises, the mean pressure rises, and pulmonary hypertension can occur. This is usually passive, but in patients with failure there can be elevation of pulmonary vascular resistance. Finally right heart failure occurs with elevation in the right ventricular diastolic and right atrial mean pressures.

In acute mitral insufficiency, severe elevation in left atrial mean pressure and large "v" waves are common. In fact the "v" wave can be so high that the pressure wave reflected back into the pulmonary artery results in a rise in pulmonary artery pressure in early diastole after the pulmonary valve has closed. It can also cause early closure of the pulmonary valve. This results in the peculiar finding of a higher pulmonary artery diastolic pressure than right ventricular systolic pressure.

Angiocardiographic measurement of the left ventricular volume in systole and diastole as well as ejection fraction and measurements of midwall left ventricular stress are possible. With high-fidelity end-tipped transducer catheters it is possible to construct pressure–volume loops. These studies are usually reserved for research and are not useful in clinical practice since they are time-consuming and at present add little to clinical management.

The quantification of mitral insufficiency can be graded in several ways.[133,139,140] The usual

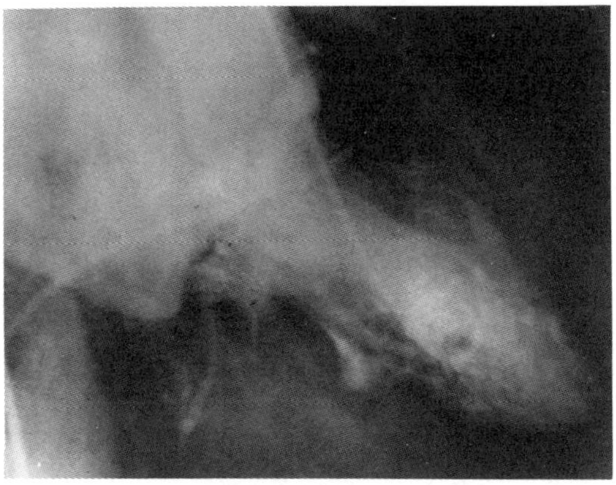

Figure 8-12 Cineangiogram in the 30-degree right anterior oblique position. Injection is in the left ventricle. The patient is a 45-year-old woman with severe mitral insufficiency. At surgery the mitral valve was myxomatous and redundant. Notice the large densely opacified left atrium. The contrast was seen to reflux into the pulmonary veins (not seen in this frame) indicating 4+ mitral regurgitation.

technique is by injection of a radiographic contrast agent into the left ventricle in the 30-degree right anterior oblique position with estimation of the severity of the regurgitated contrast into the left atrium (Figure 8-12). The severity of the regurgitation is graded from 1+ to 4+ with 1+ signifying a jet of contrast into the left atrium that disappears with the next diastole, and 4+ signifying that the entire left atrium is filled within several beats equal in opacity to the left ventricle. Usually in these patients systolic regurgitation into the pulmonary veins can be seen.

This classification of severity is the usual method for quantifying mitral insufficiency. It is possible using calculation of angiographic left ventricular volume in diastole and systole to calculate the total left ventricular stroke volume. The effective forward stroke volume can be calculated according to the Fick principle or by thermodilution techniques. By subtracting the effective forward stroke volume from the total left ventricular stroke volume, the regurgitant volume can be calculated, and expressed in millimeters per square meter surface area or, more frequently, as the fraction of total left ventricular stroke volume — the regurgitant fraction. The problem with this type of calculation is that the forward effective stroke volume and total left ventricular stroke volume are calculated by different methods and, in general, calculation of the regurgitant fraction is not very useful in clinical practice.

Other important information can be obtained by angiocardiography depending on the etiology of the mitral insufficiency.[141] For instance, prolapse of specific parts of the mitral valve can be seen and located precisely. In mitral insufficiency related to coronary disease, the extent of coronary disease and the presence and severity of regional wall motion abnormalities can be assessed. In left atrial myxoma causing mitral insufficiency, the tumor can be visualized.

Treatment

The asymptomatic patient with mitral insufficiency may need no treatment with the exception of prophylactic antibiotics at times of possible bacteremia to prevent infective endocarditis. In the workup of the patient with mitral insufficiency it is most important to identify the severity of the mitral insufficiency and the effect on the patient in terms of symptoms and left ventricular function. In certain cases it is obviously essential to identify the etiology of mitral insufficiency. For instance, it is of minor consequence as far as treatment is concerned whether the mitral insufficiency is secondary to rheumatic heart disease or to mitral valve prolapse. Here the severity of the mitral insufficiency is the main concern although there are differences in the natural history of the lesion. On the other hand, even a minor degree of mitral insufficiency caused by infective endocarditis is important, not because of the mitral insufficiency but because the infective endocarditis must be treated promptly and appropriately if the patient is to survive with the least disability.

As the patient becomes symptomatic, support of left ventricular function can be encouraged by use of digitalis, and a decrease in left atrial and pulmonary capillary pressure obtained by diuretics and preload reducing agents such as nitrates. With severe mitral insufficiency, especially acute mitral insufficiency with heart failure, both preload reduction dropping left atrial pressure, and afterload reduction decreasing peripheral vascular resistance and regurgitant fraction, can be achieved by the use of nitroprusside.[142,143] Impressive decreases in left atrial pressure and magnitude of the "v" wave and increase in effective forward stroke volume can be obtained. Whether chronic afterload reduction using hydralazine hydrochloride or other drugs will be helpful is questionable and is currently being investigated.[144,145]

In examining the factors related to the magnitude of the regurgitant volume, which is the most important factor leading to hemodynamic difficulty, it is helpful to rearrange the Gorlin equation.

$$RV \propto RA \times \sqrt{LVs - LAs} \times RP$$

Where RV = regurgitant volume. RA = regurgitant area. RP = regurgitant period. LVs = left ventricular pressure in systole, LA = left atrial pressure in systole. From this relationship it is obvious that although decreasing left ventricular systolic pressure will reduce the gradient, the decrease in regurgitant volume is only minimal. It would be more effective to decrease the regurgitant orifice area since this is related directly to the regurgitant volume. Yoran et al[146,147] have suggested in an animal model that preload reduction with nitroprusside does actually decrease the regurgitant orifice area by decreasing the left ventricular diastolic size, making the left ventricular ostium smaller and therefore allowing greater coaptation of the mitral leaflets. Since most etiologies of mitral insufficiency involve the contact surfaces of the valve leaflets, greater coaptation may well reduce the regurgitant orifice area.

In general, when a patient goes to surgery for mitral insufficiency, it must be assumed that a prosthetic valve will be needed. There are exceptions to this rule; for instance, in mitral valve prolapse, plication and resection of the redundant scallop with or without annuloplasty has been successful.[148,149] Similarly, Gerbode et al[150] have shown that valvuloplasty with plication of the unsupported portion of the leaflet in chordal rupture is successful in eliminating mitral insufficiency. When the primary problem is dilation of the mitral annulus, good long-term results have been obtained with annuoplasty and insertion of a Carpentier ring.[151–153] With technical improvements in mitral reconstruction, such operations will become more frequent and valve replacement less so.

In most cases, however, valvuloplasty is usually considered not feasible and mitral valve replacement is necessary. For this reason we believe that the patient with mitral insufficiency should be in functional class III (symptomatic on ordinary activity) on good medical management before considering valve replacement. Since most patients with valvular replacement will become functional class I or II patients, there is no question that such patients are benefited by the surgery.[148,152,154,155]

Recently there has been concern that in mitral insufficiency left ventricular contractility might decrease irreversibly while global pump function appeared to be well preserved. Since mitral insufficiency is a volume overload lesion, the left ventricular stroke volume is supported by an increase in left ventricular volume, thus compensating for a decrease in contractility. Also, because of the low resistance sink into which the left ventricle empties starting immediately with the onset of systole, the left ventricular afterload is reduced and the stroke volume and therefore the ejection fraction may be preserved as left ventricular contractility decreases.[106,107,156]

Ross[157] has indicated that in mitral insufficiency, unlike any other valve lesion, when the mitral valve is replaced and the ventricle must generate an isovolumic contraction, the left ventricular wall tension is increased and the ejection fraction is immediately decreased compared to the ejection fraction before mitral insufficiency was eliminated.[157]

Because the pump function in mitral insufficiency is supported as contractility decreases, there have been many attempts to evaluate changes in contractility separate from the preload and afterload effects. From the study of isolated heart preparations and pressure–volume loops Suga and Sagawa[158] have demonstrated that if contractility remains constant, that ventricular systolic pressure at any constant time bears a linear relationship to the corresponding volume. Therefore, for any given ventricle the end-systolic pressure–volume point falls on a line independent of the preload and the afterload. As contractility decreases, the slope of this line decreases and shifts rightward where for a given end-systolic pressure the end-systolic volume is increased.

According to this concept, as ventricular contractility decreases, the volume at end systole would increase, the end-diastolic volume would increase through the Frank-Starling mechanism to maintain stroke volume, and the ejection fraction would fall. Recently it has been shown that the evaluation of end-systolic pressure–volume relationships in man can be measured invasively with angiocardiography[159] and estimated noninvasively using echocardiographic and radioisotope volume techniques.[160–163] This has made it practical to attempt to evaluate the status of left ventricular contractility in patients with mitral insufficiency in order to identify those patients who would not improve or do poorly after valve replacement.[160,163] The goal is to find some measure of contractility that is noninvasive and can be used to follow a patient with mitral insufficiency serially. This approach is at present under active investigation, and its practical clinical importance remains to be proved by prospective studies.

For these reasons it is important to watch the patient for signs of increasing left ventricular end-diastolic volume, increasing end-systolic volume, or decreasing ejection fraction by roentgenographic, echocardiographic, or radioisotopic studies. If a trend occurs with progressive changes, then even in functional class II patients, mitral valve replacement should be considered. Certainly the ejection fraction should not be allowed to fall below 50% without consideration of mitral valve replacement.[157]

There has been a great deal written about the "asymptomatic" or mildly symptomatic patient who has had marked irreversible decrease in left ventricular contractility with apparently preserved left ventricular function and who does poorly after valve replacement because the physician waited too long to replace the valve.[160,163,164]

Borow et al[163] looked retrospectively at the preoperative left ventricular end-diastolic volume, end-systolic volume, and ejection fraction in an attempt to find the point at which the patient would not do well with surgery or, surviving surgery, would have a shortened survival due to unremittant congestive heart failure. Using postoperative M-mode echocardiography and percent left ventricular diameter change as a measure of systolic function, they showed that with increasing left ventricular end-diastolic volume, increasing end-systolic volume, and decreasing ejection fraction, there was progressively poorer postoperative function in those who survived the surgery and greater mortality at and after surgery. In their study a left ventricular end-systolic volume greater than 60 mL/m^2 predicted a poor result.[163] Schuler et al,[164] using M-mode echocardiograpy, showed that with a left ventricular end-diastolic chord greater than 7.0 cm, an end-systolic dimension greater than 5.0 cm, and a low normal or depressed ejection fraction, that postoperatively the ejection fraction fell markedly and the chamber dilatation and hypertrophy persisted.

There are studies that suggest that most patients with mitral insufficiency can be followed safely until functional class III before surgery is recommended. *Salomon* et al[153] reported on 897 consecutive patients with mitral valve replacement, half with mitral stenosis and half with mitral insufficiency. Ninety percent of these patients were functional class III and IV patients. If we presume that left ventricular function was normal in the mitral stenosis patients, it is of interest to compare the follow-up mortality in patients with mitral valve replacement for mitral stenosis with those for mitral insufficiency. When this is done mitral insufficiency patients had a higher mortality than the mitral stenosis patients over 5 to 10 years. However, on closer examination, the mitral stenosis patients all had rheumatic heart disease as the etiology whereas the mitral insufficiency patients were of several etiologies: rheumatic heart disease, prolapsed mitral valve, infective endocarditis, and arteriosclerotic heart disease. When the patients with mitral insufficiency are separated by etiology, the reason for the poor survival becomes apparent: patients with mitral insufficiency and arteriosclerotic heart disease had a poor survival. If the coronary artery disease patients are removed, patients with mitral valve prolapse and rheumatic heart disease had the same good survivel as those with mitral stenosis and presumably normal left ventricular function. It therefore appears that in those patients, 90% of whom were in functional class III or IV, that there was no inordinately great loss from congestive heart failure on follow-up and that in these patients the physician did not wait too long before surgical intervention.

In a report by Phillips et al,[155] 105 patients had mitral valve replacement for relief of isolated mitral insufficiency. There were no asymptomatic patients, 20% were functional class II patients, and the rest were functional class III or IV patients. Operative mortality was 4% and there were 12 late deaths, giving an 82% predicted 5-year survival. Of the 12 late deaths, five died suddenly and three had preoperative ejection fractions less than 40%. Only two died of congestive heart failure. One had a preoperative ejection fraction of 57% but this patient had a paravalvular leak and was 77 years old with severe noncardiac medical problems. The only other patient who died in congestive failure had a preoperative ejection fraction of 18%. The only preoperative predictors in this study correlating with decreased survival at 3 to 5 years postoperatively were aged 60 years and over with an ejection fraction of less than 40%.

These studies also suggest that it is rarely necessary to operate an asymptomatic patients with mitral insufficiency and that most patients can be safely followed until they are in functional class III on treatment before recommending valve replacement. It is our opinion, however, that if systolic pump function declines progressively as manifested by increasing end-diastolic or end-systolic volumes or decreasing ejection fraction, surgery should be considered in functional class II patients.

REFERENCES

1. Perloff JK, Roberts WC: The mitral apparatus: functional anatomy of mitral regurgitation. *Circulation* 1972;46:227–239.
2. Roberts WC: Morphologic features of the normal and abnormal mitral valve. *Am J Cardiol* 1983; 51:1005–1028.
3. Silverman ME, Hurst JW: The mitral complex. *Am Heart J* 1968;76:399–418.
4. Ranganathan N, Lam JHC, Wigle ED, et al: Morphology of the human mitral valve. II. The valve leaflets. *Circulation* 1970;41:459–467.
5. Lam JHC, Ranganathan N, Wigle ED, et al: Morphology of the human mitral valve. I. Chordae tendineae: a new classification. *Circulation* 1970;41:449–458.
6. Guthrie RB, Edwards JE: Pathology of the myxomatous mitral valve. *Minn Med* 1976; 59:637–639.
7. Ruchman RN, Van Praagh R: Anatomic types of congenital mitral stenosis: report of 49 autopsy cases with consideration of diagnosis and surgical implications. *Am J Cardiol* 1978;42:592–601.
8. Hammer WJ, Roberts WC, deLeon AC Jr: "Mitral stenosis" secondary to combined "massive" mitral annular calcific deposits and small, hypertrophied left ventricle, hemodynamic documentation in four patients. *Am J Med* 1978; 64:371–376.
9. McAllister HA, Fenoglio JJ: Cardiac involvement in Whipples's disease. *Circulation* 1975; 52:152–156.
10. Rose AG: Mitral stenosis in Whipple's disease. *Thorax* 1978;33:500–503.
11. Roberts WC, Sjoerdsma A: The cardiac disease associated with the carcinoid syndrome (cardinoide heart disease). *Am J Med* 1986;36:5–34.
12. Staub NC, Nagano H, Pearce ML: Pulmonary edema in dogs, specifically the sequence of fluid accumulation in lungs. *J Appl Physiol* 1967; 22:227–240.
13. Reed JW, Ablett M, Cotes JE: Ventilatory responses to exercise and to carbon dioxide in mitral stenosis before and after valvulotomy: causes of tachypnea. *Clin Sci Mol Med* 1978; 54:9–16.
14. Cortese DA: Pulmonary function in mitral stenosis. *Mayo Clin Proc* 1978;53:321–326.
15. Staub NC: Pulmonary edema. *Physiol Rev* 1974; 54:678–811.
16. Friedman WF, Braunwald E: Alternations in regional pulmonary blood flow in mitral valve disease studied by radioisotope scanning. *Circulation* 1966;34:363–376.
17. Giuntini C, Mariani M, Barsotti A, et al: Factors affecting regional pulmonary blood flow in left heart valvular disease. *Am J Med* 1974; 57:421–436.
18. Pain MCF, Bucens D, Cade JF, et al: Regional lung function in patients with mitral stenosis. *Aust NZ J Med* 1972;3:228.
19. Grose R, Strain J, Yipintosoi T: Right ventricular function in valvular heart disease in relation to pulmonary artery pressure. *J Am Coll Cardiol* 1983;2:225–232.
20. Gorlin R, Gorlin G: Hydraulic formula for calculation of area of stenotic mitral valve, other valves, and central circulatory shunts. *Am Heart J* 1951;41:1–29.
21. Dubin AA, March HW, Cohn K, et al: Longitudinal hemodynamic and clinical study of mitral stenosis. *Circulation* 1971;44:381–389.
22. Feinstein AR, Spagnuolo M: The clinical patterns of acute rheumatic fever: a reappraisal. *Medicine* 1962;41:279–305.
23. Tendon R, Potti S, Mathur VS, et al: Critical mitral stenosis in children. *Indian Pediatr* 1972; 9:171–173.
24. Feinstein AR, Dimassa R: Prognostic significance of valvular involvement in acute rheumatic fever. *N Engl J Med* 1959;260:1001–1007.
25. Rowe JC, Bland F, Sprague HB, et al: Course of mitral stenosis without surgery: ten and twenty year perspectives. *Ann Intern Med* 1960; 52:741–749.
26. Kalmanson D, Veyrat C, Bernier A, et al: Opening snap and isovolumic relaxation period in relation to mitral valve flow in patients with mitral stenosis: significance of the A2-0S interval. *Br Heart J* 1976;38:135–146.
27. Lees MM, Taylor SH, Scott DB, et al: A study of cardiac output at rest throughout pregnancy. *J Obstetr Gynec Br Comm* 1967;74:319–328.
28. Stott DK, Marpole DGF, Bristow JD, et al: The role of left atrial transport in aortic and mitral stenosis. *Circulation* 1970;41:1031–1041.
29. Yamaguchi T, Matsuda M, Umeda T, et al: Echocardiographic evaluation of left ventricular filling in mitral stenosis. Role of atrial contraction. *Jpn Heart J* 1978;19:698–711.
30. Thompson ME, Shaver JA, Leon DF: Effect of tachycardia on atrial transport in mitral stenosis. *Am Heart J* 1977;94:297–306.
31. Diamond MA, Genovese PD: Life-threatening hemoptysis in mitral stenosis: emergency mitral valve replacement resulting in rapid sustained sensation of pulmonary bleedings. *JAMA* 1971; 215:441–444.
32. Ferguson FC, Kobilak RE, Deitrick JE: Varices of the bronchial veins as a source of hemoptysis in mitral stenosis. *Am Heart J* 1944;28:445–456.
33. Sharma NGK, Kapoor CP, Hahambre L, et al: Ortner's syndrome. *J Indian Med Assoc* 1973; 60:427–431.
34. Olesen KH: The natural history of 271 patients with mitral stenosis under medical treatment. *Br Heart J* 1962;24:349–357.
35. Wood P: Congenital heart disease: A review of its clinical aspects in the light of experience gained by means of modern techniques. *Br Med J* 1950;2:693–698.
36. Munoz S, Gallardo J, Diaz-Gorrin JR, et al: Influence of surgery on the natural history of rheumatic mitral and aortic valve disease. *Am J*

Cardiol 1975;35:234–242.
37. Rapaport E: Natural history of aortic and mitral valve disease. *Am J Cardiol* 1975;35:221–227.
38. Chen JTT, Behar VS, Morris JJ Jr, et al: Correlation of roentgen findings with hemodynamic data in pure mitral stenosis. *Am J Roentgenol Radium Ther Nucl Med* 1968;102:280–292.
39. Carmichael JHE, Julian DG, Jones GP, et al: Radiological signs in pulmonary hypertension: the significance of lines B of Kerley. *Br J Radiol* 1954;27:393–397.
40. Moore CB, Kraus WL, Dock DS, et al: The relationship between pulmonary arterial pressure and roentgenographic appearances in mitral stenosis. *Am Heart J* 1959;58:576–581.
41. Milne ENC: Physiological interpretation of the plain radiograph in mitral stenosis, including a review of criteria for the radiological estimation of pulmonary arterial and venous pressures. *Br J Radiol* 1963;36:902–913.
42. Abedin Z, Bidwai PS, Khattri HN: Clinical, electrocardiographic and radiological evaluation of pulmonary hypertension in patients with mitral stenosis. *Jpn Heart J* 1977;18:765–776.
43. Rios JC, Goo W: Electrocardiographic correlates of rheumatic valvular disease, in Likoff W (ed): *Cardiovascular Clinics. Valvular Heart Disease.* Philadelphia, FA Davis Co, 1973 vol 5, No. 2, p 248.
44. Pridie RB, Oakley CM: Echocardiographic evaluation of the mitral valve. *Prog Cardiovasc Dis* 1978;21:92–118.
45. Fisher ML, Parisi AF, Plotnick GD, et al: Assessment of severity of mitral stenosis by echocardiographic leaflet separation. *Arch Intern Med* 1979;139:402–406.
46. Dabestani A, Skorton DJ, Child JS, et al: Mitral valve A wave and mitral stenosis. *J Clin Ultrasound* 1981;9:91–95.
47. Shiu MF, Jenkins BS, Webb-Peploe MM. Echocardiographic analysis of posterior mitral leaflet movement in mitral stenosis. *Br Heart J* 1978; 40:372–376.
48. Henry WL, Kastl DG: Echocardiographic evaluation of patients with mitral stenosis. *Am J Med* 1977;62:813–816.
49. Zanolla L, Marino P, Nicolosi GL, et al: Two-dimensional echocardiographic evaluation of mitral valve calcification sensitivity and specificity. *Chest* 1982;82:154–157.
50. Come PC, Riley MF: M mode and cross-sectional echocardiographic recognition of fibrosis and calcification of the mitral valve chordae and left ventricular papillary muscles. *Am J Cardiol* 1982;49:461–466.
51. Nichol PM, Golbert BW, Kisslo JA: Two-dimensional echocardiographic assessment of mitral stenosis. *Circulation* 1977;55:120–128.
52. Nicolosi GL, Atkins F, Dunn M: Echocardiographic evaluation of mitral stenosis in predicting mitral valve replacement vs. commissurotomy. Relation to hemodynamic measurements. *Chest* 1980;77:147–154.
53. Schweizer P, Bardos P, Krebs W, et al: Morphometric investigations in mitral stenosis using two dimensional echocardiography. *Br Heart J* 1982; 48:54–60.
54. Hatle L, Brubakk A, Tromsdale A, et al: Non-invasive assessment of pressure drop in mitral stenosis by Doppler ultrasound. *Br Heart J* 1978; 40:131–140.
55. Holen J, Aaslid R, Landmark K, et al: Determination of pressure gradient in mitral stenosis with a non-invasive ultrasound Doppler technique. *Acta Med Scand* 1976;199:455–460.
56. Holen J, Simonsen S: Determination of pressure gradient in mitral stenosis with Doppler echocardiography. *Br Heart J* 1979;41:529–535.
57. Knutsen KM, Bae EA, Sivertssen E, et al: Doppler ultrasound in mitral stenosis. *Acta Med Scand* 1982;211:433–436.
58. McDonald IG: Echocardiographic assessment of left ventricular function in mitral valve disease. *Circulation* 1976;53:865–871.
59. Ibrahim MM: Left ventricular function in rheumatic mitral stenosis. Clinical echocardiographic study. *Br Heart J* 1979;42:514–520.
60. Ahmed SS, Regan TJ, Fiore JJ, et al: The state of the left ventricular myocardium in mitral stenosis. *Am Heart J* 1977;94:28–36.
61. Gash AK, Carabello BA, Cepin D, et al: Left ventricular ejection performance and systolic muscle function in patients with mitral stenosis. *Circulation* 1983;67:148–154.
62. Effron MK, Alderman EL, Popp RL: Preoperative invasive testing in mitral stenosis: indications based on assessment of diagnostic yield. *Am J Cardiol* 1983;51:1116–1121.
63. Chun PKC, Gertz E, Davia JE, et al: Coronary atherosclerosis in mitral stenosis. *Chest* 1982; 81:36–41.
64. Meister SG, Engel TR, Feitosa GS, et al: Propranolol in mitral stenosis during sinus rhythm. *Am Heart J* 1977;94:685–688.
65. American Heart Association, Committee on Rheumatic Fever and Bacterial Endocarditis: Prevention of rheumatic fever. *Circulation* 1984; 70:1118A–1122A.
66. Shuman ST, Amren DP, Bisno AL, et al: Prevention of bacterial endocarditis. *Circulation* 1984;70:1123A–1127A.
67. Abernathy WS, Willis PW: Thromboembolic complications of rheumatic heart disease. *Cardiovasc Clin* 1973;5:132–175.
68. Fleming HA, Bailey SM: Mitral valve disease, systemic embolism and anticoagulants. *Postgrad Med J* 1971;47:599–604.
69. Neilson EH, Gales EG, Hossack KF: Thrombembolic complications of mitral valve disease. *Aust NZ J Med* 1978;8:372–376.
70. Souttar HS: The surgical treatment of mitral stenosis. *Br Med J* 1925;2:603–606.
71. Bailey CP: The surgical treatment of mitral stenosis (mitral commissurotomy). *Dis Chest* 1949;15:377–397.
72. Harken DE, Ellis LB, Ware PF, et al: The surgical treatment of mitral stenosis: I valvuloplasty. *N Engl J Med* 1948;239:801–809.
73. Houseman LB, Bonchek LI, Lambert L, et al: Prognosis of patients after open mitral commissurotomy. *J Thorac Cardiovasc Surg* 1977; 73:742–745.
74. Montoya A, Mulet J, Piffare R, et al: The advantages of open mitral commissurotomy for

mitral stenosis. *Chest* 1979;75:131–135.
75. John S, Bashi VV, Jairaj PS, et al: Closed mitral valvotomy: early results and long-term follow-up of 3724 consecutive patients. *Circulation* 1983; 68:891–896.
76. Bonchek LI: Current status of mitral commissurotomy: indications, techniques and results. *Am J Cardiol* 1983;52:411–415.
77. Smith WM, Neutze JM, Barratt-Boyes BG, et al: Open mitral valvotomy: effect of preoperative factors on results. *J Thorac Cardiovasc Surg* 1981;82:738–751.
78. Halseth WL, Elliott DP, Walker EL, et al: Open mitral commissurotomy: a modern re-evaluation. *J Thorac Cardiovasc Surg* 1980;80:842–848.
79. Bonchek LI: Indications for surgery of the mitral valve. *Am J Cardiol* 1980;46:155–158.
80. Laschinger JC, Cunningham JN Jr, Baumann FG, et al: Early open radical commisurotomy: surgical treatment of choice for mitral stenosis. *Ann Thorac Surg* 1982;34:287–298.
81. Vega JL, Fleitas M, Martinez R, et al: Open mitral commissurotomy. *Ann Thorac Surg* 1981; 31:266–270.
82. Chaffin JS, Daggett WM: Mitral valve replacement: a nine-year follow-up of risks and survivals. *Ann Thorac Surg* 1979;27:312–319.
83. Teply J, Grunkemeier G, Sutherland HD, et al: The ultimate prognosis after valve replacement: an assessment at 20 years. *Ann Thorac Surg* 1981;32:111–119.
84. Rahimtoola SH: The problem of valve prosthesis — patient mismatch. *Circulation* 1978;58:20–24.
85. Rahimtools SH: Valvular heart disease: a perspective. *J Am Coll Cardiol* 1983;1:199–215.
86. Barnhorst DA, Oxman HA, Connolly DC, et al: Long-term follow-up of isolated replacement of the aortic or mitral valve with the Starr-Edwards prosthesis. *Am J Cardiol* 1975;35:228–233.
87. Hammermeister KE, Fisher L, Kennedy JW, et al: Prediction of late survival in patients with mitral valve disease from clinical, hemodynamic and quantitative angiographic variables. *Circulation* 1978;57:341–349.
88. Procacci PM, Savran SV, Schreiter SL, et al: Prevalence of clinical mitral valve prolapse in 1,169 young women. *N Engl J Med* 1976; 294:1086–1088.
89. Davies MJ, Moore BP, Baimbridge MV: The floppy mitral valve. Study of incidence, pathology and complications in surgical, necropsy and forensic material. *Br Heart J* 1978;40:468–481.
90. Balu V, Hershowitz S, Zaki Masud AR, et al: Mitral regurgitation in coronary artery disease. *Chest* 1982;81:550–555.
91. Gahl K, Sutton R, Pearson M, et al: Mitral regurgitation in coronary heart disease. *Br Heart J* 1977;39:13–18.
92. Rostad H, Hall KV, Froysaker T: Mitral insufficiency following myocardial infarction. *Scand J Thorac Cardiovasc Surg* 1979;13:277–279.
93. Selzer A, Kelly JJ, Vannitamby M, et al: The syndrome of mitral insufficiency due to isolated rupture of the chordae tendineae. *Am J Med* 1967;43:822–836.
94. Chandraratne PAN, Aronow WS: Incidence of ruptured chordae tendineae in mitral valvular prolapse syndrome. *Chest* 1979;75:334–339.
95. Schott CR, Kotler MN, Parry WR, et al: Mitral annular calcification. Clinical and echocardiographic correlations. *Arch Intern Med* 1977; 137:1143–1150.
96. Savage DD, Garrison RJ, Castelli WP, et al: Prevalence of submitral (annular) calcium and its correlates in a seneral population-based sample (The Framinsham Study) *Am J Cardiol* 1983; 51:1375–1378.
97. Silverman ME, Hurst JW: The mitral complex: clues to its afflictions, in Likoff W (ed): *Cardiovascular Clinics. Valvular Heart Disease.* Philadelphia, FA Davis Co, 1973, vol 5, No. 2, pp 35–64.
98. DiSegni E, Edwards JE: Cleft anterior leaflet of the mitral valve with intact septa. A study of 20 cases. *Am J Cardiol* 1983;51:919–926.
99. Barlow JB, Pocock WA: Mitral valve prolapse, the specific billowing mitral leaflet syndrome or an insignificant non-ejection systolic click. *Am Heart J* 1979;97:277–185.
100. Devereaux RB, Perloff JK, Reickek N, et al: Mitral valve prolapse. *Circulation* 1976;54:3–14.
101. Burch GE, Depasquale NP, Phillips JH: The syndrome of papillary muscle dysfunction. *Am Heart J* 1968;75:399–415.
102. DeBusk RF, Harrison DC: The clinical spectrum of papillary muscle disease. *N Engl J Med* 1969; 281:1458–1467.
103. Selzer A, Katayama F: Mitral regurgitation: clinical patterns, pathophysiology and natural history. *Medicine* 1972;51:337–366.
104. Braunwald E: Mitral regurgitation: Physiological, clinical and surgical correlations. *N Engl J Med* 1969;281:425–433.
105. Bolen JL, Alderman EL: Ventriculographic and hemodynamic features of mitral regurgitation of cardiomyopathic, rheumatic, and nonrheumatic etiology. *Am J Cardiol* 1977;39:177–183.
106. Urschel CW, Covell JW, Sonnenblick EH, et al: Myocardial mechanics in aortic and valvular regurgitation: The concept of instantaneous impedance as a determinant of the performance of the intact heart. *J Clin Invest* 1968;47:867–883.
107. Eckberg DL, Gault JH, Bouchard RL, et al: Mechanics of left ventricular contraction in chronic severe mitral regurgitation. *Circulation* 1973;47:1252–1259.
108. Vokonas PS, Gorlin R, Cohn PF, et al: Dynamic geometry of the left ventricle in mitral regurgitation. *Circulation* 1973;48:786–796.
109. Cheitlin MD, Byrd RC: The click-murmur syndrome, a clinical problem in diagnosis and treatment. *JAMA* 1981;245:1357–1361.
110. Mills P, Rose J, Hollingsworth J, et al: Long-term prognosis of mitral valve prolapse. *N Engl J Med* 1977;297:13–18.
111. Rizzon P, Biasco G, Brindicei G, et al: Familial syndrome of midsystolic click and late systolic murmur. *Br Heart J* 1973;35:245–259.
112. Bon Tempo CP, Ronan JA Jr, de Leon AC Jr, et al: Radiographic appearance of the thorax in systolic click–late systolic murmur syndrome. *Am J Cardiol* 1975;36:27–31.
113. Boudoulas H, Reynolds JC, Mazzaferri E, et al: Metabolic studies in mitral valve prolapse

syndrome, a neuroendocrine-cardiovascular process. *Circulation* 1980;61:1200–1205.

114. Gaffney FA, Karlsson ES, Campbell W, et al: Autonomic dysfunction in women with mitral valve prolapse syndrome. *Circulation* 1979; 59:894.
115. Corrigall D, Popp R: Mitral valve prolapse and infective endocarditis. *Am J Med* 1977;63: 215–222
116. Swartz MH, Teichholz LE, Donoso E: Mitral valve prolapse. A review of associated arrhythmias. *Am J Med* 1977;62:377–389.
117. Jeresaty RM: Sudden death in mitral valve prolapse–click syndrome. *Am J Cardiol* 1976; 37:317–318.
118. Barnett HJM: Embolism in mitral valve prolapse. *Annu Rev Med* 1982;33:489–507.
119. Chesler E, King RA, Edwards JE: The myxomatous mitral valve and sudden death. *Circulation* 1983;67:632–639.
120. Antman EM, Angoff GH, Sloss LJ: Demonstration of the mechanism by which mitral regurgitation mimics aortic stenosis. *Am J Cardiol* 1978;42:1044–1048.
121. D'Cruz IA, Cohen HC, Prabhu R, et al: Clinical manifestations of mitral annulus calcification, with emphasis on the echocardiographic features. *Am Heart J* 1977;94:367–377.
122. Wann LS, Feigenbaum H, Weyman AE, et al: Cross-sectional echocardiographic detection of rheumatic mitral regurgitation. *Am J Cardiol* 1978;41:1258–1263.
123. Morganroth J, Mardelli TJ, Naito M, et al: Apical cross-sectional echocardiography. Standard for the diagnosis of idiopathic mitral valve prolapse syndrome. *Chest* 1981;79:23–28.
124. Mintz GS, Kotler MN, Segal BL, et al: Two-dimensional echocardiographic recognition of ruptured chordae tendineae. *Circulation* 1978; 57:244–250.
125. Quinones MA, Young JB, Waggoner AD, et al: Assessment of pulsed Doppler echocardiography in detection and quantification of aortic and mitral regurgitation. *Br Heart J* 1980;44:612–620.
126. Blanchard D, Diebold B, Peronneau P, et al: Non-invasive diagnosis of mitral regurgitation by Doppler echocardiography. *Br Heart J* 1981; 45:589–593.
127. Knutsen KM, Bae EA, Sivertssen E, et al: Detection of mitral regurgitation by Doppler ultrasound. *Acta Med Scand* 1981;210:349–351.
128. Patel AK, Rowe GG, Thomsen JH, et al: Detection and estimation of rheumatic mitral regurgitation in the presence of mitral stenosis by pulsed Doppler echocardiography. *Am J Cardiol* 1983;51:986–991.
129. Boucher CA, Okada RD, Pohost GM: Current status of radionuclide imaging in valvular heart disease. *Am J Cardiol* 1980;46:1153–1163.
130. Nicod P, Corbett JR, Firth BG, et al: Radionuclide techniques for valvular regurgitant index: comparison in patients with normal and depressed ventricular function. *J Nucl Med* 1982; 23:763–769.
131. Thompson R, Ross I, Elmes R: Quantification of valvular regurgitation by cardiac gated pool imaging. *Br Heart J* 1981;46:629–635.
132. Kress P, Geffers H, Stauch M, et al: Evaluation of aortic and mitral valve regurgitation by radionuclide ventriculography: comparison with method of Sandler and Dodge. *Clin Cardiol* 1981;4:5–10.
133. Baxley WA, Kennedy JW, Feild B, et al: Hemodynamics in ruptured chordae tendineae and chronic rheumatic mitral regurgitation. *Circulation* 1973;48:1288–1294.
134. Sasayama S, Takahashi M, Osakada G, et al: Dynamic geometry of the left atrium and left ventricle in acute mitral regurgitation. *Circulation* 1979;60:177–186.
135. Glantz SA, Misbach GA, Moores WY, et al: The pericardium substantially effects the left ventricular diastolic pressure–volume relationship in the dog. *Circulation* 1978;42:433–441.
136. Ronan JA, Steelman RB, DeLeon AC, et al: The clinical diagnosis of acute severe mitral insufficiency. *Am J Cardiol* 1971;27:284–290.
137. Friedman AW, Stein L: Pitfalls in bedside diagnosis of severe acute mitral regurgitation. Clinical and hemodynamic features. *Chest* 1980; 78:436–441.
138. Cohen LS, Mason DT, Braunwald E: Significance of an atrial gallop sound in mitral regurgitation: a clue to the diagnosis of ruptured chordae tendineae. *Circulation* 1966;35:112–118.
139. Kennedy JW, Yarnall SR, Murray JA, et al: Quantitative angiocardiography IV. Relationship of left atrial and ventricular pressure and volume in mitral valve disease. *Circulation* 1970; 41:817–824.
140. Dodge HT, Kennedy JW, Petersen JL: Quantitative angiographic methods in the evaluation of valvular heart disease. *Prog Cardiovasc Dis* 1973; 16:1–23.
141. Wexler L, Silverman JF, DeBusk RF, et al: Angiographic features of rheumatic and nonrheumatic mitral regurgitation. *Circulation* 1971; 44:1080.
142. Chatterjee K, Parmley WW, Swan HJC, et al: Beneficial effects of vasodilator agents in severe mitral regurgitation due to dysfunction of subvalvular apparatus. *Circulation* 1973;48:684–690.
143. Goodman DJ, Rosen RM, Holloway EL, et al: Effect of nitroprusside on left ventricular dynamics in mitral regurgitation. *Circulation* 1974; 50:1025–1032.
144. Greenberg BH, Massie BM, Brundage BH, et al: Beneficial effect of hydralazine in severe mitral regurgitation. *Circulation* 1978;58:273–279.
145. Greenberg BH, Demots H, Murphy E, et al: Arterial dilators in mitral regurgitation: effects on rest and exercise hemodyamics and long-term clinical follow-up. *Circulation* 1982;65:181–187.
146. Yoran C, Yellin EL, Becker RM, et al: Dynamic aspects of acute mitral regurgitation: effects of ventricular volume, pressure and contractility on the effective regurgitant orifice area. *Circulation* 1979;60:170–176.
147. Yoran C, Yellin EL, Becker RM, et al: Mechanism of reduction of mitral regurgitation with vasodilator therapy. *Am J Cardiol* 1979; 43:773–777.
148. Carpentier A, Chauvaud S, Fabiani JN, et al: Reconstructive surgery of mitral valve incom-

petence. Ten year appraisal. *J Thorac Cardiovasc Surg* 1980;79:338–348.

149. Shore DF, Wong P, Paneth M: Results of mitral valvuloplasty with a suture plication technique. *J Thorac Cardiovasc Surg* 1980;79:349–357.
150. Gerbode F, Kerth WJ, Osborn JJ, et al: Correction of mitral insufficiency by open operation. *Ann Surg* 1962;155:846–854.
151. Chopra PS, Rowe GG, Young WP, et al: Carpentier ring annuloplasty in severe noncalcific mitral insufficiency. *Arch Surg* 1977;112: 1469–1471.
152. Tandon AP, Lukacs LI, Smith DR, et al: Mitral annuloplasty: a long-term clinical and haemodynamic study. *Thorac Cardiovasc Surg* 1979; 27:39.
153. Kay JH, Zubiate P, Mendez MA, et al: Mitral valve repair for significant mitral insufficiency. *Am Heart J* 1978;96:253–262.
154. Salomon NW, Stinson EB, Griepp RB, et al: Patient related risk factors as predictors of results following mitral valve replacement. *Ann Thorac Surg* 1977;24:519–530.
155. Phillips HR, Levine FH, Carter JE, et al: Mitral valve replacement for isolated mitral regurgitation: analysis of clinical course and late postoperative left ventricular ejection fraction. *Am J Cardiol* 1981;48:647–654.
156. Ross J Jr, McCullash WH: Nature of enhanced performance of the dilated left ventricle in the dog during chronic volume overloading. *Circ Res* 1972;30:549–556.
157. Ross J Jr: Left ventricular function at the time of surgical treatment of valvular heart disease. *Ann Intern Med* 1981;94:498–504.
158. Suga H, Sagawa K: Instantaneous pressure–volume relationships and their ratio in the excised supported canine left ventricle. *Circ Res* 1974;35:117–126.
159. Pouleur H, Rousseau MF, Van Eyll C, et al: Assessment of left ventricular contractility from late systolic stress-volume relations. *Circulation* 1982;65:1204–1212.
160. Carabello BA, Nolan SP, McGuire LB: Assessment of preoperative left ventricular function in patients with mitral regurgitation: value of the end-systolic wall stress-end-systolic volume ratio. *Circulation* 1981;64:1212–1217.
161. Borow KM, Green LH, Grossman W, et al: Left ventricular end-systolic stress-shortening and stress-length relations in humans. Normal values and sensitivity to inotropic state. *Am J Cadiol* 1982;50:1301–1308.
162. Grossman W, Braunwald E, Mann T, et al: Contractile state of the left ventricle in man as evaluated from end-systolic pressure–volume relations. *Circulation* 1977;56:845–852.
163. Borow KM, Green LH, Mann T, et al: End systole volume as in predictor of postoperative left ventricular performance in volume overload from valvular regurgitation. *Am J Med* 1980; 68:655–663.
164. Schuler G, Peterson KL, Johnson A, et al: Temporal response of left ventricular performance to mitral valve surgery. *Circulation* 1979;59:1218–1231.

CHAPTER 9
Congenital Anomalies of the Aortic Valve

Dan G. McNamara

Congenital lesions of the aortic valve, including the elusive bicuspid aortic valve, occur in about 2% of the adult population,[1] far outnumbering any of the other anomalies of the cardiovascular system. The possible exception is the benign form of isolated idiopathic mitral leaflet prolapse which occurs so commonly (estimated from 10% to 20%) in the general population that many cardiologists regard it as a variation of normal.

Estimating the adult population in the United States at 147,000,000 and a 2% incidence of aortic valve anomalies, some 3 million adults have such an anomaly, not all of them functionally important, of course. Excluding aortic valve anomalies, only 0.2% of the total adult population has unoperated congenital heart defect, or about 300,000 persons.

A large number of congenital lesions of the aortic valve, both obstructive and regurgitant, produce their characteristic murmur for the first time in either late childhood, adolescence, or well into adult life.[2] This phenomenon of the late appearance of the murmur of aortic stenosis or regurgitation due to a congenital anomaly, for many years steered clinicians away from appreciating that the etiology could be a congenital anomaly of the valve. Rather, we were led to assume that the valvular disease was rheumatic, syphilitic, or else that calcific disease developed on a normal aortic valve which had been rendered vulnerable to calcific deposit by aging or a genetic predisposition to atherosclerosis.

MORPHOLOGY/PATHOLOGY

Normal aortic valve

The normal aortic valve consist of three fibrous semilunar cusps of virtually equal size located as anterior, posterior, and left portions of the valve (Figure 9-1). The cusps of the aortic valve, of course, are stronger than those of the pulmonary valve, but otherwise the cusps of both valves are similar in details of structure. The cusps are made up of a layer of fibrous tissue covered on both atrial and ventricular aspects by a layer of endocardium. The fibrous layer is much thicker at the free margin, as well as at the site of cusp attachment to the anulus. The characteristic

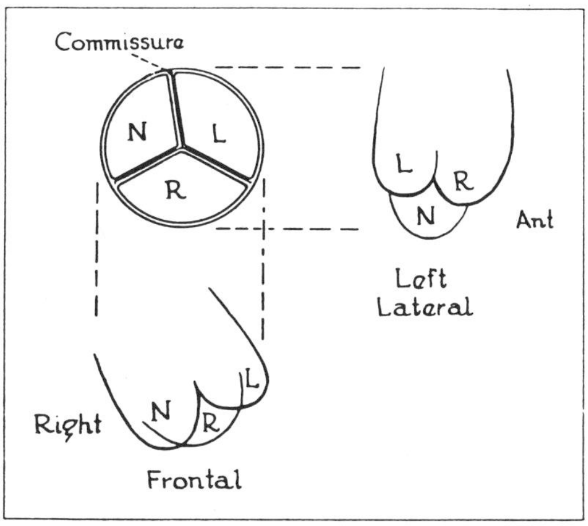

Figure 9-1 Diagram of normal aortic valve. Angiographic appearance in (upper left) horizontal view, (lower left) frontal, and (upper right) left lateral views. The three commissures divide the normal valve so that each leaflet (cusp) and each sinus of Valsalva is of equal size. In the frontal view the right coronary sinus is centrally placed between the noncoronary and left coronary sinuses and the commissure separating the noncoronary from the left sinus can be seen through the right coronary sinus. In the left lateral view the noncoronary sinus is the most inferior of the three. The anteriorly situated right coronary cusp lies slightly more inferior than the posteriorly placed left coronary sinus. (Reprinted with permission from Simon and Reis.[17])

nodule occupies the center of each free margin of the cusp. When blood is forced back toward the heart in diastole, filling the cusps, the edges meet, the nodule of each cusp comes into precise apposition and, thus, regurgitation is prevented.

Congenital anomalies of the aortic valve and left ventricular outflow tract

Congenital anomalies involving the aortic valve and the adjacent left ventricular outflow tract include the following:

1. Bicuspid aortic valve
2. Unicuspid unicommissural aortic valve
3. Tricuspid aortic valve with cusps of unequal size
4. Quadricuspid aortic valve
5. Aneurysmal dilatation of sinus(es) of Valsalva
6. Supravalvular ridge
7. Subvalvular discrete membrane
8. Subvalvular muscular ridge
9. Subvalvular left ventricular outflow tunnel

Biscuspid aortic valve In bicuspid aortic valve there may be either one anterior and one posterior cusp, or else one right and one left cusp. In about half the specimens in Roberts' series[1] (28/59) there was one anterior and one posterior cusp and both coronary arteries arose from the anterior cusp. In the other half (31/59) there was a right-left arrangement, with the right coronary artery arising from the right cusp and the left from the left. Two commissures are present in both types of bicuspid valve (Figure 9-2).

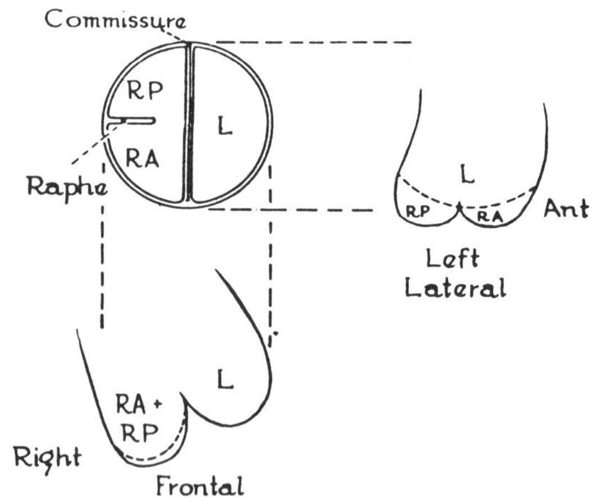

Figure 9-2 Diagram of bicuspid aortic valve of the right-left type illustrating that the right sinus (partially divided by a raphe) appears as one sinus in the frontal view, but as two slightly unequal sinuses of Valsalva with the patient in the lateral view. In the lateral view, instead of seeing the noncoronary sinus situated in the most inferior position as in the normal three-cusp valve, the left cusp margin is seen only through the shadow of the right (partially divided) sinus. (Reprinted with permission from Simon and Reis.[17])

The bicuspid aortic valve tends to be thickened from early life, even in the absence of functional disturbance, and the degree of fibrosis parallels the age of the patient. According to Campbell,[3] the bicuspid aortic valve is often thickened by 30

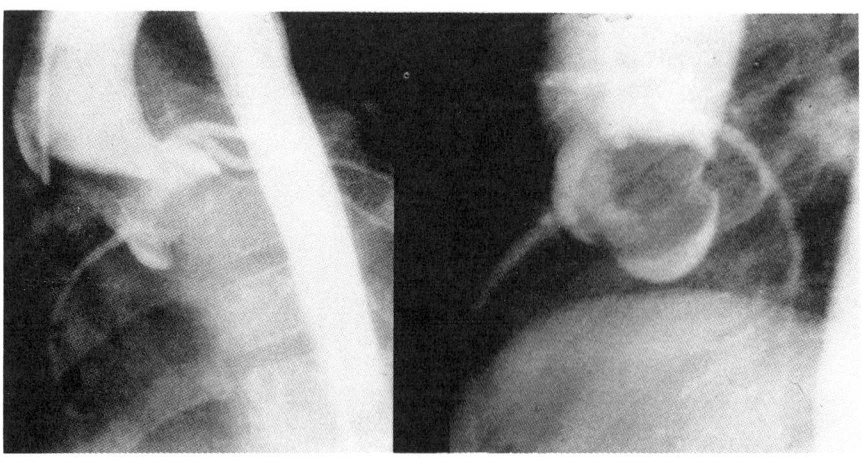

Figure 9-3 Orifice view of bicuspid aortic view not associated with coarctation and only very mild valve stenosis. In the frontal view (left) the jet is eccentrically placed. In the lateral projection (right) the dome, characteristic of some degree of stenosis, is made up of the superiorly situated and larger cusp, while the inferiorly placed sinus is the smaller of the two.

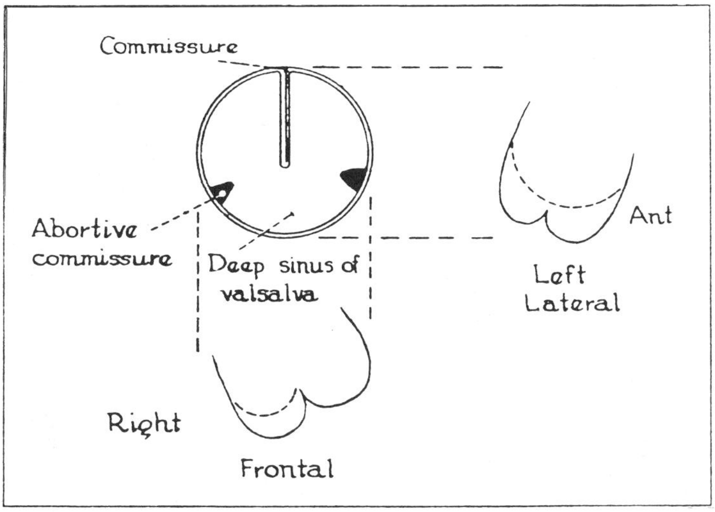

Figure 9-4 Diagram of unicommissural aortic valve. The commissure is incomplete, but because it divides the leaflet into two portions (sinuses), the frontal angiographic appearance resembles bicuspid aortic valve except tht the right portion is smaller than the left. In the left lateral view the unicommissural valve also resembles a bicuspid valve because a small abortive commissure divides the right side of the leaflet into two pouches simulating sinuses. The main difference between the bicuspid and unicommissural valve is in the lateral projection: the larger and more inferiorly placed anterior portion of the right side of the unicommissural valve points downward while the posterior half is smaller and is more superior. The jet of dye from the left ventricular angiogram is in an eccentric and posterior position; also, little tissue can be seen between the valve ring and the orifice of the stenotic area in the unicommissural valve. (Reprinted with permission from Simon and Reis.[17])

years of age and invariably so by 50 years. A similar tendency holds for calcification of the bicuspid aortic valve, which never occurs before 10 years of age, rarely so between 10 and 20 years (6%), but does occur in about one third of patients beyond 20 years of age. Among all adult patients with aortic valve stenosis, about half have a bicuspid aortic valve. Calcification is not observed in the purely regurgitant bicuspid aortic valve. Some bicuspid valves remain entirely free of calcium, even in advanced years.

Folger and Stein[4] pointed out that in bicuspid aortic valve associated with coarctation (evidently including nonobstructive mild coarctation-like anomaly of the aorta or "pseudocoarctation") the two leaflets are more or less of equal size, while in bicuspid valve unassociated with coarctation the two leaflets are more often unequal in size and thus more prone to morphologic and functional change (Figure 9-3).

Unicommissural aortic valve The unicommissural aortic valve resembles the bicuspid aortic valve, except that one commissure is fused, but there are essentially two sinuses of Valsalva (Figure 9-4 and 9-5). The difference is that the bicuspid aortic valve in the child is rarely stenotic, while the unicommissural valve virtually always produces some degree of obstruction from birth. The unicommissural valve has the same tendency to fibrosis, to calcification in adult life, and predisposition to infective endocarditis that the bicuspid aortic valve has.

Tricuspid aortic valve with cusps of unequal size Calcific aortic valve stenosis may occur on a tricuspid aortic valve. While the leaflets are three in number, they are abnormal, being of different size, and thus are subject to the hemodynamic abnormalities that lead to fibrosis and calification. About one third of the adult cases of aortic valve stenosis occur on a tricuspid valve.[1] Occasionally in childhood, stenosis of a tricuspid aortic valve may be seen (Figure 9-6).

Quadricuspid aortic valve While exceedingly rare, quadricuspid aortic valve must be considered among the congenital deformities of the aortic valve. It evidently occurs once in about 3000 consecutive autopsies in adults. It could be commoner than that, since it is a little difficult to

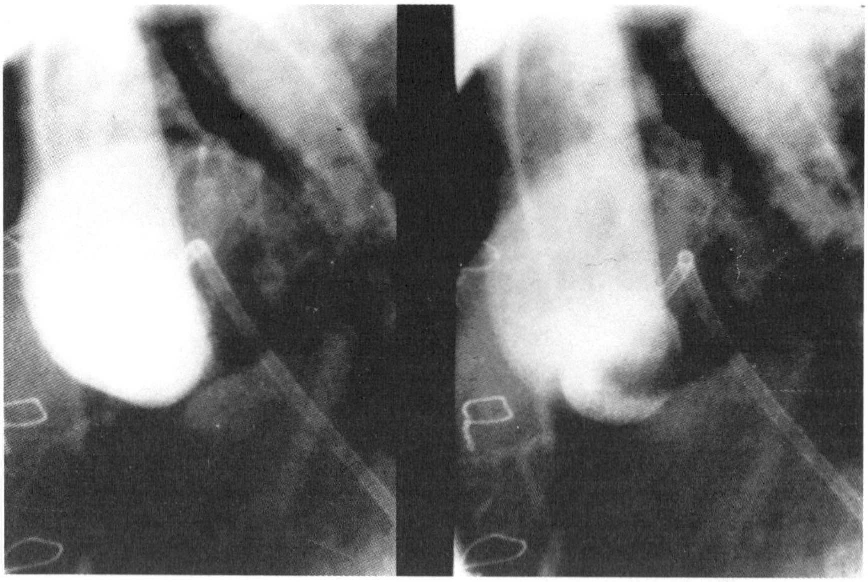

Figure 9-5 Unicommissural aortic valve; postoperative aortic valvotomy. Aortic root "barrel" view (the orifice view of Stein), showing diastole on the left and systolic view on right. The two sinuses are of unequal size, the larger one being more superiorly placed.

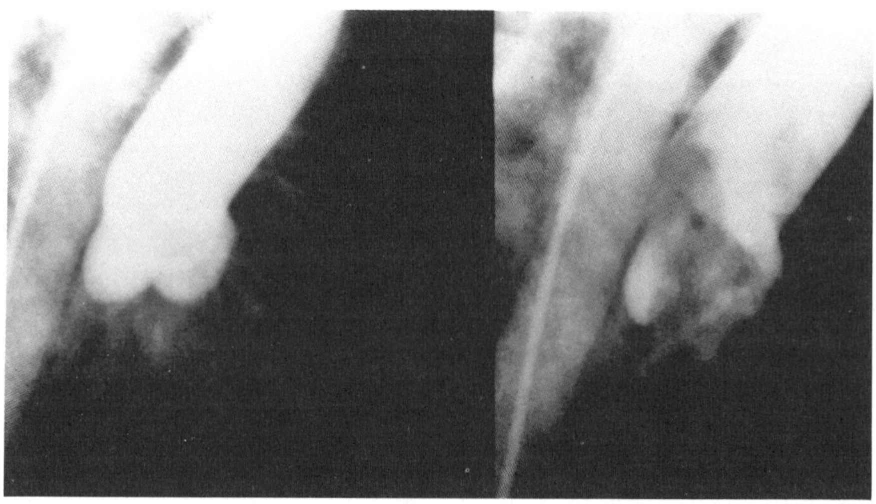

Figure 9-6 The orifice view of Stein reveals a normal appearance of the closed valve in diastole, but in systole the jet is eccentrically placed and three sinuses of slightly different size can be seen.

spot if the pathologist is not specifically looking for it. Quadricuspid *pulmonic* valve is four times more common than quadricuspid *aortic* valve, but quadricuspid pulmonic valve is usually functionally benign (96% of cases), whereas quadricuspid aortic valve is often stenotic or insufficient (46% of cases).[5] Stenosis of a quadricuspid aortic valve has occurred in the newborn infant, but regurgitation seems to develop later in the natural course of the anomaly. By contrast, stenosis of a bicuspid aortic valve is unheard of in the infant and regurgitation is rare.

The anatomy of quadricuspid aortic valve as described by Hurwitz[5] is as follows: three equal size cusps and one small cusp (found in three of seven specimens), four cusps of equal size (in

2/7), three of equal size and one large cusp (in one of seven) and four unequal size cusps (in one of seven). It was common to see small fenestrations in the cusps.

Hurwitz[5] and Roberts[1] proposed that a normally functioning quadricuspid aortic valve is not especially vulnerable to infective endocarditis. In fact, the only case of infective endocarditis on a quadricuspid aortic valve was in the patient in whom the quadricuspid aortic valve was stenotic. However, since the anomalous valve is likely to be associated with some inequality of opening of the cusps, turbulence surrounding one or more cusps could develop and predispose to infective endocarditis much as occurs in "normally functioning" bicuspid aortic valve.

Unless the quadricuspid aortic valve is stenotic or incompetent it may not be recognized clinically. Currently, no information exists as to the clinical or echocardiographic features. However, it seems likely that the quadricuspid valve would produce an abnormal appearing aortic valve on two-dimensional echocardiogram, though the echocardiographic criteria for quadricuspid aortic valve are not yet established.

Aneurysmal dilatation of sinus of Valsalva This anomaly, usually associated with Marfan's syndrome, may be associated with aortic valve regurgitation, but not invariably so. In one patient (Figure 9-7) there was neither angiographic nor auscultatory evidence of aortic valve regurgitation. Aneurysm of aortic sinus of Valsalva may be demonstrated by echocardiogram (Figure 9-8)

Bicuspid aortic valve associated with cystic medial necrosis of aorta and dissecting aneurysm Edwards et al[6] examined 119 heart specimens from patients who had died from dissecting aneurysm to determine the frequency of nonstenotic bicuspid aortic valve. They excluded six specimens in which there was aortic stenosis. There were 11 cases (9%) of congenital bicuspid aortic valve. Since the incidence of bicuspid aortic valve in the general population is only 2%, Edwards et al suggest a "causative" relationship between bicuspid aortic valve and aortic dissect-

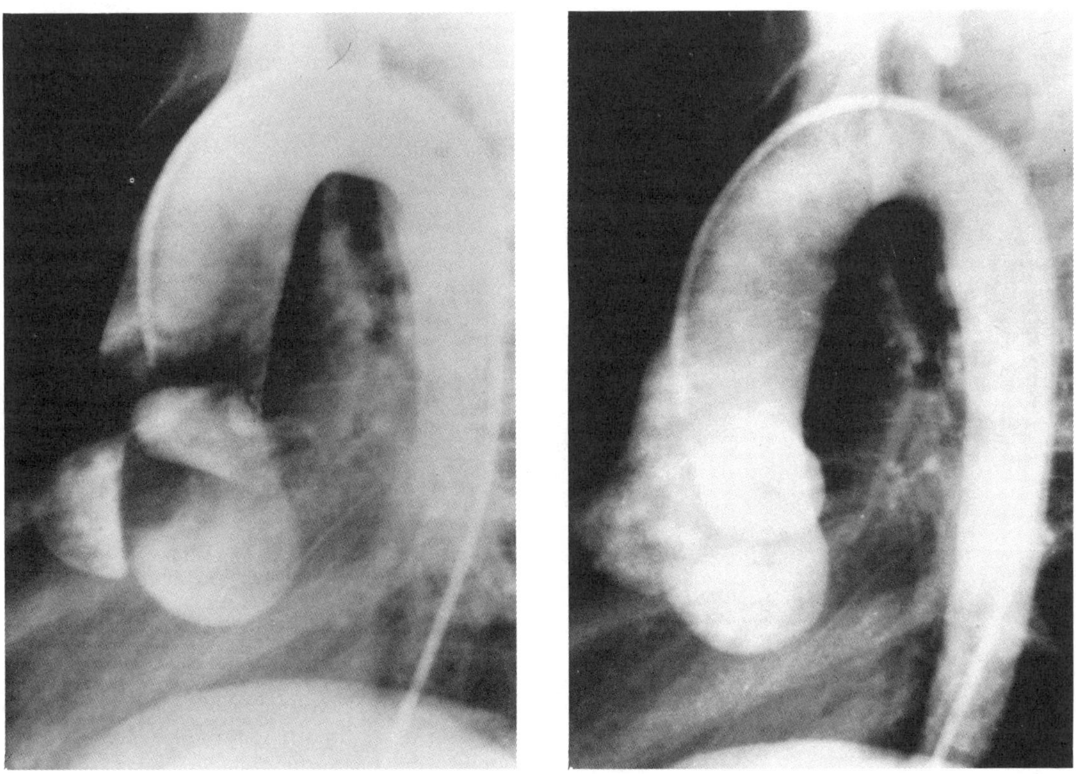

Figure 9-7A and B Aortic root angiogram demonstrating dilatation of each of the three sinuses of Valsalva, especially pronounced in the noncoronary sinus. While dissecting aneurysm may occur in the aorta of Marfan's syndrome, aneurysmal dilatation of the sinuses may remain stable and lead to no particular problem in childhood or adolescence.

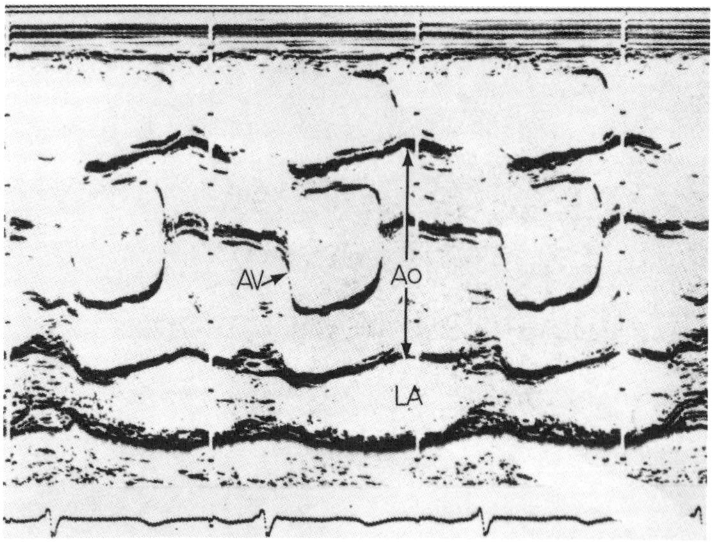

Figure 9-8 Echocardiogram of aortic root in a 6-year-old with mild aortic stenosis and aneurysm of the noncoronary sinus of Valsalva. Note the large distance between the opened valve leaflets and the posterior aortic wall. Ao = aorta, LA = left atrium, AV = aortic valve.

ing aneurysm. The age of the *11* patients ranged from 17 to 69 years and 5 of them were under 29 years of age. In only two cases (18%) was there cusp calcification. Three (27%) of the 11 cases had coarctation. According to Edwards et al,[6] the association had been reported previously in a father and son, each with bicuspid aortic valve, cystic medial necrosis, and dissecting aneurysm.

Supravalvular aortic stenosis Edwards[7] described the variable pathology of supravalvular aortic stenosis as comprising three types.

1. The hourglass type of localized constriction of the aorta just above the valve, the constriction consisting of localized medial thickening with or without intimal fibrosis
2. The membranous type in which a fibrous diaphragm lies just above the coronary artery ostia
3. The hypoplastic type in which the entire ascending aorta is lined with fibrotic material which narrows the lumen of the ascending aorta

Subvalvular aortic stenosis Subvalvular discrete membranous stenosis is often associated with acquired degenerative (sclerotic) changes in the otherwise normal aortic leaflets resulting in aortic valve insufficiency and predisposition to infective endocarditis.[8] In fact, in the patient with an aortic ejection murmur, a faint, early, high-pitched aortic diastolic murmur and no ejection click, one can suspect discrete membranous subaortic stenosis. The membrane limits movement of the aortic valve, thus no click and no closure sound is produced.[9] Once the membrane is resected, especially beyond childhood, the valve deformity is such that postoperatively the aortic insufficiency may become rather pronounced and in some cases call for aortic valve replacement. Because of this phenomenon of acquired aortic valve sclerosis secondary to the jet effect of subvalvular discrete membranous stenosis, early operation in childhood or adolescence is usually recommended for this anomaly in order to minimize the trauma to the aortic valve.

PATHOPHYSIOLOGY

Pathophysiologic consequences of aortic valve anomalies

Bicuspid aortic valve Even though the bicuspid valve in the young child usually causes no problem, it is important for the pediatrician or family physician to consider what the consequences of the anomaly could be either in childhood or in adulthood. It has long been recognized that while bicuspid aortic valve in the adult may be associated with normal valve function, the patient by 21 years of age may have developed aortic stenosis or regurgitation and the frequency of these sequelae increase with age. In addition, the bicuspid aortic valve is unusually prone to the development of infective endocarditis.

The hemodynamic consequences of bicuspid aortic valve have been studied by several investigators. In Roberts' review of 85 cases with necropsy proof, the clinical features before death were compared to the gross pathology.[10] In 61 (72%) of the 85 patients who had bicuspid aortic valve at autopsy there had been clinically apparent aortic valve stenosis; 11 (13%) had had aortic regurgitation, while in 13 (15%) of 85 patients the valve presumably had functioned normally before death.

In patients with valve stenosis, the obstruction may be due either to thickening from fibrosis or to calcification of the cusps. In the adult patient who has a stenotic bicuspid valve, calcium was present on both cusps in 59 (97%) of 61 patients. In the two who did not have cusp calcium, one patient was only 16 years old at death and had a severe transvalvular gradient of 80 mmHg, while the other patient without calcium on the bicuspid aortic valve was 44 years old and had a transvalvular gradient of 150 mmHg!

In the 13 patients with bicuspid aortic valve who had presumably normal valve function before death, the cusp in each had some slight focal thickening and in four specimens there were slight deposits of calcium in the cusps.

Aortic valve stenosis Among 105 patients (over 15 years of age) with aortic valve stenosis, 54 (51%) had bicuspid aortic valve, 13 (12%) had unicommissural unicuspid valve, 29 (28%) had tricuspid valve, three (3%) had tricuspid valve with unequally sized cusps and in six (6%) the valve was too calcified to be able to determine what the basic valve deformity might have been.[1]

To summarize the relationship of valve dysfunction in the adult patient to congenitally bicuspid aortic valve: about half the adult patients with aortic stenosis have bicuspid aortic valve, about one fourth (nine of 34) of the adult patients with aortic regurgitation have bicuspid aortic valve, about 9% (11 of 119) of adult patients with aortic dissecting aneurysm but normally functioning aortic valve have bicuspid aortic valve; and about 2% of the adult general population have bicuspid aortic valve.

While bicuspid aortic valve occurs in approximately 85% of cases of coarctation of the aorta,[11] in a review of anomalies associated with bicuspid aortic valve, Roberts found five patients (6%) with coarctation in 85 adults with bicuspid aortic valve. Including the five with coarctation, there were 11 cases (13%) of congenital heart disease among the 85 with bicuspid aortic valve.[10]

Congenitally deformed tricuspid aortic valve Roberts[1] noted that of 105 adult patients with aortic valve stenosis, three patients had tricuspid valve but cusps of unequal size and thus may have been predisposed to the same type of trauma from turbulent flow around the cusps to which the bicuspid valve is subjected. However, in 29 patients with tricuspid valve, the cusps were apparently of equal size, and thus the reason for development of thickening, fibrosis and calcification is unexplained. Perhaps some as yet unrecognized congenital deformity of these tricuspid valves renders them vulnerable to degenerative changes that lead to stenosis.

CLINICAL FEATURES AND DIAGNOSIS

Physical signs

Several congenital lesions involving the left ventricular outflow tract resemble anomalies of the aortic valve. Both definitive identification of the defect and precise assessment of severity require graphic tests, especially echocardiography, and often cardiac catheterization and angiography. However, some of the anomalies of the left ventricular outflow tract can often be distinguished from aortic valve stenosis on the basis of physical signs. They include:

1. Subaortic membranous stenosis
2. Subaortic muscular stenosis
3. Left ventricular outflow tunnel stenosis
4. Diffuse left ventricular hypertrophic obstructive cardiomyopathy
5. Lentiginosis and diffuse muscular hypertrophic cardiomyopathy
6. Supravalvular aortic stenosis, including isolated discrete stenosis and diffuse supravalvular stenosis with proximal coronary artery occlusive disease

Each of these lesions results in some degree of left ventricular-to-aortic pressure gradient. Because of this an ejection murmur and left ventricular hypertrophy are common to each of the defects and for each of them there is the same concern regarding the possible dire consequences of acute left ventricular overload with excessive exercise and the chance of life-threatening arrhythmias.

Ejection click In valvular aortic stenosis before calcification of the leaflets develops there is a characteristic ejection click heard best at the apex of the heart. In the six nonvalvular left ventricular outflow tract lesions an ejection sound does not occur. In the child with an aortic ejection murmur who is too young for calcification to have occurred, the lack of an apical ejection click should lead the clinician to suspect that the aortic stenosis is not valvular.

Thrill Both subvalvular and supravalvular aortic stenosis may produce an infraclavicular and carotid artery thrill just as occurs in valvular aortic stenosis, although the carotid thrill is much more prominent in supravalvular stenosis and the precordial thrill is more apparent in subaortic stenosis.

Pulses, blood pressure In supravalvular aortic stenosis the right carotid, right brachial, and right radial pulses are more prominent than the pulses on the left. Likewise, the right arm has a higher systolic and lower diastolic blood pressure than the left arm pressure because of the so-called choanda effect. The higher pressure generated just distal to the supravalvular stenosis is dissipated by the time the pulse wave reaches the left subclavian artery, but the higher pressure of the jet is maintained in the more proximal right subclavian artery.

In aortic valve stenosis the femoral pulse is often stronger than the brachial, especially so when the stenosis is severe and the pulse pressure is quite narrow. This phenomenon is sometimes referred to as a "reversed coarctation" — weak brachials and strong femorals. The femoral artery pulse pressure is usually wider than the brachial whether in the normal circulation or in left ventricular outflow obstruction. When the brachial pulse is severely damped from aortic stenosis, the femoral pulse pressure, being wide, may remain palpable while the brachial pulse is too damped to be felt.

Subaortic left ventricular outflow tract disorders The subaortic obstructive anomalies include discrete membrane, muscular ridge, left ventricular outflow tunnel, and diffuse (septal and left ventricular free wall) hypertrophic obstructive cardiomyopathy.

On the basis of auscultation, it would be difficult to distinguish between membrane, ridge, and tunnel, since all three have an ejection systolic murmur at the right second intercostal space, the intensity varying not so much with the location of the obstruction but with the pressure gradient across the obstruction.

None of the three anomalies produces an ejection click. A carotid artery thrill is either lacking or faint compared to valvular or supravalvular stenosis of comparable pressure gradient and cardiac output. The ejection mumur of diffuse muscular obstructive cardiomyopathy is loudest usually at the left lower sternal border and is commonly associated with an apical late systolic murmur of mitral regurgitation. The carotid pulse and brachial pulse are bounding, unlike the typical narrow pulse contour of the other forms of valvular and subvalvular aortic stenosis. In fact, the pulse contour may lead one to suspect aortic regurgitation, but there is no diastolic murmur to confirm it.

Left ventricular outflow tract disorders associated with syndromes

Elfin facies. Supravalvular aortic stenosis may be associated with the syndrome of elfin facies, mental retardation and, in early infancy, variable hypercalcemia. Beuren et al, in Germany, first identified the frequent association of peripheral pulmonary artery branch stenosis.[12] However, most patients with supravalvular aortic stenosis have normal facies and normal intelligence.

Lentiginosis. Rarely, diffuse muscular obstructive cardiomyopathy is associated with cutaneous lentiginosis.[13] The skin lesions may appear for the first time in childhood and become progressively more numerous. These may be café au lait spots ranging in size from a few millimeters to several centimeters or may be raised and resemble a pigmented nevus. They appear on face, trunk, and extremities. Lentiginosis may occur without hypertrophic cardiomyopathy and certainly most patients with hypertrophic cardiomyopathy do not have the skin lesions of lentiginosis.

Bicuspid aortic valve

Considering the high frequency of bicuspid aortic valve among all malformations of the heart, as well as the frequency in the general population, it is somewhat surprising to reflect that to the knowledge of the author no patient has been referred to our clinic by the primary care physician with the suspected clinical diagnosis of isolated bicuspid aortic valve. Among the patients who had been entered into the computer at Texas Children's Hospital from 1958 to 1983 with the diagnosis of bicuspid aortic valve, only 342 could be identified with this diagnosis out of 24,000 patients with congenital heart disease. The anomaly was recognized as an isolated defect in 124 (36%) patients (confirmed by echocardiography in 97 and by auscultation only in 24 patients), but in 183 (54%) the bicuspid aortic valve was associated with a hemodynamically important anomaly of the aorta — in 88 with stenosis of the bicuspid aortic valve, in 82 with coarctation, and in 13 with aortic regurgitation. In 17 (5%) of the 342 patients, bicuspid aortic valve was associated with a congenital heart defect that did not involve the aorta: in ten there was also a septal defect and seven were "miscellaneous". In six patients there was an arrhythmia and the bicuspid aortic valve was recognized only on routine cardiac examination in work-up for the arrhythmia. In eight patients bicuspid aortic valve was associated with Marfan's, Noonan's, Turner's, or Down's syndrome.

In considering the relatively small number of cases of bicuspid aortic valve in our diagnostic data retrieval bank, there were undoubtedly omissions as well as false-positive diagnoses of bicuspid aortic valve. The diagnosis can be made on the basis of physical examination, but the definitive diagnosis is made from either echocardiography (especially two-dimensional), angiography, or direct visualization at surgery or necropsy.

In addition to the aortic click and murmur, the presence of bicuspid aortic valve might be suspected clinically under the following circumstances: *(a)* In the patient with coarctation of the aorta in which there is an 85% chance of associated bicuspid aortic valve; *(b)* in the young or middle-aged adult (below 65 years old) with acquired calcific aortic stenosis (the development of calcific aortic stenosis beyond this age is more indicative of calcification on a tricuspid aortic valve). *(c)* in the patient who develops aortic regurgitation during the course of infective endocarditis; and *(d)* in the patient who has unexplained, isolated aortic regurgitation appearing for the first time in childhood or in adult life without a history of infective endocarditis.

Echocardiographic examination

M-mode echocardiography Nanda et al,[14] investigating the ultrasonic features of the aortic valve, recognized that in the tricuspid aortic valve the closed position of the cusps occupied the middle of the aortic lumen, but that the closed bicuspid aortic valve cusps lay in an eccentric position in diastole and could be expressed as an "eccentricity index": one half the diameter of the aortic lumen divided by the least distance of the diastolic cusp echo from the nearest aortic margin. Normals should theoretically be 1.00, but ranged up to 1.25, while bicuspid aortic valve eccentricity index ranged from 1.5 to 5.6. The index did not change after successful valvotomy in patients whose bicuspid aortic valve was stenotic (Figure 9-9). Nanda studied the M-mode echocardiogram in 21 pa-

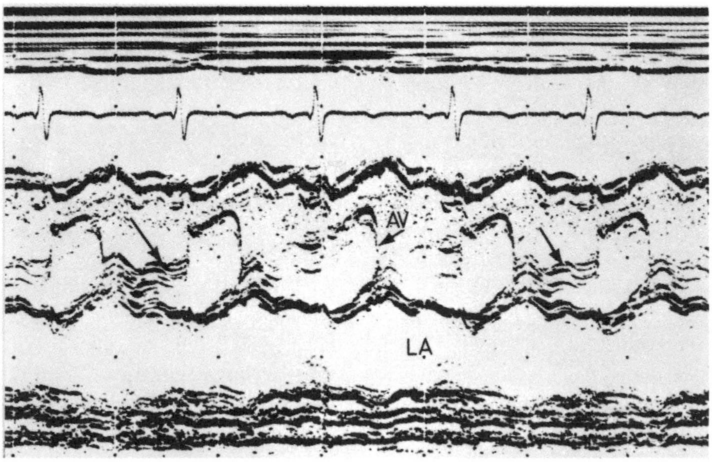

Figure 9-9 M-mode echocardiogram of aortic valve in an 8-year-old boy with mild aortic stenosis (25 mmHg gradient). There are multiple echoes from the valve in diastole (large arrows) and the leaflets open asymmetrically, typical of a bicuspid aortic valve. In this record the eccentricity index of Nanda was 2.5 (top normal 1.25). AV = aortic valve, LA = left atrium.

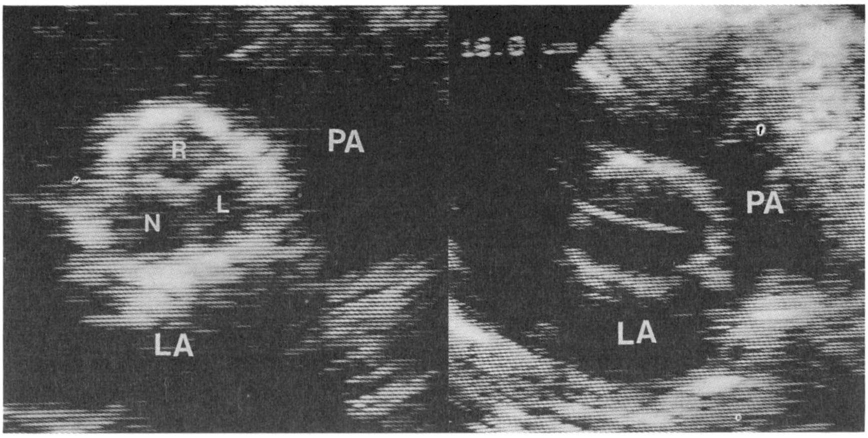

Figure 9-10 Two-dimensional echocardiograms from left parasternal short axis plane, demonstrating the difference between the normal aortic valve with three distinct leaflets (left) and a bicuspid valve with anterior-posterior cusps (right). R = right cusp, L = left cusp, N = noncoronary cusp, PA = pulmonary artery, LA = left atrium.

tients with angiographic proof of bicuspid aortic valve. In this study no false-positive or false-negative diagnosis of the valve was encountered.

However, Radford et al[15] found that the eccentricity index (using 1.3 as top normal) was abnormal in only 23 (74%) of a group of 31 patients with confirmed bicuspid aortic valve. It does not seem that M-mode echocardiography is sensitive enough for mass screening for bicuspid aortic valve.

Two-dimensional echocardiography Two-dimensional echocardiography is now the preferred method to identify and exclude bicuspid aortic valve (Figure 9-10). In a short axis two-dimensional view a demonstration of commissures in other than the normal positions at 2, 6, and 10 o'clock and demonstration of raphe by observing motions of the valve cusp, the examiner can determine whether two or three cusps are present.

In a study by Brandenburg et al [16] of patients in whom surgical or pathologic confirmation of bicuspid aortic valve could be made, the two-dimensional echo examination had a sensitivity of 78% and a specificity of 96%. In the same patients M-mode technique had a sensitivity of only 55% and a specificity of 71%.

Angiography Simon and Reis[17] studied and reported on the angiographic features of bicuspid and unicommissural aortic stenosis. The angiographic appearance of bicuspid valve depends upon the orientation of the two cusps — whether they are made up of a right and left cusp with the two commissures oriented in an anteroposterior direction or if the two cusps are made up of one anterior and one posterior cusp with the two commissures oriented in a right-to-left direction. See Figures 9-1, 9-2, 9-4, and 9-5 for angiographic features of normal aortic valve and several of the malformed valves.

Aortic valve stenosis

Aortic stenosis evokes a different image for the clinician who sees predominantly adult patients than it does for the pediatrician involved with the school age child and yet another for the neonatologist and pediatric cardiologist concerned with critical cardiopulmonary disease in the infant.

The infant with critical aortic stenosis Mild or moderately severe aortic valve stenosis is seldom recognized in the infant, but critical stenosis in the infant usually presents in the first few weeks of life as severe heart failure with signs of both pulmonary edema and low cardiac output.[18] Such an infant has barely palpable pulses, extreme pallor, and may be cyanotic from ventilatory insufficiency secondary to pulmonary edema, with resulting interference with gas exchange in the lungs. The parents will likely have noted irritability, feeding difficulty, sweating, cough, and perhaps lethargy. There is a high chance of early death in the surgically untreated patient.[19]

Influences of heart failure on typical signs of aortic stenosis If the heart failure is severe, the typical aortic stenosis murmur may be lacking. But, if carefully searched for in the primary aortic area, an ejection murmur can usually be heard, although reduced contractility may produce insufficient turbulence across the aortic

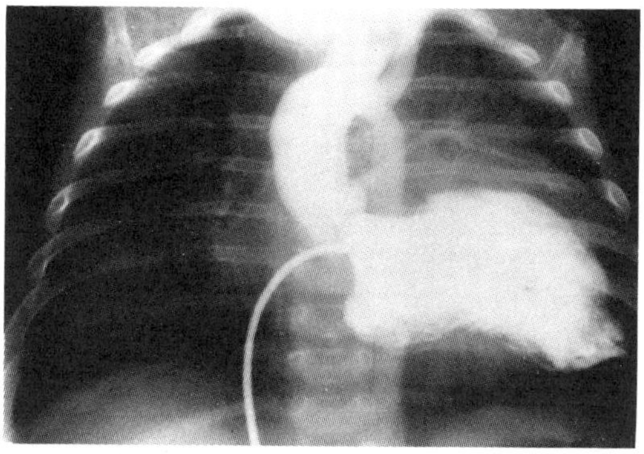

Figure 9-11 Systolic frame, frontal view, of critical isolated aortic valve stenosis in a 3-month-old infant with large-volume left ventricle, hypertrophied left ventricular wall, and thickened and domed aortic valve. The silhouette of the greatly dilated heart by routine roentgenographic examination can be seen surrounding the opacified left heart structures.

valve for the murmur to be typical of aortic stenosis. If the murmur is faint or absent, the clinician may suspect gastrointestinal (GI), pulmonary, metabolic, or neurologic disease. If cardiac enlargement is recognized by physical examination or chest roentgenogram in the absence of a murmur, then a cardiomyopathy is often suspected, including endocardial fibroelastosis, myocarditis, or, in the newborn, the hypoplastic left heart syndrome in view of the small volume pulses.

Roentgenographic and ECG signs Roentgenologically, the heart under these conditions is greatly dilated. This can be seen in Figure 9-11 which is an angiocardiogram in an infant with critical aortic stenosis. Massive enlargement of the cardiac silhouette can be seen. The ECG shows either left ventricular hypertrophy and strain or else both left and right ventricular hypertrophy if there is elevated pulmonary artery pressure.

Diagnosis by echocardiography in infants The experienced echocardiographer, using two-dimensional technique, can identify the narrowed aortic valve and abnormal motion of the cusp and will be able to determine the size of the left ventricular cavity, thickness of left ventricular wall, and percentage shortening fraction.

The importance of determining left ventricular cavity size: A small, hypoplastic left ventricle coexisting as an associated anomaly can be spotted by echocardiogram and, if present, reduces the chances of a successful outcome from operation.[19–23] Echo measured shortening fraction is reduced in these patients and, while this is an ominous sign in the adult with advanced aortic stenosis so far as recovery from operation is concerned, a large, dilated, poorly functioning left ventricle in the infant is not only a good indication for operation, but portends a better result than if the cavity is small.

Can echocardiography replace heart catheterization in infants? If the echocardiogram is typical and the patient's condition is such that heart catheterization entails a high risk, emergency aortic valvotomy can often be carried out successfully without heart catheterization. In our center it has been possible to perform heart surgery in aortic stenosis in six cases, all under 6 months of age, based upon the echocardiographic findings.[24] However, when the patient's condition permits, definitive diagnosis by heart catheterization is preferable since other defects requiring surgical attention could be present and escape notice by the echocardiographer.

Outcome of surgery in infants. Approximately two thirds of the infants with critical, life-threatening aortic stenosis operated upon at our hospital have survived operation.[19] About a third to a half of these will undoubtedly require aortic valve replacement in childhood or adolescence, but we believe that without early surgery recovery would not have been possible in any of these infants. The pathologic findings in the aortic valve in these infants will be discussed below.

The child and adolescent with aortic stenosis Unlike the infant, it is rare for the older child and adolescent with isolated aortic valve stenosis, even the very severe form, to present with heart failure. The majority of cases beyond infancy present with a heart murmur discovered on routine examination and no symptoms. Usually the patient's physician, who may have examined the patient numerous times in infancy, hears the murmur for the *first time* in early to mid- or late childhood. For this reason an acquired etiology, either rheumatic or healed infective valvulitis, may be suspected.

The ease with which a physician hears the obstructive murmur depends upon several factors. One, of course, is the pressure gradient, which influences the intensity of the murmur. In early childhood or at any age, mild aortic stenosis with left ventricular-aortic pressure gradient of only 15 to 30 mmHg produces a rather low intensity and a softer than typical aortic stenosis murmur. With age the gradient usually increases and if, for example, it increases from 15 to 30 mmHg to a range of 40 to 50 mmHg or more, the murmur becomes easy to hear and takes on the well-known characteristic features of aortic stenosis.

At 5 or 6 years of age patients are easier to examine, more cooperative, and they have fewer upper respiratory infections, feeding problems, and contagious diseases to distract the physician from a thorough cardiovascular examination. Also, once the child's body size has increased, the murmur of aortic stenosis will usually become louder because the left ventricular-to-aortic pressure gradient will have increased as a result of greater volume of blood pumped through the aortic valve with each systole. Once the murmur of aortic stenosis becomes loud enough to be easily heard, few clinicians would have any difficulty with the office diagnosis.

The difficulty in clinical assessment of aortic stenosis comes not so much in making the diagnosis but in assessing the severity and in deciding about the need for restriction of physical activity or the necessity for referral to a cardiac center and in predicting what the child's future will be, including the need for operation and anticipated complications with or without surgery. The need for restriction of physical activity is often a difficult decision to make, especially in the asymptomatic, athletically inclined teenager. In the past, the mere clinical diagnosis of aortic stenosis was considered sufficient reason to proscribe all sports or games, especially physical education classes at school, and even today evidently this is still considered by some physicians the expedient thing to do. It certainly requires less effort, as well as less responsibility, on the part of the clinician to routinely restrict all patients with aortic stenosis regardless of clinical features. However, competitive sports have an important place in the psychic as well as the physical development of the child and this author feels strongly that the physician is obligated to permit the patient as much physical activity as appears to be safe, based upon current knowleldge about the natural history of aortic stenosis as well as the availability of new technology now at our disposal to help us to assess severity both at rest and under conditions of exercise.

Estimating severity based upon peripheral pulse contour and blood pressure — differences in child and adult In the adult patient a slow rising pulse almost invariably characterizes very severe aortic stenosis, but in the child, because the aorta is more compliant than in the adult, the pulse contour is changed during transmission from the root of the aorta to the peripheral pulses. Hawker et al[25] studied both the central and peripheral aortic pressure pulse in 38 patients ranging in age from 3 to 16 years. Twenty-eight of the patients had not had surgery for aortic stenosis and ten patients were postoperative. Patients with aortic insufficiency were excluded. There were nine normals studied. He found that neither the central nor peripheral arterial pulse pressure correlated with the severity of aortic stenosis in children. Likewise, the blood pressure may be normal in mild to moderately severe stenosis in the child, whereas in the adult the pulse pressure correlates well with severity of stenosis. The reverse is also true. The author has seen several children who, inexplicably, despite a rather narrow pulse pressure and small volume pulse, proved to have only a mild pressure gradient. Nevertheless, a small volume pulse can indicate severe obstruction and the finding calls for a special effort to determine if severe obstruction might be present.

Chest Roentgenogram In both the child and the adolescent, including both the mild and severe forms of aortic valve stenosis, the silhouette of the ascending aorta appears slightly dilated. Otherwise, a normal cardiac silhouette is virtually the rule in aortic stenosis in childhood and adolescence, whether the anomaly be mild, moderate, or severe. While the infant with critical aortic stenosis develops a dilated left ventricle roentgenologically, cardiac chamber dilatation in the child or adolescent suggests that a reason other than aortic valve stenosis exists for the enlargement. The addition of aortic valve insufficiency plus stenosis is one common cause for cardiac dilatation. Associated mitral regurgitation is another. An associated left-to-right shunt (eg, patent ductus arteriosus) is yet another.

The electrocardiogram In evaluating the patient with aortic stenosis and attempting to judge the severity using noninvasive diagnostic aids, the clinician intuitively relies to a large extent on the ECG. However, this time-honored diagnostic aid is not so reliable for this purpose as one might expect.

In order to assess the reliability of the ECG, Hohn et al[26] in a multicenter natural history study compared the ECG with the measured peak systolic pressure gradient across the stenosis in 175 patients. In patients who had only mild stenosis by cardiac catheterization (peak systolic left ventricular-to-aortic pressure gradient of less than 50 mmHg), one third of them had left ventricular hypertrophy on the ECG (a false-positive

Table 9-1
ECG Findings Related to the Peak Systolic Gradient

Gradient (mmHg)	No. of Cases	Normal ECG (%)	LVH (%)	LVH and Strain (%)
< 30	15	10(67)	5(33)	—
30–49	34	20(60)	10(29)	1(11)
50–100	88	25(28)	29(33)	34(39)
> 100	38	2(5)	6(16)	30(79)

Data compiled from Hohn et al.[26]

ECG), while among the patients with severe stenosis (gradients 50 to 120 mmHg) the ECG was normal in 21% (a false-negative). However, left ventricular hypertrophy and strain pattern with ST and reversed polarity of T wave in the patient with aortic valve stenosis is an indication of severe obstruction about 90% of the time.[12] (see Table 9-1)

In Hugenholtz's[27] comparison of the ECG with the spatial vectorcardiogram, 28 of the 29 patients with severe aortic stenosis had an abnormal spatial vector, but only 18 of the 29 had an abnormal ECG. In view of the superiority of the vectorcardiogram over the ECG in identifying patients with severe aortic stenosis, it is curious that vectorcarchiography is rarely used today in pediatric cardiology centers. Perhaps it is because obtaining an artifact-free vectorcardiogram which can be reliably reproduced is technically difficult. Also, differences in measuring techniques and recording techniques have rendered the method less useful than one would have anticipated from the Hugenholtz study.

Multivariate analysis In order to determine if the features of the history and physical examination will be of help to the clinician in predicting which patients have severe stenosis, Wagner et al[28] applied multivariate analysis of history and physical findings in 44 patients more than 2 years of age with four different levels of severity of aortic stenosis. The patients were classified as *(a)* trivial stenosis (a left ventricular-to-aortic pressure gradient less than 25 mmHg), *(b)* mild stenosis (25 to 50 mmHg), *(c)* moderate stenosis (50 to 80 mmHg), and *(d)* severe stenosis (pressure gradient more than 80 mmHg). In considering five symptoms, there was, as one might expect, a higher chance of symptoms in the patients with severe obstruction, but a small percentage of patients with only trivial stenosis had symptoms. True angina occurred only in patients with severe stenosis. Among patients in the severe category, 60% were entirely free of symptoms.

Similarly, Wagner et al studied elements of the physical examination of the heart and found that a precordial thrill was present in all severity groups. Likewise, there were patients with a high-intensity murmur (grades 5 to 6) as well as those with a low intensity murmur (grades 1 to 2) in each of the four severity groups. It was rare (2% to 3%), however, to have a faint (grade 1 to 2) murmur in severe or moderate stenosis, but it did occur, and it was uncommon to have a very loud (grades 5 to 6) murmur in trivial or mild stenosis (1% and 6% respectively), but this paradox also was observed.

A loud murmur and palpable thrill clearly exclude trivial stenosis, but do not separate mild from moderate or severe stenosis. Likewise, chest pain with effort excludes trivial stenosis, but the presence or absence of fatigue, dyspnea, or syncope fail to help the clinician to distinguish in the individual patient mild, moderate, and severe forms of aortic stenosis. So, from a statistical standpoint, considering a large number of patients, the history and physical examination were helpful in the group as a whole, but in dealing with an individual patient exceptions occur often enough that neither the history nor physical examination can be used with *total* confidence to indicate if the patient has mild, moderate, or severe disease, thus leading the clinician to rely upon cardiac catheterization data. Now it would appear that the Doppler ultrasound technique is often reliable (see below)

The heart size on chest film was usually normal in all four levels of severity, but statistically more often normal in trivial and mild (90% and 94% respectively) than in moderate or severe disease (84% and 77% respectively). The clinician dealing with one patient has to keep in mind that there is this wide range among the severity groups. Probably in the patients with moderate enlargement of the heart some aortic regurgitation existed to account for this. The authors do not indicate that, but state that aortic regurgitation was heard more often in those with smaller gradients.

Most cardiologists now would agree that it is risky in the care of the individual patient with aortic stenosis to assume that the lesion is mild because the ECG is normal. On the other hand, a left ventricular strain pattern is a reliable indicator of severe disease and justifies definitive study even in the absence of subjective symptoms.

Response to exercise test Alpert et al[29] studied

the blood pressure response to exercise in 29 children with aortic stenosis and 116 children without heart disease. In the normal children, systolic blood pressure rose by an average of 43 mmHg, while in the patients with aortic stenosis, systolic blood pressure rose by an average of only 30 mmHg. This was highly significant statistically, although in one patient with severe stenosis the blood pressure rose by 65 mmHg and in four patients with an inadequate blood pressure rise with exercise the stenosis proved to be very mild. Therefore, in only 16 of the 29 patients did the blood pressure response with exercise correctly reveal the level of severity of aortic stenosis. For this reason, this author feels uneasy using a negative or a positive rise in blood pressure with total reliance in judging the patient's suitability for unlimited exercise or the need for operation. However, the development of chest pain or syncope (including dizziness) with exercise or the appearance of distinct ST and T wave changes must be regarded as evidence of severe disease and justifies heart catheterization.

M-mode echocardiography Johnson et al[30] devised an M-mode method for estimating left ventricular pressure in patients with left ventricular outflow tract obstruction using the formula:

$$\text{left ventricular pressure (mmHg)} = 225 \times \frac{\text{systolic wall thickness (mm)}}{\text{systolic internal diameter of left ventricle}}$$

In 57 children aged 2 to 22 years with fixed aortic stenosis, the left ventricular pressure estimated by this method compared favorably with that demonstrated at cardiac catheterization ($r = .89$), but there were eight important *underestimates* of pressure ranging from 30 to 50 mmHg and there were seven important *overestimates* of pressure ranging from 30 to 50 mmHg. One could hardly rely totally on the Johnson formula derived from the M-mode echocardiogram in referring a patient for operation, but taking into account the other components of the clinical and graphic examination, a pressure estimate might influence the decision for performing cardiac catheterization.

The recognition by ultrasound of aortic stenosis is especially sensitive and highly specific when the obstruction is severe and associated with thickening of the valve leaflets (Figure 9-12).

Two-dimensional echocardiography Using cross-sectional echocardiographic technique, Weyman et al[31,32] studied 28 children ranging in age from $1\frac{1}{2}$ to 16 years with an average age of 9 years, and 22 normal subjects of comparable age. The diagnosis of aortic valve stenosis was readily made in each using cross-sectional echocardiography on the basis of: (1) an increase in echo production, (2) abnormal leaflet motion, and (3) abnormal systolic position of the leaflets. Measurement of the maximum aortic cusp separation correlated well with the calculated valve area. Maximum aortic cusp separation was corrected for the size of the aortic root diameter. The ratio of maximum aortic cusp separation to aortic diameter compared to the peak systolic pressure gradient gave an r value of .88 and this ratio related to the aortic valve area gave an r value of .80. Currently, echocardiographers find the cross-sectional echocardiogram far superior to the M-mode technique in identifying aortic valve stenosis as well as in assessing severity (Figure 9-13).

Doppler echocardiography The work of Hatle et al[33] in estimating valve gradients has made noninvasive estimation of severity in lesions such as aortic valve stenosis an approachable reality. If the angle of the ultrasound beam is close to that of the angle of the maximal velocity of the jet, a close correlation can be obtained between the gradient measured directly with that from Doppler study analysis. This is especially successful in young subjects. Doppler echocardiography tends to underestimate the pressure gradient and the estimates are reproducible. Errors are more likely to occur when the Doppler signal is very weak. Underestimate of pressure drop was within 25% in 17 of 18 patients.

Kosturakis et al,[34] studied three patients with aortic stenosis and 11 with pulmonic stenosis. They compared stenotic orifice area by catheterization data (Gorlin method) to that obtained from a pulsed Doppler-derived formula and demonstrated close correlation with r value of .97.

NATURAL COURSE OF AORTIC STENOSIS

Child and adolescent

At Texas Children's Hospital, Houston, we followed 37 patients with four different types of aortic stenosis for periods averaging 4 years (range 1 to 10 years) in whom two cardiac catheterizations were performed.[35] There were 18 patients with valvular stenosis, ten with both

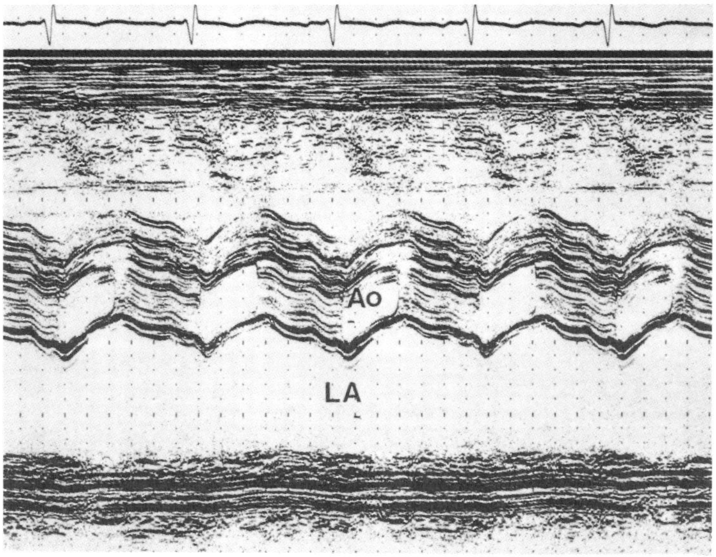

Figure 9-12 Severe aortic valve stenosis. M-mode echocardiogram showing multiple echoes filling aortic root in diastole, suggestive of pronounced thickening of the aortic valve leaflets. Ao = aorta, LA = left atrium.

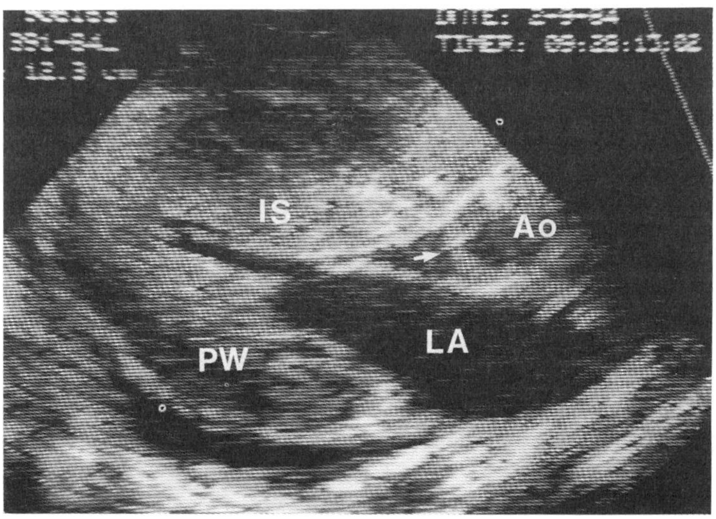

Figure 9-13 Two-dimensional echocardiogram in long axis projection demonstrating a thickened aortic valve (arrow) and marked concentric left ventricular hypertrophy. IS = interventricular septum. PW = posterior wall, Ao = aorta, LA = left atrium.

valvular stenosis and insufficiency, six with discrete subvalvular stenosis, and three with supravalvular stenosis. Except for those patients with associated aortic insufficiency, there was an increase in left ventricular peak systolic pressure, the left ventricular-to-aortic peak systolic gradient, and an increase in arteriovenous oxygen difference. Also, there was a significant decrease in cardiac index and in stenotic orifice area index. Only two patients had become symptomatic between catheterization at (average age) 7 years and second catheterization at (average age) 11 years. One patient developed chest pain and the other, fatigue with exercise. In four patients a pronounced decrease in stenotic orifice area indexed exceeded that expected for only a small change in body size, indicating that an actual narrowing of the stenotic orifice area must have occurred and accounted for the pressure rise, while in two others, despite a large increase in growth, the stenotic orifice area indexed actually was larger.

Clinical features can be misleading in following the child with aortic stenosis. The murmur, heart sounds, and pulse tracings have been unreliable indicators of the severity. The ECG may remain normal in the presence of rising left ventricular-to-aortic gradient, although an increase in left ventricular hypertrophy with strain on the ECG should be taken as an indication of increased severity of obstruction. In our study the progression of subvalvular aortic stenosis and supravalvular stenosis was more pronounced than that of aortic valvular stenosis. Our findings demonstrate that aortic stenosis in childhood and adolescence tends to progress, usually due to increased flow (secondary to increased body growth) across the stenotic orifice, although in a few patients an actual decrease in orifice area adds to the progression. In the adult the progression of severity relates to a decrease in stenotic orifice area.

In 1965 Hohn et al[26] reported progression from mild to severe stenosis in 19 (50%) of his 38 patients with aortic stenosis and three (8%) of 38 patients who were clinically considered to be unchanged were found to have, to the authors' surprise, a high left ventricular-to-aortic pressure gradient.

In 1977, as part of a multicenter natural history study in which the natural course of several malformations of the heart was studied, Wagner et al[18] described the course of 473 children under 21 with aortic valve stenosis. This remains the largest and only prospective analysis published on this subject.

The male to female ratio was 4 to 1, which confirms the long-suspected and still unexplained predilection that aortic stenosis has for the male. Only 25 (5%) of the 473 patients were under 2 years of age; 285 (60%) were between 2 and 11 years old, and 163 (34%) were between 11 and 21 years of age. Of the 25 infants, 20 (80%) were classified as having either critical, severe, or moderately severe stenosis. Only five of the infants had so-called mild (left ventricular-to-aortic gradient 25 to 50 mmHg) and none had trivial stenosis (gradient <25 mmHg). By contrast, less severe forms of the anomaly begin to be recognized in early to midchildhood; among patients 2 to 11 years of age one fourth had trivial stenosis and one third had mild stenosis. So half of the children 2 to 11 years of age had mild or trivial stenosis, whereas only 20% of the infants did. Likewise, in 46% of the older children and adolescents, the aortic stenosis was only mild or trivial. This last finding confirms in a large number of patients what many of us had long suspected, that mild aortic stenosis is simply not recognized as often in the infant as it is in the child. Whether the diagnosis is missed or mild stenosis does not occur in the child is not known.

While four of the 25 infants had marked cardiac enlargement and two had frank congestive failure, among the older children the only patient who developed congestive heart failure was one who died during treatment for subacute bacterial endocarditis. Thus, while the adult patient often appears with congestive heart failure, it is extremely rare for this to be seen in the child, yet it is common in the infant who is referred to a cardiac center.

The clinical course of 294 patients treated medically was reviewed. Nine of these patients died during the 8-year period of observation and in seven (2.3%) of the 294, death was from a cardiac cause and in two additional patients from a noncardiac cause. In two of the seven deaths the patients were infants and both had been in congestive failure; one died after heart catheterization. Of the five patients beyond infancy who died of cardiac cause, three deaths were sudden, presumably from arrhythmia, and two occurred during treatment for subacute bacterial endocarditis.

Recatheterization in 112 patients treated medically showed that in one third of the patients the gradient had increased during the period of follow-up by more than 10 mmHg, plus 20% of the gradient noted at the first cardiac catheterization. But in 10% of patients the gradients had actually decreased significantly. In three of the 12 patients whose pressure decreased, the gradient at the first catheterization was more than 70 mmHg and these patients might well have been considered for operation. These gradients were as follows: 70, 75, and 80 mmHg and they decreased to 38, 40, and 40 mmHg respectively. The authors believe this apparent "improvement" was not so much an increase in stenotic orifice size, but rather a difference in hemodynamic state of the patient at the two catheterizations. While these examples of apparent if not real improvement are isolated, anecdotal, and unusual occurrences, the clinician cannot help but recall that this phenomenon may occur in the process of managing the individual patient.

Wagner et al categorized the clinical state of the patient as either excellent, good, fair, or poor. The "excellent" category indicated a trivial pressure gradient, no symptom, and no ECG or roentgenographic abnormality. Of the six infants, two died, three were in poor conditions, and only one was classified clinically as good at the time of follow-up. Of the 213 older children, five died from cardiac causes and each of these had been classified from fair to poor initially. Only 26 (50%) of the 52 patients in the so-called excellent category initially remained stable on follow-up. The other patients were fair or poor. Half of those in the good category remained so and two thirds of the fair patients remained stable while one third deteriorated, including four of the five patients who died. In summary, during an 8-year follow-up of the six infants, one was better, one was the same, two were worse, and two died. Of the older children 14% were better, 44% were the same, 39% were worse, and 3% had died.

Adult

In 1982 Wagner & Selyer[36] reported on the course of aortic stenosis in the adult patient, pointing out that in the adult, progression of aortic stenosis is much more rapid than in the child. Fifty adult (56 years average) patients were followed for a period ranging from 2 to 14 years. In 36 (72%) of the 50 patients there was progression in severity, in 13 there was no change, and in one patient there was actual improvement. The authors noted that of the patients who progressed in severity, one half progressed rapidly and the other half slowly. Degenerative calcific aortic stenosis was present in 14/21 (67%) of the rapid progressors and in only 7/29 (24%) of the slow progressors.

Many other investigators have confirmed that aortic valve stenosis is known to progress and at a more rapid rate in adults than in children. Campbell[3] observed that half the patients he followed did very well in the first three decades of life; one fourth had minor symptoms and one fourth had severe symptoms. But by the fourth or fifth decade only one fourth were doing well and three fourths were doing poorly or had died. The annual death rate rose steadily from early childhood through the fifth decade from 1.2% per year from 1 year of age to 20 years, and to 3%, 3.5%, 6%, and 8.5% respectively for the third through sixth decades.

Cheitlin et al[37] reviewed 29 patients 20 years of age or older with aortic stenosis who had had two cardiac catheterizations. None of these patients had had operation or subacute bacterial endocarditis between the two procedures. The average time between studies was 4 years. Half of the patients increased their gradient by 50% or more and in half there was no increase in gradient.

The pathogenesis of progression of severity of aortic stenosis

Stein et al[38] proposed that organized microthrombi that develop upon a deformed valve tend to calcify. Turbulent flow occurs at a deformed valve, even if stenosis is not severe. Turbulence leads to hemolysis which causes a release of adenosine diphosphate (ADP) which in turn causes platelet aggregation. The RBCs also release partial thromboblastin when hemolysis occurs which in turn forms thrombin and renders the aggregates of platelets irreversible. Initially, in childhood and adolescence, the bicuspid aortic valve although not stenotic does not open fully, creating turbulence that can start this process of valve cusp trauma. Turbulent flow with its effect on the cellular elements of the blood produces microthrombi that organize and lead to the deformity that progresses to calcific aortic stenosis.

In an effort to reduce the development of calcific aortic stenosis, a long-term clinical trial is needed to evaluate the effect of drugs aimed at platelet aggregation inhibition started in the young individual who is at risk to develop aortic valve calcification.

Sudden death

Sudden death has long been the dreaded complication of aortic valve stenosis in the child and adolescent. This possible outcome is often cited as the justification for cardiac catheterization in the patient with clinical signs of only very mild aortic stenosis; it is the reason given for surgical repair simply on the basis of a left ventricular-to-aortic pressure gradient in the range of only moderate severity (eg, 50 to 60 mmHg) in the aysmptomatic patient without other evidence of cardiac dysfunction. Because of the chance of sudden death, some clinicians caution against sports for all patients with clinical signs of aortic valve stenosis.

In the study of Wagner et al[18] of the natural course of 294 patients with aortic valve stenosis followed for an average of 8 years, five cardiac deaths occurred in patients beyond infancy and three of these deaths were sudden, presumably due to arrhythmia. Each patient had been in the hemodynamic category of fair to poor and, while the deaths were sudden, they were not regarded as totally unexpected.

Many pediatric cardiologists following a large number of patients with congenital heart disease find that sudden death due to aortic valve stenosis is less common now than it was 30 to 40 years ago. The difference is believed to be due to earlier recognition of aortic stenosis by the primary care physician, improved methods of assessing severity by the pediatric cardiologist, and the referral of patients for valvotomy for even a moderate left ventricular-to-aortic pressure gradient despite lack of symptoms or ECG changes.

Doyle et al[39] described in detail the four sudden deaths she had seen among 92 children with aortic stenosis followed for a period ranging from 1 to 22 years (average 7 years). The patients who died suddenly were 7, 10, 14 and 20 years of age. Each had severe left ventricular hypertrophy and strain on ECG. Only one, the 14-year-old girl, denied any symptoms. This patient had been taking digitalis while awaiting operation at the time of death. This, plus the fact that her death occurred during sleep, makes one wonder if the inotropic drug may have had an adverse effect on the left ventricular aortic gradient and could have predisposed the patient to arrhythmia. This event occurred in 1959, well before anyone questioned the advisability of using digitalis in patients with left ventricular outflow tract obstruction.

Doyle reviewed 35 published reports of sudden death in young patients (range 2 to 23 years) in whom an ECG was available for review. In 25 (70%) of the 35 patients the ECG had shown left ventricular strain, in seven (21%) the ECG showed left ventricular hypertrophy, and in three (9%) the ECG was reported to be normal!

Garson et al[40] found only two instances of aortic stenosis among 101 patients who had sudden death in the patients registered in the cardiology service at Texas Children's Hospital during the 25-year period from 1958 to 1983. Both patients had been symptomatic, had clinical features of aortic stenosis, and were certainly candidates for operation but had not yet been scheduled for it.

This relatively low incidence of sudden death due to aortic stenosis may be the result of a long-standing policy to refer patients for surgery without delay if there is hemodynamically important aortic stenosis (left ventricle-to-aortic gradient of 60 mmHg or more), whether or not there are symptoms or ECG signs of left ventricular strain.

Driscoll and Edwards[41] reviewed 61 cases of sudden death in children which were reported in 13 different publications. Six (10%) of the 61 deaths were in patients with aortic stenosis and only one of these six patients had a prior history of syncope. In considering syncope as a risk factor for sudden death in children, the high incidence of syncope in healthy adolescents was considered. As many as 12% to 15% of healthy adolescents have been reported to have a benign type of vasodepressor syncope. This type of syncope often occurs with emotional stress or following pain and may occur in patients who are in a hot, crowded room in an upright or sitting position, but it does not usually occur with exercise as does the high-risk type of syncope. Exercise-induced syncope in the patient with aortic stenosis must be regarded as an ominous sign. It is a marker for potential sudden death. Incidentally, the same can be said for exercise-induced syncope in the individual without known heart disease.

McHenry et al [42] reported on sudden death in patients with aortic stenosis who had associated pulmonary hypertension. They reported four patients who died within 24 hours of heart catheterization — patients who admittedly had severe aortic stenosis but who were reasonably well off and awaiting surgery within a few days but not as an emergency. Each patient at catheterization had left ventricular failure and elevated pulmonary artery pressure. In three additional patients their condition deteriorated rapidly after catheterization and they were sent for emergency surgery. Because of this experience the investigators reviewed the hemodynamic data of 72 adult patients with congenital aortic stenosis. Pulmonary artery mean pressure was elevated for the entire group (27 mmHg) but in those who died suddenly and in those who required emergency surgery the mean pulmonary artery pressure was 47 mmHg.

Pulmonary hypertension complicating isolated aortic valve stenosis is virtually never a problem in the child or adolescent and in fact must be fairly uncommon in the adult. The age of the 15 patients in the review by McHenry et al[42] ranged from 49 to 67 years. Considering that each of the patients with pulmonary hypertension had left ventricular failure with elevated left ventricular end-diastolic pressure and elevated left atrial pressure, the pulmonary hypetension is no surprise and merely reflects the severity of the left ventricular failure. It should be a reminder to the cardiologist and surgeon, however, that the patient with aortic stenosis and left ventricular failure is fragile and if surgery is to be performed it should be carried out as soon after the heart catheterization as possible — preferably on the same day.

PHYSICAL ACTIVITY IN PATIENTS WITH AORTIC STENOSIS

At a recent conference on cardiovascular abnormalities in the athlete, the following recommendations were made for aortic stenosis[43]:

For patients with trivial aortic stenosis (resting left ventricular-to-aortic gradient less than 20 mmHg), full sports participation may be allowed if there is no enlargement of heart by physical examination, ECG or chest roentgenogram, a normal exercise stress test, and no arrhythmia at rest, with exercise, or on 24-hour ambulatory monitor. Since mild aortic stenosis may progress, yearly evaluation is recommended for continued sports participation. Only mild forms of physical activity are permitted for patients in whom the left ventricular-to-central aortic pressure gradient is 40 mmHg or more (moderate or severe stenosis) or if in the absence of heart catheterization there is either any enlargement of the heart by physical examination. ECG, or roentgenographic means. Likewise, active sports are limited for the patient with positive exercise stress test, and arrhythmia at rest, with exercise, or on 24-hour ambulatory monitor, or if there is aortic regurgitation of more than mild degree.

SURGICAL TREATMENT

Indications

The left ventricular–aortic pressure gradient The resting left ventricular-to-central aortic peak systolic pressure gradient serves as the standard by which severity of the stenosis can be judged. Cases are usually categorized by the classification of Wagner et al[28]:

1. Trivial stenosis (left ventricular-to-aortic pressure gradient less than 25 mmHg)
2. Mild stenosis (25 to 50 mmHg)
3. Moderate stenosis (50 to 80 mmHg)
4. Severe stenosis (gradient more than 80mmHg)

Based upon pressure gradient alone, patients in the severe category are clearly candidates for operation at any age and those in the trivial group are clearly not candidates in childhood or adolescence, but may become candidates as adults when fibrosis and calcification further narrow the aortic valve orifice. Those in the mild category are usually not surgical candidates in childhood, but fully half of this group will develop more severe obstruction by adolescence and will be ready for operation before adulthood. As referred to earlier, among patients with aortic stenosis studied twice at Texas Children's Hospital with a 4-year interval between studies, half demonstrated more severe obstruction at the second catheterization.[32] This change was related to increase in body growth in approximately half of the patients but in the others the change was clearly out of proportion to body growth. Neither fibrosis nor calcification had developed by direct inspection at the time of operation to account for the change.

Aortic valve stenosis plus regurgitation When mild aortic stenosis is associated with clinically apparent aortic regurgitation, an increase in severity of the pressure gradient from childhood to adolescence is less likely. The aortic regurgitation may progress, but the left ventricular-to-aortic pressure gradient usually does not increase. Perhaps dilatation of the aortic root and anulus protects against progressive narrowing of the stenotic area. Furthermore, there seems to be less tendency to calcification when there is an important degree of valvular regurgitation.[10]

In the absence of symptoms or strain pattern on ECG, patients with aortic stenosis in the moderate category in infancy and childhood may usually be followed medically. However, in the opinion of the author, the patient with moderate stenosis should be seriously considered for operation even without symptoms or strain on the ECG. When operation is performed after 21 years of age, aortic valve replacement is usually always necessary, while the stenotic valve can usually be salvaged by valvotomy in the adolescent patient.

Noncorrelative pressure gradient and clinical data It often happens that the clinical and hemodynamic findings are divergent. If the clinical findings indicate that the stenosis is probably more severe than the pressure gradient would indicate, it may be that the "mild" pressure gradient is explainable by one of the following reasons:

1. The cardiac output was depressed at the time that the pressure was recorded. This could have been due to excessive sedation, the action of a cardiac depressant drug, or unrecognized hypovolemia.

2. A peripheral artery (femoral or brachial) was used for comparison with left ventricular pressure rather than the central aorta. In the normal circulation the femoral artery peak systolic pressure measures 5 to 10 mmHg higher than aortic root pressure, but in aortic stenosis the femoral pressure may in some cases measure as much as 15 to 20 mmHg higher than central aorta pressure. Thus, if the peripheral artery is used to calculate the left ventricular-to-aortic pressure gradient, the result may be falsely low.

3. A falsely low gradient could be obtained because of an improperly balanced strain gauge in the catheterization laboratory.

4. Partial damping of a fluid-filled catheter is another possible source of error.

The same can be said for cases in which the gradient reported at heart catheterization seems to be unreasonably high. This could be caused by several conditions:

1. Catheter overshoot on ventricular pressure tracing is a recognized phenomenon that can mislead the person responsible for measuring the pressure from a record or from the oscilloscope screen.

2. Catheter entrapment, due to the catheter tip being partially embedded between the papillary and left ventricular muscle, will produce a characteristic narrow and peaked pressure curve, which experienced staff will recognize as artifact.

3. A high cardiac output may produce a falsely high pressure gradient. This could result from a drug effect (atropine or sympathomimetic agent), anxiety, or a sudden increase in blood volume (eg, from rapid intravenous (IV) infusion). These points should be considered when the pressure gradient reported from heart catheterization seems unreasonably high.

It may be necessary to review the actual pressure record to consider if any of these artifacts could account for a disparity of clinical and hemodynamic information.

Symptoms We have already learned that the most disturbing symptom is exertional angina and this in the presence of even mild stenosis would be a strong indication for surgical repair in the adult or adolescent or moderate stenosis in the child. It should be recalled, however, that lack of symptoms does not indicate a lack of severe stenosis. In the patients of Wagner et al in the severe category, 60% were entirely free of symptoms.[28] On the other hand, a small percentage of patients with only trivial stenosis had symptoms which were evidently not truly related to the cardiovascular anomaly. None of these symptoms included exertional angina, however.

Age and body size If surgery is contemplated in the third decade of life in a patient with moderate or even severe stenosis, this author feels that the operation is better carried out before 20 or 21 years of age in order to avoid valve replacement. Most patients in adolescence still have a freely mobile, nonfibrotic, and noncalcified valve which can readily be opened by valvotomy. Surgery in childhood should be avoided if possible, but in severe stenosis operation may have to be carried out in childhood to avoid sudden death. In infancy, surgery is carried out only for patients who have congestive heart failure. In the adult patient, since valvotomy is virtually never possible, whether the stenosis be mild, moderate, or severe, strict indications for operation are adhered to in order to avoid valve replacement.

Results

Both early and late results of surgical treatment of aortic stenosis vary considerably with the age group under consideration: (1) infancy, (2) childhood and adolescence, (3) adulthood.

Infancy The immediate surgical mortality in the infant less than 1 year of age is about 50% in most centers. This mortality is much higher than that for most of the other types of definitive surgery in the infant for critical heart disease. The mortality in such complicated and severe malformations as tetralogy of Fallot and transposition of the great arteries ranges from 5% to 15%.

Hamman et al[23] reported an operative mortality of 53% in 19 infants who had surgery for critical aortic valve stenosis. As was noted by other investigators, the size of the left ventricular cavity was a consistent determinant of the outcome. The left ventricular end-diastolic volume was small (89% of predicted normal) in nonsurvivors and the volume was larger than normal (159% of predicted normal) in the survivors.

In the review of Wagner et al,[18] of the 13 infants who had surgical treatment, seven (54%) died, four (31%) improved, and two (15%) were unchanged. Of the 127 older children, 5 (4%) died, 71 (56%) were improved, and 41 (32%) were the same as before surgery, while 10 (8%) were worse than preoperatively. In their series one additional death resulted postoperatively from a car accident.

Childhood and adolescence Sandor et al[44] reviewed the early and late results of surgery for aortic valve stenosis in 187 infants and children operated upon at the Hospital for Sick Children in Toronto. There was a 52% early mortality within 1 month of operation in the infants (13 of 25 patients) and a 1.9% early mortality in patients 1 year to 20 years old. The surviving infants were followed for 4 years on average and the older patients for 7 years. Two infants had a second operation with no late death, but 13.5% (20/148) of the children required reoperation with 20% mortality. Another five patients reviewed by Sandor et al died late postoperatively (two were sudden, two from infective endocarditis, and one was related to an accident). Most of the patients had either no symptoms or else very minor exercise intolerance (New York Heart Association functional class I or II). The authors conclude that, while the operation is palliative, it does offer considerable symptomatic improvement and reduces the chance, though it does not eliminate the possibility, of sudden death. There is apparently little or no influence on the occurrence of infective endocarditis. In patients between 1 and 21 years of age, Sandor et al cited an operative mortality ranging from 0% to 7% in other centers; in their experience mortality was 1.9% in 161 patients in this age group.[44]

Orsmond et al[45] studied the hemodynamics in 18 children before and after aortic valvotomy. The patients had had operation at a mean age of 10 years and were studied between 2 years and 10 years postoperation. The average cardiac output was normal, both before and after surgery. The mean left ventricular-to-aortic pressure gradient was reduced from 60 mmHg preoperatively to 20 mmHg postoperatively, but three patients had an inadequate relief of the gradient. Before surgery, five patients had only very mild aortic regurgitation, but postoperatively all but two patients had angiographic evidence of aortic regurgitation. In ten of the 18 patients, exercise hemodynamics were measured before and after valvotomy. The left ventricular-to-aortic gradient with peak exercise was 73 mmHg preoperatively and 24 mmHg postoperatively. (Recall that the resting gradient was 60 mmHg preoperatively and 20 mmHg postoperatively.) The left ventricular systolic pressure during peak exercise had been 230 mmHg preoperatively, but was only 175 mmHg postoperatively.

Orsmond recommended that physicians allow normal exercise tolerance in children after aortic valvotomy when the residual gradient is minor and when there is minimal aortic regurgitation.[45]

Complications and long-term follow-up

Late postoperative complications included residual left ventricular outflow tract obstruction, important aortic regurgitation, need for reoperation, occurrences of infective endocarditis, and late death.

Considering all these adverse events in patients 5 to 14 years after operation, a satisfactory outcome was observed in 54% of adult patients with aortic valve stenosis (281/522), in 54% of patients with subvalve aortic stenosis (120/222), and in 78% of patients with idiopathic hypertrophic subaortic stenosis (14/18). About half of the problems that occurred in long term follow-up were observed 1 year postoperatively.[44]

Reoperation

In the report of Jones et al,[46] seven (17%) of 41 patients who had valvotomy for aortic valve stenosis required reoperation 1 to 19 years later — four patients for aortic regurgitation and three patients for persistent stenosis. In published reports reviewed by Jones et al, reoperation was required in 66 (18%) of 365 patients who had aortic valvotomy after follow-up over 5 to 15 years. Jones et al reported that 5 (12%) of 41 postoperative patients had subacute bacterial endocarditis 6 to 13 years after operation. In the published series reviewed by Jones et al, 20 (6%) of 320 postoperative patients had bacterial endocarditis after operation. Late deaths occurred in 20% of patients, but two were noncardiac. Of the six cardiac deaths, five were sudden and unexpected; one of those five had severe, persistent obstruction and four had aortic regurgitation. Late survival in the published reports was also about 80% of all postoperative patients and almost all late deaths were related to the aortic valve problem.

AORTIC REGURGITATION DUE TO CONGENITAL ANOMALY IN THE CHILD

While isolated aortic regurgitation in Asiatic and Eastern European children is often due to rheumatic fever, this is a rare etiology for isolated aortic regurgitation in children in the Western world. In fact, isolated rheumatic aortic regurgitation was rare 30 years ago when rheumatic fever was more common in the United States than it is now. Rheumatic aortic regurgitation may accompany rheumatic mitral regurgitation in the United States, but new cases of rheumatic heart disease fortunately have become rarities in this country.

When the physician hears the murmur of aortic regurgitation in the child or adolescent for the first time, one can suspect that it is probably due to one of the congenital anomalies of either the aortic valve, the left ventricular outflow tract, or the aorta itself, but for a variety of reasons the murmur did not make its appearance earlier in infancy.

The murmur of pulmonary regurgitation in the presence of pulmonary hypertension sounds almost identical to that of aortic regurgitation and both are heard best along the left sternal border. Differentiating aortic from pulmonary regurgitation on physical examination may not be so easy since the wide pulse pressure characteristic of moderate to severe aortic regurgitation is not always present in congenital aortic regurgitation, especially in the presence of associated aortic stenosis. Right ventricular hypertrophy by physical examination or ECG points toward pulmonary rather than aortic regurgitation, of course, but there are exceptions. Aortic regurgitation may accompany lesions which result in right ventricular hypertrophy. For example, a fistulous connection of a ruptured sinus of Valsalva to the right atrium or right ventricle, and pulmonary regurgitation may occur in the absence of right ventricular hypertrophy (eg, bicuspid pulmonary valve or other deformity).

The low-frequency diastolic murmur of relative mitral stenosis heard at the mitral area in the severe form of aortic regurgitation (Austin Flint murmur) has a similar sound to the low-frequency diastolic murmur of relative tricuspid valve stenosis heard in the tricuspid valve area due to the severe form of pulmonary valve regurgitation. The simplest and most expedient noninvasive test to differentiate aortic from pulmonic valve regurgitation is the echocardiographic demonstration of fluttering of the mitral valve in aortic valve regurgitation. The actual semilunar valve leaflet regurgitation may not be demonstrable by echocardiographic visualization of either semilunar valve.

A number of congenital anomalies can lead to aortic regurgitation. They include the following:

1. *Bicuspid aortic valve* In an autopsy series of adult patients with bicuspid aortic valve in whom the antemortem clinical features were known, 13% had pure aortic regurgitation, an equal number had normally functioning aortic valve, and all the rest had aortic stenosis.[10]

Among patients referred to the Texas Children's Hospital pediatric cardiology clinic, 342 proved to have bicuspid aortic valve. Thirteen of them, or 4%, had clinically apparent aortic regurgitation and 88, or 26% of patients had aortic stenosis.

2. *Unicommissural aortic stenosis* About one third of our pediatric patients with the diagnosis of aortic stenosis confirmed by cardiac catheterization and presumed to have unicommissural aortic stenosis proved to have aortic regurgitation on clinical examination. This meant that at least an aortic regurgitation murmur was present. In the course of cardiac catheterization in the patient with aortic stenosis who has no aortic regurgitation murmur, an aortic root angiogram may reveal a mild degree of aortic regurgitation despite lack of clinical signs of valve insufficiency.

3. *Aneurysmal dilatation of the sinus(es) of Valsalva* When the dilatation is mild it is a silent anomaly. However, progressive dilatation in the adult may lead to rupture of the right anterior sinus or noncoronary sinus into the right atrium or right ventricle; the left anterior sinus ruptures into the left atrium or into the pericardium. The clinical features include the abrupt onset of chest pain, right heart failure, a systolic-diastolic to-and-fro murmur over the precordium, and bounding peripheral pulses. This clinical picture suggesting acute aortic insufficiency calls for prompt definitive diagnosis by aortography followed by immediate surgical repair. If promptly carried out, the results are good. Children, however, rarely develop rupture of a dilated sinus of Valsalva. In Marfan's syndrome usually all three aortic sinuses of Valsalva are dilated. the dilatation may remain stable or progress, leading to aortic regurgitation, but rupture rarely occurs.

4. *Mucopolysaccharide deposits on the aortic valve* Mucopolysaccharide deposits on the aortic valve in Hurler's syndrome and Hunter's syndrome may be seen as part of the genetic disorder; however, mitral valve regurgitation is more common. In Morguio's syndrome and Scheie's syndrome, aortic regurgitation is a characteristic cardiovascular lesion due to mucopolysaccharide deposit. Aortic regurgitation has been reported in association with Ehlers-Danlos syn-

drome, presumably from aneurysmal dilatation of the aortic sinus of Valsalva similar to that in Marfan's syndrome, but this lesion is far less common in Ehlers-Danlos than in Marfan's syndrome.

5. *Aortic regurgitation associated with ventricular septal defect* About 5% of patients with ventricular septal defect have associated aortic regurgitation. It occurs most often when the ventricular septal defect is supracristal. In this situation the right coronary cusp can herniate through the ventricular septal defect. Herniation of either the right or the noncoronary cusp may occur in infracristal ventricular septal defect. Aortic regurgitation murmur may appear in infancy, but more often is first heard in childhood. The regurgitation characteristically becomes progressively more severe over a period of several years. Surgical repair of the ventricular septal defect may sometimes correct the aortic valve regurgitation, but operation may require plication of the leaflet.

It is not known if the insufficient cusp begins as a redundant cusp and gradually increases in severity or if, because of an unusual position of the ventricular septal defect, the cusp which is originally normal prolapses into the ventricular septal defect.

6. *Aortic regurgitation associated with aortic stenosis* Among the 37 patients with one of the forms of aortic stenosis, about one third had clear clinical signs of aortic regurgitation.[35] During the 4-year period of follow-up between two heart catheterizations, the patients with valvular, supravalvular, and subvalvular stenosis all had an increase in the left ventricular-to-aortic pressure gradient, but this was not the case for the patients with valvular aortic stenosis and associated aortic regurgitation determined by physical examination. Thus the patient with moderate or mild aortic valve stenosis who has clear auscultatory and echocardiographic signs, and not merely angiographic evidence of aortic regurgitation, can be followed medically with more confidence in childhood and early adolescence than the patient with pure aortic stenosis. Furthermore, calcification on the regurgitant aortic valve compared to the stenotic aortic valve appears to be infrequent in the adult.

REFERENCES

1. Roberts WC: The structure of the aortic valve in clinically isolated aortic stenosis: an autopsy study of 162 patients over 15 years of age. *Circulation* 1970;42:91–97.
2. Falcone MW, Roberts WC, Morrow AG: Congenital aortic stenosis resulting from a unicommissural valve. Clinical and anatomic features in twenty-one adult patients. *Circulation* 1971;44: 272–280.
3. Campbell M: The natural history of congenital aortic stenosis. *Br Heart J* 1968;30:514–526.
4. Folger GM, Stein PD: Bicuspid aortic valve morphology when associated with coarctation of the aorta. *Cathet Cardiovasc Diagn* 1984; 10:17–25.
5. Hurwitz LE: Quadricuspid semilunar valve. *Am J Cardiol* 1973;31:623–626.
6. Edwards WD, Leaf DS, Edwards JE: Dissecting aortic aneurysm associated with congenital bicuspid aortic valve. *Circulation* 1978;57:1022–1025.
7. Edwards JE: Pathology of left ventricular outflow obstruction. *Circulation* 1965;31:586–599.
8. Morrow AG, Lynn F, Roberts WC, et al: Discrete subaortic stenosis complicated by aortic valvular regurgitation. Clinical, hemodynamic and pathologic studies and the results of operative treatment. *Circulation* 1965;31:163–171.
9. Oakley CM, Halladie-Smith KA: Assessment of site and severity in congenital aortic stenosis. *Br Heart J* 1967;29:367–379.
10. Roberts WC: The congenitally bicuspid aortic valve: a study of 85 autopsied patients. *Am J Cardiol* 1970;26:72–79.
11. Edwards JE: The congenital bicuspid aortic valve, editorial. *Circulation* 1961;23:485–488.
12. Beuren AJ, Schulze C, Eberle P, et al: The syndrome of supravalvular aortic stenosis, peripheral pulmonary stenosis, mental retardation and similar facial appearance. *Am J Cardiol* 1964;13: 471–483.
13. Somerville J, Bonham-Carter RE: The heart in lentiginosis. *Br Heart J* 1972;34:1–9.
14. Nanda NC, Gramiak R, Manning J, et al: Echocardiograph recognition of the congenital bicuspid aortic valve. *Circulation* 1974;49:870–875.
15. Radford AJ, Bloom KR, Izukawa T, et al: Echocardiographic assessment of bicuspid aortic valves. *Circulation* 1976;53:80–85.
16. Brandenburg RO Jr, Tajik AJ, Edwards WD, et al: Accuracy of two-dimensional echocardiographic diagnosis of congenitally bicuspid aortic valve: echocardiographic anatomic correlation in 115 patients. *Am J Cardiol* 1983;51:1469–1473.
17. Simon AL, Reis RL: The angiographic features of bicuspid and unicommissural aortic stenosis. *Am J Cardiol* 1971;28:353–358.
18. Wagner HR, Ellison RC, Keane JF, et al: Clinical course in aortic stenosis. *Circulation* 1977;56 suppl 1:47–56.
19. Kugler JD, Campbell E, Vargo TA, et al: Results of aortic valvotomy on infants with isolated aortic valvular stenosis. *J Thorac Cardiovasc Surg* 1979; 78:553–558.
20. Latson LA, Cheatham JP, Gutgesell HP. Relation of the echocardiographic estimate of left ventricular size to mortality in infants with severe left ventricular outflow obstruction. *Am J Cardiol.* 1981;48:887–891.
21. Lakier JB, Lewis AB, Heymann MA, et al:

Isolated aortic stenosis in the neonate. Natural history and hemodynamic considerations. *Circulation* 1974;50:801–808.
22. Keane JF, Bernard WF, Nadas AS: Aortic stenosis surgery in infancy. *Circulation* 1975;52: 1138–1143.
23. Hamman JW, Parrish MD, Graham TP. Risk factors for infants undergoing aortic valvotomy for critical aortic valvar stenosis, abstracted. *J Am Coll Cardiol* 1984;3:585.
24. Huhta JC, Latson LA, Gutgesell HP, et al: Echocardiography in the diagnosis and management of symptomatic aortic valve stenosis in infants. *Circulation* 1984;70:438–444.
25. Hawker RE, Seara CA, Krovetz LJ: Distalward modification of the arterial pulse wave in children with congenital aortic stenosis. *Circulation* 1974; 50:181–187.
26. Hohn AR, VanPraagh SV, Moore AAD, et al: Aortic stenosis. *Circulation* 1965;31–32 suppl 3:4.
27. Hugenholtz PG, Lees MM, Nadas AS: The scalar electrocardiogram, vectorcardiogram, and exercise electrocardiogram in the assessment of congenital aortic stenosis. *Circulation* 1962;26:79–91.
28. Wagner HR, Weidman WH, Ellison RC: Indirect assessment of severity in aortic stenosis. *Circulation* 1977;56 suppl 1:20–23.
29. Alpert BS, Kartodihardjo W, Harp R: Exercise blood pressure response — a predictor of severity of aortic stenosis in children. *J Pediatr* 1981; 98:763–765.
30. Johnson GL, Meyer RA, Schwartz DC: Echocardiographic evaluation of fixed left ventricular outlet obstruction in children. *Circulation* 1977; 56:299–304.
31. Weyman AE, Feigenbaum H, Dillon JC: Cross-sectional echocardiography in assessing the severity of valvular aortic stenosis. *Circulation* 1975; 52:828–834.
32. Weyman AE, Feigenbaum H, Hurwitz RA: Cross-sectional echocardiographic assessment of the severity of aortic stenosis in children. *Circulation* 1977;55:773–778.
33. Halte L, Augelson BA, Trousdal A: Non-invasive assessment of aortic stenosis by Doppler ultrasound. *Br Heart J* 1980;43:284–292.
34. Kosturakis D, Allen HD, Goldberg SJ: Doppler quantitation of stenotic semilunar valve area, abstracted. *J Am Coll Cardiol* 1984;3:494.
35. El-Said G, Galioto FM, Mullins CE, et al: Natural hemodynamic history of congenital aortic stenosis in childhood. *Am J Cardiol* 1972;30:6–12.
36. Wagner S, Selyer A: Patterns of progression of aortic stenosis: a longitudinal hemodynamic study. *Circulation* 1982;65:709–712.
37. Cheitlin MD, Gertz EW, Brundage BH: Rate of progression of severity of valvular aortic stenosis in the adult. *Am Heart J* 1979;98:689–700.
38. Stein PD, Sabbah HN, Pitha JV: Continuing disease process of calcific aortic stenosis: role of microthrombi and turbulent flow. *Am J Cardiol* 1977;39:159–163.
39. Doyle EF, Arumugham P, Lara E: Sudden death in young patients with congenital aortic stenosis. *Pediatrics* 1974;53:481–489.
40. Garson A, Gillette PC, McVey P, et al: Sudden death in pediatric cardiovascular patients, abracted. *J Am Coll Cardiol* 1984;3:484.
41. Driscoll DJ, Edwards WD: Sudden unexpected death in children and adolescents. *J Am Coll Cardiol* 1985;5:118–121.
42. McHenry MM, Rice J, Matlof HJ, et al: Pulmonary hypertension and sudden death in aortic stenosis. *Br Heart J* 1979;41:463–467.
43. McNamara DG, Bricker JT, Galioto FM, et al: Cardiovascular abnormalities in the athlete: Recommendations regarding eligibility for competition. *J Am Coll Cardiol* 1985;6:1200–1208.
44. Sandor GGS, Olley PM, Trusler GA, et al: Long-term follow-up of patients after valvotomy for congenital valvular aortic stenosis in children. *J Thorac Cardiovasc Surg* 1980;80:171–176.
45. Orsmond GS, Bessinger FB, Moller JH: Rest and exercise hemodynamics in children before and after aortic valvotomy. *Am Heart J* 1980;99: 76–86.
46. Jones M, Barnhart GR, Morrow AG: Late results after operations for left ventricular outflow tract obstruction. *Am J Cardiol* 1982;50:569–579.

CHAPTER 10
Acquired Aortic Valve Disease

Barry Greenberg

Situated, as it is, between the main pumping chamber of the heart and the systemic circulation, the aortic valve plays an important role in maintaining cardiac performance. Abnormalities of the valve may result in both a decrease in the amount of blood flow from the heart to the periphery as well as an increase in the pressure or volume load that is imposed on the left ventricle. In general, the natural history of aortic valve disease is determined by two factors. The first is the severity of the valve lesion. The second (but no less important) factor is the status of the left ventricle and its ability to compensate for the altered loading conditions. Neither of these factors is static and, depending on the specific lesion, one or both may evolve considerably during the course of the disease. As we shall see, it is the ability of the left ventricle to develop compensatory changes over time that explains the prolonged clinical course that is characteristic of chronic aortic valve disease.

In this chapter, acquired diseases of the aortic valve will be considered. However, some aspects of the congenitally bicuspid valve will also be discussed. This lesion is included because its effects on left ventricular structure and function are similar to those caused by the acquired valve lesions. In addition, clinically important disease due to a bicuspid aortic valve is usually not seen until the patient reaches adulthood. Although some aspects of acute aortic insufficiency are discussed, this condition is covered more extensively in the chapter on valvular emergencies.

AORTIC STENOSIS

Etiology and Pathology

Obstruction to left ventricular outflow may occur at the valvular, subvalvular, or supravalvular level. The lesions which cause subvalvular (including the dynamic obstruction seen in patients with hypertrophic cardiomyopathy) and supravalvular stenosis are almost always congenital and will not be discussed in this chapter. In considering valvular aortic stenosis the most common etiologies by far are congenital malformations, degenerative calcific disease, and rheumatic disease.[1–4] Severe, widespread atherosclerosis in association with type II hyperlipoproteinemia may result in some degree of aortic stenosis. Other causes, such as ochronosis, are extremely uncommon. Roberts[1] has presented evidence that congenital malformations, particularly a bicuspid valve, are the predominant cause of aortic stenosis in the adult. In his autopsy series of 105 patients above 14 years of age with anatomically isolated aortic stenosis, 13 had a unicuspid valve, 54 a bicuspid valve, 32 a tricuspid valve, and in 6 the structure was uncertain.[1] However, in patients over 65 years of age senile calcification of a tricuspid valve is the cause in over 90%.[2] Rheumatic disease, which usually causes multivalve involvement or mixed stenosis and regurgitation, rarely results in isolated aortic stenosis.[1]

The development of stenosis in a bicuspid valve is characterized by thickening and loss of flexibility of the valve leaflets. The valve usually has a "fish-mouth" appearance and there is no evidence of commissural fusion. The development of important stenosis is almost always accompanied by heavy calcification of the valve in adult patients.[3,4] It is believed that the abnormal architecture of the bicuspid aortic valve leads to turbulent flow which, in turn, increases the stresses on the valve and ultimately leads to degenerative changes and calcification. Stein et al have postulated that turbulence in flow due to a structural abnormality may lead to the deposition and subsequent organization of microthrombi on the valve surface.[5] A bicuspid aortic valve is probably the most common congenital cardiac malformation (if one excludes a prolapsing mitral valve) and may be present in up to 2% of births.[3] Malformations of the aortic valve have been associated with coarction of the aorta and other congenital abnormalities in 13% of cases.[3] It has been estimated that about a third of the population born with a bicuspid valve will develop stenosis, a third will develop insufficiency (often in association with infectious endocarditis), and a third will not develop hemodynamically important disease.[6] A bicuspid valve may result in clinically important disease during any decade of life. However, the incidence of aortic stenosis in patients with a bicuspid valve increases with age. Fenoglio et al found that 46% of patients above 50 years and 73% above 70 years with a bicuspid valve had some degree of stenosis.[6]

In patients older than 65 years of age, aortic stenosis is most often due to calcification of a tricuspid valve which was either structurally normal or in which there was a mild abnormality in the size of the individual leaflets. The continued stress faced by the aortic valve during the lifetime of the individual apparently results in structural changes in the leaflets which diminish their flexibility and predispose to later calcification. Commissural fusion is usually minimal or absent and heavy calcification which inhibits leaflet mobility is present in virtually all cases.[2] The calcification often involves the mitral anulus and may even extend into the coronary arteries. Rheumatic disease causes vascularization of the valve leaflets and, later in the course, commissural fusion, leaflet thickening, retraction, and loss of flexibility. Most commonly the rheumatic aortic valve has a reduced, fixed central orifice which is both stenotic and regurgitant.[1]

Pathophysiology

In adults, the cross-sectional area of the normal aortic valve is 3.0 cm^2 or greater. As the valve orifice narrows, the transvalvular gradient must increase in order to maintain cardiac output in the normal range. The interrelationship of aortic valve gradient, flow and orifice size is shown in Figure 10-1. With mild degrees of stenosis, flow at rest, which is usually around 250 mL/s of systole, can be maintained with development of a small gradient. Even during exercise, when flow is increased several-fold, the increase in gradient is minimal. Further reductions in orifice size at this stage of the disease will have minimal effects on hemodynamics. However, by the time that the valve area has been reduced to 1.0 cm^2 the gradient at rest will be around 50 mmHg and any increase in flow will result in a substantial increase in gradient. At a

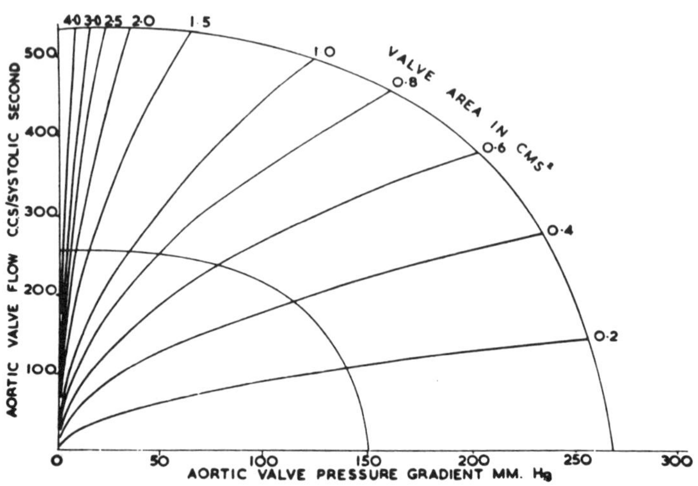

Figure 10-1 Relationship between aortic valve area, transvalvular gradient, and flow. As the valve orifice narrows, progressively larger increments in the transvalvular gradient are required to maintain normal flow. (Reproduced with permission from Herman MV, et al: Resistance to blood flow in stenotic valves: Calculation of orifice area, in Grossman W: *Cardiac Catheterization and Angiography*. Philadelphia, Lea & Febiger, 1976, p 93.)

valve area of 0.6 cm^2, a gradient of 75 to 80 mmHg is required to maintain normal flow at rest. Thus, as the stenosis becomes more severe, further reductions in valve area will cause progressively larger increases in both the resting and exercise gradients that are required to maintain flow. This relationship explains why patients can tolerate aortic stenosis for years before the onset of symptoms. In addition, the development of hypertrophy helps the left ventricle generate adequate pressure so that flow can be maintained during the prolonged asymptomatic phase of the disease. However, pressure cannot be generated to an infinite level and, at some point, flow must be compromised. This occurs first during exercise and, with severe disease, flow may be reduced even at rest. In general, critical impedance to flow occurs when the cross-sectional area of the aortic valve is reduced to a fourth of normal or less than 0.7 cm^2.

The increase in left ventricular systolic pressure, which occurs as aortic stenosis progresses, is a potent stimulus for the development of left ventricular hypertrophy. On gross examination of the heart there is a substantial increase in left ventricular muscle mass which, in the absence of failure, occurs with minimal or no increase in the overall chamber size. Typically, the heart in aortic stenosis may weigh between 400 and 1000 g or more. The myocardial fibers show evidence of substantial increase in the transverse diameter of the cell with an increase in both myofibrils and mitochondria.[7] As pointed out by Grossman et al, the increase in left ventricular wall thickness serves to normalize systolic wall stress which would otherwise be increased by the rise in left ventricular systolic pressure.[8]

Left ventricular failure is a late complication of aortic stenosis and may be due to a variety of mechanisms. When the increased pressure load imposed on the left ventricle by the stenotic aortic valve overwhelms myocardial reserve, failure may develop on the basis of what Ross has termed "afterload mismatch."[9] Gunther and Grossman have demonstrated in patients that impaired cardiac performance may be due to inappropriately high end-systolic wall stress (eg, afterload) rather than depressed contractility.[10] Other mechanisms include ischemia of the hypertrophied left ventricle, which is potentially reversible, and the development of chronic fibrotic changes, which are probably permanent.

The hypertrophied left ventricle in patients with aortic stenosis has been shown to have increased diastolic stiffness.[11–13] Consequently, a forceful, appropriately timed left atrial contribution is an important factor in producing adequate end-diastolic fiber stretch so that stroke volume can be maintained.[14] At the same time, the forceful atrial kick protects the pulmonary capillaries from the sustained increases in intravascular pressure which would otherwise be necessary to insure filling of the stiff ventricular chamber. When the atrial contribution is lost, as in atrial fibrillation, a substantial reduction in cardiac output, along with an increase in pulmonary capillary pressure, often occurs.

One of the key features of aortic stenosis is that clinical symptoms tend to develop late in the course of the disease. This can be explained on the basis of a number of the factors mentioned above. The relationship between valve area, transvalvular gradient, and flow explains why large gradients are seen only after considerable narrowing of the valve has occurred. The compensatory changes in left ventricular architecture are an effective means of maintaining wall stress within normal limits, and the overall performance of the left ventricle is greatly aided by a forceful, appropriately timed atrial kick which helps maintain stroke volume and keeps pulmonary capillary pressure in an acceptable range.

Diagnosis

Symptoms The classical triad of symptoms that occurs in patients with aortic stenosis are angina pectoris, syncope or presyncope, and congestive heart failure. The prevalence of angina in adult patients with aortic stenosis varies in the medical literature (probably as a result of the age, sex, and severity of the disease in the population under scrutiny), but overall it appears to be around 50%.[15–20] Wood has observed that both the characteristics of the pain and the response to nitroglycerin are similar to that seen in patients with coronary artery disease.[15] The presence of chest pain cannot be used to predict whether or not the patient has coronary disease. However, Paquay et al[18] who evaluated 76 patients with documented aortic stenosis found that when typical angina was present,[23] (64%) of the 36 patients had significant coronary disease. They also found that in the absence of chest pain, only one of 19 patients had significant coronary disease. Similar findings were reported by Basta et al[20] who found that none of the 19 patients without angina who were studied had significant coronary disease. However, in older patients silent coronary artery disease appears to be more prevalent.[16] The reason why patients with aortic stenosis develop myocardial ischemia in the absence of coronary artery disease is not certain. Although the increase in myocardial mass in aortic stenosis causes an increase in myocardial oxygen demands (MVO_2), estimates of myocardial mass have been shown to be unrelated to the presence of angina.[20,21] However, when hypertrophy is not adequate for the pressure or volume load, the resultant increase in systolic wall stress would be expected to increase MVO_2 and increase the likelihood of developing ischemia. As mentioned previously, the hypertrophic ventricle is stiffer than normal. The increase in left ventricular end-diastolic pressure may be a factor in reducing coronary flow to the subendocardial region. Patients with critical aortic stenosis may also have insufficient coronary reserve. Recently, Marcus et al[22] have demonstrated that the hyperemic blood flow response (which is a measure of coronary reserve) to ischemia induced by a 20-second occlusion off the left anterior descending coronary artery was decreased substantially in 14 patients with left ventricular hypertrophy due to aortic stenosis as compared to a group of control patients. Whether the reason for the decreased flow is inadequate microvascularization, compression of small intramyocardial vessels, or some other· cause is uncertain. A further discussion of this topic is included in chapter 13.

Syncope, or near syncope may be the presenting symptom in aortic stenosis. The syndrome usually occurs either during or immediately following exercise. Several mechanisms may be involved. As discussed previously, when critical stenosis develops, the pressure necessary to increase flow during exercise may become enormous. Thus, even the nonfailing ventricle may be unable to maintain cardiac output during times of increased demands. When the increase in cardiac output fails to keep pace with the reduction in systemic vascular resistance that accompanies dynamic exercise, the net result is a reduction in arterial perfusion pressure. In addition, when exercise is terminated, the forceful muscle contractions in the periphery are no longer available to push blood back to the heart. If left ventricular diastolic volume is reduced, left ventricular stroke volume would be expected to be diminished according to the Frank-Starling mechanism. Schwartz et al[23] have provided evidence that, in some patients with aortic stenosis, an abrupt decrease in left ventricular systolic pump function (perhaps caused by myocardial ischemia) is responsible for the drop in arterial pressure during exercise. The occurrence of atrial or ventricular arrhythmias during exercise may also contribute to the reduction in cardiac output. Mark et al[24] have demonstrated that the normal forearm vasoconstrictor response to leg exercise was inhibited or reversed in patients with aortic stenosis. They postulated that this was due to a activation of left ventricular baroreceptors.[24] Thus, the reduction in perfusion pressure could be due to inappropriate vasodilation in the vascular bed of nonexercising muscle groups. Finally, there is evidence showing that abnormalities of the conducting system are common in patients with aortic stenosis, particularly when heavy calcification of the aortic valve is present. Dhingra et al[25] demonstrated prolonged distal conduction, as manifest by an abnormally long HV interval in 12 of 24 patients with aortic stenosis. This abnormal finding was associated with transvalvular gradients greater than 40 mmHg and the presence of valvular calcification.[25] These workers postulated that transient episodes of heart block may be the cause of the syncopal episodes in some patients with aortic stenosis.

Exertional dyspnea and other manifestations of heart failure are probably the most common symptoms reported by patients with aortic stenosis. As discussed previously, they are caused by a failure of the adaptive mechanisms to compensate fully for the hemodynamic burdens imposed on the left ventricle by the valve lesion. The onset of atrial fibrillation, which abruptly takes away the forceful atrial kick and also reduces the diastolic filling period that is needed to fill the stiff ventricle, may precipitate fulminant, life-threatening pulmonary edema. As will be discussed, patients who develop left-sided failure have a markedly shortened natural history. Consequently, the later development of right-sided failure is an uncommon occurrence in aortic stenosis.

Physical Examination The physical examination of patients with aortic stenosis varies somewhat depending on the age of the patient, pathology of the valve lesion, stage of the disease, and whether or not aortic regurgitation is also present. For instance, physical findings that are dependent on the magnitude of flow across the valve, such as the intensity of the aortic systolic murmur and the presence of a systolic thrill, are magnified when there is coexistent aortic insufficiency and a large stroke volume. These findings are usually considerably less prominent in the patient who has heart failure and a reduced stroke volume. Differentiation between valvular obstruction and other forms of left ventricular outflow obstruction has been the topic of a review by Perloff.[26]

Aortic stenosis is predominantly a disease of middle-aged to elderly males, although younger males and females are by no means excluded. Aside from the cardiovascular abnormalities, the patient often has a normal physical examination. The blood pressure is usually unremarkable but may be somewhat reduced in patients with critical disease who have low cardiac output. The presence of systolic hypertension should not be used to exclude the possibility of significant aortic stenosis, since the left ventricle is capable of generating pressures up to and even beyond 300 mmHg. Systolic hypertension, when present with this disease, is more commonly seen in older patients. In a survey of patients with critical aortic stenosis who were older than 60 years of age, which was conducted at our institution, the prevalence of systolic hypertension was 39%.[16] The carotid pulses have both reduced volume and a slow upstroke — the so-called parvus et tardus pulse. An anacrotic shoulder (or hump) may be appreciated during the upstroke and is often followed by a shudder or thrill. The level of the anacrotic shoulder on the pulse wave gives a rough approximation of the severity of stenosis. In general, the lower the shoulder, the more severe the stenosis. This physical finding may sometimes be mistaken for the bisferiens pulse of aortic insufficiency or the dual component pulse of idiopathic hypertrophic subaortic stenosis (IHSS). In aortic insufficiency, the two peaks of the pulse wave are approximately equal in height, and the pulse characteristically has a brisk upstroke and rapid run-off. In IHSS, the pulse is described as having a "spike and dome" configuration in which there is a relatively normal initial upstroke followed by a delayed, slow-rising second component. The classical carotid pulse tracing of aortic stenosis may be altered when the valve is incompetent as well as stenotic. Elderly patients who have stiff, noncomplaint vessels may also have a relatively normal-appearing pulse despite the presence of critical disease.

In the absence of right heart failure the neck veins appear normal. However, a prominent "a" wave may be seen in the jugular venous pulse tracing. This is believed to result from the hypertrophic left ventricle impinging on the right ventricular cavity and effectively altering the complaince characteristics of that chamber. Since aortic stenosis results in concentric hypertrophy of the left ventricle, the apical impulse is not displaced laterally until late in the disease when left heart failure develops. The apical impulse is usually forceful and sustained. A late diastolic filling or "a" wave, due to the forceful atrial contribution, can be palpated over the apex. The first heart sound is usually normal in intensity. An ejection click heard shortly after S_1 suggests the presence of a bicuspid valve. The intensity of the ejection click may be diminished as the disease progresses and is often absent in adult patients with critical stenosis due to reduced valve mobility. In the presence of critical aortic stenosis the second heart sound is usually single because of the diminished mobility of the valve leaflets. In some cases, paradoxical splitting of the second heart sound caused by delay in left ventricular ejection may be appreciated. Little helpful information is gained when a fourth heart sound is heard, but not palpated, since the presence of an audible S_4 has been noted in a high percentage of patients with less than critical aortic stenosis as well as in normal subjects.[27]

The murmur of aortic stenosis begins shortly after the first heart sound and immediately following the ejection click when it is present. Classically, the murmur is heard best over the right second intercostal space or the left third intercostal space and radiates upward toward the neck. The murmur is crescendo-decrescendo in nature. It reaches peak intensity early when the stenosis is mild and will peak progressively later in systole as the severity of stenosis increases. Neither the presence nor the intensity of a systolic thrill correlates well with the severity of stenosis since this finding is highly dependent on the magnitude of the left ventricular stroke volume.

In elderly patients, the murmur may be best appreciated at the cardiac apex.[2,28,29] In such cases it is often higher pitched than usual and may have a musical component. It often resembles the sound of plywood being sawed against the grain. Roberts has postulated that the murmur of calcific aortic stenosis in elderly patients may be heard better at the apex for three reasons: (1) Changes in chest wall configuration (as in emphysema) obscure the intensity of the murmur at the base; (2) The pathophysiology of the valve disease results in flow between the rigid valve leaflets rather than through a central jet as in either rheumatic or congenital disease. In this case, vibrations of the valve leaflets are radiated back toward the cavity of the ventricle and are heard best at the cardiac apex. (3) Calcification of the mitral anulus may result in some degrees of mitral valve incompetence.[2]

The murmur of aortic stenosis may be difficult to differentiate from that of mitral regurgitation, particularly in elderly patients. When in doubt, the source of the murmur can often be determined by cautiously administrating amyl nitrate to the patient.[28,30] The reduction in systemic vascular resistance caused by this drug increases the murmur of aortic stenosis and reduces the intensity of the mitral regurgitation murmur. The sensitivity and specificity of this maneuver in differentiating between these two valve lesions is good[31]; however, the test should be done with great care (eg, patient in the supine position, single whiff of amyl to begin with) since a dramatic fall in arterial pressure may occur.

Patients with IHSS often have physical findings that are similar to those seen in aortic stenosis. Isometric exercise, which tends to increase afterload and left ventricular diastolic volume, will result in a marked reduction in the intensity of the murmur of IHSS but may also diminish the intensity of the murmur due to valvular aortic stenosis. The holding phase of the Valsalva maneuver reduces left ventricular volume and intensifies both murmur and gradient in IHSS and usually diminishes the murmur of aortic stenosis. If the patient is having premature beats, assessment of pulse pressure is often quite helpful in differentiating the lesions. In IHSS, the increased contractility of the postpremature beat increases outflow obstruction so that stroke volume and pulse pressure are reduced. Both the murmur and pulse are slightly increased in the postpremature beat in valvular stenosis.

When patients present with classical physical findings, the diagnosis of valvular aortic stenosis can be made with a great deal of certainty. Thus, in the presence of a sustained apical impulse and palpable fourth heart sound, a late peaking, grunting systolic murmur at the base, a single or paradoxically split second heart sound, and a slowly rising, low-volume carotid pulse with a prominent low anacrotic shoulder, the likelihood of critical aortic stenosis is extremely high. However, the findings in an individual patient are often equivocal and the clinician may have difficulty in separating critical from subcritical disease.

Electrocardiogram Left ventricular hypertrophy with secondary ST and T wave changes have been noted in 80% to 90% of patients with critical aortic stenosis.[15,16,29] Evidence of left atrial enlargement may also be seen. The remaining 10% to 20% will have a left bundle-branch block pattern or nonspecific repolarization abnormalities. Only rarely will the patient with critical aortic stenosis have a completely normal ECG. The rhythm is usually sinus, but around 20% of patients will be in atrial fibrillation.[17]

Chest Roentgenogram Since concentric hypertrophy without an increase in chamber volume is the usual response to a pressure load, the cardiac silhouette in aortic stenosis is of normal size on the chest film until late in the course of the disease. The left heart border may be somewhat boot-shaped as a result of left ventricular hypertrophy. Left atrial enlargement is seen occasionally. An important finding is the presence of aortic valvular calcium. As shown in Figure 10-2, this is best seen in the lateral film. When there is uncertainty regarding the presence of aortic valvular calcium the issue can often be resolved by use of image-intensified fluoroscopy. Glancy et al have reported that severe aortic stenosis was extremely rare in patients in whom calcium could not be demonstrated either fluoroscopically or on chest film.[32] These workers also showed that the extent of aortic valve calcification correlated with the peak systolic gradient across the valve. When heavy calcification is present, extension into the mitral anulus and even into the coronary vessels may be seen. Another useful roentgenographic finding is the presence of an enlarged aortic root due to poststenotic dilation of the vessel. This is most commonly seen in patients with rheumatic disease or a biscuspid valve. It is caused by the central jet of blood striking the wall of the aorta. It is less commonly seen in elderly patients who have degenerative calcific changes in a tricuspid valve.

Echocardiography Over the past decade there has been considerable interest in the use of noninvasive techniques as a means of confirming the diagnosis of aortic valve disease and in determining the severity of the lesion. Both M-mode and two-dimensional echocardiography have been useful in detecting abnormalities of the aortic valve, particularly, in defining the presence of a congenital malformation.[33,34] Brandenburg et al found that two-dimensiónal echocardiography had a 78% sensitivity, 96% specificity, and 93% accuracy in detecting the presence of a bicuspid valve.[34] However, adequate visualization was not possible in 25% of patients. Because of its ability to improve spatial

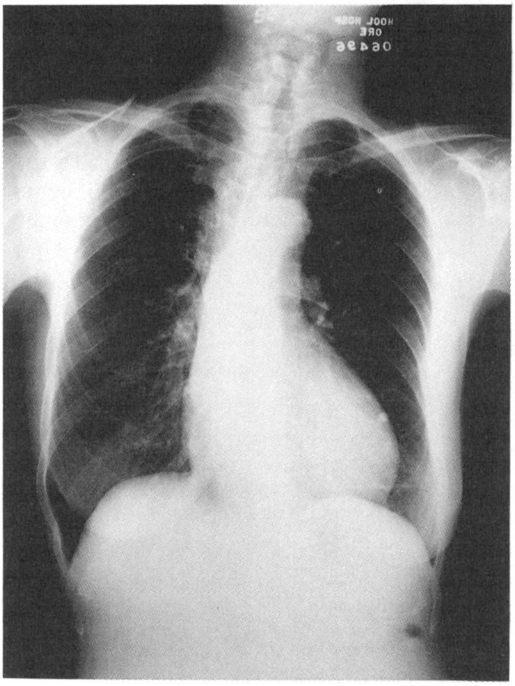

Figure 10-2A

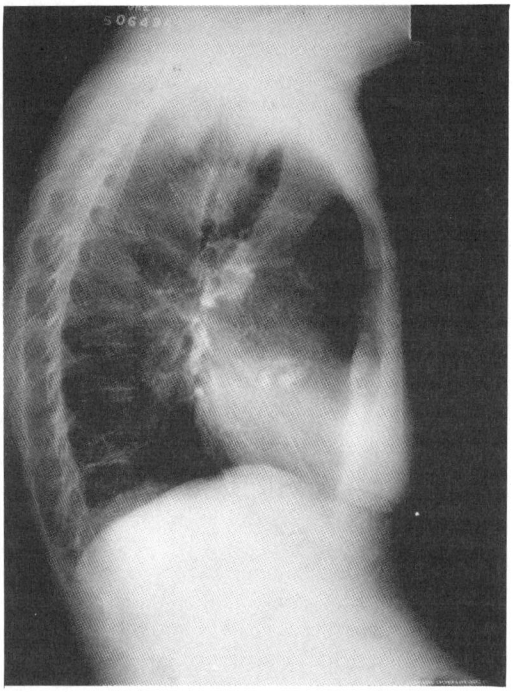

Figure 10-2B

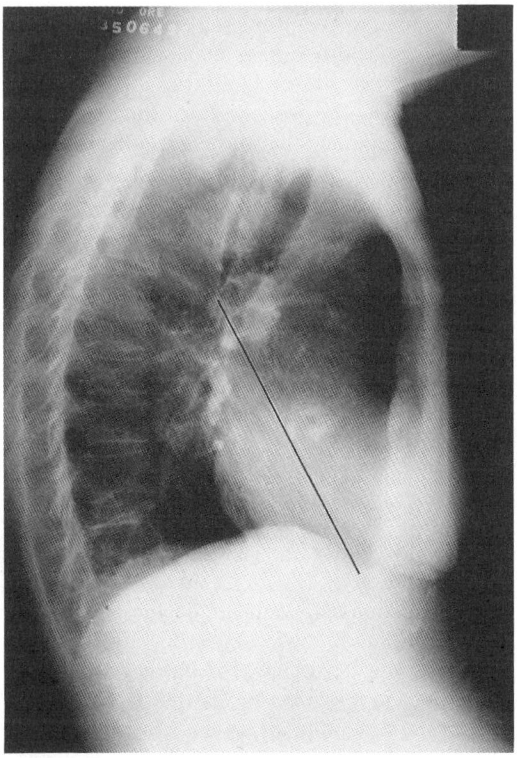

Figure 10-2C

Figure 10-2 Chest film of a patient with critical aortic stenosis. A Posteroanterior projection. Borderline cardiac enlargement is present and the apex of the heart is tilted upward as is seen with concentric hypertrophy of the left ventricle. B Lateral projection. Heavy calcification in the form of a ring is seen in the area of the aortic valve. C Lateral projection. When the cardiac silhouette is bisected by a line extending from the carina of the trachea to the cardiac apex, the plane of the aortic valve will be seen above the line while the mitral valve plane will be seen below.

orientation so that maximal cusp separation can be evaluated, two-dimensional echocardiography is preferred when the severity of aortic stenosis is to be assessed.[35] However, although this method appears to be a sensitive means of detecting the presence of valvular aortic stenosis, its ability to discriminate between critical and subcritical disease is limited.[36,37] The reason for this has to do with the fact that valvular calcification, which accompanies virtually all cases of aortic stenosis in adults, significantly impairs image quality and leads to an overestimation of the degree of stenosis. In aortic stenosis the valve orifice is often deformed and irregular making it difficult to visualize and accurately planimeter. In addition, orifice size is influenced by left ventricular stroke volume as well as the mobility of the leaflets. When left ventricular dysfunction is present and stroke volume is low, leaflet separation may be reduced leading to an overestimation of the severity of stenosis.

Although the echocardiogram cannot be used to quantitate the severity of stenosis, it can distinguish mild from severe disease and does give useful information concerning the presence of left ventricular chamber size, wall thickness, and systolic pump function. The echocardiogram can also be used to rule out other forms of left ventricular outflow obstruction such as subvalvular or supravalvular stenosis. Early reports that left ventricular systolic pressure could be derived by echocardiogram[38] if one assumed that peak systolic wall stress was constant have not been confirmed by more recent investigations.[39] This method does not appear to be a reliable means of assessing aortic stenosis in adults.

Recently, there has been considerable interest in the use of Doppler ultrasound to assess the severity of aortic stenosis. This technique uses reflected sound waves to measure the velocity of blood flow in the ascending aorta just distal to the valve. It is based on the Bernoulli principle which states that the pressure drop across an area of obstruction varies directly with the increase in velocity of flow across that orifice. A close correlation between measured transvalvular gradient and the estimate obtained using Doppler ultrasound has been reported.[40,41] However, the angle of incidence between the ultrasound beam and aortic blood flow is critical and is a possible source of error. The accuracy of this method to distinguish critical from subcritical disease is uncertain at present.

Catheterization Cardiac catheterization remains the most reliable way of determining the severity of valvular aortic stenosis and for separating critical from subcritical disease. In order to measure the transvalvular gradient, a catheter must be introduced into the left ventricle either retrograde across the aortic valve or by the transseptal technique. Left ventricular systolic pressure is then compared with simultaneously measured aortic pressure. Cardiac output and the systolic ejection period of the left ventricle must also be measured so that the flow per unit time across the valve can be calculated. This information is then used in the hydraulic formula of Gorlin where K is a constant:

$$\text{Aortic valve area} = \frac{\text{flow/unit time}}{K\sqrt{\text{gradient}}}$$

Potential errors in the calculation of valve area are discussed in chapter 9. Evaluation of the coronary vessels, mitral valve, and of left ventricular systolic pump function can also be undertaken at the time of catheterization, although the latter can also be reliably measured noninvasively by radionuclear techniques.

Although catheterization can be undertaken safely in most patients with aortic stenosis, the procedure is not without risks. In particular, systemic blood pressure is exquisitely sensitive to the reduction in intravascular volume which often occurs both during and immediately following the procedure. Careful attention to fluid balance during the postcatheterization period has helped to minimize the frequency and severity of hypotension in our laboratory.

Natural History

As already mentioned, symptoms occur late in the course of aortic stenosis. Although sudden cardiac death may be the initial presentation, this is probably uncommon in the truly asymptomatic patient. Once symptoms appear, the patient can be thought of as having entered a new, more ominous phase of the disease. For instance, in symptomatic patients, the average survival at 5 years appears to be less than 50% and at 10 years it is only 10% to 20%.[42–44] Ross and Braunwald[45] have suggested that once heart failure occurs the average survival is only 1.5 years. Mortality appears to be increased when a combination of symptoms develop and also following the occurrence of atrial fibrillation.[17] As shown in Figure 10-3, patients with critical aortic stenosis appear to have a substantially different natural history than do patients with other left heart valvular lesions.

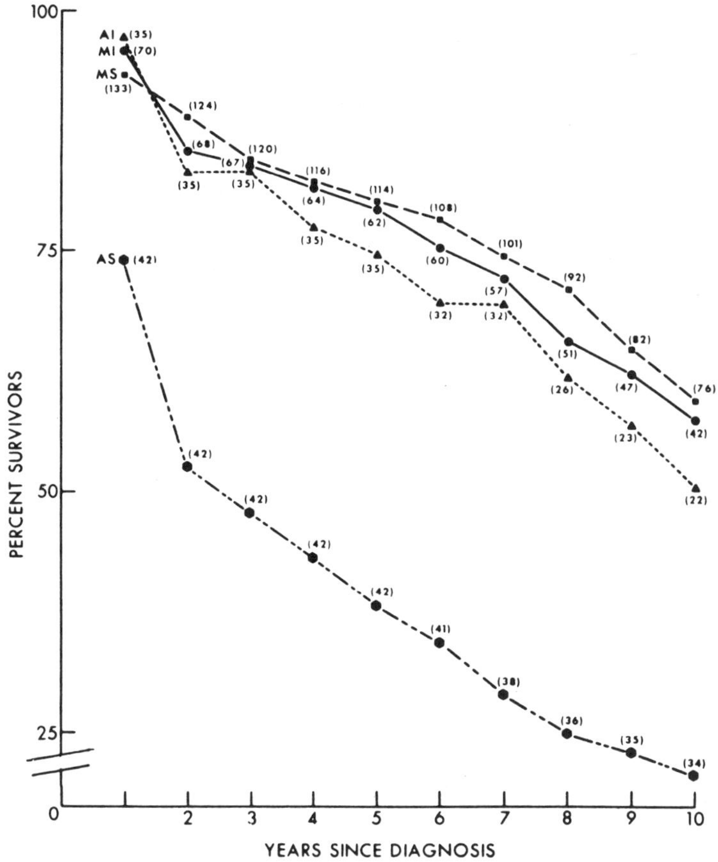

Figure 10-3 Survival of patients with valvular heart disease treated medically. The poor prognosis of patients with aortic stenosis compared to other left heart valvular lesions is noted. AI = aortic insufficiency, MI = mitral insufficiency, MS = mitral stenosis. (Reproduced with permission from Rapaport.[42])

Some patients are identified early in the course of the disease, before symptoms due to critical narrowing of the valve have occurred. Recently, information about the rate of progression of stenosis in these patients has been reported. Cheitlin et al,[46] in a retrospective study, evaluated 29 patients with known aortic stenosis who had at least two cardiac catheterizations. In the 16 patients in whom the peak systolic gradient increased, the average rate of increase was 1.3 mmHg per month with the most rapid gradient increase being 3.8 mmHg per month. In the remaining 15 patients the changes in peak systolic gradient were considerably less. These workers correlated the onset of angina pectoris and the development of left ventricular hypertrophy on ECG with progression of transvalvular gradient.[46] Other studies have shown similar variability in the rate of progression of stenosis over time.[47–49] Wagner and Selzer have suggested that patients with degenerative calcific aortic stenosis progress more rapidly than do patients with aortic stenosis caused by either congenital or rheumatic disease.[49]

Management

Patients with known aortic valve disease should receive endocarditis prophylaxis for procedures associated with a bacteremia regardless of the severity of disease. Other aspects of the management of the asymptomatic patient with critical aortic stenosis are controversial. The dilemma comes about because the initial clinical manifestation of the disease may be sudden death. The incidence of this dreaded complication is not known but is probably low in the truly asymptomatic patient. It should be remembered that early surgical intervention exposes the patient to a finite risk of cardiac death during operation, as well as the continued risk of complications from the valve prosthesis. Therefore, it has been my practice to refrain from advising prophylactic surgery in this subset of patients. Strenuous exercise should be limited and careful and frequent follow-up is mandatory. Some clinicians favor catheterizing the asymptomatic patient who has evidence of critical aortic stenosis by examination or noninvasive testing in order to determine the severity of the disease. Patients with large transvalvular gradients are then often sent to surgery. However, studies in support of this approach (or the more conservative approach) are lacking.

Since symptoms do not occur until late in the course of the disease, it is not uncommon for aortic stenosis to be discovered as part of a routine physical examination or during work-up of another, unassociated medical problem. When there is evidence to suggest that critical aortic stenosis is present in a patient who is scheduled to undergo a major surgical procedure, diagnostic evaluation to confirm the presence and severity of the lesion must be undertaken prior to operation since the patient (even if he is asymptomatic) is likely to be at increased risk for cardiovascular events during the perioperative period.[50] If critical aortic stenosis is found, the potential risks and benefits of the noncardiac surgery should be re-evaluated with this in mind. When the noncardiac surgery is still considered to be necessary, the author has recommended that valve replacement be performed in some patients. This decision is based on the magnitude of the noncardiac procedure, the severity of the stenosis, and the overall condition of the patient at the time.

Asymptomatic patients with valvular aortic stenosis are usually seen half-yearly or yearly depending on the severity of the disease. The development of left ventricular hypertrophy with ST-T wave changes on the ECG is often the earliest indicator that there has been a significant increase in the severity of the disease. Once symptoms of angina, syncope, or heart failure appear, valve replacement is indicated. Although there have been no randomized, controlled trials of medical versus surgical management of symptomatic patients with critical aortic stenosis, the natural history of medically managed patients[42–45] compares so poorly to that of patients who have undergone valve replacement that such a trial will not be performed.

Whether or not all patients suspected of having critical aortic stenosis should undergo preoperative catheterization is a controversial topic. Some authors feel that this may not be necessary in all patients.[51,52] However, this point has been contested by others.[53–55] Although physical findings and noninvasive tests may provide the correct diagnosis in most patients, the accuracy of this approach in differentiating subcritical from critical disease remains uncertain. Since the consequences of either over- or underestimation of the severity of disease are major, it is my practice to recommend routine preoperative catheterization. In addition to defining the severity of the aortic valve lesion, the presence of other valve lesions and the status of the coronary vessels can be assessed as part of the procedure. In poorly compensated or unstable patients, the risks of catheterization may outweigh the benefits. Such patients should be taken directly to surgery when the diagnosis of aortic stenosis seems straightforward.

In patients with critical aortic stenosis, the presence of severe left ventricular dysfunction is not a reason to defer surgical intervention as it may be in patients with coronary disease or chronic left-sided valvular regurgitation. There is considerable information showing that even in patients with advanced left ventricular dysfunction, valve replacement for aortic stenosis often results in marked improvement in left ventricular systolic pump function. Many of these patients will also experience relief of symptoms as well as improved survival.[56–60] The reason why the long-term outlook for this condition is better than that for other left-sided valvular lesions is that left ventricular dysfunction in critical aortic stenosis is not necessarily caused by irreversible damage to heart muscle. In many cases it is due to excessive afterload imposed by the obstructive lesion as discussed earlier in this chapter.

In general, aortic stenosis is a disease of the elderly. With improvement in operative techniques and the widespread use of cold cardioplegia to aid in myocardial preservation, the operative mortality in elderly patients has improved considerably over the past several years. Murphy et al have reported the results of surgery for critical aortic stenosis in a group of 99 consecutive patients who were above age 60.[16] There was a 16% operative mortality and the projected 10-year survival was 58%. Symptomatic improvement occurred in virtually all patients and the results of surgery were not adversely influenced by preoperative ejection fraction. Other studies support these encouraging results.[61–65] Therefore, in patients with critical aortic stenosis, age alone should not be a limiting factor in the decision regarding surgery.

Since aortic stenosis is more frequent in males and tends to occur in older patients, it is not surprising that a high proportion of patients who are surgical candidates have been found to have evidence of coronary artery disease on catheterization. When coronary artery bypass grafting of involved vessels is combined with valve replacement, operative mortality is not adversely affected.[66–69] However, there is some controversy over whether or not coronary bypass should be performed routinely since it has not been shown that long-term survival is favorably affected by combining this procedure with valve replacement.[70] In the absence of clear-cut guidelines, most cardiologists perform coronary angiography prior to valve surgery in patients above 40 years of age and in those with angina. Bypass surgery is then usually undertaken in patients with left main and/or multivessel disease.

AORTIC INSUFFICIENCY

Etiology and Pathology

Diseases which cause dilatation of the ascending aorta, disruption of the substructure supporting the valve, or damage to the leaflets themselves may result in aortic insufficiency (AI).[71] Specific conditions are summarized in Table 10-1. Over the past several decades the frequency with which some of these diseases are seen has changed considerably. Rheumatic valvular disease is considerably less common now than it was 30 years ago due to the virtual eradication of acute rheumatic fever in the United States. Although the prevalence of rheumatic disease was 49% and 37% respectively in two large recently published series,[72,73] our own experience in Oregon suggests that for newly diagnosed cases the number is much lower. Rheumatic disease still needs to be considered in older patients in this country, and in patients who were raised in countries where acute rheumatic fever remains a serious health problem. Luetic disease, which was also a common etiology of AI in past years, is now seen with decreasing frequency. Infective endocarditis has emerged as one of the most frequent causes of AI. This is particularly true in urban areas with large populations of intravenous (IV) drug abusers. Until recently, congenital abnormalities of the aortic valve were thought to result almost exclusively in valve stenosis. However, it appears that AI can be the predominant lesion as the congenitally abnormal valve deteriorates over time.[72] Roberts et al have suggested that approximately one fourth of patients with a bicuspid valve eventually develop pure AI.[72]

Rheumatic disease which involves the aortic

Table 10-1
Etiology of Aortic Insufficiency

Etiology	Pathology		
	Leaflet Abnormality	Aortic Root Disease	Loss of Commissural Support
A. Common			
Rheumatic disease[71]	+	−	−
Congenital abnormalities[71,72]	+	−	?
Endocarditis[71]	+	−	±
B. Less common			
Luetic disease[71]	probably 2°	+	−
Connective tissue disease[71,74–77] (eg, Marfan's syndrome)	+	+	−
Aortic dissection[71,77]	−	+	+
Postaortic commissurotomy	+	−	−
C. Uncommon			
Sinus of Valsalva aneurysm[71,77]	−	+	−
Trauma[71,77]	+	+	−
In association with ventricular septal defect[71,77]	−	−	+
Hypertrophic obstructive cardiomyopathy	+	−	−
Systemic hypertension[78]	?	?	?
Chronic renal disease	?	?	?
In association with systemic disease[79–81] (eg, ankylosing spondylitis, Reiter's syndrome, Whipple's syndrome)	+	+	−

valve leads to scarring and retraction of the valve leaflets with prominent commissural fusion.[71,72] The end result is often a valve with a central orifice that is both stenotic and incompetent. Endocarditis causes AI by destroying the valve leaflets. In some patients, scarring and retraction, which is initiated during the acute phase of the disease, progresses after the infection has been treated. This accounts for the late development of severe AI in patients who have been "cured" bacteriologically. Prolapse of the aortic valve leaflets may be due to an intrinsic structural abnormality such as myxomatous degeneration or may develop in a normal valve which is suddenly exposed to an increase in aortic diastolic pressure. The latter may occur as a result of nonpenetrating trauma or as a consequence of rapid deceleration (as in a motor vehicle accident). Some varieties of ventricular septal defect which involve the aortic valve substructure may also result in AI due to leaflet prolapse. Aortic root dilatation caused by aortic dissection or aortic root disease due to syphilis or Marfan's syndrome may cause AI by stretching the valve leaflets apart so that full apposition during diastole does not occur.

Since both infective endocarditis and aortic dissection figure prominently in the differential diagnosis, it is important to define the etiology of acute AI. In patients with chronic disease, accurate identification of the cause is often difficult. Fortunately, this is not as important as it is in the acute setting. Two-dimensional echocardiography may be of considerable value in defining the cause of AI.[82] In particular, this technique is useful in defining abnormalities of the aortic root such as aortic dissection or aneurysm of the sinus of Valsalva. Two-dimensional echocardiography may also identify a bicuspid valve, the characteristic changes of rheumatic disease, and the presence of vegetations in patients with infectious endocarditis. Computed tomography (CT) is also helpful in assessing the size of the aortic root and the presence of an aortic aneurysm.

Pathophysiology

The topic of acute aortic insufficiency is discussed in detail in chapters 2 and 15. In brief, when AI develops acutely, mechanisms that can effectively compensate for the reduction in forward cardiac output and for the diastolic volume overload imposed on the left ventricle are limited.[83] Both the structure of the left ventricle and the restraining effect of the pericardial sac prohibit abrupt increases in left ventricular size. Thus, when the left ventricle is acutely volume-loaded, diastolic filling pressure is increased. When the lesion is severe, left ventricular and aortic pressures equalize late in diastole. Left ventricular diastolic pressure may exceed left atrial pressure and cause premature closure of the mitral valve.[84,85] Mitral valve preclosure has the beneficial effect of protecting the left atrium and pulmonary circuit from the extremes of diastolic pressure that develop acutely in the left ventricle. Although sympathetic stimulation of the heart increases contractility and heart rate, these effects may still not be sufficient to maintain forward cardiac output in the normal range when regurgitation is severe. When cardiac output is reduced, there will be a compensatory increase in systemic vascular resistance (SVR) in an effort to maintain arterial perfusion pressure. Unfortunately, the increase in SVR has the unwanted effect of worsening regurgitant flow.

As discussed in the chapter 2, chronic AI results in substantial modification in left ventricular structure and function.[86–88] Both the left ventricle and the pericardium dilate allowing the increased volume load to be accommodated at a lower diastolic filling pressure than is possible in the acute setting. The increase in chamber size also enables total left ventricular stroke volume to be increased[78–80] while the low impedance state that exists in the arterial vascular bed has a beneficial effect on left ventricular systolic pump function.[89] An additional compensatory change that takes place in response to the change in left ventricular loading conditions is an increase in left ventricular wall thickness and muscle mass. As suggested by Grossman et al,[8] left ventricular hypertrophy develops in response to an increased pressure or volume load and serves to normalize wall stress which would otherwise be increased. In patients with chronic AI, the ratio of wall thickness to cavity size is preserved. The cardiac enlargement that occurs can be thought of as a magnified but proportional version of the normal organ. This is different from the situation seen in patients with chronic aortic stenosis who develop disproportionate thickening of the myocardium in relation to cavity size. Another reason that chronic AI is well tolerated is that many of the cardiovascular adaptations to exercise have a favorable effect on the regurgitation.[90–94] By decreasing the diastolic flow period, an increase in heart rate will reduce the amount of regurgitant flow. The reduction in systemic vascular resistance that occurs with dynamic exercise also serves to redistribute total left ventricular stroke volume so that forward cardiac output is increased at the expense of regurgitation flow.

The factors that cause the eventual deterioration of the left ventricle in patients with chronic AI are poorly understood. However, both the severity of the regurgitation and the duration of disease are important in this regard. There is recent evidence to suggest that failure of left ventricular hypertrophy to match loading conditions (which leads to an increase in systolic wall stress) may be an early indicator that the left ventricle is no longer able to compensate for the volume load. Some investigators have shown that preoperative evidence of increased wall stress is associated with a poor response to valve replacement.[95,96] We, along with other workers in this area, have demonstrated an association between increased systolic wall stress and evidence of abnormal cardiac performance as evidenced by a reduction in ejection fraction during exercise.[97–99] As will be discussed later in this chapter, no matter what the cause, once left ventricular systolic pump dysfunction becomes manifest, the likelihood of a good long-term result following corrective surgery is reduced.

Evaluation

History The medical history is often the best way to define the etiology of aortic insufficiency. Thus, information regarding the presence of fever, chills, night sweats, malaise, myalgias, or history of IV drug abuse, recent dental work, chest trauma, hypertension, arthritis, or urethritis should be sought from the patient.

The predominant symptom of acute AI is shortness of breath. Acute severe regurgitation may result in chest pain due to myocardial ischemia even in patients who do not have coronary artery disease. When aortic valvular regurgitation develops over a longer period of time, the compensatory mechanisms previously reviewed enable the patient to continue normal activities (which may include strenuous exercise) without symptoms for many years despite the presence of severe disease.[97,100–102] On close questioning there is often a history of atypical chest pain[102] thought to be due to the expansion of the ascending aorta and great vessels during systole. Patients often complain of palpitations and may describe an uncomfortable fullness in the throat following a premature beat due to the increased stroke volume of the postpremature beat. Many patients are aware of a forceful apical impulse which is most noticeable at night, particularly when they sleep on their left side or on their stomach. The onset of more pronounced symptoms in patients with aortic insufficiency may be due to either deterioration of underlying left ventricular systolic pump function, worsening valvular regurgitation, or the effects of other cardiac diseases, such as coronary artery disease, which limit the ability of the left ventricle to compensate for the volume overload. The most common symptoms are exertional dyspnea and fatigue. Orthopnea and paroxysmal nocturnal dyspnea develop later in the course. Angina and syncope are uncommon in patients with chronic AI.[102] A recent report by Olshausen et al demonstrates that ventricular arrhythmias are common in patients with AI and that the frequency and severity tend to be related to left ventricular performance.[103] However, sudden cardiac death appears to be rare, particularly in patients with normal systolic pump function.

Physical Examination[104] As outlined in the chapter describing valvular emergencies, patients who develop acute AI often do not have the characteristic physical findings that are associated with chronic AI. In patients with acute disease, a narrow pulse pressure, diminished first heart sound, and prominent third heart sound are common. Even when the lesion is severe, the diastolic murmur may be short and unimpressive. The reason for this is that as the aortic and left ventricular diastolic pressures approach diastasis there is little pressure gradient to cause blood to regurgitate back across the incompetent valve. A fourth heart sound is almost always absent since the atrial contribution to left ventricular filling is minimal. Resting tachycardia, signs of peripheral hypoperfusion, and chest congestion are seen in severe cases. The peripheral pulses rarely exhibit the characteristic changes seen in patients with chronic AI.

In patients with chronic AI, systolic blood pressure is usually elevated while diastolic pressure tends to be low. In some patients, diastolic sounds may be audible even after the pressure cuff is toally deflated. However, since intra-arterial pressure is rarely below 40 to 50 mmHg, diastolic blood pressure should be determined by muffling rather than disappearance of the heart sounds. The carotid pulse is usually forceful and has a brisk upstroke and rapid run-off. In chronic AI, the tidal wave is accentuated and a bisfiriens contour of the carotid and other pulses may be appreciated. The wide pulse pressure results in the characteristic peripheral manifestations which include head-bob, water hammer pulse[105] (accentuation of the radial pulse upon elevation of the arm), and pulsations in the peripheral capillary beds (often made visible by light compression of finger or toenails). Blood pressure in the legs, which usually exceeds that in the arms by 10 to 20 mmHg in normal subjects, is often 40 to 50 mmHg greater in patients with AI. A to-and-fro murmur may be appreciated when the stethoscope head is used to gently compress the femoral artery.

Although the composite picture gained from the physical examination is a reasonably good indicator of the severity of disease, it must be remembered that these physical signs are affected by factors in addition to the severity of regurgitation. Elderly patients, whose arteries are stiff, may exhibit a pulse pressure that is greatly in excess of the severity of the regurgitant lesion. Many of the characteristic peripheral manifestations can be seen in normal subjects when peripheral resistance is reduced as on a hot and humid day or following exercise. In addition, when left ventricular failure occurs, the characteristic changes in the pulses may become less prominent due to the combined effects of a reduction in stroke volume and an increase in systemic vascular resistance. In fact, an increase in diastolic pressure, in a previously stable patient with chronic AI, may be an early sign of deterioration.

The apical impulse in the patient with chronic AI is usually displaced laterally towards the axilla and occasionally downward to the sixth or seventh intercostal space. It is often diffuse and quite forceful. A markedly sustained apical impulse suggests the presence of left ventricular systolic pump dysfunction or associated aortic stenosis. The first and second heart sounds[106] are often reduced in intensity. The second heart sound may appear to be single or absent when the pulmonic component is immersed in the aortic diastolic murmur. A fourth heart sound is common. The presence of a third heart sound in chronic AI often indicates the presence of left ventricular dysfunction.[107] An aortic ejection click can often be appreciated in patients with a dilated aortic root or bicuspid aortic valve. A systolic murmur is common and may be accompanied by a systolic thrill. The presence of either systolic murmur or thrill do not indicate that the patient has coexistent aortic stenosis since these findings are often a reflection of the marked increase in total left ventricular stroke volume rather than actual obstruction to flow. When the murmur is mid- to late-peaking an associated aortic stenosis is more likely.

The aortic diastolic murmur begins immediately after A_2. It is usually high-pitched and blowing but may be musical when AI is due to prolapse or a tear in the leaflets. The murmur is usually best appreciated along the left sternal border and can be brought out by listening with the patient sitting forward and at full exhalation. When AI is due to disease of the aortic root, the murmur may be loudest at the upper right sternal border. Maneuvers such as handgrip and squatting, which increase systemic vascular resistance, promote regurgitant flow and increase the intensity of the murmur. Administration of amyl nitrate lowers resistance and reduces the intensity of the murmur. Because the intensity of the murmur is dependent on peripheral vascular tone, it is not uncommon for it to vary considerably from one examination to the next. In general, the severity of the valve lesion is more closely related to the duration of the murmur rather than to its intensity.

A second, lower pitched diastolic murmur known as the Austin Flint murmur may be heard at the cardiac apex. The Austin Flint murmur appears to be caused by turbulence in the antegrade mitral flow stream due to mixing with retrograde aortic flow.[108,109] Although vibrations of the anterior leaflet of the mitral valve may also contribute, this does not appear to be a major factor since the Austin Flint murmur has been heard in patients with a mitral valve prosthesis.[110] Because of its location and pitch, the Austin Flint murmur can be mistaken for the murmur of mitral stenosis. Associated findings on the physical examination which argue against the presence of mitral stenosis are the presence of a soft S_1 and the absence of an opening snap. Further differentiation can be obtained by administering amyl nitrate. This agent reduces the intensity of the Austin Flint murmur, and either increases or causes no change in the intensity of the murmur of mitral stenosis.

Chest Roentgenogram Acute, severe AI often results in the roentgenographic picture of pulmonary congestion with a normal-appearing cardiac silhouette. The presence of aortic root dilatation in a patient with acute AI should raise the possibility of aortic dissection or an aneurysm of a sinus of Valsalva.

The most prominent feature of chronic AI on the chest film is the presence of left ventricular enlargement (Figure 10-4).[111] The apex of the heart is often displaced downward in the postero-

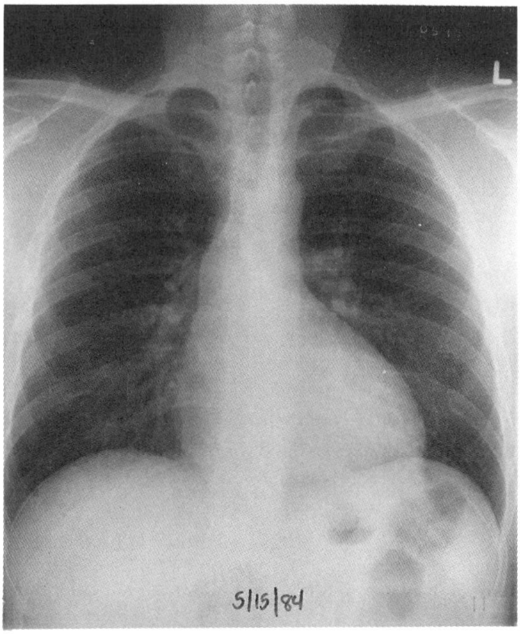

Figure 10-4A

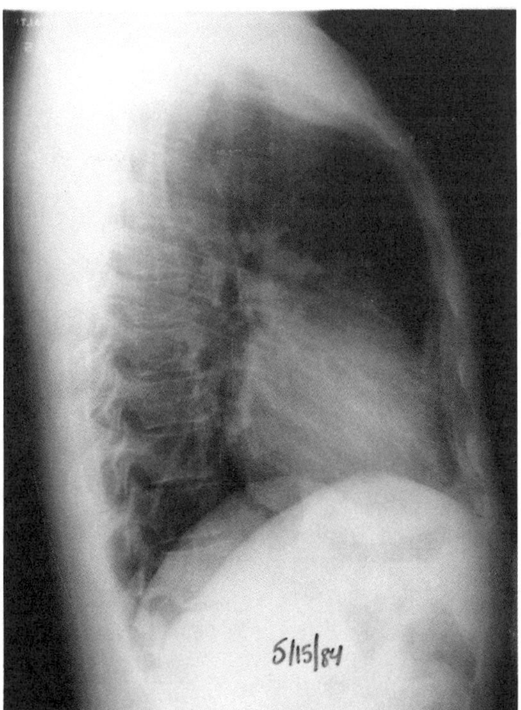

Figure 10-4B

Figure 10-4 Chest film of a patient with chronic severe aortic insufficiency. A Posteroanterior projection. There is cardiomegaly and prominence of the ascending aorta. B Lateral projection. Posterior projection of the left ventricular silhouette is prominent.

anterior view since the left ventricle tends to elongate in this disease. Cardiac enlargement may be best seen in the lateral projection in some cases. Signs of left atrial enlargement may also be present. Although an increase in the cardiac thoracic (CT) ratio is common, neither quantification of regurgitation nor accurate determination of left ventricular chamber size is possible by this measurement. In a group of 42 patients with chronic AI studied in our laboratory, the correlation between left ventricular end-diastolic volume determined angiographically and CT ratio was only 0.41 and considerable scatter around the regression line was seen.[112] Engorgement of upper lobe pulmonary veins, Kerley-B lines and pulmonary infiltrates indicate the presence of heart failure. Aortic root enlargement is common in patients with chronic severe AI even in the absence of disease involving the aortic root. Enlargement of the ascending aorta can be secondary to the marked increase in total left ventricular stroke volume that is characteristic of the disease. The presence of marked aortic root dilatation suggests that aortic root disease may be the primary problem, but differentiation between primary and secondary aortic root enlargement is often difficult by chest film alone.

Electrocardiogram Patients with acute AI may have a normal ECG, but sinus tachycardia and nonspecific ST-T wave changes are commonly seen. When acute, severe disease results in an imbalance between myocardial oxygen supply and demand, ischemic changes may be seen.

The most frequent ECG abnormality in patients with chronic aortic insufficiency is left ventricular hypertrophy (LVH) with strain, which is present in 60% to 80% of patients.[101,102,112] The development of this pattern depends on the severity of the regurgitation, its duration, and the presence of coexistent aortic stenosis. Early in the course of chronic AI, a pattern of diastolic volume overloading consisting of small Q waves and large R and tall T waves in the left precordial leads may be seen. We have observed that left ventricular end-diastolic volume is significantly larger in patients with LVH than in those without this abnormality.[112] P wave prolongation of 0.12 second or greater in lead II or a biphasic P wave in lead V_1 suggests the presence of left atrial enlargement. Premature atrial and ventricular beats are common.[103] Conduction system abnormalities are unusual except in patients with ankylosing spondylitis or Reiter's syndrome.

Echocardiography Echocardiography has been used to: (1) detect the presence of aortic insufficiency, (2) define its severity, (3) assess aortic root and valve leaflet pathology to determine etiology, and (4) evaluate left ventricular chamber size and systolic pump function. As will be discussed below, echo measurements of chamber size and wall thickness can also be used in the derivation of other prognostically useful indicators of left ventricular performance. Both M-mode and two-dimensional echocardiography are used in evaluating patients with AI.[35] In general, the M-mode technique is preferred for quantitating left ventricular size and function while two-dimensional echocardiography has proved most valuable in assessing structure. Often, the information obtained by one study is used to confirm or complement data from the other. In acute AI, echocardiography is helpful in evaluating the etiology of the valve lesion, and has been especially useful in diagnosing aortic valve vegetations, leaflet prolapse, or aortic root pathology. Preclosure of the mitral valve prior to the onset of ventricular systole can be assessed by either M-mode or two-dimensional study. When present, it usually indicates that regurgitation is severe. This finding has been useful in identifying patients who are at risk for subsequent clinical deterioration.[113–115]

In patients with chronic disease, the echocardiogram provides indirect evidence of regurgitant flow by demonstrating diastolic fluttering of the anterior mitral leaflet or interventricular septum.[35] Two-dimensional imaging has also been helpful in determining whether the primary problem is in the valve leaflets or aortic root. Although echocardiography has been used to assess left ventricular chamber size and systolic pump function, both M-mode and two-dimensional imaging have their limitations. Several investigators have demonstrated a strong correlation between echo measurements and left ventricular volumes.[112,116,117] However, each study has also demonstrated that there is a considerable scatter of individual values around the regression line so that prediction of volumes cannot be made with certainty. Abdulla et al[117] have postulated that the inaccuracy in measuring left ventricular volumes by M-mode echocardiography may be due to the fact that elongation of the subvalvular apparatus in AI leads to multiple different measurements of dimension that are technically accurate. It has been estimated that differences in angulation of the transducer head may alter assessment of chamber dimension by as much as 20%.[118] Although more accurate assessment of volume may in time be possible using two-dimensional echocardiography, problems with accurate definition of endocardial surface on stop-frame analysis have not yet been fully resolved.

Although echo evaluation of left ventricular chamber size and systolic function may not be entirely accurate in an individual patient at any single point in time, the use of serial studies has proved to be a useful way of following the progression of disease.[119] However, as we have recently noted, there may be considerable interstudy variability in echo measurements which may be difficult to differentiate from clinically important changes in structure or function.[120] Interstudy variability can be minimized substantially by evaluating serial tests side by side rather than independently. We have shown that when tests are read separately, changes in end-diastolic dimension of less than 8 mm cannot be ascribed to a clinically important change in ventricular size with a high degree of certainty. However, when studies are read together, changes in dimension in excess of 3 mm have a high likelihood of representing a real change in chamber size. Similarly, fractional shortening would have to decrease by as much as 11% on separate readings and only 5% on simultaneous readings before the physician could be confident that a change in systolic function had occurred.

Recently, Doppler ultrasound techniques have been used to detect both the presence and severity of regurgitant flow.[121,122] Ciobanu et al[121] reported the Doppler technique sensitivity to be 96% in the detection of aortic insufficiency. The method was specific in the small number of patients who were studied and, in general, the noninvasive assessment of the severity of AI correlated with the results of angiography (r = .88).[121]

Radionuclide Angiography This technique has enjoyed considerable popularity in the evaluation of chronic AI. The patient's own red blood cells are labelled with technetium 99m and imaging is performed during either first-pass or gated equilibrium studies. Left ventricular ejection fraction and volumes can be calculated by a counts-based nongeometric method using commercially available computer software. A close correlation between radionuclide angiography and conventional contrast angiography for both left ventricular volumes and ejection fraction has been demonstrated.[123–125] As with echocardiography, changes in radionuclide angiographic determination of left ventricular volumes and ejection fraction should be evaluated in the context of the inherent study to study variability in these measurements.

The changes in left ventricular volumes and ejection fraction (EF) during exercise have also been evaluated. Borer et al were the first to assess the exercise EF response in AI patients.[126] These workers showed that, unlike normal control subjects who uniformly increase their EF during exercise, symptomatic patients with AI usually had a reduction in EF. In addition, several groups of investigators have shown that asymptomatic patients have a heterogeneous exercise EF response.[127–133] Bonow et al, who followed a large cohort of patients with chronic AI, have presented evidence that late deterioration was more likely to occur in patients whose EF fell during exercise.[134] We have recently evaluated the EF response in a group of 56 patients with chronic AI. All of these patients were asymptomatic, had preserved resting EF, and evidence of left ventricular dilatation.[97] During exercise 18 patients increased EF by at least 0.05 unit, 18 patients remained within 0.05 unit of the rest value, and 20 patients decreased EF by at least 0.05 unit. As shown in Figure 10-5, patients who experienced a reduction in EF had evidence of diminished exercise capacity. We also showed that patients whose EF fell had increased levels of end-systolic wall stress at rest, and that during exercise wall stress increased even further. These observations suggest that afterload excess may play an important role in the abnormal EF response that is seen in some patients with chronic AI. Since left ventricular hypertrophy is the usual means of normalizing wall stress, these observations also raise the interesting possibility that the abnormal exercise response is caused by a failure of the usual compensatory mechanisms to respond fully to the abnormal loading conditions.

Another use of radionuclide angiography is in the assessment of regurgitant flow. Measurement of stroke counts, which is analogous to stroke volume, can be obtained from the right and left ventricles by subtracting end-systolic from end-diastolic counts. In the absence of an intracardiac shunt or valvular regurgitation, right and left ventricular stroke counts should be equal. In practice, a stroke count ratio (SCR), comparing left to right ventricles, which ranges from 0.9 to 1.3, is measured in normal subjects. Patients with aortic regurgitation will eject a greater stroke volume from the left ventricle with each beat so that the SCR will be elevated. In general, the higher the SCR, the more severe the regurgitation. Several laboratories have demonstrated a reasonably good correlation between the SCR and conventional angiographic techniques.[135–138] This method is probably most useful in detecting relative changes in stroke volume following interventions that alter the severity of the regurgitation.

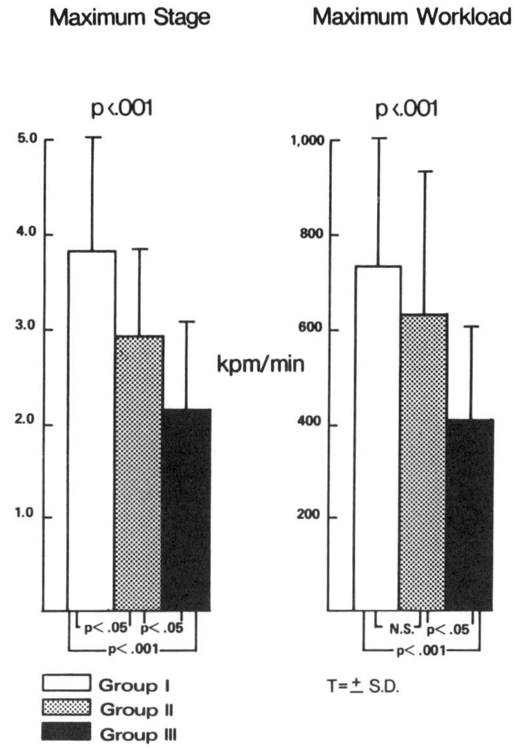

Figure 10-5 Association between exercise capacity and exercise ejection fraction (EF) response in 56 patients with chronic aortic insufficiency. All patients were asymptomatic and had preserved resting EF. Group I patients (n = 18) increased EF ⩾ 0.05 unit; group II (n = 18) changed < 0.05 unit in either direction; group III (n = 20) decreased EF ⩾ 0.05 unit. An abnormal EF response was associated with diminished exercise capacity as manifest by completion of fewer stages and a lower maximal workload.

Natural History For reasons already discussed, compensatory mechanisms in the left ventricle enable the patient with chronic AI to tolerate the volume overload state with minimal or no symptoms for a prolonged period. It is not unusual for patients with "free" AI to be fully active and to engage in strenuous physical activity without difficulty during this period.[100,102] The duration of the compensated phase is unpredictable but appears to depend on the severity of the volume overload, occurrence of events such as endocarditis which further damage the valve, and the coexistence of other valve lesions or coronary disease. However, even after important AI is noted, most patients remain without symptoms for 10 years or longer.[101] Goldschlager et al have shown that limiting symptoms are unusual, despite the presence of severe disease, in patients below age 40.[102] Unfortunately, serious deterioration in underlying left ventricular performance may occur even in the absence of symptoms.

Considerable mortality data have been collected over the years in patients with aortic insufficiency. Hegglin et al have pointed out that mortality in patients with mild to moderate AI probably does not exceed that seen in the population in general.[139] Much of the natural history data for severe disease was collected several decades ago when the vast majority of cases were caused by rheumatic disease. In some series, antibiotic prophylaxis for rheumatic fever and endocarditis were not yet available, and many of the currently used potent diuretics had not yet been discovered. Nonetheless, Bland and Wheeler reported a 38% 10-year mortality and a 56% 20-year mortality in patients with free AI.[100] More recently, Rapaport has reported that three fourths of patients with free AI who are followed medically will be alive at 5 years and half will still be alive at 10 years.[42]

The natural history of asymptomatic patients with chronic severe AI has recently been described by Bonow et al from the National Institutes of Health (NIH).[134] They followed the clinical course of 77 patients, all of whom had preserved resting EF, for an average of 49 months (range 6 to 114 months). Despite the presence of severe AI on initial examination there were no deaths recorded during this period. Only patients who developed symptoms or evidence of left ventricular dysfunction were taken to surgery for valve replacement. As shown in Figure 10-6, the percentage of patients not requiring surgery was 90%±3% at 3 years, 80%±6% at 5 years, and 75%±7% at 7 years. Thus, prognosis in this group of patients was excellent with less than 4% per year requiring valve replacement. Factors predictive of deterioration included left ventricular end-diastolic dimension of 70 mm, end-systolic dimension of 50 mm, and an abnormal ejection fraction response to exercise. For instance, when the end-systolic dimension exceeded 50 mm at baseline, only 31% of patients had not become symptomatic or developed left ventricular dysfunction by 4.5 years. The outcome of surgery was quite favorable in the patients who required valve replacement. In the

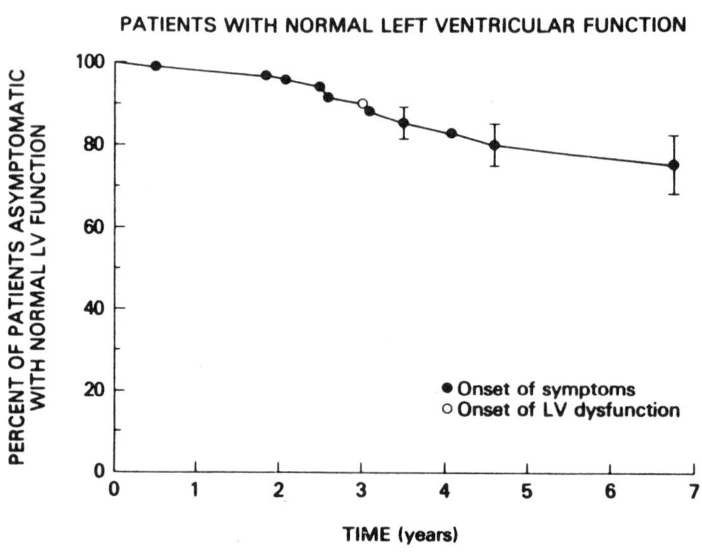

Figure 10-6 Natural history of patients with aortic insufficiency. The 77 patients surveyed had a normal resting ejection fraction (EF) on entry. The two end points were evidence of left ventricular dysfunction (as manifest by a fall in resting EF) or the onset of symptoms. LV = left ventricular. (Reproduced with permission from Bonow RO, et al[134] and the American Heart Association.)

12 patients who underwent surgery, there was no operative mortality. Follow-up evaluation showed evidence of substantial regression of left ventricular dilatation and improvement in EF in all of these patients.

Once symptoms develop, the downhill course accelerates considerably. Again, much of the available data was collected in an earlier era, and thus should be interpreted with caution. However, diminished work capacity, angina, and in particular the development of right heart failure have all been associated with a poor prognosis.[100,101,139]

Management

The management of acute AI is outlined in chapter 15. In patients with chronic AI, functional disability and mortality are influenced by both the amount of regurgitation and the status of the left ventricle. Therefore, therapeutic interventions should be aimed at maintaining the integrity of the valve and in preserving left ventricular function. Once aortic insufficiency is diagnosed, efforts should be made to prevent worsening valvular incompetence. Endocarditis prophylaxis for all procedures associated with bacteremia should be recommended regardless of the severity of the AI. In patients with rheumatic disease, antibiotic prophylaxis against recurrent bouts of rheumatic fever through the fourth decade is probably of value, particularly when there is a high risk of exposure to streptococcus infections, as occurs in health professionals, and persons residing in underdeveloped areas of the world. Since systemic hypertension increases regurgitant flow, control of blood pressure should be pursued aggressively. However, systolic pressure, which is almost always elevated in AI, usually does not require treatment. The author has relied on the level of diastolic pressure to define the presence of hypertension and has reserved therapy for patients whose diastolic pressure exceeds 90 mmHg.

Aortic insufficiency is correctable by surgically removing the valve and replacing it with a prosthetic device. In the 25 years that this procedure has been available, the survival and functional capacity of thousands of patients has been improved. However, valve replacement is not without risks. Operative mortality, although improved from the past, averages around 4% to 8% in most experienced centers.[140–144] The operative risk appears to be proportional to the severity of symptoms and left ventricular dysfunction. Recent reports have shown that selected patients can undergo the procedure at a lower risk.[134,145] In addition, the ideal valve prosthesis is not yet available. Complications related to the prosthetic device, including dysfunction or deterioration, infection, hemolysis, thromboembolic complications, and bleeding secondary to anticoagulation, have a major impact on the subsequent morbidity and mortality of patients who survive aortic valve replacement (AVR).[145] When there is evidence of marked impairment of left ventricular systolic pump function, the likelihood that AVR will improve survival, increase functional capacity, or result in regression of left ventricular dilatation and hypertrophy is considerably less than in patients with preserved left ventricular function.[144,145,147–150] As shown in Figure 10-7, Greves et al from our institution demonstrated a significant difference in 5-year survival post-AVR in 45 patients with isolated AI based on preoperative EF.[144] To insure a good result, AVR should be undertaken prior to the development of irreversible left ventricular dysfunction, but not so early as to prematurely expose the patient to the risks of surgery and from the prosthesis. Consequently, there has been a great deal of interest in recent years in defining the optimal timing for AVR.

As discussed above, the clinical course of asymptomatic patients with normal left ventricular function appears to be quite good. The data collected at the NIH by Bonow et al suggest that observation rather than early intervention should be the approach in these patients.[134] Some authors have argued that the indications for surgery should include a left ventricular end-systolic dimension of 55 mm by M-mode echocardiography.[151] This view has been contested by others who have pointed out the technical problems inherent in this measurement.[115] In addition, the data of Bonow et al[134] and Fioretti et al from Rotterdam[152] have shown convincingly that an excellent operative result (eg, low operative mortality and high likelihood of a decrease in left ventricular size) is possible in patients whose ventricles exceeded 55 mm in end-systolic dimension. Asymptomatic patients with AI should have an ECG, chest film, and echocardiogram obtained at baseline. These tests, when used in combination, are highly accurate in detecting patients with severe left ventricular dilatation and the presence of systolic pump dysfunction.[112] Patients who have abnormalities on these tests should undergo noninvasive measurement of EF by radionuclide angiography. If

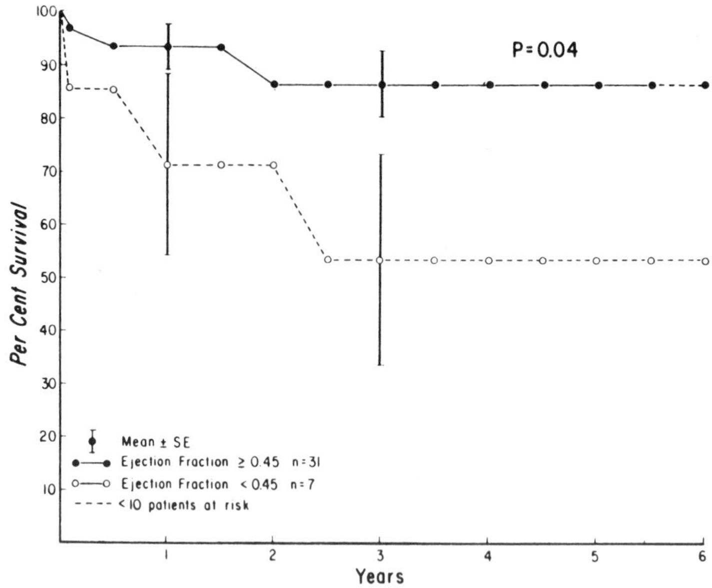

Figure 10-7 Preoperative ejection fraction (EF) as a determinant of survival following surgery for chronic aortic insufficiency. A significant difference in the survival of patients with an EF ≥ 0.45 as compared to those with an EF < 0.45 is seen. (Reproduced with permission from Greves J, et al.[144])

EF is within the normal range, valve replacement is not indicated. Follow-up evaluation should be performed on a yearly basis (or more frequently in patients with an end-systolic dimension in excess of 50 mm) with EF measurement repeated in patients who show significant changes in the other noninvasive measurements. Valve replacement should be considered only in those patients who become symptomatic or, as discussed below, in those who develop evidence of left ventricular dysfunction.

Some patients with AI may develop evidence of left ventricular dysfunction prior to the development of symptoms.[102] The following information is helpful in making decisions in the management of these patients: (1) The asymptomatic period appears to be short-lived in this subset and most patients become symptomatic within 2 to 3 years.[134,141] (2) Patients who are symptomatic and have evidence of left ventricular dysfunction appear to have a higher operative mortality and are less likely to show evidence of clinical improvement or regression of left ventricular dilatation and hypertrophy.[144,145,147–151] (3) There is also some evidence to suggest that asymptomatic patients with left ventricular dysfunction (particularly those with good exercise tolerance as assessed by treadmill testing[153]) have a better long-term outcome following surgery than do symptomatic patients.[145] These data support early operative intervention in asymptomatic patients with chronic AI who develop evidence of left ventricular dysfunction and the author usually recommends surgery in such cases.

The occurrence of symptoms in a previously asymptomatic patient usually heralds the onset of a new phase of the disease. If left ventricular function is normal and the symptoms are mild, a trial of medical therapy (eg, a diuretic ± digitalis) may enable the patient to regain his asymptomatic status. However, a prolonged trial of medical management that fails to improve symptoms should be avoided since this may lead to deterioration in left ventricular systolic pump function.

Symptomatic patients with left ventricular dysfunction are, as mentioned previously, less likely to demonstrate symptomatic improvement and/or regression of left ventricular dilatation and hypertrophy following surgery. This is true despite advances in surgical techniques that have both reduced operative mortality and helped in the intraoperative protection of myocardium. Presumably, irreversible changes in the left ventricle have occurred. Although the long-term outcome is not favorable in this group, there is evidence that valve replacement will lead to regression of left ventricular hypertrophy and dilatation and recovery of systolic function in some patients.[144,154,155] Differentiation of those who are likely to improve from those who are not cannot be made with a high degree of certainty. Since some patients will improve and the natural history of medically treated patients is poor once both symptoms and left ventricular dysfunction appear, surgery is usually recommended for patients who fall into this category. Factors suggesting a poor result following AVR include more severe left ventricular dysfunction,[133,156] marked increase in end-systolic volume, and evidence of inadequate hypertrophy for the degree of volume overload (eg, increased wall stress).[95,96] Patients who are markedly symptomatic (eg, functional class III and IV),[144] and those with preoperative evidence of reduced exercise tolerance also appear to do less well following surgery.[153]

Vasodilator Therapy in Chronic Aortic Regurgitation

Arterial dilating agents such as nitroprusside,[157,158] hydralazine hydrochloride,[159,160] and nifedipine[161] have been shown to improve cardiac performance in AI by favorably redistributing total left ventricular stroke volume. When these agents are given, forward flow is increased and regurgitant flow is reduced. Data from our laboratory show that the acute administration of hydralazine results in an increase in cardiac output and a reduction in pulmonary capillary wedge pressure both at rest and during exercise. The acute hemodynamic effects of hydralazine in a group of patients with severe AI are summarized in Figure 10-8.

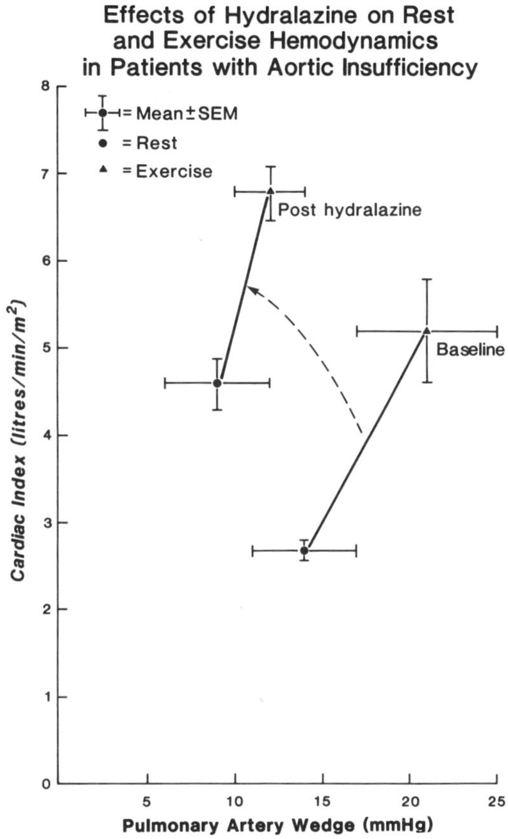

Figure 10-8 The acute effects of arterial dilator therapy (hydralazine hydrochloride) on rest and exercise hemodynamics in a group of ten patients with chronic severe aortic insufficiency. A reduction in left ventricular filling pressure and an increase in cardiac index is seen both at rest and during peak bicycle exercise.

Although clinical trials are currently underway, there is little available information describing the long-term effects of vasodilator therapy in patients with chronic AI. The results from a patient treated with hydralazine over a period of 14 months are summarized in Figure 10-9.[162]

The author has found that a trial of vasodilator therapy is of value in symptomatic patients who are either unwilling or unable (due to intercurrent medical problems) to undergo AVR, and as a means of improving cardiac performance prior to surgery in patients with severe disease. Such therapy might also be considered in patients with advanced left ventricular dysfunction since the surgical results are so poor in this group. The drug of choice is hydralazine hydrochloride given orally in divided doses so that the total is approximately 3 mg/kg body weight over a 24-hour period. Flushing, headache, nausea, anorexia, and tachycardia are common during the initiation of therapy. These side effects can usually be minimized by slow titration of the drug up to the desired daily dose. More severe long-term side effects, which may necessitate discontinuation of hydralazine, include the appearance of a drug rash, drug fever, or development of a lupus-like syndrome. The possibility that prophylactic vasodilator therapy initiated at an early stage of the disease might alter the natural history by reducing the volume overload faced by the left ventricle is an intriguing one. If prophylactic arterial dilation had this effect, then surgery might be delayed or even

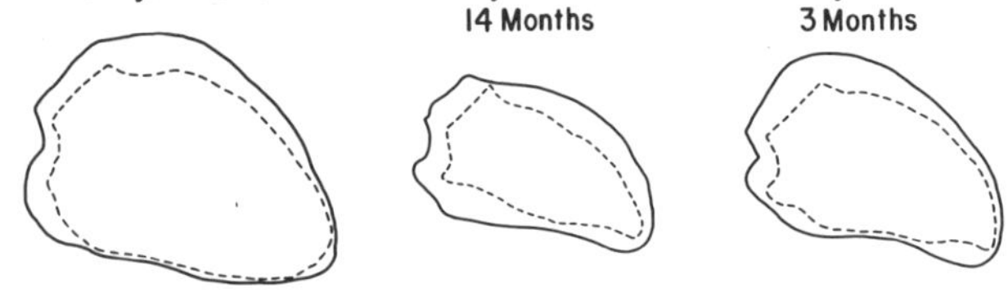

E.C.54♀	Pre-Hydralazine 4/78	On Hydralazine 14 Months 6/79	Off Hydralazine 3 Months 9/79
LEFT VENTRICULAR VOLUMES			
End Diastolic (cc/m^2)	181	121	138
End Systolic (cc/m^2)	118	46	73
Stroke (cc/m^2)	63	75	73
EJECTION FRACTION	.35	.62	.47
LEFT VENTRICULAR MASS (gm/m^2)	197	120	---

Figure 10-9 Long-term effects of vasodilator therapy in a 54-year-old female patient with chronic aortic insufficiency. The patient was maintained on hydralazine hydrochloride for 14 months. During this period she experienced substantial clinical improvement. There was evidence of regression of left ventricular dilatation and hypertrophy as well as recovery of systolic pump function. However, 3 months after therapy had been discontinued, due to troublesome side effects, evidence of deterioration was noted. (Reproduced with permission from Greenberg B, Rahimtoola SH: Vasodilator therapy for valvular heart disease. *JAMA* 1981;246:269–272.)

avoided in many patients with chronic AI. We are currently in the midst of a clinical trial designed to assess the long-term effects of arterial dilation in chronic AI.

REFERENCES

1. Roberts WC: Anatomically isolated aortic valvular disease: The case against its being of rheumatic etiology. *Am J Med* 1970;49:151–159.
2. Roberts WC, Perloff JK, Costantino T: Severe valvular aortic stenosis in patients over 65 years of age: A clinicopathologic study. *Am J Cardiol* 1971;27:497–505.
3. Roberts WC: The congenitally bicuspid aortic valve: A study of 85 autopsy cases. *Am J Cardiol* 1970;26:72–84.
4. Mills P, Leech G, Davies M, et al: The natural history of the bicuspid aortic valve. *Br Heart J* 1978;40:951–957.
5. Stein PD, Sabbah HN, Pitha JV: Continuing disease process of calcific aortic stenosis. *Am J Cardiol* 1977;39:159–163.
6. Fenoglio JJ Jr, McAllister HA Jr, DeCastro CM, et al: Congenital bicuspid aortic valve after age 20. *Am J Cardiol* 1977;39:164–169.
7. Maron BJ, Ferrans VJ, Roberts WC: Myocardial ultrastructure in patients with chronic aortic valve disease. *Am J Cadiol* 1975;35:725–738.
8. Grossman W, Jones D, McLaurin LP: Wall stress and patterns of hypertrophy in the human left ventricle. *J Clin Invest* 1975;56:56–64.
9. Ross J Jr: Afterload mismatch and preload reserve: a conceptual framework for the analysis of ventricular function. *Prog Cardiovasc Dis* 1976;18:255–264.
10. Gunther S, Grossman W: Determinants of ventricular function in pressure-overload hypertrophy in man *Circulation* 1979;59:679–688.
11. Peterson KL, Tsuji J, Johnson AI, et al: Diastolic left ventricular pressure–volume and stress-strain relations in patients with valvular aortic stenosis and left ventricular hypertrophy. *Circulation* 1978;58:77–89.
12. Schwarz F, Flameng W, Schaper J, et al: Correlation between myocardial structure and diastolic properties of the heart in chronic aortic valve disease: Effects of corrective surgery. *Am J Cardiol* 1978;42:895–903.
13. Hess OM, Ritter M, Schneider J, et al: Diastolic stiffness and myocardial structure in aortic valve disease before and after valve replacement. *Circulation* 1984;69:855–865.
14. Stott DK, Marpole DGF, Bristow JD, et al: The role of left atrial transport in aortic and mitral stenosis. *Circulation* 1970;41:1031–1041.
15. Wood P: Aortic stenosis. *Am J Cardiol* 1958; 1:553–571.
16. Murphy ES, Lawson RM, Starr A, et al: Severe aortic stenosis in patients 60 years of age and older: Left ventricular function and 10-year survival after valve replacement. *Circulation* 1981;64(suppl 2):II:184–188.
17. Bergeron J, Abelmann WH, Vazquez-Milan M, et al: Aortic stenosis: clinical manifestations and course of the disease. *Arch Intern Med* 1984; 94:911–924.
18. Paquay PA, Anderson G, Diefenthal H, et al: Chest pain as a predictor of coronary artery disease in patients with obstructive aortic valve disease. *Am J Cardiol* 1976;38:863–869.
19. Hancock EW: Aortic stenosis, angina pectoris, and coronary artery disease. *Am Heart J* 1977; 93:382–393.
20. Basta LL, Raines D, Najjar S, et al: Clinical,

haemodynamic, and coronary angiographic correlates of angina pectoris in patients with severe aortic valve disease. *Br Heart J* 1975;37:150–157.
21. Nadell R, DePace NL, Ren JF, et al: Myocardial oxygen supply/demand ratio in aortic stenosis: Hemodynamic and echocardiographic evaluation of patients with and without angina pectoris. *J Am Coll Cardiol* 1983;2:258–262.
22. Marcus ML, Doty DB, Hiratzka LF, et al: Decreased coronary reserve: A mechanism for angina pectoris in patients with aortic stenosis and normal coronary arteries. *N Engl J Med* 1982;307:1362–1366.
23. Schwartz LS, Goldfischer J, Sprague GJ, et al: Syncope and sudden death in aortic stenosis. *Am J Cardiol* 1969;23:647–658.
24. Mark AL, Kioschos JM, Abboud FM, et al: Abnormal vascular responses to exercise in patients with aortic stenosis. *J Clin Invest* 1973; 52:1138–1146.
25. Dhingra RC, Amat-y-Leon F, Pietras RJ, et al: Sites of conduction disease in aortic stenosis: Significance of valve gradient and calcification. *Ann Intern Med* 1977;87:275–280.
26. Perloff JK: Clinical recognition of aortic stenosis: The physical signs and differential diagnosis of the various forms of obstruction to left ventricular outflow. *Prog Cardiovasc Dis* 1968; 10:323–352.
27. Kavalier MA, Stewart J, Travel ME: The apical A wave versus the fourth heart sound in assessing the severity of aortic stenosis. *Circulation* 1975; 51:324–327.
28. Davison ET, Friedman SA: Significance of systolic murmurs in the aged. *N Engl J Med* 1968; 279:225–230.
29. Finegan RF, Gianelly RE, Harrison DC: Aortic stenosis in the elderly. *N Engl J Med* 1969;281: 1261–1264.
30. Barlow J, Shillingford J: The use of amyl nitrate in differentiating mitral and aortic systolic murmurs. *Br Heart J* 1958;20:162–166.
31. Rothman A, Goldberger AL: Aids to cardiac auscultation. *Ann Intern Med* 1983;99:346–353.
32. Glancy DL, Freed TA, O'Brien KP, et al: Calcium in the aortic valve: Roentgenologic and hemodynamic correlations in 148 patients. *Ann Intern Med* 1969;71:245–250.
33. Nanda NC, Gramiak R, Manning J, et al: Echocardiographic recognition of the congenital bicuspid aortic valve. *Circulation* 1974;49: 870–875.
34. Brandenburg RO Jr, Tajik AJ, Edwards WD, et al: Accuracy of 2-dimensional echocardiographic diagnosis of congenitally bicuspid aortic valve: Echocardiographic-anatomic correlation in 115 patients. *Am J Cardiol* 1983;51:1469–1473.
35. Green SE, Popp RL: Role of echocardiography in diagnosis and management of valvular heart disease. *Mod Concepts Cardiovasc Dis* 1981; 50:31–36.
36. Weyman AE, Feigenbaum H, Dillon JC, et al: Cross-sectional echocardiography in assessing the severity of valvular aortic stenosis. *Circulation* 1975;52:828–834.
37. DeMaria AN, Bommer W, Joye J, et al: Value and limitations of cross-sectional echocardiography of the aortic valve in the diagnosis and quantification of valvular aortic stenosis. *Circulation* 1980;62:304–312.
38. Schwartz A, Vignola PA, Walker HJ, et al: Echocardiographic estimation of aortic-valve gradient in aortic stenosis. *Ann Intern Med* 1978; 89:329–335.
39. DePace NL, Ren JF, Iskandrian AS, et al: Correlation of echocardiographic wall stress and left ventricular pressure and function in aortic stenosis. *Circulation* 1983;67:854–859.
40. Stamm RB, Martin RP: Quantification of pressure gradients across stenotic valves by Doppler ultrasound. *J Am Coll Cardiol* 1983;2:707–718.
41. Berger M, Berdoff RL, Gallerstein PE, et al: Evaluation of aortic stenosis by continuous wave Doppler ultrasound. *J Am Coll Cardiol* 1984; 3:150–156.
42. Rapaport E: Natural history of aortic and mitral valve disease. *Am J Cadiol* 1975;35:221–229.
43. Frank S, Johnson A, Ross J Jr: Natural history of valvular aortic stenosis. *Br Heart J* 1973; 35:41–46.
44. Schwarz F, Baumann P, Manthey J, et al: The effect of aortic valve replacement on survival. *Circulation* 1982;66:1105–1110.
45. Ross J Jr, Braunwald E: Aortic stenosis. *Circulation* 1968;37,38:V–61–67.
46. Cheitlin MD, Gertz EW, Brundage BH, et al: Rate of progression of severity of valvular aortic stenosis in the adult. *Am Heart J* 1979;98: 689–700.
47. Bogart DB, Murphy BL, Wong BYS, et al: Progression of aortic stenosis. *Chest* 1979;76: 391 396.
48. Nestico PF, DePace NL, Kimbiris D, et al: Progression of isolated aortic stenosis: Analysis of 29 patients having more than one cardiac catheterization. *Am J Cardiol* 1983;52: 1054–1058.
49. Wagner S, Selzer A: Patterns of progression of aortic stenosis: A longitudinal hemodynamic study. *Circulation* 1982;65:709–712.
50. Goldman L, Caldera DL, Nussbaum SR, et al: Multifactorial index of cardiac risk in non-cardiac surgical procedures. *N Engl J Med* 1977;297: 845–850.
51. Sutton MGS, Sutton MSJ, Oldershaw P, et al: Valve replacement without preoperative cardiac catheterization. *N Engl J Med* 1981;305: 1233–1238.
52. Brandenburg RO: No more routine catheterization for valvular heart disease? *N Engl J Med* 1981;305:1277–1278.
53. Roberts WC: Reasons for cardiac catheterization before cardiac-valve replacement. *N Engl J Med* 1982;306:1291–1293.
54. Rahimtoola SH: The need for cardiac catheterization and angiography in valvular heart disease is not disproven. *Ann Intern Med* 1982; 97:433–439.
55. Parisi AF, Polland ED: Are non-invasive tests sufficient for preoperative evaluation of aortic stenosis. *J Am Coll Cardiol* 1984;3:1092–1095.
56. Pantely G, Morton M, Rahimtoola SH: Effects of successful, uncomplicated valve replacement on ventricular hypertrophy, volume, and per-

formance in aortic stenosis and in aortic incompetence. *J Thorac Cardiovasc Surg* 1978;75: 383–391.
57. Schwarz F, Flameng W, Thormann J, et al: Recovery from myocardial failure after aortic valve replacement. *J Thorac Cardiovasc Surg* 1978;75:854–864.
58. O'Toole JD, Geiser EA, Reddy PS, et al: Effect of preoperative ejection fraction on survival and hemodynamic improvement following aortic valve replacement. *Circulation* 1978;58: 1175–1184.
59. Smith N, McAnulty JH, Rahimtoola SH: Severe aortic stenosis with impaired left ventricular function and clinical heart failure: Results of valve replacement. *Circulation* 1978;58:258–264.
60. Henry WL, Bonow RO, Borer JS, et al: Evaluation of aortic valve replacement in patients with valvular aortic stenosis. *Circulation* 1980; 61: 814–825.
61. Hochberg MS, Morrow AG, Michaelis LL, et al: Aortic valve replacement in the elderly: Encouraging postoperative clinical and hemodynamic results. *Arch Surg* 1977;112:1475–1480.
62. Copeland JG, Griepp RB, Stinson EB, et al: Isolated aortic valve replacement in patients older than 65 years. *JAMA* 1977;237:1578–1581.
63. Stephenson LW, Vaugh HM, Edmunds LH: Surgery using cardiopulmonary bypass in the elderly. *Circulation* 1978;58:250–254.
64. Jamieson WRD, Dooner J, Munro I, et al: Cardiac valve replacement in the elderly: A review of 320 consecutive cases. *Circulation* 1981; 64(suppl 2):177–183.
65. Austen WG, DeSanctis RW, Buckley MJ, et al: Surgical management of aortic valve disease in the elderly. *JAMA* 1970;211:624–626.
66. Macmanus Q, Grunkmeier G, Lambert L, et al: Aortic valve replacement and aorta-coronary bypass surgery: Results with perfusion of proximal and distal coronary arteries. *J Thorac Cardiovasc Surg* 1978;75:865–869.
67. Richardson JV, Kouchoukos NT, Wright JO III, et al: Combined aortic valve replacement and myocardial revascularization: Results in 220 patients. *Circulation* 1979;59:75–81.
68. Lytle BW, Cosgrove DM, Loop FD, et al: Replacement of aortic valve combined with myocardial revascularization: determinants of early and late risk for 500 patients, 1967–1981. *Circulation* 1983;68:1149–1162.
69. Kirklin JW, Kouchoukos NT: Aortic valve replacement without myocardial revascularization, editorial. *Circulation* 1981;63:243–251.
70. Bonow RO, Lent KM, Rosing DR, et al: Aortic valve replacement without myocardial revascularization in patients with combined aortic valvular and coronary artery disease. *Circulation* 1981;63:243–251.
71. Edwards JE: Pathologic aspects of cardiac vascular insufficiencies. *AMA Arch Surg* 1958;77: 634–649.
72. Roberts WC, Morrow AC, McIntosh CL, et al: Congentially bicuspid aortic valve causing severe, pure aortic regurgitation without superimposed infective endocarditis. *Am J Cardiol* 1981;47: 206–208.
73. Stone PH, Clark RD, Goldschlager N, et al: Determinants of prognosis of patients with aortic regurgitation who undergo aortic valve replacement. *J Am Coll Cardiol* 1984;3: 1118–1126.
74. Read RC, Thal AP, Wendt VE: Symptomatic valvular myxomatous transformation. *Circulation* 1965;32:897–910.
75. Davis Z, Pluth JR, Giuliani ER: The Marfan syndrome and cardiac surgery. *J Thorac Cardiovasc Surg* 1978;75:505–509.
76. Emanuel R, Marcomichelakis J, Moores EC, et al: Formes frustes of Marfan's syndrome presenting with severe aortic regurgitation. *Br Heart J* 1977;39:190–197.
77. Carter JB, Sethi S, Lee GB, et al: Prolapse of semilunar cusps as causes of aortic insufficiency. *Circulation* 1971;43:922–932.
78. Waller BF, Zoltick JM, Rosen JH, et al: Severe aortic regurgitation from systemic hypertension (without aortic dissection) requiring aortic valve replacement. *Am J Cardiol* 1982;49:473–477.
79. Stewart SR, Robbins DL, Castles JJ: Acute fulminant aortic and mitral insufficiency in ankylosing spondylitis. *N Engl J Med* 1978;299: 1148–1149.
80. Bostwick DG, Bensch KG, Burke JS, et al: Whipple's disease presenting as aortic insufficiency. *N Engl J Med* 1981;305:995–998.
81. Roberts WC, Hollingsworth JF, Bulkley BH, et al: Combined mitral and aortic regurgitation in ankylosing spondylitis. *Am J Med* 1974;56: 237–243.
82. Imaizumi T, Orita Y, Koiwaya Y, et al: Utility of two-dimensional echocardiography in the differential diagnosis of the etiology of aortic regurgitation. *Am Heart J* 1982;103:887–896.
83. Morganroth J, Perloff JK, Zeldis SM, et al: Acute, severe aortic regurgitation: Pathophysiology, clinical recognition, and management. *Ann Intern Med* 1977;87:223–232.
84. Pride RB, Benham R, Oakley CM: Echocardiography of the mitral valve in aortic valve disease. *Br Heart J* 1971;33:296–304.
85. Botvinick EH, Schiller NB, Wickermasekaren R, et al: Echocardiographic demonstration of early mitral valve closure in severe aortic insufficiency — Its clinical implications. *Circulation* 1975;51: 836–846.
86. Ross J Jr, McCullagh WH: Nature of enhanced performance of the dilated left ventricle in the dog during chronic volume overloading. *Circ Res* 1972;30:549–556.
87. McCullagh WH, Covell JW, Ross J Jr: Left ventricular dilatation and diastolic compliance changes during chronic volume overloading. *Circulation* 1972;45:943–951.
88. Ross J Jr: Adaptations of the left ventricle to chronic volume overload. *Circ Res* 1974; 34, 35(suppl 2):II-64–II-70.
89. Urschel CW, Covell JW, Sonnenblick EH, et al: Myocardial mechanics in aortic and mitral valvular regurgitation: the concept of instantaneous impedance as a determinant of the performance of the intact heart. *J Clin Heart* 1968;47:867–883.
90. Lewis RP, Bristow JD, Griswold HE: Exercise hemodynamics in aortic regurgitation. *Am Heart*

J 1970;80:171–176.
91. Ettinger PO, Frank MJ, Levinson GE: Hemodynamics at rest and during exercise in combined aortic stenosis and insufficiency. *Circulation* 1972;45:267–276.
92. Judge TP, Kennedy JW, Bennett LJ, et al: Quantitative hemodynamic effects of heart rate in aortic regurgitation. *Circulation* 1971;44:355–367.
93. Levinson GE, Frank MJ, Schwarz CJ: The effect of rest and physical effort on the left ventricular burden in mitral and aortic regurgitation. *Am Heart J* 1970;80:791–801.
94. Firth BG, Dehmer GJ, Nicod P, et al: Effect of increasing heart rate in patients with aortic regurgitation: Effect of incremental atrial pacing on scintigraphic, hemodynamic and thermodilution measurements. *Am J Cardiol* 1982;49:1860–1867.
95. Kumpuris AG, Quinones MA, Waggoner AD, et al: Importance of preoperative hypertrophy, wall stress and end-systolic dimension as echocardiographic predictors of normalization of left ventricular dilatation after valve replacement in chronic aortic insufficiency. *Am J Cardiol* 1982;49:1091–1100.
96. Gaasch WH, Carroll JD, Levine HJ, et al: Chronic aortic regurgitation: Prognostic value of left ventricular end-systolic dimension and end-diastolic radius/thickness ratio. *J Am Coll Cardiol* 1983;1:775–782.
97. Greenberg BH, Massie B, Thomas D, et al: Association between the exercise ejection fraction response and systolic wall stress in patients with chronic aortic insufficiency. *Circulation* 1985;71:458–465.
98. Lewis SM, Riba AL, Berger JH, et al: Radionuclide angiographic exercise left ventricular performance in chronic aortic regurgitation: Relationship to resting echographic ventricular dimensions and systolic wall stress index. *Am Heart J* 1982;103:498–504.
99. Goldman ME, Packer M, Horowitz SF, et al: Relation between exercise-induced changes in ejection fraction and systolic loading conditions at rest in aortic regurgitation. *J Am Coll Cardiol* 1984;3:924–929.
100. Bland EF, Wheeler EO: Severe aortic regurgitation in young people: A long-term perspective with reference to prognosis and prosthesis. *N Engl J Med* 1957;256:667–672.
101. Segal J, Harvey WP, Hufnagel C: A clinical study of one hundred cases of severe aortic insufficiency. *Am J Med* 1956;2:200–210.
102. Goldschlager N, Pfeifer J, Cohn K, et al: The natural history of aortic regurgitation: A clinical and hemodynamic study. *Am J Med* 1973;54:577–588.
103. Olshausen K, Schwarz F, Apfelbach J, et al: Determinants of the incidence and severity of ventricular arrhythmias in aortic valve disease. *Am J Cardiol* 1983;51:1103–1109.
104. Reichek N, Shelburne JC, Perloff JK: Clinical aspects of rheumatic valvular disease. *Prog Cardiovasc Dis* 1973;15:491–537.
105. Warnes CA, Harris PC, Fritts HW: Effect of elevating the wrist on the radial pulse in aortic regurgitation: Corrigan revisited. *Am J Cardiol* 1983;51:1551–1553.
106. Sabbah HN, Khaja F, Anbe DT, et al: The aortic closure sound in pure aortic insufficiency. *Circulation* 1977;56:859–863.
107. Abdulla AM, Frank MJ, Erdin RA Jr, et al: Clinical significance and hemodynamic correlates of the third heart sound gallop in aortic regurgitation. *Circulation* 1981;64:464–471.
108. Fortuin NJ, Craige E: On the mechanism of the Austin Flint murmur. *Circulation* 1972;45:558–570.
109. Laniado S, Yellin EL, Yoran C, et al: Physiologic mechanisms in aortic insufficiency. I. The effect of changing heart rate on flow dynamics II. Determinants of Austin Flint murmur. *Circulation* 1982;66:226–232.
110. Schaefer RA, McAnulty JH, Starr A, et al: Diastolic murmurs in the presence of Starr-Edwards mitral prosthesis: With emphasis on the genesis of the Austin Flint murmur. *Circulation* 1975;51:402–409.
111. Carlsson E, Gross R, Holt RG: The radiological diagnosis of cardiac valvar insufficiencies. *Circulation* 1977;55:921–933.
112. Karaian CH, Greenberg BH, Rahimtoola SH: Non-invasive assessment of the left ventricle in chronic aortic insufficiency. *Circulation* 1980;62(suppl 3):187.
113. DeMaria AN, King JF, Salel AF, et al: Echography and phonography of acute aortic regurgitation in bacterial endocarditis. *Ann Intern Med* 1975;82:329–335.
114. Wann LS, Dillon JC, Weyman AE, et al: Echocardiography in bacterial endocarditis. *N Engl J Med* 1976;295:135–139.
115. Mann T, McLaurin L, Grossman W, et al: Assessing the hemodynamic severity of acute aortic regurgitation due to infective endocarditis. *N Engl J Med* 1975;293:108–113.
116. Johnson AD, Alpert JS, Francis GS, et al: Assessment of left ventricular function in severe aortic regurgitation. *Circulation* 1976;54:975–979.
117. Abdulla AM, Frank MJ, Canedo MI, et al: Limitations of echocardiography in the assessment of left ventricular size and function in aortic regurgitation. *Circulation* 1980;61:148–155.
118. O'Rourke RA, Crawford MH: Timing of valve replacement in patients with chronic aortic regurgitation, editorial. *Circulation* 1980;61:493–495.
119. Clark RD, Korcuska K, Cohn K: Serial echocardiographic evaluation of left ventricular function in valvular disease, including reproducibility guidelines for serial studies. *Circulation* 1980;62:564–575.
120. Massie B, Greenberg B, Cheitlin M, et al: Intertest variability of echo and x-ray assessments: Implications for decision making in patients with valvular regurgitation. *J Am Coll Cardiol* 1984;3:493.
121. Ciobanu M, Abbasi AS, Allen M, et al: Pulsed doppler echocardiography in the diagnosis and estimation of severity of aortic insufficiency. *Am J Cardiol* 1982;49:339–343.
122. Boughner DR: Assessment of aortic insufficiency by transcutaneous doppler ultrasound. *Circula-*

tion 1975;52:874–879.

123. Slutsky R, Karliner J, Ricci D, et al: Left ventricular volumes by gated equilibrium radionuclide angiography: A new method. *Circulation* 1979; 60:556–564.
124. Dehmer GJ, Lewis SE, Hillis LD, et al: Nongeometric determination of left ventricular volumes from equilibrium blood pool scans. *Am J Cardiol* 1980;45:293–300.
125. Massie BM, Kramer BL, Gertz EW, et al: Radionuclide measurement of left ventricular volume: Comparison of gometric and counts based methods. *Circulation* 1981;65:725–730.
126. Borer JS, Bacharach SL, Green MV, et al: Exercise-induced left ventricular dysfunction in symptomatic and asymptomatic patients with aortic regurgitation: Assessment with radionuclide cineangiography. *Am J Cardiol* 1978; 42:351–357.
127. Dehmer GJ, Firth BH, Hillis LD, et al: Alterations in left ventricular volumes and ejection fraction at rest and during exercise in patients with aortic regurgitation. *Am J Cardiol* 1981; 48:17–27.
128. Iskandrian AS, Hakki AH, Kane SA, et al: Quantitative radionuclide angiography in assessment of hemodynamic changes during upright exercise: Observations in normal subjects, patients with coronary artery disease and patients with aortic regurgitation. *Am J Cardiol* 1981;48: 239–246.
129. Peter CA, Jones RH: Cardiac response to exercise in patients with chronic aortic regurgitation. *Am Heart J* 1982;104:85–91.
130. Steingart RM, Yee C, Weinstein L, et al: Radionuclide ventriculographic study of adaptation to exercise in aortic regurgitation. *Am J Cardiol* 1983;51:483–488.
131. Huxley RL, Gaffney A, Corbett JR, et al: Early detection of left ventricular dysfunction in chronic aortic regurgitation as assessed by contrast angiography, echocardiography, and rest and exercise scintigraphy. *Am J Cardiol* 1983;51: 1542–1550.
132. Johnson LL, Powers ER, Tzall WR, et al: Left ventricular volume and ejection fraction response to exercise in aortic regurgitation. *Am J Cardiol* 1983;51:1379–1385.
133. Iskandrian AS, Hakki AH, Manno B, et al: Left ventricular function in chronic aortic regurgitation. *J Am Coll Cardiol* 1983;1:1374–1380.
134. Bonow RO, Rosing DR, McIntosh CL, et al: The natural history of asymptomatic patients with aortic regurgitation and normal left ventricular function. *Circulation* 1983;68:509–517.
135. Sorenson SG, O'Rourke RA, Chaudhuri TK: Non-invasive quantitation of valvular regurgitation by gated equilibrium radionuclide angiography. *Circulation* 1980;63:1089–1098.
136. Konstam MA, Wynne J, Holman BL, et al: Use of equilibrium (gated) radionuclide ventriculography to quantitate left ventricular output in patients with and without left-sided valvular regurgitation. *Circulation* 1981;64:578–585.
137. Bough E, Gandsman EJ, North DL, et al: Gated radionuclide angiographic evaluation of valve regurgitation. *Am J Cardiol* 1980;46:423.
138. Janowitz WR, Fester A: Quantitation of left ventricular regurgitant fraction by first pass radionuclide angiocardiography. *Am J Cardiol* 1982;49:85–92.
139. Hegglin R, Scheu H, Rothlin M: Aortic insufficiency. *Circulation* 1968;37,38(suppl 5): V77–V92.
140. Murphy ES, Kloster FE: Late results of valve replacement surgery. *Mod Concepts Cardiovasc Dis* 1979;48:53–58.
141. Bonow RO, Rosing DR, Kent KM, et al: Timing of operation for chronic aortic regurgitation. *Am J Cardiol* 1982;50:325–336.
142. McGoon MD, Fuster V, McGoon DC, et al: Aortic and mitral valve incompetence: Long-term follow-up (10–19 years) of patients treated with the Starr-Edwards prosthesis. *J Am Coll Cardiol* 1984;3:930–938.
143. Richardson JV, Kouchoukos NT, Wright JO III, et al: Combined aortic valve replacement and myocardial revascularization: Result in 220 patients. *Circulation* 1979;59:75–81.
144. Greves J, Rahimtoola SH, McAnulty JH, et al: Preoperative criteria predictive of late survival following valve replacement for severe aortic regurgitation. *Am Heart J* 1981;101:300–308.
145. Murphy ES, Kloster FE: Late results of valve replacement surgery. *Mod Concepts Cardiovasc Dis* 1979;48:59–66.
146. Toussaint C, Cribier A, Cazor L, et al: Hemodynamic and angiographic evaluation of aortic regurgitation 8 and 27 months after aortic valve replacement. *Circulation* 1981;64:456–463.
147. Henry WL, Bonow RO, Borer JS, et al: Observations on the optimum time for operative intervention for aortic regurgitation. *Circulation* 1980;61:471–483.
148. Hirshfeld JW Jr, Epstein SE, Roberts AJ, et al: Indices predicting long-term survival after valve replacement in patients with aortic regurgitation and patients with aortic stenosis. *Circulation* 1974;50:1190–1199.
149. Smith HJ, Neutzer JM, Roche AHG, et al: The natural history of rheumatic aortic regurgitation and the indications for surgery. *Br Heart J* 1976; 38:147–154.
150. Samuels DA, Curfman GD, Friedlich AL, et al: Valve replacement for aortic regurgitation: Long-term follow-up with factors influencing the results. *Circulation* 1979;60:647–654.
151. Henry WL, Bonow RO, Rosing DR, et al: Observations on the optimum time for operative intervention for aortic regurgitation II. Serial echocardiographic evaluation of asymptomatic patients. *Circulation* 1980;61:484–492.
152. Fioretti P, Roelandt J, Bos RJ, et al: Echocardiography in chronic aortic insufficiency. Is valve replacement too late when left ventricular end-systolic dimension reaches 55 mm? *Circulation* 1983;67:216–220.
153. Bonow RO, Borer JS, Rosing DR, et al: Preoperative exercise capacity in symptomatic patients with aortic regurgitation as a predictor of postoperative left ventricular function and long-term prognosis. *Circulation* 1980;62:1280–1290.
154. Schuler G, Peterson KL, Johnson AD, et al: Hypertrophy and function after surgical correc-

tion of aortic regurgitation. *Am J Cardiol* 1979; 44:585–594.
155. Kennedy JW, Doces J, Stewart DK: Left ventricular function before and following aortic valve replacement. *Circulation* 1970;56:944–950.
156. Boucher CA, Bingham JB, Osbakken MD, et al: Early changes in left ventricular size and function after correction of left ventricular volume overload. *Am J Cardiol* 1981;47:991–1004.
157. Bolen JL, Alderman EL: Hemodynamic consequences of afterload reduction in patients with chronic aortic regurgitation. *Circulation* 1976; 53:879–883.
158. Miller RR, Vismara LA, DeMaria AN, et al: Afterload reduction therapy with nitroprusside in severe aortic regurgitation: Improved cardiac performance and reduced regurgitant volume. *Am J Cardiol* 1976;38:564–567.
159. Greenberg BH, DeMots H, Murphy E, et al: Mechanism for improved cardiac performance with arteriolar dilators in aortic insufficiency. *Circulation* 1981;63:263–268.
160. Greenberg BH, DeMots H, Murphy E, et al: Beneficial effects of hydralazine on rest and exercise hemodynamics in patients with chronic severe aortic insufficiency. *Circulation* 1980;62: 49–54.
161. Fioretti P, Benussi B, Scardi S, et al: Afterload reduction with nifedipine in aortic insufficiency. *Am J Cardiol* 1982;49:1728–1732.
162. Greenberg BH, Rahimtoola SH: Long-term vasodilator therapy in aortic insufficiency: Evidence for regression of left ventricular dilatation and hypertrophy and improvement in systolic pump function. *Ann Intern Med* 1980;93: 440–442.

CHAPTER 11
Multivalvular Heart Disease

Henry DeMots

Patients with abnormal function of more than one cardiac valve often present special problems in diagnosis and management. The physician must determine the extent to which each valve contributes to the patient's symptoms and also estimate the effect of coexisting myocardial dysfunction.

The incidence of multivalvular heart disease has declined in the United States because of successful public health measures directed against rheumatic fever, a major cause of multivalvular disease, and because of successful early interventions intended to prevent chronic ventricular overload and dilatation.

ETIOLOGY

Multivalvular heart disease occurs when a systemic disease simultaneously affects the tissue of several valves, when an overload condition produced by one valve or by myocardial dysfunction affects a second valve, or when two different disease processes affect different valves.

Specific etiologies

Rheumatic heart disease commonly affects more than one cardiac valve and rarely affects only the aortic or the tricuspid valve.[1] Approximately one half of patients with rheumatic heart disease have involvement of more than one valve.[1,2]

Patients with Marfan's syndrome frequently have abnormalities of the mitral and the aortic valves. Echocardiographic evidence of abnormalities were found in 97% of Marfan's patients examined in one study. Both the mitral and the aortic valves showed echocardiographic abnormalities in 60% of the patients.[3] Mitral valve prolapse and myxomatous proliferation produce the mitral valve dysfunction and dilatation of the aortic root with cystic medionecrosis and myxomatous proliferation of valve leaflets cause aortic valve dysfunction (Figure 11-1).

Infective endocarditis may involve more than one valve, but is usually found on one valve only. Instances of endocarditis involving two valves usually occur where preexisting valvular abnormalities were present.

Patients with congenital heart disease may have coexisting lesions of two valves.

Secondary lesions

A chronic pressure or volume overload produced by one valve may affect the function of valves proximal to it. Increased ventricular pressure and changes in the geometry of the cardiac chambers produced by ventricular overload and by pulmonary hypertension produce regurgitation in a previously normally functioning valve.

Pulmonary hypertension caused by mitral valve disease may lead to pulmonic and tricuspid regurgitation. Tricuspid regurgitation is usually preceded by right ventricular dysfunction and dilatation of the right ventricle and tricuspid annulus.

PATHOPHYSIOLOGY

An abnormality in one valve can induce abnormal function in a previously normal valve. Figure 11-2 is a schema outlining the effects that a functional abnormality of one valve may produce in another.

It is a controversial point whether annular

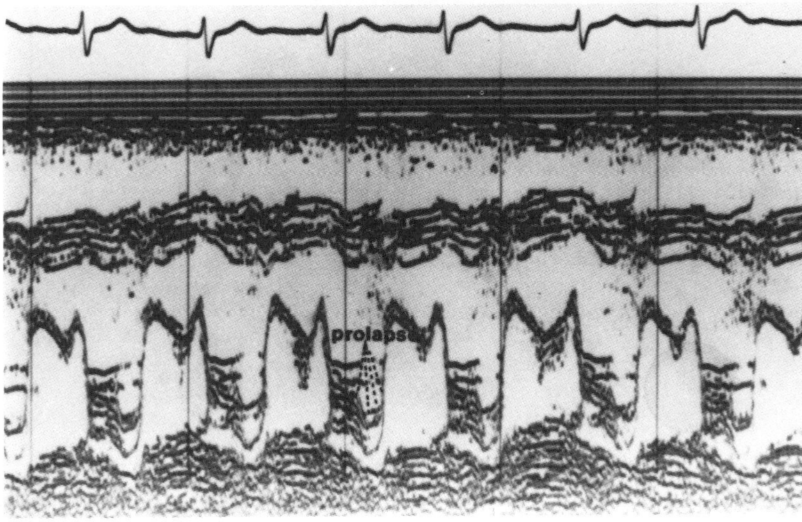

Figure 11-1A Marked prolapse of the posterior leaflet of the mitral valve in a patient with Marfan's syndrome. RV = right ventricle, IVS = interventricular septum, MV = mitral valve, LAw = left atrial wall.

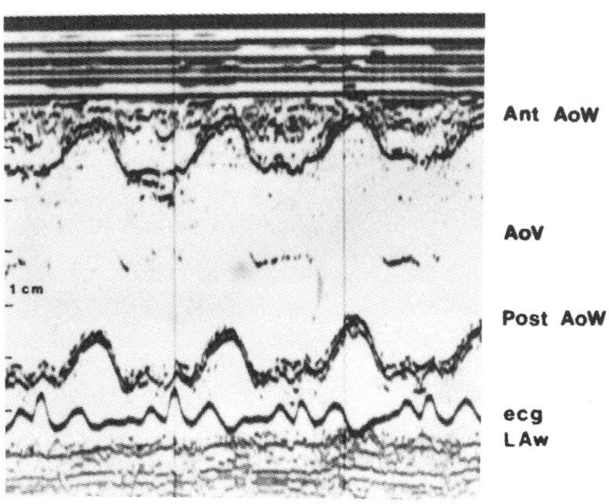

Figure 11-1B Aortic annular dilatation in a patient with Marfan's syndrome. Abnormalities of both valves are found in a majority of patients with Marfan's syndrome. Ant AoW = anterior aortic wall, AoV = aortic valve, Post AoW = posterior aortic wall, LAw = left atrial wall. (Reproduced with permission from Brown et al.[3])

dilatation occurs in atrioventricular valves to cause valvular regurgitation or whether abnormalities induced in the function of the subvalvular mechanism are completely responsible for secondary valvular abnormalities. Bulkley and Roberts[4] have measured the annular circumferences in a number of these patients and found them to be normal. Carpentier et al,[5] however, have promoted the use of annuloplasty for the surgical therapy of both tricuspid and mitral regurgitation which they believe to be caused by dilatation of the nonseptal portions of the annuli.

Mitral regurgitation may also occur because of lateral displacement of the base of the papillary muscles when left ventricular dilatation occurs and the leaflets of the valve are no longer able to coapt.[6,7]

When there is organic disease in two valves the first may transform a nonsignificant functional abnormality into a significant abnormality. Two functionally abnormal valves which would not cause problems alone may together be responsible for significant disability.

Aortic regurgitation produces left ventricular dilatation which may aggravate mitral regurgitation that is already present, or may result in mitral regurgitation if none is present. Since both mitral and aortic regurgitation produce volume overload of the left ventricle, ventricular dilatation may be observed with only moderately severe disease of each of the two valves. The inefficiency of this combination of lesions is dramatized when angiographic contrast material is observed reaching the left atrium from an aortic supravalvular injection.

In acute aortic regurgitation (Figure 11-3), a normal mitral valve will close early in diastole. This limits forward flow from the left atrium, but also limits regurgitant flow which might other-

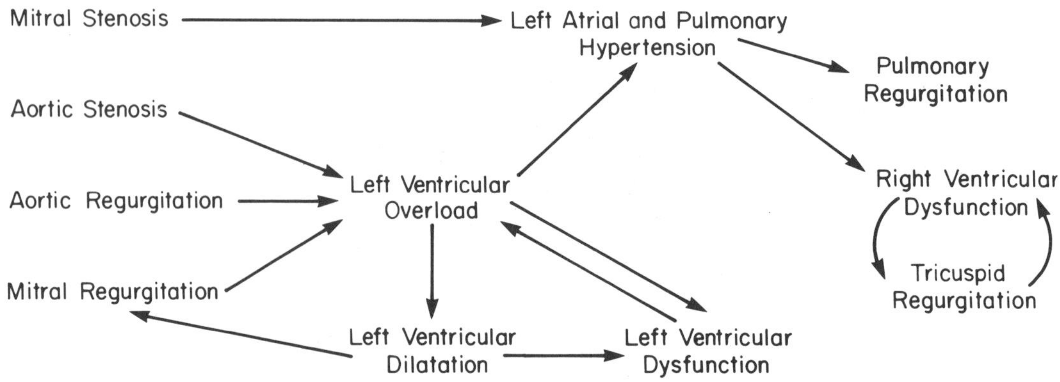

Figure 11-2 Abnormalities of one valve may produce functional abnormalities or structural changes in a second valve. Though the etiologies are varied, chronicity is usually required before these effects occur.

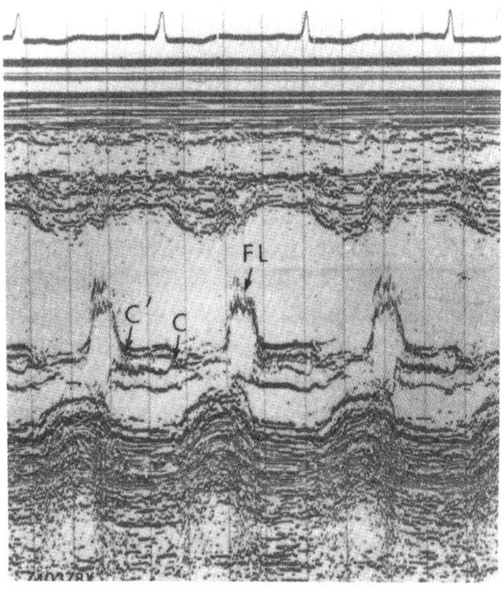

Figure 11-3 Acute severe aortic valve regurgitation produces fluttering (FL) of the anterior leaflet of the mitral valve and causes nearly complete closure of the mitral valve (C′) before ventricular systole (C). (Reproduced with permission from Feigenbaum H: *Echocardiography*, ed 3. Philadelphia, Lea & Febiger, 1981, p 282.)

wise occur. When the aortic regurgitation is severe, the left ventricular end-diastolic pressure is higher than the left atrial pressure. An incompetent mitral valve allows this high pressure to be transmitted to the left atrium and pulmonary circulation.[8] Early mitral valve closure is evident on an echocardiogram in cases of severe aortic regurgitation. If the mitral valve subvalvular mechanism is not normal or there is intrinsic disease of the mitral leaflets, early closure may not be possible.

Aortic stenosis may aggravate mitral regurgitation because the impedance to outflow through the aortic valve becomes high relative to the impedance to regurgitant flow through the mitral valve.[9] Consequently, the volume of blood which regurgitates to the left atrium increases. Much of the regurgitant flow crosses the mitral valve early in systole and reduces the ventricular preload. Since the cardiac output is dependent on a high preload in patients with aortic stenosis, the cardiac output cannot be maintained at normal levels if mitral regurgitation is added to aortic stenosis because the left ventricular preload cannot be adequately increased. Mitral stenosis also limits left ventricular preload by limiting diastolic filling. The poor manner in which patients with mitral stenosis tolerate rapid heart rates is aggravated if there is coexisting aortic stenosis since patients with aortic stenosis are sensitive to small changes in preload.[10]

Chronic mitral valve disease will induce changes in the pulmonary vascular bed resulting in sustained pulmonary hypertension. This, in turn, may produce pulmonary valvular regurgitation due to annular dilatation.

Pulmonary hypertension will also lead to tricuspid regurgitation. The mechanisms for the development of secondary tricuspid regurgitation are similar to the mechanisms for the development of mitral regurgitation in patients with left ventricular overload.

The development of the combination of pulmonary hypertension, right ventricular dilatation, and tricuspid regurgitation has significant implications for the patient with multivalvular disease. When the function of the right side of the heart becomes the limiting factor in changes in cardiac output, surgical correction of left heart valve lesions may fail to improve the functional status of the patient. Because a fixed right heart output limits left ventricular preload, these patients are limited by fatigue and are less likely to experience symptoms of pulmonary congestion.

EVALUATION OF THE PATIENT

History

The clinical history in most patients with multivalvular disease is similar to the clinical history in patients with single valve disease. In multivalvular disease the amount of disability reported by the patient may be greater than the physical examination would suggest. This may be because the importance of some valve lesions are masked by the presence of others or because the patient's disability is due to the sum of the effects of several minor abnormalities.

The history may be particularly misleading in patients with combined aortic and mitral stenosis[11–15] Patients with severe aortic stenosis in whom the predominant symptoms might usually include dizziness and angina may not have them if mitral stenosis is also present. The symptoms of mitral stenosis predominate in most of these patients.

Particular attention should be given to a history compatible with right heart failure in a patient who does not have primary tricuspid or pulmonic valve disease. This finding suggests chronicity of the valvular heart disease and damage to the right side of the heart as a result of chronic overload of the right ventricle.

When there is evidence of multivalvular disease a review of those systemic conditions associated with multivalvular disease is in order to establish the etiology.

An important function of the history in patients with multivalvular disease is to determine the chronicity of the illness and the sequence of events. The changes in functional status often occur slowly with valvular heart disease and the patient is often unaware of them. A recitation of the progress of symptoms is not adequate unless it is coupled with information regarding the patient's activity level. Patients with slowly developing disability may subconsciously forgo activities which produce symptoms and be incompletely aware of the extent to which their disability has progressed.

The symptoms which limit exercise must also be established. In some patients a history of progression of symptoms can be elicited beginning with dyspnea on exertion in the early stages and proceeding to easy fatiguability without significant dyspnea in the late stages. It may be postulated that the patient is initially limited by symptoms of left heart failure and then develops secondary pulmonary hypertension and right heart failure. This leads to a low, relatively fixed cardiac output associated with the symptoms of fatigue.

If there is intrinsic disease of the pulmonic or tricuspid valve, symptoms of right heart failure would occur early in the course of the illness.

An accurate assessment of the extent of the patient's disability is crucial in the determination of the timing of surgery. Deterioration of the functional status of the patient to the point where he experiences symptoms during the performance of his usual activities is an indication for cardiac catheterization in a patient with multivalvular disease even though the physical examination suggests that the two lesions are mild.

Physical examination

A knowledge of the pathophysiology of multivalvular disease is helpful in interpreting the significance of the physical findings. Listening to the individual sounds and portions of the cardiac cycle serially rather than all at once is especially crucial. The technique of inching from the apex to the base to distinguish changes in the timing and quality of murmurs is helpful in distinguishing between murmurs occurring during the same portion of the cardiac cycle.[16] This may be the only way to be sure whether or not a murmur of mitral regurgitation is present in some patients with a loud murmur of aortic stenosis.

The significance of a murmur of aortic stenosis in a patient who has coexisting mitral stenosis may be underestimated because of the low stroke volume found in patients with mitral stenosis.[11–15,17] The fourth heart sound and the double apical impulse often found in aortic stenosis may be absent because these findings require more rapid filling of the left ventricle than is possible in patients with mitral stenosis.

Aortic regurgitation may coexist with mitral stenosis in patients with rheumatic heart disease.[18] This combination of lesions may produce diagnostic confusion because a diastolic murmur simulating mitral stenosis may be produced by aortic regurgitation. Differentiation of this murmur from organic mitral stenosis may be difficult. The absence of other auscultatory signs of mitral stenosis such as a loud first heart sound and the disappearance or softening of the murmur following amyl nitrate inhalation favor the diagnosis of the Austin Flint murmur; their presence favors organic mitral stenosis.

When organic mitral stenosis is present the physical findings of aortic regurgitation may be less prominant so that the severity of the lesion will be underestimated. An unexpectedly large left ventricular size should alert the physician to the importance of the aortic regurgitation.

Patients with mitral stenosis are prone to the development of pulmonary hypertension and pulmonary valvular regurgitation. Therefore, whenever a diastolic decreascendo murmur is heard along the left sternal border, the possibility of regurgitation of either semilunar valve must be considered. The response of the murmur to amyl nitrate may be helpful in distinguishing the two since the murmur of aortic regurgitation is decreased and the murmur of pulmonic regurgitation is increased by this maneuver. Usually, findings associated with pulmonary hypertension, such as a loud pulmonic second sound, will also be present.

Tricuspid regurgitation may often be difficult to detect by physical examination because it is often due to functional changes on the left side of the heart. The findings on the left side of the heart may ask the findings of the abnormalities on the right side of the heart. A murmur of tricuspid regurgitation is often found in association with a murmur of mitral regurgitation. Though the former is said to increase and the later to decrease with inspiration, these changes are often too small to be interpreted. The diagnosis of tricuspid regurgitation can often be made by detecting large "v" waves in the neck veins or pulsation of the liver. However, since the changes in right heart function occur slowly, the right atrium may be dilated and compliant. In those instances the amplitude of the "v" waves due to the regurgitation are not large. Whenever there is peripheral edema and an elevated jugular venous pressure the possibility of tricuspid regurgitation must be considered.

Chest Roentgenogram

The chest film is helpful in assessing chamber size, in assessing the amount of pulmonary venous congestion, in corroborating the physical findings of pulmonary hypertension, and in the detection of valvular calcification. It is a simple and safe way to monitor interval changes.

The specific roentgenologic findings of individual valve lesions have been described elsewhere in this volume. The chest film can be of great help in determining the significance of a second murmur or in alerting the physician to the presence of an occult second valvular abnormality.

When chamber enlargement occurs it may be due either to volume overload related to increasing regurgitation through a valve or to ventricular dysfunction. An examination of the chest film does not allow this distinction to be made but it does alert the physician to the fact that there is an additional problem to be evaluated.

When mitral stenosis is present, left ventricular enlargement may not be great, even in the face of significant aortic regurgitation. Enlargement of the left ventricle may be prominant with combined aortic and mitral regurgitation, even when the murmurs of the two lesions are unimpressive. Enlargement of the left ventricle in a patient with aortic stenosis is not expected unless the aortic stenosis is both severe and chronic or unless mitral or aortic regurgitation has also developed.

Enlargement of the main pulmonary artery should suggest the possibility that a diastolic decrescendo murmur signifies pulmonary valvular regurgitation rather than aortic regurgitation. It may also signify the presence of pulmonary hypertension.

Enlargement of the heart to the right of the spine may be due either to massive left atrial enlargement or to right atrial enlargement. The later is usually associated with roentgenographic signs of right ventricular enlargement. This deserves careful attention because it indicates the onset of right heart failure which is usually accompanied by tricuspid regurgitation. It suggests an ominous and occasionally irreversible degree of progress in the patient's illness.

Electrocardiography

The uses of the ECG are similar in single and multivalve disease. Clues to the presence of an occult second lesion may be found on the ECG. For example, left ventricular hypertrophy may not occur despite severe aortic stenosis if the patient also has mitral stenosis. The ECG will reflect the absence of hypertrophy. In this instance the ECG may indicate the presence of otherwise occult mitral stenosis by demonstrating left atrial enlargement.

Nuclear cardiology and echocardiography

Echocardiography will identify abnormalities of valves that might otherwise go undetected.

Identification of or exclusion of occult rheumatic mitral valve disease and of aortic valve disease in the patient with a low cardiac output can be of great clinical usefulness. In patients with aortic regurgitation the echocardiogram may be of considerable aid in distinguishing an Austin Flint murmur from the murmur of organic mitral stenosis by showing the characteristic diastolic anterior motion of the posterior mitral leaflet in rheumatic heart disease or the fluttering of the anterior mitral leaflet and early mitral closure that may accompany the Austin Flint murmur.[19] The echocardiogram represents a sensitive means of detecting the aortic and mitral valve abnormalities of patients with Marfan's syndrome even before the lesions are clinically significant.[4]

Doppler studies are useful in distinguishing between mitral and tricuspid regurgitation and between pulmonic and aortic regurgitation provided one is aware of the great sensitivity of these techniques in detecting small amounts of turbulance.

Both the echocardiogram and the nuclear-gated blood pool examination may be used to measure the function and size of the ventricles. From these data inferences may be made about the function of the valves. Echocardiography provides the most accurate method of assessing left atrial size. Nuclear techniques provide a method for estimating the significance of mitral regurgitation by comparing the output of the left and right ventricles. The method assumes that only the mitral valve is functioning abnormally and the technique must, therefore, be used with caution.

Cardiac catheterization

Multivalvular disease occasionally imposes technical problems to be overcome in the course of cardiac catheterization. Multichamber enlargement makes the catheter manipulations more difficult. Valvular regurgitation complicates the use of indicator dilution techniques for measuring cardiac output. Catheterization of the left ventricle may be difficult if there is stenosis of both the mitral and aortic valves. In most circumstances, however, either the retrograde or transeptal technique will be successful. Referral of a patient to cardiac surgery for the treatment of multivalvular disease without catheterization of the left ventricle is hazardous and consideration of transcutaneous left ventricular puncture should be seriously considered if the usual techniques fail.[20–21] If the pericardium has been previously opened this may be performed with an 18-gauge needle, which allows angiography of the left ventricle, but if the pericardium has not been previously opened, the threat of pericardial tamponade exists and a 21-gauge needle should be used.

Evaluation of valves requires careful, simultaneous measurement of the pressures on each side of each valve and the cardiac output. When recordings of pressures and flows have been made, the Gorlin formula[22] is highly useful in integrating the information to determine the significance of gradients. Severe aortic stenosis may be present with a gradient of only 20 mmHg if cardiac output is low because of coexisting mitral or tricuspid disease.[17]

The importance of mitral regurgitation that is demonstrated angiographically in a patient with significant aortic stenosis must be carefully evaluated. If the amount of mitral regurgitation is small it is likely to disapppear following replacement of the aortic valve. A number of factors may be considered in determining whether mitral valve replacement is needed or whether the regurgitation is likely to regress after aortic valve replacement. These considerations include an assessment of the severity of the regurgitation and a determination of whether the regurgitation is associated with intrinsic disease of the valve leaflets. The history and physical examination can be helpful by suggesting etiologic diagnoses associated with intrinsic valve disease. The echocardiogram can occasionally demonstrate intrinsic valve disease, and in some cases intraoperative assessment may be required.

The measurement of left ventricular volume allows an assessment of the significance of combined aortic and mitral regurgitation. Though each regurgitant lesion may be only moderately severe, the combined effect will be reflected by changes in left ventricular end-diastolic volume.

Performance of supine bicycle exercise in the course of cardiac catheterization is often helpful in elucidating the mechanism of exercise limitation, quantitating the severity of disability, and predicting the extent of improvement to be expected following surgical intervention. A patient with mitral stenosis and tricuspid regurgitation who also develops marked elevation of the left ventricular end-diastolic pressure during exercise may have occult left ventricular dysfunction which will continue to limit him following surgery. Failure to increase the cardiac output or elevate the pulmonary artery wedge pressure suggests that the limiting factor resides in the function of the right side of the heart.

THERAPY

Surgical therapy

There are several factors which make the decision to perform valve replacement a difficult one in patients with multivalvular disease. The physician may not have the option of treating each valve separately by waiting until each reaches a critical level of severity. Each additional operation carries risk and the number of procedures must be kept to a minimum. It may also be necessary to replace a second valve that would not usually require replacement in order to wean the patient from cardiopulmonary bypass.

Though patients often show improvement following multivalve replacement,[23] many patients fail to improve symptomatically because prosthetic valves do not function as well as a normal natural valve. Following surgery the patient is left with two mildly obstructed valves in series. The problem is compounded if one of the valves has an effective orifice which is relatively small for the size of the patient.[24]

Frequently, patients with multivalvular disease have relatively mild disease of each involved valve so that the diseased valves are functioning nearly as well as the prosthetic valves that would be inserted in their place. In these circumstances a chronic, though mild, condition of overload is placed on the ventricle. This eventually causes dysfunction of that ventricle. When surgery is finally recommended the patient is left with two mildly obstructed prosthetic valves and mild left ventricular dysfunction. The improvement in functional status in these circumstances may be negligible. Surgery may, nevertheless, be indicated to halt or slow the rate of progression of disability.

Though it may occasionally be necessary to replace some valves that would not ordinarily require replacement, great care must be given to avoiding replacement of valves that are dysfunctional secondary to dysfunction of another valve. The most frequently encountered example of this is the patient with severe aortic valve disease who has mitral regurgitation because of left ventricular dilatation. Mitral regurgitation will usually regress if there is no organic disease of the mitral leaflets. Occasionally mitral annuloplasty may be useful in reversing some of the effects of dilatation.[5,25]

The decision whether to replace the mitral valve or not is critical because a wrong decision may result in the need for reoperation at a later date. Replacement of the mitral valve is technically more difficult when an aortic prosthesis has already been implanted. The decision may be aided by knowing the etiology of and the likelihood of progression of the mitral valve disease.

Operative mortality in most centers is higher for multivalve replacement than for single valve replacement.[26,27] Most reports describe the experience with patients operated upon before current myocardial protection techniques were widely used[28–37] and thus current operative risks are probably somewhat lower.[38–39] The increased risk of surgery is related to the complexity of the surgery and the longer bypass times, to the severity of illness of the patient, to secondary abnormalities in cardial performance which have developed over time, or because the patient is left with prosthetic valves in series. Several series of operative mortalities reported after 1970 are shown in Table 11-1. Two reports that give operative mortalities for single valve replacement in the same institution are also shown so that the relative risk of double valve replacement can be compared to the risk of single valve replacement.

Triple valve replacement is performed rarely because rheumatic heart disease is encountered less frequently and because timely operation for mitral and aortic valve disease may have reduced the frequency of secondary tricuspid valve regurgitation. Tricuspid annuloplasty has emerged as a good alternative to tricuspid valve replacement in many patients. Though operative risk is high,[28,32,34,36,37] functional improvement may follow triple valve replacement.[36–37]

The optimal time for surgical intervention in a patient with multivalvular disease is when the severity of the lesions is such that prosthetic valve replacement will improve hemodynamic performance and ventricular dysfunction has not yet occurred. Unfortunately, this conjunction of circumstances does not always occur and compromises must be made. If a general rule must be invoked it would be that irreversible changes in ventricular function should not be allowed to occur because of untreated valvular dysfunction. This rule, unfortunately, is often difficult to obey because the identification of the point at which changes occur is often difficult or impossible. Echocardiography, which allows serial noninvasive determinations of left ventricular dimensions and function, may be of valve in determining the optimal time for surgery.[40]

Medical therapy

The medical therapy of patients with multival-

Table 11-1
Mortalities for Valve Replacement

Study/Yr	AVR	MVR	A & M	M & T	TVR
Midell and DeBoer, 1972[28]			6/61(10%)	2/17(17%)	3/12(25%)
Melvin et al, 1973[29]			22/100(22%)		
Nitter-Hauge et al, 1979[30]			2/23(9%)		
Rufilanchas et al, 1976[31]			4/42(10%)		
Sanfellippo et al, 1976[32]				14/61(23%)	15/62(25%)
Stephenson et al, 1975,[33] 1977[34]			32/251(12%)		9/38(24%)
Aberg et al, 1977[35]		7/75(9%)			
Oyer et al, 1977[27]	46/686(7%)	79/853(9%)	18/209(9%)		
Rhodes et al, 1977[36]					6/26(24%)
Isom, 1977[26]	42/470(9%)	39/362(11%)	24/129(19%)	19/112(17%)	
McManus et al, 1978[37]					9/48(19%)
Parr et al, 1979[38*]			7/33(21%)		
Stephenson et al, 1984[39*]			9/150(6%)		

The table shows operative mortality rates for multivalve replacement published after 1970. Two studies which also reported mortality rates for single valve replacement are shown for comparison. AVR = aortic valve replacement, MVR = mitral valve replacement, A & M = aortic and mitral valve replacement, M & T = mitral and tricuspid valve replacement, TVR — triple valve replacement.
* Mortalities were less than 2% when potassium arrest cardioplegia was used.

vular disease requires application of the same principles that apply to patients with single valve disease. Afterload reduction with vasodilators, which has proved effective in improving hemodynamic performance in a number of valvular lesions, deserves special mention because the physician often wishes to delay the use of surgical therapy when treating a patient who has more than one lesion that is producing only mild hemodynamic impairment. The potential benefit from vasodilators is greatest in patients who have mitral or aortic regurgitation with or without left ventricular dysfunction. The regurgitant fraction is reduced, exercise performance is increased, filling pressures are reduced, and cardiac output is increased both at rest and exercise.[41–43]

Benefit from vasodilators can also be shown in patients with mild aortic stenosis.[44] The likelihood of benefit will depend on the relative contribution of the arteriolar and valvular impedance to outflow.

REFERENCES

1. Robbins SL, Cotran RS: *Pathologic Basis of Disease*. Philadelphia, WB Saunders Co, 1979.
2. Roberts WC, Anatomically isolated aortic valve disease: The case against its being of rheumatic etiology. *Am J Med* 1970;49:151–159.
3. Brown OR, DeMots, H, Kloster FE, et al: Aortic root dilatation and mitral valve prolapse in Marfan's syndrome. *Circulation* 1975;52:651–657.
4. Bulkley BH, Roberts WC: Dilatation of the mitral annulus: A rare cause of mitral regurgitation. *Am J Med* 1975;59:457–463.
5. Carpentier A, DeLoche A, Dauptain J: A new reconstructive operation for correction of mitral and tricuspid insufficiency. *J Thorac Cardiovasc Surg* 1971;61:1–13.
6. Burch GE, DePasquale NP, Phillips JH: The syndrome of papillary muscle dysfunction. *Am Heart J* 1968;75:399–415.
7. Kremkau EL, Gilbertson PR, Bristow JD: Acquired, non-rheumatic mitral regurgitation: Clinical management with emphasis on evaluation of myocardial performance. *Prog Cardiovasc Dis* 1973;15:403–425.
8. Welch GH Jr, Braunwald E, Sarnoff SJ: Hemodynamic effects of quantitatively varied experimental aortic regurgitation. *Circ Res* 1957;5: 546–551.
9. Braunwald E, Welch GH Jr, Sarnoff SJ: Hemodynamic effects of quantitatively varied experimental mitral regurgitation. *Cir Res* 1957;5: 539–545.
10. Stott DK, Marpole DGF, Bristow JD, et al: The role of left atrial transport in aortic and mitral stenosis. *Circulation* 1970;41:1031–1041.
11. Honey M: Clinical and hemodynamic observations on combined mitral and aortic stenosis. *Br Heart J* 1961;23:545–555.
12. Katznelson G, Hreissaty RM, Levinson GE, et al: Combined aortic and mitral stenosis: A clinical and physiologic study. *Am J Med* 1960;29: 242–256.
13. Reid JM, Stevenson JG, Barclay RS, et al: Combined aortic and mitral stenosis. *Br Heart J* 1962;24:509–515.
14. Zitnik RS, Piemme TE, Messer RJ, et al: The masking of aortic stenosis by mitral stenosis. *Am Heart J* 1965;69:22–30.
15. Morrow AG, Awe WC, Braunwald E: Combined mitral and aortic stenosis. *Br Heart J* 1962;24: 606–612.
16. Levine SA, Harvey WP: *Clinical Auscultation of the Heart*, Philadelphia, WB Saunders Co, 1959.
17. Schattenberg TT, Titus JL, Parkin TW: Clinical findings in acquired aortic valve stenosis. Effect of

disease of other valves. *Am Heart J* 1967;73: 322–325.
18. Segal J, Harvey WP, Hufnagel CA: Clinical study of 100 cases of severe aortic insufficiency. *Am J Med* 1956;21:200–210.
19. Pridie RB, Benham R, Oakley CM: Echocardiography of the mitral valve in aortic valve disease. *Br Heart J* 1971;33:296–304.
20. Baxley WA, Soto B: Hemodynamic evaluation of patients with combined aortic and mitral prostheses. *Am J Cardiol* 1980;45:42–47.
21. Greves J, DeMots H, Murphy E, et al: Transthoracic left ventricular puncture and angiography in patients with double valve disease. *Circulation* 1979;60(II):99.
22. Gorlin R, Gorlin SG: Hydraulic formula for calculation of the area of the stenotic mitral valve, other cardiac valves and central circulatory shunts. *Am Heart J* 1951;41:1–29.
23. Bristow JD, Farrehi C, McCord CW, et al: Clinical and hemodynamic observations after combined aortic and mitral replacement. *Circulation* 1965;31:67–79.
24. Rahimtoola SH: The problem of valve prosthesis-patient mismatch. *Circulation* 1978;58:20–24.
25. Chopra PS, Rowe GG, Young WP: Carpentier ring annuloplasty in severe noncalcific mitral insufficiency. *Am Heart J* 1978;96:253–262.
26. Isom OW, Spencer FC Glassman E, et al: Long term results in 1375 patients undergoing valve replacement with the Starr-Edwards cloth covered steel ball prosthesis. *Ann Surg* 1977;186:310–323.
27. Oyer PE, Steinson EB, Griepp RB, et al: Valve replacement with the Starr-Edwards and Hancock prostheses: Comparative analysis of late morbidity and mortality. *Ann Surg* 1977;186:301–309.
28. Midell D, DeBoer A: Multiple valve replacement. *Arch Surg* 1972;104:471.
29. Melvin DB, Tecklenberg PL, Hollingsworth JF, et al: Computer based analysis of preoperative and postoperative prognositic factors in 100 patients with combined aortic and mitral valve replacement. *Circulation* 1973;48(suppl 3):56–62.
30. Nitter-Hauge S, Froysaker T, Enge I, et al: Clinical and hemodynamic observations after combined aortic and mitral valve replacement with the Bjork-Shiley tilting disc valve prosthesis: Early and late results in 25 patients. *Scand J Thorac Cardiovasc Surg* 1979;13:25–31.
31. Rufilanchas JJ, Maronas JM, Agosti J, et al: Combined aortic and mitral replacement with the Bjork-Shiley prosthesis. *Scand J Thorac Cardiovasc Surg* 1976;10:193–196.
32. Sanfellippo PM, Guiliani ER, Danielson GK, et al: Tricuspid valve replacement: Early and late results with the Starr-Edwards prosthesis. *J Thorac Cardiovasc Surg* 1976;71:441–445.
33. Stephenson LW, Kouchoukas NT, Kirlin JW, et al: Combined aortic and mitral valve replacement: Results in 251 patients. *Circulation* 1975;51(II):31.
34. Stephenson LW, Kouchoukas NT, Kirklin JW: Triple valve replacement: An analysis of eight years' experience. *Ann Thorac Surg* 1977;23: 327–332.
35. Aberg B, Henze A, Bjork VO: Combined aortic and mitral valve replacement with the Bjork-Shiley tilting disc valve prosthesis. *Scand J Thorac Cardiovasc Surg* 1977;11:1–10.
36. Rhodes GR, McIntosh CL, Redwood DR, et al: Clinical and hemodynamic results following triple valve replacement: Mechanical vs. porcine xenograft prostheses. *Circulation* 1977;56(suppl 2): 122–127.
37. McManus Q, Grunkemeier G, Starr A: Late results of triple valve replacement: A 14 year review. *Ann Thorac Surg* 1978;25:402–406.
38. Parr GVS, Fox S, Waldhausen JA, et al: Improving results in combined aortic and mitral valve replacement using cold potassium cardioplegia *J Cardiovasc Surg* 1979;20:457–461.
39. Stephenson LW, Edie RN, Harken AH, et al: Combined aortic and mitral valve replacement: Changes in practice and prognosis. *Circulation* 1984;69:640–644.
40. Henry WL, Bonow RO, Borer JJ: Observations on the optimum time for the operative intervention for aortic regurgitation: Evaluation of the results of aortic valve replacement in symptomatic patients. *Circulation* 1980;61:471–483.
41. Greenberg BH, DeMots H. Murphy ES, et al: Arterial dilators in mitral regurgitation: Effects on rest and exersize hemodynamics and long term clinical followup. *Circulation* 1982;65:181–187.
42. Greenberg BH, DeMots H, Murphy ES, et al: Mechanism for improved cardiac performance with arteriolar dilators in aortic insufficiency. *Circulation* 1981;63:263–268.
43. Greenberg BH, DeMots H, Murphy ES, et al: Beneficial effects of hydralazine on rest and exersize hemodynamics in patients with chronic severe aortic insufficiency. *Circulation* 1980;62: 49–55.
44. Greenberg BH, Massie B: Beneficial effects of afterload reduction therapy in patients with congestive heart failure and moderate aortic stenosis. *Circulation* 1980;61:1212–1216.

CHAPTER 12
Effects of Pregnancy in Patients with Valvular Heart Disease

James Metcalfe
John McAnulty

This chapter will emphasize two essential concepts. First, the use of any diagnostic or therapeutic technique in a pregnant woman must take into consideration the health of both the mother and her child. The presence of a "second patient" — the developing fetus — mandates avoidance whenever possible of invasive diagnostic procedures, drugs, and surgery. However, when any of these is considered essential for the well-being of the mother, it should be utilized. The second basic concept is that the rational management of pregnancy in a woman with heart disease requires an understanding of the effects of pregnancy upon the normal cardiovascular system.

This chapter will discuss the choice of diagnostic and therapeutic procedures in pregnant women with valvular disease, review the hemodynamic changes characteristic of pregnancy, and consider their interaction with specific valve deformities.

CARDIOVASCULAR DIAGNOSIS DURING PREGNANCY

Some procedures for the diagnosis of heart disease are potentially dangerous. In addition, overutilization is an appropriate concern, especially during pregnancy. The risk of inaccurate interpretation is compounded by ignorance of the changes expected in normal pregnancy. Accordingly, in discussing diagnostic procedures, the variations in normal findings which can be encountered during pregnancy in women without heart disease will be reviewed.

Procedures Resulting in Radiation Exposure

Exposure to ionizing radiation should be minimized during pregnancy. Several general rules are worthy of adoption. First, when a procedure involving ionizing radiation is being considered for a woman of childbearing age, the test should not be performed during the second half of the menstrual cycle. Second, every woman of childbearing age should be carefully questioned about the possibility of pregnancy before an elective procedure involving ionizing radiation is performed. When uncertainty about pregnancy exists, an elective procedure should be deferred until the situation is clarified. Third, when a procedure involving radiation exposure is warranted, the procedure that gives the least amount of radiation should be selected. In addition, shielding of the uterus should always be performed.

The timing of x-ray exposure affects the incidence of cogenital anomalies.[1] The highest incidence of congential anomalies results when exposure is received during weeks 3 through 10 of gestation. The danger lessens between the tenth and 20th weeks, and congenital anomalies resulting from radiation received after mid-pregnancy are rare.

Films of the chest for evaluating the size and shape of the heart and for estimating pulmonary vascularity result in radiation doses of less than 1 rad. At this dose level, no statistically significant increase in the incidence of congenital malformations can be demonstrated even when exposure occurs during the first trimester of pregnancy.[2] When a chest film is taken without recognizing the presence of an early pregnancy, interruption of the pregnancy need not be considered because of that procedure.[3]

If maternal health dictates the need for cardiac catheterization or abdominal angiography, the risk of fetal abnormality is increased. The increased risks must be weighed against the expected benefit of the procedure.

A chest film is the radiographic procedure most likely to be ordered. Even during a normal pregnancy, findings can be altered in women without heart disease. The heart can appear enlarged as a result of elevation of the hemidiaphragm and because of cardiac chamber enlargement. The expected increase in blood volume can also result in apparent pulmonary vascular engorgement.

The use of radionuclides for cardiac diagnosis is associated with minimal radiation exposure to the fetus since most of them are bound to proteins that do not cross the placenta. Nevertheless, avoidance of these procedures during pregnancy is advisable because release of the nuclide from the protein occurs, and defects in the placental barrier may result in significant exposure.[4]

Electrocardiography

The ECG is not predictably altered by pregnancy. In general, the rules of interpretation that apply in young women are applicable during pregnancy.[5] The axis of the QRS complex may shift toward the left, and some observers have reported nonspecific abnormalities of the ST segment and T wave. However, because these changes do not occur in all pregnant women, they cannot be dismissed when other evidence of heart disease is present.

Echocardiography

There are no recognized risks to the fetus from the use of cardiac ultrasound. When echocardiography promises to give important diagnostic information, it is the procedure of choice. The changes of normal pregnancy must be taken into account when interpreting echocardiagraphic studies.[6,7] The most important of these is an increase in the end-diastolic dimension of the left ventricle.

CARDIAC THERAPY DURING PREGNANCY

Most of the therapeutic measures that are of proven usefulness in patients with valvular disease can be employed during pregnancy. Normal activity during pregnancy is well tolerated by most women with heart disease. If symptoms of pulmonary congestion occur in a woman with valvular disease during pregnancy, reduction of activity is a reasonable first recommendation. Restriction of activity is properly augmented by restriction of fluid and sodium. Unless carried to extremes, these dietary restraints are unlikely to cause adverse effects.

Whenever possible, drugs should be avoided during pregnancy, but many can be used with reasonable safety. Pregnancy does not change the indications for digitalis therapy. Digoxin is most frequently used although it, like digitoxin, does cross the placental barrier. There is no evidence that either has any teratogenic effect or adversely affects the baby.[8–10] High digoxin levels can be achieved in fetal blood by maternal administration, particularly late in pregnancy, a fact that has implications for the treatment of fetal arrhythmias. During pregnancy, increased doses of digoxin are required to achieve the usual therapeutic levels because its volume of distribution is increased by expansion of the maternal and fetal fluid spaces. Digoxin has an oxytocic action that may initiate uterine contractions, and it has been suspected of shortening labor; however, these are not considered as important contraindications. Both digoxin and digitoxin are secreted in maternal milk.[11]

When orally administered diuretics first became available, they were used to limit fluid retention during pregnancy and as prophylaxis against toxemia.[12] Experience has shown that pedal edema is a harmless and common accompaniment of pregnancy and that long-term diuretic use does not lower the incidence of toxemia.[13,14] Indeed, "prophylactic" diuretics may obscure early evidence of preeclampsia and may aggravate it by causing depletion of extracellular fluid.[15,16] For these reasons, diuretic agents should be used only when a clear indication exists. The least controversial of these is pulmonary congestion caused by heart disease that cannot be controlled by restriction of sodium and activity. Thiazide diuretics cross the placental barrier but no teratogenic effect has been established. Furosemide also enters the fetal circulation and, like the thiazides, is found in maternal milk. Furosemide is such a potent diuretic that its use, especially during pregnancy, requires careful monitoring of intravascular volume and electrolyte levels.

Less information is available concerning the

effects of vasodilator agents in pregnant women. All of them may affect the volume and distribution of intravascular fluid, changes that may result in hypotension or a fall in cardiac output. Since pregnant women are particularly prone to sudden changes in venous return, the use of vasodilators should be carefully supervised; however, there is no objective evidence that they are intolerant of these drugs and their judicious use during pregnancy in carefully selected individuals appears appropriate.

An antiarrhythmic drug is occasionally required during pregnancy in a woman with heart disease. Experience is limited but any of them can be used during pregnancy according to standard routines.[8,10,17–19]

β-Blocking agents are being used with increasing frequency. All of them have an oxytocic action and the potential of jeopardizing the adaptation of the newborn child to its extrauterine environment[8,16,20–22]; however, they have been used frequently in pregnancy without adverse effects.[10,17,23] We recommend that these agents be used during pregnancy when no safer alternative is available. When they are used, regional anesthesia for labor and delivery must be carefully supervised and preparation should be made for tentative monitoring of the neonate for bradycardia, respiratory depression, hyperglycemia, and hyperbilirubinemia.

Drugs that affect the movement of calcium into and within endothelial and myocardial cells have been introduced into the therapeutic armamentarium so recently that little information is available concerning their effects on uterine blood flow, fetal health and development, or the well-being of the neonate. All may result in hypotension and all may cause bradycardia; verapamil has a particular propensity for the latter action. These calcium-channel blockers have been used in some pregnant women without demonstrable adverse effects on the fetus.[10] Until more is learned about the safety of these agents during pregnancy, their long-term use should be avoided as a matter of principle. However, verapamil may be the best choice for the acute therapy of a life-threatening supraventricular tachycardia.

Some women with valvular disease require long-term anticoagulation. Although successful pregnancies have been reported in women taking warfarin sodium derivatives,[24,25] the use of these agents is contraindicated during pregnancy.[16,26–28] As many as 25% of the offspring of women taking oral anticoagulants will develop an embryopathy that includes abnormalities of the CNS. The danger of this complication is greatest when oral anticoagulants are used during the first trimester of pregnancy. In addition, the risks of abortion and stillbirth resulting from peri-placental bleeding are increased.[16,26,27] When oral anticoagulants are used near term, there is a 5% to 10% risk of perinatal hemorrhage with the attendant danger of permanent injury to the fetus. Accordingly, heparin is the anticoagulant of choice during pregnancy. This drug does not cross the placenta; however, it does increase the risk of maternal bleeding and of abortion and stillbirth.[28]

Antiplatelet agents disturb the coagulation mechanisms of both mother and fetus. The most commonly used, aspirin, is associated with an increased incidence of abortions, stillbirth, and decreased infant birth weight.[29–31]

Cardiac surgery can be performed during pregnancy and is justified when indicated for maternal safety. Temporary and permanent pacemakers may be inserted, but radiation exposure must be minimized. In general, surgical procedures are best performed before conception or deferred until after delivery. The selection of an anesthetic agent requires careful consideration and depends to some degree upon the experience of the anesthesiologist. The anesthetic approach that minimizes changes in blood pressure and heart rate is preferable, especially in women with valvular disease.

GENERAL MANAGEMENT OF THE PREGNANT WOMAN WITH HEART DISEASE

Although specific valve abnormalities and complications require individual management, some generalizations are appropriate. First, the diagnosis of heart disease should be made only when its presence is certain. It is inappropriate to frighten a woman, to alter pregnancy, or to impose the risks of medical therapy unless the diagnosis of heart disease is established. Second, although concerns about fetal health are appropriate, maternal health should be given the higher priority. Third, both prospective parents should be counselled as accurately as possible concerning the potential risks of maternal heart disease to both the mother and fetus. Fourth, the health of a woman contemplating pregnancy should be optimal before gestation begins. This precaution is especially important in women with heart disease. For example, cigarette smoking should be discontinued, a good program of nutrition, activity and rest adopted, and optimal hemodynamic status achieved. In addition, some measures can be taken to minimize the risk of pregnancy. For example, women should be immunized against influenza and pneumococci prior to conception because superimposed infection may jeopardize the ability of some women with valvular disease to complete pregnancy safely. Once pregnancy has begun, vaccination with live organisms is inadvisable.[32] In addition, general measures to avoid infections are warranted. These precautions emphasize the general principle that women with heart disease can frequently undertake pregnancy safely if they are protected against additional cardiac burdens such as anemia, infection, overwork, and anxiety.

Finally, some generalizations concerning antibiotic prophylaxis are appropriate. Women with valvular disease are at increased risk of infective endocarditis. Although the efficacy of antibiotic prophylaxis to prevent this complication has not been demonstrated, we recommend its use during delivery and at other times when bacteremia occurs, using the antibiotic regimen outlined by the American Heart Association.[33] The American Heart Association does not recommend antibiotic prophylaxis during uncomplicated labor and delivery; however, since bacteremia has been documented as occurring at that time, the authors routinely begin antibiotic prophylaxis at the onset of labor, a recommendation made by other clinicians who follow large numbers of women with cardiac deformities.[34] There is less disagreement concerning the use of antibiotic prophylaxis against rheumatic fever. Although there is no agreement concerning the effect of pregnancy upon susceptibility to rheumatic recurrences, motherhood implies increased exposure to streptococci. Furthermore, pregnant women are unusually future-oriented, and compliant, and instruction concerning long-term prophylaxis is readily accepted. Certainly patients already receiving rheumatic fever prophyalxis should continue their programs during and following pregnancy.

HEMODYNAMIC CHANGES DURING PREGNANCY

Important changes in maternal cardiovascular physiology occur during normal pregnancy and explain why some women with valvular disease are at increased risk. Cardiac output increases by approximately 40% by mid-pregnancy.[35] This hemodynamic change is associated with a fall in peripheral vascular resistance of similar magnitude, so maternal systemic arterial blood pressures remain substantially unchanged. Initially, the rise in cardiac output occurs as a result of an increased stroke volume and this continues into the second trimester. As term approaches, maternal heart rate increases progressively and stroke volume tends to fall. In the latter half of pregnancy, maternal cardiac output is increasingly sensitive to changes in body position which alter venous return. Maternal cardiac output may fall below nonpregnant values during supine recumbency in the third trimester.[36]

The rate of oxygen consumption at rest increases steadily throughout pregnancy, reaching 20% above the nonpregnant average by term. Because maternal cardiac output increases earlier and proportionately more than oxygen consumption, resting arteriovenous oxygen difference narrows early in pregnancy, then widens as term approaches.

During labor, venous return is augmented as a result of blood expelled from the uterus with each contraction. This causes a transient increase in cardiac output.[37] Depending upon the method of delivery and the amount of blood loss, maternal cardiac output may increase by as much as 80% above term values following delivery. It then returns to baseline levels over the course of several weeks postpartum. Maternal cardiac output is probably maintained above nonpregnant levels during lactation, but measurements have not been made.

The fall in peripheral vascular resistance that occurs during pregnancy is due to vasodilation of specific vascular beds leading to redistribution of cardiac output (Figure 12-1).

These hemodynamic changes are accompanied by, and are partly attributed to, changes in sodium and water balance. Plasma volume begins to increase during the first trimester of pregnancy reaching values 50% above normal by the 20th week.[38] Total red cell volume increases later, and proportionally less than plasma volume. As a result, a dilutional anemia normally occurs, reaching its maximum at about the 30th week of pregnancy. Total extracellular fluid volume increases steadily with an overall accumulation of 6 to 8 L by term. Sodium retention during pregnancy amounts to between 500 and 900 mEq.[15]

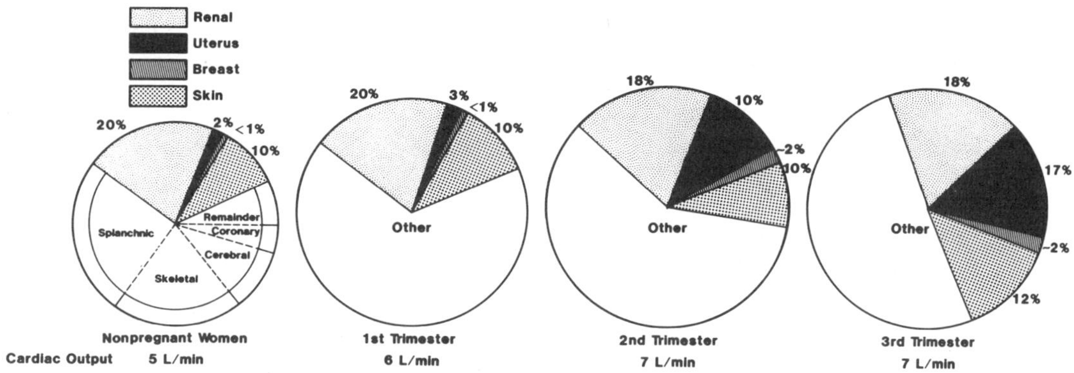

Figure 12-1 Cardiac output and its distribution at rest during pregnancy. The data used for this diagram are incomplete, especially early in pregnancy. Values for each organ system are given as a percentage of total cardiac output. Changes in blood flow to "Other" areas during pregnancy are not well defined. The graphs demonstrate that: (1) resting cardiac output increases by 40% during pregnancy; (2) uterine blood flow increases progressively during pregnancy, reaching a value at term approximately tenfold greater than that of the nonpregnant uterus; (3) although the increase in uterine blood flow is substantial, the increased flow to the remaining tissues during pregnancy taxes the heart more heavily; and (4) renal blood flow increases early during pregnancy and the increase is maintained until delivery. The value given for uterine blood flow at term is substantially greater than those previously reported[56] and is based upon radionuclide imaging[57] with subjects in left lateral recumbency.

The mechanism that causes the increased stroke volume of early pregnancy has not been adequately defined, but current evidence supports a fundamental change in myocardial dynamics. The susceptibility to sudden changes in venous return is attributed to venous relaxation combined with obstruction of the inferior vena cava by the enlarging uterus, especially in the supine position.

SPECIFIC VALVE LESIONS

Mitral Stenosis

Stenosis of the mitral valve is increasingly less common in the United States because of the progressive decline in the incidence of rheumatic fever.[39,40] However, it is still one of the common valve lesions encountered in young women, even in the United States, and remains a major cause of maternal morbidity from heart disease in much of the world.[40,41]

Mitral stenosis impedes blood flow from the left atrium to the left ventricle during diastole. When the degree of mitral stenosis reaches a critical level, cardiac output is reduced and pulmonary vascular pressures are increased. Because pregnancy is normally associated with increases in heart rate (with reduction in diastolic filling time) and cardiac output, the hemodynamic impediment imposed by mitral stenosis is particularly dangerous and the danger is increased by anything (especially physical activity) that causes further augmentation of heart rate or cardiac output.[42] Tachycardia is particularly dangerous because it limits the time available for diastolic forward flow.

The hemodynamic demands of pregnancy may result in symptoms of pulmonary vascular congestion in women with significant mitral stenosis. Dyspnea and orthopnea may occur, even at rest, particularly when cardiac output reaches its peak at the 20th week. Additionally, the elevated left atrial pressure increases the tendency for atrial arrhythmias, a complication that compounds the danger of reduced blood flow through the mitral valve.

An occasional patient with mitral stenosis develops dizziness and syncope without evidence of pulmonary vascular congestion.[43] This is taken as evidence of reduced cardiac output resulting from volume depletion. In order for the woman with mitral stenosis to maintain her cardiac output, an elevated left atrial pressure is required. During pregnancy, there is increased danger of blood entrapment in the venous system, particularly in the veins of the legs.[44,45] When venous return drops, cardiac output falls and syncope may result.

Management The dangers associated with pregnancy for a woman with mitral stenosis depend upon the severity of the valve lesion and the presence of complications including pulmonary valvular disease, right ventricular damage, and atrial fibrillation. Women who are completely asymptomatic prior to pregnancy usually tolerate childbearing uneventfully. Women in New York Heart Association functional classes II or III prior to pregnancy are at increased risk from the hemodynamic changes associated with gestation. The prognosis for women in functional class IV is so poor that pregnancy should be discouraged. Women who have symptoms of pulmonary congestion when not pregnant should not undertake pregnancy until careful evaluation and, when indicated, surgical correction is accomplished. If women with this degree of limitation become pregnant, early interruption should be considered with the prospect of reconsidering pregnancy following surgical correction of the valve abnormality.

Pregnancy should not be undertaken for at least 6 months following valve surgery. A careful re-evaluation of cardiac function is desirable before the decision to conceive is made. Unfortunately, surgical correction of mitral stenosis does not always enable women to undertaken pregnancy successfully.[46] The dangers of anticoagulation during pregnancy constitute a persuasive argument for placement of a tissue prosthesis when childbearing is planned.

For the pregnant woman with mitral stenosis, the goal of management is to maintain an adequate cardiac output without intolerable elevation of pulmonary capillary pressure. Restriction of activity is effective in achieving these objectives and is usually adequate. When symptoms persist, however, sodium restriction and the cautious use of diuretics are appropriate. Tachyarrhythmias are a particular danger and should be treated aggressively. Experience with verapamil during pregnancy is leading to increased use of that agent for controlling the ventricular rate when atrial fibrillation occurs, but digoxin remains the drug of choice for long-term control of ventricular rate. Electrical cardioversion is not contraindicated during pregnancy and, if necessary, an antiarrhythmic drug can be used to prevent recurrence.

When dangerous pulmonary congestion persists despite intensive medical therapy, corrective valve surgery can be considered.[47] Maintenance of augmented levels of systemic blood flow by the extracorporeal circulation should theoretically minimize the danger of pregnancy loss and fetal deformities. Whenever possible, surgery should be deferred until pregnancy is completed.

Because mitral stenosis is almost always caused by rheumatic fever, antibiotic prophylaxis against rheumatic recurrence is recommended. The indications for antibiotic prophylaxis against bacterial endocarditis are the same as in the nonpregnant individual and, as noted previously, antibiotics are advised at the time of labor and delivery.

Anxiety and pain should be minimized during delivery. Vaginal delivery, using epidural anesthesia without epinephrine, appears to be associated with minimal hemodynamic changes.

Decrements in venous return may result from hypovolemia secondary to vigorous diuresis and may compromise cardiac output. When excessive fatigue or syncope occurs, re-evaluation of the therapeutic regimen is essential.

Patients with mitral valve disease often develop pulmonary hypertension. Whatever its cause, the existence of this complication is a relative contraindication to pregnancy.[48–50] This injunction is particularly important in patients with mitral valve disease because correction of the valve lesion often results in a reduction of pulmonary hypertension, thus decreasing the risk of subsequent pregnancy.

Mitral Regurgitation

Mitral regurgitation is better tolerated during pregnancy than is mitral stenosis and there are good theoretical reasons to explain the different prognoses of the two lesions. The fall in peripheral vascular resistance that normally occurs during pregnancy should beneficially affect the distribution of left ventricular stroke volume in the presence of mitral regurgitation, improving forward flow into the aorta and lessening regurgitant flow into the left atrium.[47]

Management Patients with mitral regurgitation as their predominant valve lesion who are asymptomatic prior to pregnancy seldom develop symptoms during pregnancy. If fatigue or evidence of pulmonary congestion develop, the therapeutic approach is similar to that for patients with symptomatic mitral stenosis. Limitation of activity and of sodium intake are the first steps. If these do not control pulmonary congestion, digitalis and diuretics are employed. If symptoms persist despite these measures, vasodilator therapy may be beneficial; however, the effects of venous and arteriolar dilators on uterine blood flow and fetal oxygenation have not been accurately defined. In an extreme situation, if surgical correction of mitral regurgitation is required, it may be performed during pregnancy but risk of fetal loss or deformity is not negligible. From this, it follows that the rare woman with mitral regurgitation who is symptomatic prior to pregnancy should have surgical correction of her valve deformity prior to beginning gestation.

Aortic Valve Stenosis

Aortic valve stenosis occurs more frequently in men than in women and is unusual as an isolated lesion. In the United States, it is now almost always congenital. When congenital, it is often associated with other abnormalities of the cardiovascular system.

When aortic valve stenosis reduces cardiac output, easy fatigability is a common presenting symptom. When syncope, pulmonary congestion, or angina are noted, the risk of sudden death is appreciable and corrective surgery is indicated.

The demand for increased cardiac output which accompanies pregnancy may result in an increase in left-sided filling pressures and resultant pulmonary congestion. Some observers have suggested that this lesion is poorly tolerated during pregnancy: four deaths were reported among 23 women with aortic stenosis in association with a total of 38 pregnancies. In addition, four of those pregnancies ended in spontaneous abortion and five in therapeutic abortion.[51] In another large series, however, maternal mortality was not observed,[34] but congenital cardiac abnormalities were found in 20% of children born to mothers with lesions that obstructed left ventricular outflow. The incidence of congenital heart disease in the children was less when surgical relief of outflow obstruction was accomplished prior to pregnancy. Although this experience was not limited to patients with aortic valve stenosis, it is another reason to consider surgery prior to pregnancy in a woman with significant valve stenosis, even if asymptomatic.

Management When aortic stenosis is recognized prior to pregnancy, hemodynamic investigation is justified even in the absence of symptoms. If significant stenosis is documented, surgical intervention before pregnancy is recommended. When aortic stenosis is recognized early in pregnancy in an asymptomatic woman, close supervision is essential, but interruption of pregnancy is not justified in our opinion. Whenever the ominous symptoms of syncope, angina or pulmonary congestion occur, prompt investigation is appropriate. However, in patients who are already pregnant, we would defer cardiac catheterization and attempt to relieve symptoms by medical management. Restriction of activity is essential and if congestive heart failure develops, limitation of sodium intake and initiation of digitalis are important. Diuretics should be employed cautiously because sudden reductions in cardiac output due to inadequate filling may result. If symptoms persist despite these therapeutic interventions, cardiac catheterization is appropriate so that aortic valve surgery can be considered objectively.

Whenever valve surgery is required during pregnancy, peripheral perfusion should be maintained by the heart-lung machine at levels at least 40% greater than those employed for non-pregnant women. Although a mechanical prosthesis is ordinarily preferred for valve replacement in a young woman, the hazards of long-term anticoagulation are considered a relative indication for insertion of a heterograft prosthesis despite the possible need for recurrent surgery in the future.

Aortic Regurgitation

Aortic regurgitation is more likely to be encountered in young women than is isolated aortic stenosis. Nevertheless, it is an unusual valve deformity. In a large series of pregnant patients with valvular disease evaluated when rheumatic valvular deformities were more prevalent than they are now, aortic insufficiency was recognized in less than 10%.[47,52] The etiology of isolated aortic regurgitation is controversial.

As is the case with mitral regurgitation, the reduction of peripheral vascular resistance that occurs during pregnancy should have beneficial hemodynamic effects for patients with aortic regurgitation. This is not well documented by experience but patients with insufficiency of the aortic valve appear, in general, to tolerate pregnancy well.

Management If severe aortic regurgitation is recognized prior to surgery, consideration of valve surgery is appropriate, even in asymptomatic patients. The disadvantages of this approach are that it subjects women to the dangers of prosthetic valve insertions and chronic anticoagulation. If the abnormality is recognized during pregnancy in an asymptomatic patient, surgery is not indicated. If symptoms appear, medical management is attempted but vasodilator therapy assumes a higher priority with this lesion than in those previously discussed. When aortic regurgitation develops suddenly, particularly as a result of bacterial endocarditis or dissection of the aorta, and causes hemodynamic deterioration, emergency surgery is required, even when the patient is pregnant; mortality with medical management exceeds 50% in this situation.[53–55]

Tricuspid Valve Disease

Significant tricuspid valve disease is so uncommon that there is little information concerning tolerance during pregnancy. The most common cause of significant tricuspid regurgitation in the United States is the use and abuse of intravenous (IV) drugs. As with mitral regurgitation, it seems likely that pregnancy will be well tolerated and that if symptoms occur, medical therapy is indicated.

Tricuspid stenosis is even more rare than tricuspid regurgitation. The authors have no experience with this valve lesion during pregnancy and our recommendations as to management would be individualized according to the presentation.

Pulmonic Valve Disease

Pulmonic valve abnormalities are not unusual, but significant lesions that have not been surgically corrected are uncommon in women of childbearing age. If significant pulmonic stenosis is suspected prior to pregnancy, hemodynamic evaluation for consideration of corrective surgery is recommended; if the lesion is recognized during pregnancy and the woman is asymptomatic, evaluation should be deferred until she has delivered. Symptoms, particularly transient neurologic episodes compatible with a low cardiac output, but also chest pain or fatigue, call for strict limitation of activity. Persistence of symptoms despite these measures is a reasonable indication for cardiac catheterization and possible cardiac surgery, even during pregnancy.

Pulmonic stenosis is almost exclusively a congenital abnormality. It is associated with a 25% chance of spontaneous abortion and another 25% of newborn infants will have cardiac abnormalities.[34] Previous maternal surgery for pulmonic stenosis does not appear to affect the incidence of cardiac abnormalities in the offspring.

Primary pulmonic insufficiency is too rare to discuss in relation to pregnancy. As more women who have undergone surgery for congenital heart disease (particularly tetralogy of Fallot) reach childbearing age, pulmonic insufficiency will be encountered more frequently. Presently there is no clear evidence that it is poorly tolerated and, as with aortic insufficiency, it is expected that major therapeutic interventions during pregnancy will be unnecessary.

REFERENCES

1. Dekaban A: Abnormalities in children exposed to x-radiation during various stages of gestation: Tentative timetable of radiation injury to the human fetus, p 1. *J Nucl Med* 1968;9:471–477.
2. Capizzi RL: Hematologic neoplasms during pregnancy, in Brodsky I, Kahn SB, Moyer JH (eds): *Cancer Chemotherapy II. 22nd Hahnemann Symposium.* New York, Grune & Stratton, Inc, 1972, pp 131–146.
3. Bonebrake CR, Noller KL, Loehnen CP, et al: Routine chest roentgenography in pregnancy. *JAMA* 1978;240:2747–2748.
4. Mitchell MS, Capizzi RL: Neoplastic diseases, in Burrow GN, Ferris TF (eds): *Medical Complications during Pregnancy*, ed 2. Philadelphia, WB Saunders Co, 1982, pp 510–537.
5. Schwartz DB, Schamroth L: The effect of pregnancy on the frontal plane QRS axis. *J Electrocardiol* 1979;12:279–281.
6. Rubler S, Damani PM, Pinto ER: Cardiac size and performance during pregnancy estimated with echocardiography. *Am J Cardiol* 1977;40:534–540.
7. Katz R, Karline JS, Resnik R: Effects of a natural volume overload state (pregnancy) on left ventricular performance in normal human subjects. *Circulation* 1978;58:434–441.
8. Brinkman CR III, Woods JR Jr: Effects of cardiovascular drugs during pregnancy. *Cardiovasc Med* 1976;1:231–251.
9. Rogers MC, Willerson JT, Goldblatt A, et al: Serum digoxin concentrations in human fetus, neonate and infant. *N Engl J Med* 1972;287:1010–1013.
10. Rotmensch HH, Elkayam U, Frishman W: Antiarrhythmic drug therapy during pregnancy. *Ann Intern Med* 1983;98:487–497.
11. Weaver JB, Pearson JF: Influence of digitalis on time of onset and duration of labor in women with cardiac disease. *Br Med J* 1973;3:519–520.
12. Finnerty FA, Betko FJ: Lowering the perinatal mortality and the prematurity rate: The value of prophylactic thiazides in juveniles. *JAMA* 1966;195:429–432.
13. Gray MJ: Use and abuse of thiazides in pregnancy *Clin Obstet Gynecol* 1968;11:568–578.
14. Kraus GW, Marchese JR, Yen SSC: Prophylactic use of thiazides in pregnancy. *JAMA* 1966;198:1150–1154.
15. Lindheimer MD, Katz AI: Sodium and diuretics in pregnancy *N Engl J Med* 1973;288:891–894.
16. Ueland K, McAnulty JH, Ueland FR, et al: Special considerations in the use of cardiovascular drugs. *Clin Obstet Gynecol* 1981;24:809–823.
17. Tamari I, Eldar M, Rabinowitz B. et al: Medical treatment of cardiovascular disorders during pregnancy. *Am Heart J* 1982;104:1357–1363.
18. Hill LM, Malkasin GD Jr: The use of quinidine

sulfate throughout pregnancy. *Obstet Gynecol* 1979;54:366–368.
19. Mendelson CL: Discorders of heartbeat during pregnancy. *Am J Obstet Gynecol* 1956;72:1268–1301.
20. Cottrill CM, McAllister RG Jr, Gettes L, et al: Propranolol therapy during pregnancy, labor and delivery: Evidence of transplacental drug transfer and impaired neonatal drug disposition. *J Pediatr* 1977;91:812–814.
21. Datta S, Kitzmiller JL, Ostheimer GW, et al: Propranolol and parturition. *Obstet Gynecol* 1978; 51:577–581.
22. Gladstone GR, Hordof A, Gersony WM: Propranolol administration during pregnancy: Effects on the fetus. *J Pediatr* 1975;86:962–964.
23. Rubin PC: Beta-blockers in pregnancy. *N Engl J Med* 1981;305:1323–1326.
24. Casanegra P, Avilés G, Maturana G, Dubernet J: Cardiovascular management of pregnant women with a heart valve prosthesis. *Am J Cardiol* 1975;36:802–806.
25. Fillmore SJ, McDevitt E: Effects of coumarin compounds on the fetus. *Ann Intern Med* 1970;73: 731–735.
26. Stevenson RE, Burton M, Ferlauto GJ, et al: Hazards of oral anticoagulants during pregnancy. *JAMA* 1980;243:1549–1551.
27. Hall JG, Pauli RM, Wilson KM: Maternal and fetal sequelae of anticoagulation during pregnancy. *Am J Med* 1980;68:122–140.
28. Merrill LK, VerBrug DJ: The choice of long-term anticoagulants for the pregnant patient. *Obstet Gynecol* 1976;47:711–714.
29. Corby DG: Aspirin in pregnancy: Maternal and fetal effects. *Pediatrics* 1978;62:930–937.
30. Bleyer WA, Breckenridge RT: Studies on the detection of adverse drug reactions in the newborn: II. The effects of prenatal aspirin on newborn hemostasis. *JAMA* 1970;213:2049–2053.
31. Corby DG, Schulman I: The effects of antenatal drug administration on aggregation of platelets of newborn infants. *J Pediatr* 1971;79:307–313.
32. Rubella vaccime — recommendation of the Public Health Service Advisory Committee on Immunization Practices, Center for Disease Control, US Dept of Health, Education, and Welfare, Atlanta. *Ann Intern Med* 1978;88:543–545.
33. Shulman ST, Amren DP, Bisno AL, et al: Prevention of bacterial endocarditis. *Circulation* 1984;70:1123A–1127A.
34. Whittemore R, Hobbins JC, Engle MA: Pregnancy and its outcome in women with and without surgical treatment of congenital heart disease. *Am J Cardiol* 1982;50:641–651.
35. Metcalfe J, Ueland K: Maternal cardiovascular adjustments to pregnancy. *Prog Cardiovasc Dsi* 1974;16:363–374.
36. Lees MM, Taylor SH, Scott DB, et al: A study of cardiac output at rest throughout pregnancy. *J Obstet Gynaecol Br Commonw* 1967;74:319–328.
37. Ueland K, Hansen JM: Maternal cardiovascular dynamics. III. Labor and delivery under local and caudal analgesia. *Am J Obstet Gynecol* 1969;103: 8–18.
38. Chesley LC: Plasma and red cell volumes during pregnancy. *Am J Obstet Gynecol* 1972;112:440–450.
39. Bisno AL: Worldwide control of rheumatic fever. *Ann Intern Med* 1979;91:918–919.
40. Padmavati S: Rheumatic fever and rheumatic heart disease in developing countries. *Bull WHO* 1978;56:543–550.
41. Krause RM: The influence of infection on the geography of heart disease. *Circulation* 1979;60: 972–976.
42. Ueland K, Novy, MJ, Metcalfe J: Cardiorespiratory responses to pregnancy and exercise in normal women and patients with heart disease. *Am J Obstet Gynecol* 1973;115:4–10.
43. Szekely P, Turner R, Snaith L: Pregnancy and the changing pattern of rheumatic heart disease. *Br Heart J* 1973;35:1293–1303.
44. Kerr MG: The mechanical effects of the gravid uterus in late pregnancy. *J Obstet Gynaecol Br Commonw* 1965;72:513–529.
45. Kerr MG, Scott DB, Samuel E: Studies of the inferior vena cava in late pregnancy. *Br Med J* 1964;1:532–533.
46. Ibarra-Perez C, Arevalo-Toledo N, Alvarez-De la Cadena O, et al: The course of pregnancy in patients with artificial heart valves. *Am J Med* 1976;61:504–512.
47. Szekely P, Snaith L: *Heart Disease and Pregnancy*, Edinburgh, Churchill Livingstone Inc, 1974.
48. Dresdale DT, Schultz M, Michtom RJ: Primary pulmonary hypertension. I. Clinical and hemodynamic study. *Am J Med* 1951;11:686–705.
49. Nielsen NC, Fabricius J: Primary pulmonary hypertension with special reference to prognosis. *Acta Med Scand* 1961;170:731–741.
50. McCaffrey RN, Dunn LJ: Primary pulmonary hypertension in pregnancy. *Obstet Gynecol Surv* 1964;19:567–591.
51. Arias F, Pineda J: Aortic stenosis and pregnancy. *J Reprod Med* 1978;20:229–232.
52. Burwell CS, Metcalfe J: *Heart Disease and Pregnancy*. Boston, Little Brown & Co, 1958.
53. McAnulty JH, Rahimtoola SH: Surgery for infective endocarditis. *JAMA* 1979;242:77–79.
54. Wilson WR, Danielson GK, Giulani ER, et al: Valve replacement in patients with active infective endocarditis. *Circulation* 1978;58:585–588.
55. Richardson JV, Karp RB, Kirklin JW, et al: Treatment of infective endocarditis: A 10-year comparative analysis. *Circulation* 1978;58:589–597.
56. Metcalfe J, Romney SL, Ramsey LH, et al: Estimation of uterine blood flow in normal human pregnancy at term. *J Clin Invest* 1955;34:1632–1638.
57. Lunnell NO, Nylund LE, Lewander R, et al: Uteroplacental blood flow in pre-eclampsia measurements with indium 113m and a computer-linked gamma camera. *Clin Expl Hypertens* 1982; 1:105–117.

CHAPTER 13
Interaction of Coronary Artery Disease and Valvular Heart Disease

George A. Pantely

PHYSIOLOGY OF THE CORONARY CIRCULATION

The heart is unique compared to other organs: it is a highly metabolic, continuously contracting muscle that requires a constant supply of oxygen. In a steady state, various factors determine the oxygen consumption of the heart. A small, relatively constant amount of oxygen is required to maintain cell viability and for electrical activation and depolarization of cells. The major determinants of myocardial oxygen consumption are the heart rate, wall stress, myocardial fiber shortening, and inotropic state. The wall stress is determined by the volume and the pressure developed by the ventricle. Increases in these variables increase myocardial oxygen consumption. At rest, the oxygen consumption of the heart is 6 to 8 mL/min/p 100 g tissue. Coronary flow is 60 to 80 mL/min/p 100 g tissue, and oxgyen extraction is 12 to 15 mL of oxygen/p 100 mL blood. During activity, myocardial oxygen consumption increases three- to fourfold. Since little additional oxygen extraction is possible, coronary flow must increase to meet the oxygen requirements of the heart. A high premium is, therefore, placed on the normal function of the coronary vascular bed. Many factors regulate coronary flow to ensure a continuous and adequate supply of oxygen at rest and during exertion.

Regulation of the Coronary Circulation

Coronary flow is related directly to the pressure gradient between the proximal coronary artery and the right atrial or coronary sinus pressure and inversely related to coronary vascular resistance. Coronary flow is regulated predominantly by changes in resistance. Coronary vascular resistance is affected by several variables.

Physical factors. An important part of coronary vascular resistance is the compressive resistance of intramyocardial vessels due to ventricular systole.[1-3] Compressive resistance accounts for the flow pattern seen in the epicardial coronary arteries (Figure 13-1). Despite the higher driving pressure during systole, the compressive resistance is so great that most of coronary flow occurs during diastole when compressive force is lower. In the left coronary artery, 70% to 80% of flow occurs during diastole: the diastolic/systolic flow ratio is about 6/1.[4] In humans and swine, the right coronary supplies the posterior interventricular septum and the posterior left ventricular wall as well as the right ventricle. The coronary flow pattern in the dominant right coronary artery of swine is similar to the left coronary artery (Figure 13-1). The right coronary artery in the dog usually supplies only the right ventricle; due to the smaller developed tension in the right ventricle, a greater proportion of flow in this nondominant right coronary artery occurs during systole.

Extrinsic (neurohumeral) factors. Coronary resistance and, hence, flow are regulated by autonomic mechanisms. The coronary bed contains β-adrenergic receptors which cause vasodilation when stimulated and α-adrenergic receptors which cause vasoconstriction when stimulated.[5] Parasympathetic vasodilator receptors are also

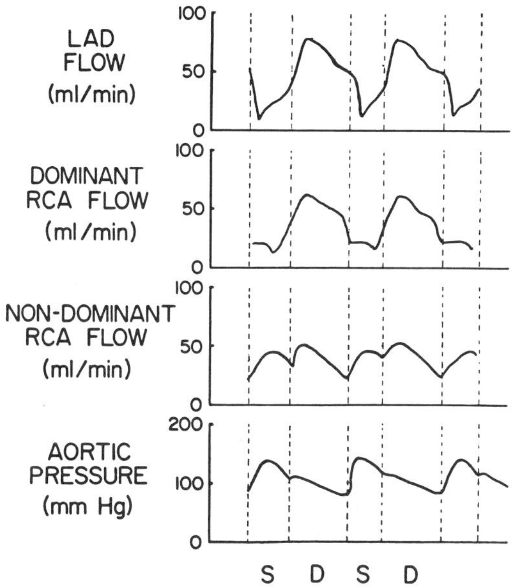

Figure 13-1 Phasic flow in the left anterior descending coronary artery (LAD), a dominant right coronary artery (RCA) in swine and a nondominant right coronary artery in dogs with aortic pressure. Left anterior descending flow is greatest during diastole and lowest during systole. Phasic flow in a dominant right coronary artery is similar to the left anterior descending flow. Since the nondominant right coronary artery supplies only the low pressure right ventricle, more flow occurs during systole. Date from Oregon Health Sciences University.

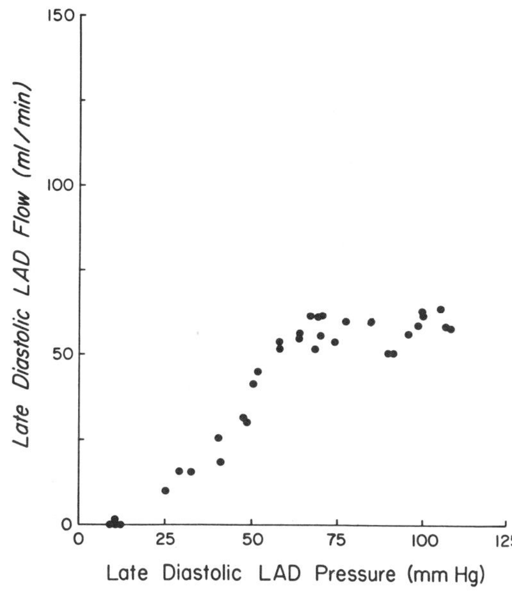

Figure 13-2 Coronary artery pressure–flow relationship showing autoregulation. LAD = left anterior descending coronary artery. Data from Oregon Health Sciences University.

present.[6] There does appear to be resting sympathetic vasoconstrictor tone in the coronary bed; coronary vasodilation results from a reduction in this resting sympathetic tone.[7,8]

While regulation of coronary resistance and flow by autonomic mechanisms has been demonstrated, its importance is controversial because of difficulty in sorting out the principal effects of neural control from secondary effects which simultaneously modify other determinants of coronary flow and myocardial oxygen consumption. Although neural control may not play a major role in regulation of the normal coronary circulation, it may play a role in disease states such as coronary artery spasm.[9]

Intrinsic (autoregulatory) factors. Coronary flow is clearly linked to myocardial oxygen consumption over a wide range of arterial pressures and cardiac outputs. This matching of flow to oxygen consumption is called autoregulation.[10–12] If myocardial oxygen consumption is constant and mean coronary pressure is increased, coronary flow will increase transiently and then return to its original level over the next 15 to 30 seconds. Coronary artery constriction keeps flow constant despite the increased driving pressure. At about a pressure of 150 mmHg, coronary flow will remain elevated because the increased driving pressure exceeds the ability of the coronary artery to keep flow constant by vasoconstriction. If mean coronary pressure is reduced while myocardial oxygen consumption is constant, coronary flow will decrease transiently and then gradually return to the control level. Flow is maintained despite the lower perfusion pressure by a reduction in coronary resistance (vasodilation). When mean coronary artery pressure is reduced below 50 mmHg, the coronary artery has exhaused its vasodilatory reserve (ie, it cannot reduce resistance further) and flow is then linearly related to pressure. Figure 13-2 illustrates this coronary artery pressure-flow relationship during autoregulation.

Autoregulatory control is linked to local metabolism that alters resistance in the small arterioles.[13] Tissue hypoxia, carbon dioxide, potassium, prostaglandins, lactic acid, and adenosine have all been suggested as the regulators. While the most systematic evidence has been advanced for adenosine,[13,14] the mechanisms controlling autoregulation are still not fully understood.

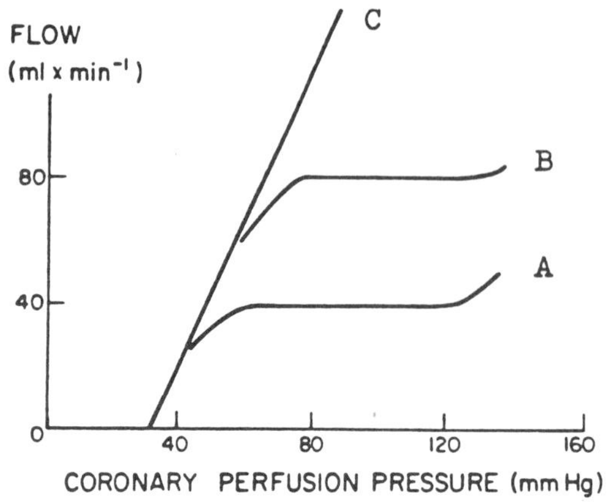

Figure 13-3 Pressure-flow relationship during maximum vasodilation (line C) and during autoregulation in basal state (line A) and with increased cardiac oxygen consumption (line B). See text. (Adapted with permission from Hoffman.[15])

In Figure 13-3, the straight line (line C) represents the pressure-flow relationship when all the coronary vessels are maximally dilated; this can be achieved by an infusion of adenosine. At a given pressure, the difference between autoregulatory flow (line A) and the maximum vasodilation flow is a measure of the coronary flow reserve; ie, how much flow can increase by additional reductions in coronary vascular resistance.

The coronary circulation will function along a given autoregulation plateau as long as myocardial oxygen consumption is constant. Increases or decreases in myocardial oxygen consumption will change the position of the plateau.[11,15] For example, when myocardial oxygen consumption increases, coronary flow increases and the coronary circulation functions on a higher autoregulatory plateau (Figure 13-3, line B). If the heart is functioning along autoregulatory plateau B, it has less coronary reserve than if it is functioning along plateau A.

Difficulties arise during attempts to construct such pressure-flow relationships in humans. A less direct way to evaluate coronary reactive hyperemic response is possible. Intense myocardial ischemia produces maximal coronary dilation. If a coronary artery is occluded for 10 to 30 seconds, release of the occlusion and restoration of normal perfusion pressure will be followed by a marked increase in coronary flow which dissipates over the next 30 to 60 seconds.[16–18] The difference between the resting flow and the peak flow that occurs after the induced reactive hyperemia is an estimate of the coronary vascular reserve.

The normal coronary reserve is three to four times resting flow, that is, flow can increase three- to fourfold above basal flow at a constant pressure. If flow does not increase that much, the vessel is utilizing more of its vasodilatory reserve during the basal state to maintain adequate flow. The amount that flow can increase to meet increased oxygen demands is limited. Determining vasodilatory reserve is a way to see the relative position of one point on the autoregulatory plateau compared to one point on the maximum vasodilation pressure-flow relationship at a given pressure as shown in Figure 13-3.

Distribution of Coronary Flow

Under resting conditions, flow to the endocardial portion of the left ventricular wall is about the same or slightly greater than flow to the epicardial portion of the wall.[19–21] While mean transmural flow is the same, the portion of flow to reach each level differs in systole and diastole.[22] As discussed earlier, increased pressure during systole inhibits blood flow. Systolic tissue pressure increases from epicardium to endocardium and flow during systole varies inversely with pressure; systolic flow in the endocardial portion is lower than systolic flow in the epicardial portion of the wall. The opposite is true during diastole — diastolic flow to the endocardium is higher than diastolic flow to the epicardium. A smaller vasodilatory reserve, therefore, is present in the endocardium. This may not cause problems under normal conditions; however, if coronary perfusing pressure decreases to the lower end of the autoregulatory range, vasodilatory reserve is exhausted first in the subendocardium. This makes the subendocardium at greatest risk for ischemia.[15]

Many studies have shown that reduced coronary perfusion pressure does cause endocardial ischemia. Attempts have been made to use noninvasive measurements to determine when endocardial ischemia is likely to be present.[15,23] In animal experiments, relative subendocardial perfusion (ratio of flow per gram in endocardium compared to the epicardium) can be predicted from the ratio of two pressure-time areas: The diastolic pressure time index (DPTI), the area between coronary and left ventricular pressure in diastole, and the systolic pressure time index (SPTI), the area beneath the left ventricular systolic pressure. Results from animal studies indicate that subendocardial ischemia is likely when this ratio is less than 0.4.[15]

CORONARY FLOW IN VALVULAR HEART DISEASE

The occurrence of chest pain in patients with valvular heart disease and normal coronary arteries on angiography indicates that coronary flow may be adversely affected by the valvular lesion or by the induced left ventricular hypertrophy. In addition, ECG abnormalities suggestive of ischemia are frequently noted in patients with valvular heart disease. These important clinical observations have led to studies of the consequences of valvular lesions on the determinants of myocardial oxygen consumption and on coronary flow.

Coronary Flow in Aortic Stenosis

Angina is more frequent with aortic stenosis than with any other valve lesion; it occurs in over 50% of patients.[24] The angina occurs with and without coronary artery disease. The effect of aortic stenosis on myocardial oxygen consumption and coronary flow has been studied extensively in animals and humans (Table 13-1). When the aorta is suddenly constricted in experimental animals, left ventricular pressure rises and wall stress is increased while the extent and velocity of shortening declines; this results in a reduction in cardiac output. The increase in wall stress, if prolonged, leads to concentric hypertrophy of the left ventricle and a return of peak wall stress and cardiac output toward normal. Similar events occur in human hearts with aortic outflow obstruction. However, since the obstruction usually develops gradually, cardiac function remains normal at rest, despite a severe pressure gradient across the valve.[25] The increased muscle mass, the elevated systolic pressure, and prolonged ejection of the left ventricle all elevate myocardial oxygen requirements at rest.

Studies in experimental animals utilize two models: supracoronary or subcoronary osteal stenosis. In animals with chronic supracoronary osteal stenosis, total resting coronary flow is increased, however, when flow is adjusted per unit weight of left ventricle, flow per unit weight is normal. Thus, pressure-induced hypertrophy increases total coronary flow, but it does not increase flow per unit weight of the left ventricle.[26–28] The transmural distribution of flow is normal. Reductions in resting coronary flow and evidence of a reduction in endocardial flow have been reported during severe pressure overload or if compensatory adaptions are inadequate.[29] The decrease was due to a reduction in the systolic component of flow with no change in the diastolic component. With severe hypertrophy, retrograde flow can occur during late systole.

Studies of animals with subcoronary osteal stenosis more closely approximates the hemodynamics of valvular aortic stenosis in man. Pyle et al[30] studied a small number of dogs with congenital subaortic stenosis. Each dog had marked left ventricular hypertrophy. Mean left circumflex flow was quite low compared to a group of normal dogs studied by the same techniques. The coronary flow pattern was altered with a marked reversal of flow during almost all of systole. The diastolic flow pattern was similar to normal dogs. The magnitude of reactive hyperemia in the dogs with the congenital stenosis was similar to that in normal dogs, but the same abnormal pattern of flow persisted. Similar results were noted during exercise. At autopsy, many of the intramural coronary arteries were thickened due to increased connective tissue and smooth muscle proliferation in the intima and media.

Attarian et al[27] studied 14 dogs with chronic left ventricular hypertrophy induced by surgically

Table 13-1
Myocardial Oxygen Consumption and Supply in Aortic Stenosis

Consumption	Supply
Increased by:	*Increased by:*
Increased systolic pressure	Increased oxygen extraction
Increased left ventricular mass	Reduced by:
Prolonged left ventricular ejection time	High intraventricular pressure which interferes with systolic coronary flow
	Diminished vasodilatory reserve, especially subendocardium

created subcoronary valvular stenosis. Epicardial flow was normal, but endocardial flow was low, resulting in a low endocardial/epicardial flow ratio. Subendocardial high energy phosphate content and respiratory control indices for NAD-linked substrate were significantly lower than in normal dogs. Griggs et al[31] previously showed similar results in dogs with acute pressure overload.

The key difference between these two animal models is that in subcoronary osteal stenosis, the coronary artery has a lower perfusion pressure than the left ventricle. The abnormalities in animals with supracoronary osteal stenosis are similar to those noted in animals with subcoronary osteal stenosis, but in subcoronary osteal stenosis, the magnitude of the abnormalities is greater. Subcoronary osteal stenosis is associated with a lower coronary flow per unit weight of myocardium. This appears to be due to a greater reduction or even absence of flow during systole, presumably because systolic compressive forces interfere with or interrupt flow. This deficit cannot be made up during diastole because of a limited coronary vascular reserve. Subosteal stenosis also causes a greater impairment in subendocardial flow and metabolism.[32]

Feldman et al[33] have looked at the effect of coronary artery constriction on coronary flow in dogs with aortic stenosis. They produced gradients of almost 50 mmHg acutely by inflation of a balloon in the outflow tract; since the outflow tract obstruction was produced acutely, left ventricular hypertrophy was not present. Aortic stenosis altered coronary hemodynamics and increased the hemodynamic importance of a coronary artery narrowing. The degree of aortic stenosis that was induced in this study altered coronary flow hemodynamics similar to a 60% coronary artery narrowing without aortic stenosis. Peak reactive hyperemia with 60% or greater coronary artery narrowing was consistently lower when aortic stenosis was present. Aortic stenosis plus a 60% coronary narrowing caused a reduction in coronary vascular reserve that was similar to that caused by an 80% coronary narrowing without valve stenosis. The endocardial/epicardial flow ratio did not change significantly until 90% coronary artery stenosis was present; then the ratio decreased only when aortic stenosis was present. The etiology of these changes in coronary flow is a complex interaction of increased left ventricular intramyocardial pressure, a lower aortic systolic pressure, marked left ventricular hypertrophy, and thickening of the intramural coronary arteries.

Human studies. Studies have been performed in patients with aortic stenosis and normal coronary arteries[34,35] and in children with supravalvular aortic stenosis.[36] Flow per gram of left ventricle was normal at rest. Coronary reserve, assessed by ischemia-induced reactive hyperemia, was greatly impaired in coronary vessels that supplied the hypertrophied left ventricle. Coronary reserve was also impaired in the nonhypertrophied right ventricle, but less so than in the left ventricle. The abnormalities in coronary reserve did not resolve immediately after the valve replacement. Other studies have also reported decreased vasodilatory reserve in patients with aortic stenosis.[37,38] The mechanism is uncertain, but it could be due to inadequate growth of coronary circulation during hypertrophy leading to an increase in minimal coronary vascular resistance. It may not be related directly to the high pressures because the abnormality did not resolve when the pressure overload was released, at least not early after the release of the pressure.

Coronary flow has been shown to increase during isometric exercise[39] and during supine bicycle exercise[40] in patients with aortic stenosis. While the exercise was not severe, the increase in flow was judged to be appropriate by the hemodynamic variables measured and by the DPTI/SPTI ratio.

Metabolic studies in patients with aortic stenosis have reported normal coronary sinus lactate at rest. Lactate production has been demonstrated during β-adrenergic receptor stimulation with isoproterenol in a group of patients with valvular aortic stenosis with no evidence of coronary artery disease.[41] Similar results have been reported during pacing in patients with aortic stenosis.[42] These results suggest that subendocardial ischemia may occur in patients with aortic stenosis and normal coronary arteries when myocardial oxygen consumption is increased.

Mechanism of angina in aortic stenosis (Table 13-1). In patients with aortic stenosis, the high intraventricular pressure compared to coronary artery pressure interfere with systolic flow. Since mean flow per unit weight of myocardium is normal at rest, an increase in diastolic flow occurs to compensate for the reduction in systolic flow. Thus, a portion of diastolic vasodilatory reserve is utilized to maintain flow normal at rest. Coronary flow increases during moderate exercise. With more severe exertion, coronary flow cannot increase sufficiently to meet the increased myocardial oxygen demand. Subendocardial ischemia results despite normal coronary arteries. This pathophysiologic sequence seems to be related to the extent of the hypertrophy and the difference between left ventricular pressure and coronary driving pressure. If coronary disease is present, the hemodynamic significance of a given stenotic lesion is magnified by the presence of aortic stenosis, and ischemia is even more likely to occur.

Coronary Flow in Aortic Regurgitation

Patients with severe aortic insufficiency may have angina in the absence of coronary disease.[43] This valvular lesion, as the clinical experience suggests, adversely affects coronary flow.

Effect of aortic regurgitation on myocardial metabolism and oxygen consumption (Table 13-2). Studies of changes in coronary flow have been performed during acute regurgitation in animals. Acute hemodynamic changes include increases in heart rate, stroke volume, and systolic arterial pressure, while diastolic and mean arterial pressure decrease. Retrograde diastolic flow in the femoral artery and the central aorta are noted with induction of the regurgitation. The degree of these changes depends on the severity of the lesion.[44,45]

With acute, severe aortic regurgitation, preload, wall stress, and myocardial oxygen consumption rise substantially. The increased volume leads to dilation of the ventricle and, in accord with Laplace's law, increased left ventricular wall stress. Ventricular hypertrophy results to normalize wall stress.[45–47]

Effect of aortic regurgitation on coronary flow (animal studies). Changes in coronary flow occur at the onset of valvular regurgitation. Mean coronary flow falls to very low levels initially, but as regurgitation continues for several minutes, mean flow returns to just below or near normal levels, and coronary sinus oxygen content decreases and myocardial oxygen consumption increases slightly.[45]

The pattern of coronary flow also changes significantly. Flow during diastole decreases and flow during systole increases. As the regurgitation continues, diastolic flow remains low, or may become negative transiently, and systolic flow remains high. This leads to a reversal of the normal diastolic/systolic coronary flow ratio.

When normal aortic valve function is restored, the pattern of flow returns to normal and mean coronary flow increases, gradually returning toward normal. This reactive hyperemia indicates that despite some increase in myocardial oxygen consumption, flow was not adequate to prevent some myocardial ischemia, particularly of the subendocardium.[48]

Feldmen et al[49] looked at coronary flow during acutely induced aortic regurgitation with different degrees of coronary artery narrrowing in dogs. During moderate regurgitation without any coronary narrowing, flow during peak reactive hyperemia was reduced to the same degree as when a 70% coronary artery narrowing without regurgitation was present. If a 60% coronary narrowing was present during aortic regurgitation, peak flow during reactive hyperemia was reduced to the same degree as when an 80% coronary narrowing without regurgitation was present. Thus, during acute aortic regurgitation, coronary flow reserve is diminished and a given coronary artery narrowing has hemodynamic properties similar to higher degrees of narrowing when no aortic regurgitation is present.

The hemodynamic findings in chronic regurgition are similar to acute regurgitation, but do not appear to be quite as severe for comparable degrees of valvular incompetence.[50] Myocardial oxygen consumption is increased due to an increase in total coronary flow as well as flow

Table 13-2
Myocardial Oxygen Consumption and Supply in Aortic Regurgitation

Consumption	Supply
Increased by:	*Increased by:*
Elevated preload	Increased oxygen extraction
Increased left ventricular volume	*Reduced by*
Increased left ventricular mass	Low diastolic perfusion pressure with reduction (or reversal) of diastolic flow
Increased fiber shortening	Diminished vasodilatory reserve, especially subendocardium

per weight of myocardium and an increase in the arterial–coronary sinus oxygen difference. The increase in coronary flow in chronic aortic regurgitation contrasts with the low to near control flow in acute regurgitation. A similar increase in the systolic and decrease in the diastolic component of flow was noted, but the changes were not as great as in acute regurgitation.[51]: under control conditions, the systolic component of flow was 23%; it increased to 75% in acute regurgitation, but was 45% to 50% in chronic regurgitation. Reversal of coronary diastolic flow was not noted in chronic regurgitation. Coronary reserve was diminished in chronic as it was in acute regurgitation.[51]

To summarize the information in experimental studies in animals, aortic regurgitation changes the predominant phase of coronary flow toward systole. The degree of the shift is related inversely to the diastolic pressure and to the acuteness of the insufficiency. Total coronary flow is unchanged or falls during acute regurgitation, but in chronic lesions, when ventricular chamber enlargement and an increase in wall thickness occurs, total coronary flow is increased; however, flow per unit weight of myocardium is normal. Coronary vasodilatory reserve is decreased in aortic regurgitation, more so during the acute phase. The hemodynamic significance of a coronary artery stenosis is accentuated by aortic insufficiency.

Human studies. Studies of coronary flow in humans have been performed in patients with chronic aortic regurgitation. Folts et al[52] studied coronary flow in the dominant right coronary artery before and after surgical repair of aortic regurgitation. Prior to correcting the regurgitation, the diastolic/systolic flow ratio was .88 and coronary flow was 116 mL/min. Shortly after valve replacement, right coronary flow increased to 180 mL/min and the diastolic/systolic flow ratio increased to 2.18 which is similar to the normal value. The increase in coronary flow was probably due to a higher diastolic perfusion pressure. Thus, the same reversal of the normal coronary flow pattern as seen in experimental animals is present in humans and correction of the aortic regurgitation restores the flow pattern toward normal.

Coronary reserve in patients with chronic aortic regurgitation is reduced compared to people without this valve lesion.[53,54] Pichard et al[53] reported that the patients that had angina with normal coronary arteries had the lowest coronary reserve. This suggests that these patients may have subendocardial ischemia because they may not be able to increase coronary flow to adequate levels during increased myocardial oxygen demand.

Two studies have looked at coronary flow in patients with aortic regurgitation during moderate exercise. Rowe et al[40] studied patients during supine bicycle exercise. They found that at rest, coronary flow was in the normal range per unit weight of myocardium while total flow was increased. Oxygen consumption, coronary flow, and left ventricular oxygen consumption increased during moderate supine bicycle exercise.[40] This increase in coronary flow was appropriate for the amount of exercise performed. Bertrand et al[39] studied patients with chronic aortic regurgitation and found that total coronary sinus flow was two to three times above normal, but was in the normal range when corrected per unit weight. During isometric exercise, coronary sinus flow increased significantly to 180% of the resting value. The DPTI/SPTI ratio (a measure of myocardial oxygen supply and demand) showed that there was no discrepancy between the increased myocardial oxygen demand and the increase in coronary flow. They did not find any significant differences in coronary flow at rest or during exercise between patients with and without angina.[39]

Mechanism of altered coronary flow and angina in aortic regurgitation. The coronary flow pattern is altered significantly in patients with acute and chronic aortic regurgitation with an increase in flow during systole and a reduction in, or reversal of, flow during diastole. The cause of the reversal of the normal systolic/diastolic flow pattern and even retrograde diastolic flow in aortic regurgitation is not completely understood. In studies of dogs with shock[55] and arteriovenous fistualas[56] with diastolic pressures as low as are seen in aortic regurgitation, the diastolic flow is low, but is above zero. While resistance in coronary arteries decreases during diastole, it may be that the resistance to backflow into the left ventricle is so low that flow down the coronary arteries is reduced or even becomes retrograde, ie, the course of least resistance is retrograde into the left ventricle. If retrograde flow into the left ventricle is rapid, by Bernoulli's principle, pressure in the supravalvular area will be lower than in the coronary arteries. This may result in the decrease or retrograde diastolic coronary artery flow. Systolic flow probably increases because of the higher systolic pressure in a vasodilated vascular bed.

The mechanisms of angina in patients with

aortic regurgitation, as in patients with aortic stenosis, appears to be due to subendocardial ischemia. Vasodilatory reserve is utilized to maintain mean flow per unit weight of myocardium within normal range at rest. Since maximum vasodilatory reserve is reduced, coronary flow cannot increase sufficiently to meet increased myocardial oxygen demand during strenuous exertion[39] and subendocardial ischemia results. The abnormalities in coronary flow appear to be related to the severity of the regurgitant lesion. If coronary artery disease is present, aortic regurgitation can magnify the hemodynamic significance of the obstruction. The abnormal coronary flow pattern returns to normal after correction of the regurgitant lesion.

Coronary Flow in Mitral Valve Disease

Myocardial oxygen consumption and coronary flow in mitral regurgitation. Few studies of coronary flow have been done in volume overload due to mitral regurgitation because of the difficulty in inducing this valve lesion experimentally and because it does not appear to have a major adverse effect on myocardial oxygen consumption and coronary flow. Acute mitral regurgitation produces only a minimal increase in myocardial oxygen consumption because the increased myocardial fiber shortening does not greatly increase oxygen consumption. The major determinants of myocardial oxygen consumption — wall stress, contractility, and heart rate — are little affected with this lesion. In addition, the duration of left ventricular systolic tension is reduced, also leading to a reduction in oxygen consumption.[45,57] Coronary flow per unit weight, coronary vascular resistance and the transmural distribution of flow in dogs with volume overload hypertrophy induced by chronic complete heart block were similar to values in normal dogs.[58] During vasodilation induced by adenosine, coronary flow increased to over five times the control value, indicating that coronary reserve was normal.

A preliminary report showed that coronary vasodilatory reserve was diminished mildly in humans with volume overload hypertrophy associated with mitral regurgitation.[59] These studies were performed during valve replacement surgery in eight patients with severe mitral regurgitation and normal coronary arteries. While available data are limited, it does appear that volume overload due to mitral regurgitation does not have an extremely detrimental effect on left ventricular myocardial oxygen consumption and coronary flow.

The effect of mitral valve disease on right ventricular coronary flow. Whereas mitral regurgitation does not appear to have an extraordinary effect on left ventricular performance and coronary flow, mitral stenosis appears to have even less. However, these two valvular lesions may have a greater effect on right ventricular coronary flow by increasing left atrial pressure, resulting in secondary pulmonary hypertension, and right ventricular pressure-induced hypertrophy.

The effects of pressure-induced right ventricular hypertrophy have been investigated in lamb and calves shortly after birth.[60,61] Hypertension was induced by supravalvular pulmonary obstruction. Coronary flow per unit weight and coronary vascular reserve were normal. Murray and Vatner[62,63] studied right ventricular hypertrophy induced in adult dogs. They found that right ventricular coronary flow per unit weight was increased and the transmural distribution of flow was not significantly altered. In contrast to the neonatal animals, right ventricular coronary reserve was markedly diminished. Thus, if right ventricular pressure overload is induced early in life, its coronary circulation can compensate appropriately, while if the pressure overload first occurs later, the coronary circulation cannot compensate adequately.

Studies in humans have been performed in patients with right ventricular hypertrophy secondary to congenital heart disease. It appears that with right ventricular hypertrophy due to volume overload[64] and pressure overload[65], the coronary reactive hyperemic response in the vessels perfusing the hypertrophied ventricle is markedly diminished. It is not clear how severe the pressure overload has to be in order to produce the abnormalities noted. One must be cautious in extrapolating these data from neonates and children with congenital heart disease to adults with mitral valve disease. Nevertheless, right ventricular hypertrophy secondary to left-sided valvular lesions could cause some reduction in right ventricular coronary vascular reserve and angina secondary to right ventricular ischemia.

MANAGEMENT OF ANGINA AND CORONARY ARTERY DISEASE IN PATIENTS WITH VALVULAR HEART DISEASE

Angina occurs in 50% to 70% of adults with aortic stenosis while documented coronary artery disease occurs in about 25% of patients. The frequency of anginal chest pain in adults with aortic regurgitation varies from 3% to 50% and, in contrast to patients with aortic stenosis, is usually associated with coronary artery disease.[66–69] This reflects the adverse effect of aortic valve disease on coronary flow and determinants of myocardial oxygen supply and demand.

Medical therapy for angina in patients with significant aortic stenosis is limited. Nitroglycerin appears to be beneficial if systemic hypotension is avoided. Basta et al[66] treated 36 patients with aortic valve disease and angina with nitroglycerin. About half had relief of the angina; the benefit occurred in patients with and without coronary artery disease. The nitroglycerin decreased left ventricular and aortic systolic pressures and reduced systolic work. These changes lead to a net reduction in myocardial oxygen consumption.[70] Nifedipine would be expected to have a similar effect, but this has not been established.

In patients with aortic regurgitation, reducing impedance to left ventricular ejection by arterial dilation leads to an increase in cardiac output and stroke work, and a reduction in regurgitant fraction, left ventricular diastolic volume, and wall stress; the net effect is a reduction in myocardial oxygen consumption and improvement in symptoms of angina.[71] The same benefits occur in patients with mitral regurgitation.[72] While the reduction in regurgitant fraction might be expected to restore the pattern of flow toward normal and thus increase coronary flow, this has not been confirmed.

Since the imbalance between myocardial oxygen supply and demand in aortic valve disease is due mostly to the mechanical abnormalities, symptoms of angina, with or without associated coronary artery disease, are relieved or improved by surgical correction of the valvular abnormality. Because of this, the need for saphenous vein bypass graft implantation in patients undergoing surgery for valvular heart disease is still debated.[73–75] Proponents of the combined procedure argue that patients with aortic valve replacement and no coronary artery disease have a better survival than patients with aortic valve replacement and coronary artery disease who did not have associated bypass surgery.[76] Also, the operative risk of associated bypass surgery plus valve replacement is the same as aortic valve replacement alone.[77–81] Since the operative risk is not increased by additional bypass surgery if the general condition of the patient is good and left ventricular function is not severely depressed, combined valve replalcement and myocardial revascularization is usually recommended in patients with valvular disease and significant coronary artery disease.

SUMMARY

While resting coronary flow is normal in most patients with valvular heart disease, abnormalities are noted in coronary vascular reserve in the absence of coronary artery disease. These patients are unable to increase flow during activity or stress to meet increased myocardial oxygen consumption. Angina pectoris secondary to subendocardial ischemia results. The extent of the abnormality does vary with the type and severity of the valvular lesion. In addition, the hemodynamic significance of coronary artery stenoses are enhanced by the associated valvular lesion.

Patients with aortic stenosis have the greatest reduction in coronary vascular reserve. The high intraventricular systolic pressure reduces or abolishes systolic coronary flow. Diastolic vasodilation is utilized to make up for the reduced systolic flow. While this may keep resting flow near normal, it diminishes coronary vascular reserve during increased myocardial oxygen consumption and may lead to subendocardial ischemia.

Patients with aortic insufficiency also have a reduction in coronary vascular reserve, but their abnormality is not as severe as it is in patients with aortic stenosis. While mean coronary flow is unchanged at rest, the flow pattern during the cardiac cycle is altered. The regurgitant lesion is associated with a dramatic reduction in diastolic coronary flow and an increase in systolic coronary flow, the opposite of what is found in aortic stenosis. Coronary vasodilatory reserve is utilized to maintain mean flow normal at rest; this limits the ability of the heart to meet myocardial oxygen demand during strenuous exertion and leads to subendocardial ischemia.

Mitral regurgitation has little effect on left ventricular coronary flow. Coronary vascular reserve is mildly reduced, but this limitation is rarely significant enough to cause subendocardial ischemia. Mitral stenosis does not appear to have any significant adverse effect on left ventricular coronary flow.

Mitral regurgitation or stenosis, if severe, may

lead to pressure-induced right ventricular hypertrophy. This may result in a reduction in coronary vascular reserve to the right ventricle, and right ventricular ischemia during increased oxygen demand.

The abnormalities in the coronary flow pattern noted in aortic stenosis and regurgitation resolve after correction of the lesion. However, it is not known whether valve replacement restores the coronary vascular reserve to normal.

In patients with coronary artery disease who will be undergoing surgery for valvular heart disease, associated bypass graft surgery at the time of valve replacement is usually recommended.

REFERENCES

1. Sabiston DC Jr, Gregg DE: Effect of cardiac contraction on coronary flow. *Circulation* 1975; 15:14–20.
2. Downey JM, Downey HF, Kirk ES: Effects of myocardial strains on coronary blood flow. *Circ Res* 1974;34:286–292.
3. Snyder R, Downey JM, Kirk ES: The active and passive components of extravascular coronary resistance. *Cardiovasc Res* 1975;9:161–166.
4. Khouri EM, Gregg DE, Rayford CR: Effect of exercise on cardiac output, left coronary flow and myocardial metabolism in the unanesthetized dog. *Circ Res* 1965;17:427–437.
5. Feigl EO: Sympathetic control of coronary circulation. *Circ Res* 1967;20:262–271.
6. Feigl EO; Parasympathetic control of coronary flow in dogs. *Circ Res* 1969;25:509–519.
7. Brachfeld N, Monroe RG, Gorlin R: Effect of pericoronary denervation on coronary hemodynamics. *Am J Physiol* 1960;199:174–178.
8. Vatner SF, Franklin D, Van Critters RL, et al: Effects of carotid sinus nerve stimulation on the coronary circulation of the conscious dog. *Circ Res* 1970;27:11–21.
9. Hillis LD, Braunwald E: Coronary artery spasm. *N Engl J Med* 1978;229:695–702.
10. Berne RM: Cardiodynamics and the coronary circulation in hypothermia. *Ann NY Acad Sci* 1959;80:365–383.
11. Mosher P, Ross J Jr, McFate PA, et al: Control of coronary blood flow by an autoregulatory mechanism. *Circ Res* 1964;14:250–259.
12. Rouleau J Boerboom LE, Surjadhana A, et al: The role of autoregulation and tissue diastolic pressures in the transmural distribution of left ventricular blood flow in anesthetized dogs. *Circ Res* 1979;45:804–815.
13. Berne RM, Rubio R: Coronary circulation, in Berne RM, Sperelakis N, Geiger SR (eds): *Handbook of Physiology, Section 2: The Cardiovascular System*. Baltimore, Williams & Wilkins Co, 1979, vol 1, pp 873–952.
14. Rubio VR, Wiedmeier T, Berne RM: Nucleoside phosphorylase: Localization and role in the myocardial distribution of purines. *Am J Physiol* 1972;222:550–555.
15. Hoffman JIE: Determinants and prediction of transmural myocardial perfusion. *Circulation* 1978;58:381–391.
16. Olsson RA, Gregg DE: Myocardial reactive hypermia in the unanesthetized dog. *Am J Physiol* 1965;208:224–230.
17. Bache RJ, Cobb FR, Greenfield JC Jr: Limitations of the coronary vascular response to ischemia in the awake dog. *Circ Res* 1974;35:527–535.
18. Marcus M, Wright C, Doty D, et al: Measurements of coronary velocity and reactive hyperemia in the coronary circulation of humans. *Circ Res* 1981;49:877–891.
19. Fedor M, McIntosh DM, Rembert JC, et al: Coronary and transmural myocardial blood flow responses in awake domestic pigs. *Am J Physiol* 1978;235:H435–H444.
20. Hoffman JIE, Buckberg GD: Transmural variations in myocardial perfusion, in Yu PN, Goodwin JF (eds): *Progress in Cardiology*. Philadelphia, Lea & Febiger, 1976, pp 37–88.
21. Cobb FR, Bache RJ, Greenfield JC Jr: Regional myocardial blood flow in awake dogs. *J Clin Invest* 1974;53:1618–1625.
22. Hess DS, Bache RJ: Transmural distribution of myocardial blood flow during systole in the awake dog. *Circ Res* 1976;38:5–15.
23. Marcus M: Transmural distribution of myocardial perfusion, in Marcus M (ed): *The Coronary Circulation in Health and Disease*. New York, McGraw-Hill Book Co, 1983, pp 113–128.
24. Wood P: Aortic stenosis. *Am J Cardiol* 1958; 1:553–571.
25. Sasayama S, Ross J Jr: Franklin D, et al: Adaptations of the left ventricle to chronic pressure overload. *Circ Res* 1976;38:172–178.
26. Einzig S, Leonard JJ, Tripp MR, et al: Changes in regional blood flow and variable development of hypertrophy after aortic banding in puppies. *Cardiovasc Res* 1981;15:711–723.
27. Attarian DE, Jones RN, Currie WD, et al: Characteristics of chronic left ventricular hypertrophy induced by subcoronary valvular aortic stenosis. 1. Myocardial blood flow and metabolism. *J Thorac Cardiovasc Surg* 1981; 81:382–388.
28. Marcus ML, Mueller TM, Eastham CL: Effects of short- and long-term left ventricular hypertrophy on coronary circulation. *Am J Physiol* 1981;241: H358–H362.
29. Malik AB, Tomio A, O'Kane H, et al: Cardiac function, coronary flow, and oxygen consumption in stable left ventricular hypertrophy. *Am J Physiol* 1973;225:186–191.
30. Pyle RL, Lowensohn HS, Khouri EM, et al: Left circumflex coronary artery hemodynamics in conscious dogs with congenital subaortic stenosis. *Circ Res* 1973;33:34–38.
31. Griggs DM, Chen CC, Tchokoev VV: Subendocardial anaerobic metabolism in experimental aortic stenosis. *Am J Physiol* 1973;224:607–612.
32. Vinten-Johansen J, Weiss HR: Oxygen consumption in subepicardial and subendocardial regions of the canine left ventricle. *Circ Res* 1980; 46:139–145.

33. Feldman RL, Nichols WW, Edgerton JR, et al: Influence of aortic stenosis on the hemodynamic importance of coronary artery narrowing in dogs without left ventricular hypertrophy. *Am J Cardiol* 1983;51:865–871.
34. Marcus ML, Doty DB, Hiratzka LF, et al: Decreased coronary reserve. A mechanism for angina pectoris in patients with aortic stenosis and normal coronary arteries. *N Engl J Med* 1982;307: 1362–1366.
35. Pichard AD, Gorlin R, Smith H, et al: Coronary flow studies in patients with left ventricular hypertrophy of the hypertensive type. *Am J Cardiol* 1981;47:547–553.
36. Doty DB, Eastham CL, Hiratzka LF, et al: Determination of coronary reserve in patients with supravalvular aortic stenosis. *Circulation* 1982; 66 (pt 2):1-186–1-192.
37. Strauer BE: *Hypertensive Heart Disease*, New York, Springer-Verlag, 1980.
38. Tauchert M, Hilgar HH: Application of the coronary reserve concept to the study of myocardial perfusion, in Shaper W (ed): *The Pathophysiology of Myocardial Perfusion*. Amsterdam, Elsevier North Holland Inc, 1979, pp 141–167.
39. Bertrand ME, Lablanche JM, Tilmant PY, et al: Coronary sinus blood flow at rest and during isometric exercise in patients with aortic valve disease. *Am J Cardiol* 1981;47:199–205.
40. Rowe GG, Afonso S, Lugo JE, et al: Coronary blood flow and myocardial oxidative metabolism at rest and during exercise in subjects with severe aortic valve disease. *Circulation* 1965;32:251–257.
41. Fallen EL, Elliott WC, Gorlin R: Mechanisms of angina in aortic stenosis. *Circulation* 1967;36: 480–488.
42. Trenouth RS, Phelps NC, Neill WA: Determinants of left ventricular hypertrophy and oxygen supply in chronic aortic valve disease. *Circulation* 1976;53:644–650.
43. Segal J, Harvey WP, Hufnagel C: A clinical study of one hundred cases of severe aortic insufficiency. *Am J Med* 1956;21:200–210.
44. Folts JD, Rowe GG: Coronary and hemodynamic effects of temporary acute aortic insufficiency in intact anesthetized dogs. *Circ Res* 1974;35: 238–246.
45. Urschel CW, Covell JW, Graham TP, et al: Effects of acute valvular regurgitation on oxygen consumption of canine heart. *Circ Res* 1968; 23:33–43.
46. Kennedy JW, Twiss RD, Blackman JR, et al: Quantitative angiocardiography. III. Relationship of left ventricular pressure, volume and mass in aortic valve disease. *Circulation* 1968;38: 838–845.
47. Grossman W, Jones D, McLaurin LD: Wall stress and patterns of hypertrophy in the human left ventricle. *J Clin Invest* 1975;56:56–64.
48. Vinten-Johansen J, Weiss HR: Regional oxygen consumption in canine left ventricular myocardium in experimental acute valvular insufficiency. *Cardiovasc Res* 1981;15:305–312.
49. Feldman RL, Nichols WW, Pepine CJ, et al: Influence of aortic insufficiency on the hemodynamic significance of a coronary artery narrowing. *Circulation* 1979;60:259–268.
50. West JW, Wendel H, Foltz EL: Effects of aortic insufficiency on circulatory dynamics of the dog. *Circ Res* 1959;7:685–692.
51. Karp RB, Roe BB: Effect of aortic insufficiency on phasic flow patterns in the coronary artery. *Ann Surg* 1966;164:959–966.
52. Folts JD, Rowe GG, Kahn DR, et al: Phasic changes in human right coronary blood flow before and after repair of aortic insufficiency. *Am Heart J* 1979;97:211–215.
53. Pichard AD, Smith H, Holt J, et al: Coronary vascular reserve in left ventricular hypertrophy secondary to chronic aortic regurgitation. *Am J Cardiol* 1983;51:315–320.
54. Heiss HW, Wink K, Barmeyer, J, et al: Myocardial oxygen consumption and substrate uptake in man during physiological and pathologic volume load. *Basic Res Cardiol* 1977;72:293–298.
55. Gregg DE, Fischer LC: Blood supply to the heart, in Dow P, Hamilton WF (eds): *The Handbook of Physiology*. Washington, DC, American Physiology Society, 1963, vol 2, pp 1517–1584.
56. Rowe GG, Castillo CA, Afonso S, et al: Systemic and coronary hemodynamic effect of arteriovenous fistulas. *Am Heart J* 1962;64:44–49.
57. Braunwald E: Control of myocardial oxygen consumption: Physiologic and clinical considerations. *Am J Cardiol* 1971;27:416–432.
58. Gascho JA, Mueller TM, Eastham C, et al: Effect of volume-overload hypertrophy on the coronary circulation in awake dogs. *Cardiovasc Res* 1982; 16:288–292.
59. Eastham CL, Doty DB, Hiratzka LF, et al: Volume-overload left ventricular hypertrophy impairs coronary reserve in humans, abstracted. *Circulation* 1981;64(suppl 4):26.
60. Archie JP, Fixler DE, Ulloyt DJ, et al: Regional myocardial blood flow in lambs with concentric right ventricular hypertrophy. *Circ Res* 1974;34: 143–154.
61. Manohar M, Thurmon JC, Tranquilli WJ, et al: Regional myocardial blood flow and coronary vascular reserve in unanesthetized young calves with severe concentric right ventricular hypertrophy. *Circ Res* 1981;48:785–796.
62. Murray PA, Vatner SF: Reduction of maximal coronary vasodilator capacity in conscious dogs with right ventricular hypertrophy. *Circ Res* 1981; 48:25–33.
63. Murray PA, Vatner SF: Abnormal coronary vascular response to exercise in dogs with severe right ventricular hypertrophy. *J Clin Invest* 1981; 67:1314–1323.
64. Doty D, Wright AC, Eastham C, et al: Coronary reserve in atrial septal defect, abstracted. *Circulation* 1980;62:III–115.
65. Marcus ML, Doty D, Hiratzka L, et al: Impaired coronary reserve in children with cyanotic congenital heart disease, abstracted. *Circulation* 1981;64:127.
66. Basta LL, Raines D, Najjar S, et al: Clinical, haemodynamic, and coronary angiographic correlates of angina pectoris in patients with severe aortic valve disease. *Br Heart J* 1975;37: 150–157.
67. Bonchek LI, Anderson RP, Rosch J: Should coronary arteriography be performed routinely before valve replacement? *Am J Cardiol* 1973;31:

462–466.

68. Vieweg WJR, Tretheway DG, Alpert JS, et al: Distribution of coronary artery disease in patients with isolated aortic valve disease. *Cardiovasc Surg* 1976;17:9–12.
69. Paquay PA, Anderson G, Viefenthal H, et al: Chest pain as a predictor of coronary artery disease in patients with obstructive valve disease. *Am J Cardiol* 1976;38:863–869.
70. Perloff JG, Ronan JA, deLeon AC: The effect of nitroglycerin on left ventricular wall tension in fixed orifice aortic stenosis. *Circulation* 1965;32: 204–213.
71. Greenberg BH, DeMots H, Murphy E, et al: Beneficial effects of hydralazine on rest and exercise hemodynamics in patients with chronic severe aortic insufficiency. *Circulation* 1980;62: 49–54.
72. Greenberg BH, DeMots H, Murphy E, et al: Arterial dilators in mitral regurgitation: effects on rest and exercise hemodynamics and long term clinical follow-up. *Circulation* 1982;65:181–187.
73. St. John Sutton MG, St. John Sutton M, Oldershaw P, et al: Valve replacement without preoperative cardiac catheterization. *N Engl J Med* 1981;305:1233–1238.
74. Bonow RO, Kent KM, Rosing DR, et al: Aortic valve replacement without myocardial revascularization in patients with combined aortic valvular and coronary artery disease. *Circulation* 1981;63: 243–251.
75. Kirklin JW, Kouchoukos NT: Aortic valve replacement without myocardial revascularization, editorial. *Circulation* 1981;63:252–253.
76. Copeland JG, Griepp RB, Stinson ED, et al: Long-term followup after isolated aortic valve replacement. *J Thorac Cardiovasc Surg* 1977;74: 875–885.
77. MacManus Q, Grunkemeier G, Lambert L, et al: Aortic valve replacement and aorto-coronary bypass surgery. Results with perfusion of proximal and distal coronary arteries. *J Thorac Cardiovasc Surg* 1978;75:865–869.
78. Richardson JV, Kouchoukos NT, Wright JO, et al: Combined aortic valve replacement and myocardial revascularization. Results in 220 patients. *Circulation* 1979;59:75–81.
79. Loop FD, Phillips DF, Roy M, et al: Aortic valve replacement combined with myocardial revascularization. *Circulation* 1977;55:169–173.
80. Lacey JP, Goodin RR, McMartin D, et al: Coronary atherosclerosis in valvular heart disease. *Ann Thorac Surg* 1977;23:429–435.
81. Lytle BW, Cosgrove DM, Loop FD, et al: Replacement of aortic valve combined with myocardial revascularization: determinants of early and late risk for 500 patients, 1967–1981. *Circulation* 1983;68:1149–1162.

CHAPTER 14
The Role of Exercise Measurements in the Evaluation of Valvular Heart Disease

Ali Nusrat
Barry M. Massie

Exercise testing and exercise hemodynamic measurements have played an important role in the understanding of the pathophysiology of valvular heart disease and continue to be useful in patient management. As a result of our increasing experience with the selection of patients for valve surgery and the diminishing risks of valve replacement, as well as the availability of noninvasive techniques for evaluating valvular anatomy and left ventricular size and function, exercise hemodynamics are now less commonly performed. However, these measurements continue to have a role, particularly in the evaluation of difficult patients, and noninvasive measurements of cardiac function during exercise as well as assessments of exercise capacity are being employed more frequently.

The objectives of exercise hemodynamic measurements in valvular heart disease are as follows:

1. To determine the significance of the valve lesion
2. To evaluate discrepancies between symptons and rest hemodynamics
3. To assess prognosis
4. To evaluate medical and surgical therapy

In the end, indications for exercise measurements reflect the continuing difficulty in determining the need and the most appropriate time for valve surgery in some patients. For instance, there is little need for such testing in patients with symptomatic aortic stenosis or clear-cut symptom-limiting mitral stenosis. However, in a sedentary patient with mitral stenosis complaining mostly of fatigue, who has normal pressures and a small transmitral gradient but low cardiac output, the finding of a dramatic increase in the gradient with even limited exercise might confirm the need for surgery. Similarly, as a result of vigorous diuresis or a very compliant left atrium, patients with regurgitant lesions and dyspnea may have normal resting pulmonary artery, left atrial and left ventricular pressures in the catheterization laboratory. During exercise, however, such patients may exhibit dramatic deterioration, thus confirming the need for surgical intervention. In fact, discrepancies between symptomatology and measured resting hemodynamics are perhaps the best indication for exercise measurements.

Exercise evaluations by both invasive and noninvasive techniques have also been used as a measure of compensation in patients with borderline indications or without any current need for surgery. In that setting, which usually involves patients with regurgitant lesions, the objective is to obtain prognostic information. Further applications of exercise measurements have been to evaluate the outcome of medical therapy, such as vasodilation in mitral or aortic insufficiency, or the function of prosthetic valves.

In this chapter, we will review some relevant aspects of exercise physiology and then consider the types of exercise measurements available and their role in different valvular lesions. We will only address the adult patient, since the role of exercise evaluation may be different in children with congenital valve disease, and consequently we will deal only with mitral and aortic valve disease.

PHYSIOLOGIC RESPONSE TO EXERCISE

In normal individuals, and to a lesser extent in patients with valvular heart disease, the hemodynamic response to exercise is a product of both the cardiac response and changes in the periphery.[1–3] The physiologic goal of these adaptations is to increase oxygen delivery to the exercising muscles without accompanying deleterious effects. Cardiovascular responses differ markedly for isotonic and isometric exercise, and since the former is most prevalent in daily activities and in testing procedures, our comments will be confined to isotonic exercise.

In normal subjects, the heart functions essentially as an externally regulated pump, increasing its output two- to fivefold during exercise. The major increment in cardiac output reflects a two- to nearly fourfold rise in heart rate. In order to maintain this increase in output, venous return must increase proportionately and this is accomplished by both a "milking" action of contracting muscle and an adrenergically mediated increase in venous return. The extent to which an increase in left ventricular preload (eg, end-diastolic volume) occurs is variable, and probably reflects the type of exercise, the degree of cardiac reserve, and the conditioning status of the individual. Patients with poor left ventricular function may dilate their left ventricle with stress and highly trained athletes may also sustain an increase in end-diastolic volume to take advantage of the Frank-Starling effect, but most individuals will not undergo significant changes in chamber size. Cardiac contractility is enhanced by sympathetic nervous system stimulation and hormonally mediated responses as well as by a facilitating effect of tachycardia. Thus, whether end-diastolic volume remains constant or rises, an increase in ejection fraction will provide a larger stroke volume. Finally, it should be noted that all of these responses which lead to a rise in cardiac output are facilitated by a reduction in impedance to aortic ejection which results from profound peripheral vasodilation.

This latter response and the increase in venous return are two of the changes in working muscle which are vital to the physiologic adaptation to exercise and which link the heart to the periphery. There is also an increase in oxygen extraction, due to increased blood-tissue oxygen gradients and shifts in the oxygen-hemoglobin dissociation curve. Finally, local factors, the sympathetic nervous system, and circulating neurohumoral mediators all selectively alter vascular tone to optimize the distribution of blood flow to working muscle.

Patients with valvular heart disease exhibit both important similarities and striking differences in their response to exercise when compared to normal subjects.[4] The first factor to consider is cardiac performance, and the most obvious differences occur when mechanical obstruction is present. Irrespective of all other factors, severe aortic stenosis will limit the increase in flow across the valve, limiting cardiac output and increasing the transvalvular gradient. Left ventricular volume, and hence left atrial pressure, may rise considerably, increasing left ventricular wall tension and oxygen requirements. Since coronary artery flow may not rise appropriately, and may even fall if peripheral vasodilation leads to a drop in aortic diastolic pressure, myocardial ischemia may result. In mitral stenosis, diastolic flow is limited leading to a rise in left atrial pressure which may be severely exacerbated by a rise in heart rate that impinges on the diastolic filling period. Patients with valvular insufficiency perform relatively better during exercise, exhibiting greater capacity with relatively less hemodynamic deterioration, since the ratio of forward to total left ventricular output may be favorably affected by the lower peripheral vascular resistance. This is particularly the case in aortic insufficiency, when the diastolic "regurgitant period" is shortened. Nonetheless, some degree of regurgitation usually persists and limits the maximal rise in cardiac output. The third cardiac factor in patients with valvular disease is the status of the myocardium. Particularly in long-standing volume overload, myocardial contractility or contractile reserve may be depressed. Hence, the normal rise in ejection fraction or stroke volume may not occur and the left ventricle may dilate in response to the added venous return, producing left atrial hypertension.

Thus, measurements of maximal forward cardiac output and left atrial pressure (usually reflected by pulmonary capillary wedge pressure) differentiate normals from most patients with clinically significant valvular disease and also reveal a spectrum of severity of abnormal responses. Noninvasive measurements, such as the ejection fraction response to exercise, may not provide an indication of rising intracardiac pressures or accurately reflect changes in forward cardiac output.

A final but very important consideration is the

Table 14-1
Positional Differences in Hemodynamic Measurements in Normal Subjects and Patients with Heart Disease

	Normal		CHF		CAD	
	R	Ex	R	Ex	R	Ex
Heart rate	↑	↑	→	↑	→	↑
Mean arterial pressure	→	→	→	↓	↑	↑
Left ventricular filling pressure	↓	↓	→	↓	→	↓
Cardiac index	↓	→	→	→	↓	↑
Stroke index	↓	↓	↓	→	↓	→
Double product	↑	↑	↑	→	↑	↑
Workload		→		↑		↑

Abbreviations: ↑ = significantly higher upright *v* supine; ↓ = significantly lower upright *v* supine; → = no significant difference upright *v* supine; CHF = congestive heart failure; CAD = coronary artery disease; R = rest; Ex = exercise.

type of exercise performed.[5] Most commonly, isotonic exercise is employed. Bicycle ergometry is preferable to a treadmill because the lesser degree of body motion facilitates measurements. However, important differences between upright and supine exercise have been noted, both in normals and patients with cardiac disease (Table 14-1).[6–8] In general, heart rate increases are greater in the upright position, and blood pressure rises more with the patient supine. Maximal cardiac output may not differ substantially in the two positions, but it reflects a lesser change in stroke volume in the sitting position. Pulmonary artery and pulmonary capillary wedge pressure tend to rise more and left ventricular volume is more likely to increase during supine exercise. These differences may account for some of the varying results reported in both catheterization and radionuclide studies. Unless otherwise indicated, the findings discussed in this article relate to supine bicycle exercise.

INVASIVE EXERCISE HEMODYNAMIC MEASUREMENTS

Mitral Stenosis

Perhaps because surgical therapy for mitral stenosis became available before other valve lesions, much of the early interest in exercise hemodynamics was in this area. In 1951, Gorlin et al reported their hemodynamic findings during exercise in mitral stenosis, noting some increase in cardiac output and marked rises in pulmonary capillary wedge, pulmonary artery, and right ventricular pressures in eight patients.[9] These findings have been duplicated by others.[10,11] The rise in cardiac output in relation to the magnitude of exercise (the "exercise factor") is commonly depressed below the normal valve of 600 mL/min for each 100 mL/min increase in oxygen consumption.

The marked increase in transmitral gradient made exercise measurements particularly useful in quantifying the severity of stenosis in patients with small gradients and borderline-calculated valve areas. Accurate measurements of pressure gradients and variability in cardiac output determinations may make such calculations inacurate, particularly in low output states. The marked dependence of the transmitral gradient, reflected by the pulmonary capillary wedge pressure, on diastolic flow is illustrated in Figure 14-1. In patients with borderline-calculated valve area in the range of 0.8 to 1.6 cm^2, wedge pressure rises dramatically with flow and even modest exercise will produce diastolic flow increases by increasing heart rate and cardiac output. Of note is that calculated valve areas may be somewhat larger during exercise than at rest, perhaps as a result of a lessening of the obstruction due to the greater flow and higher left atrial pressure.

Mitral stenosis remains one of the clinical settings in which there is sometimes considerable discrepancy between the patient's symptoms and both the physical findings and resting hemodynamic measurements. There are a number of potential reasons for these discrepancies, and exercise hemodynamic evaluation may be useful in delineating them. In patients with low cardiac output, left atrial pressure may be nearly normal at rest despite severe stenosis. As mentioned previously, even minimal exercise will dramatically demonstrate the gradient in these individuals. Conversely, some active patients with moderate or even relatively mild mitral stenosis will become symptomatic with strenuous exertion despite normal resting hemodynamics. In these patients, exercise measurements will often demonstrate that at rapid heart rates or high cardiac outputs, left atrial pressures rise to potentially symptomatic levels. A most intriguing group of patients are those who have a hyperactive pulmonary vasculature.[11] They raise their pulmonary artery pressure and calculated pulmonary arteriolar resistance disproportionately and may become severely symptomatic. Exercise hemodynamic measurements are the only way to detect these individuals, whose abnormality is surgically reversible.

In a large study designed to relate the clinical

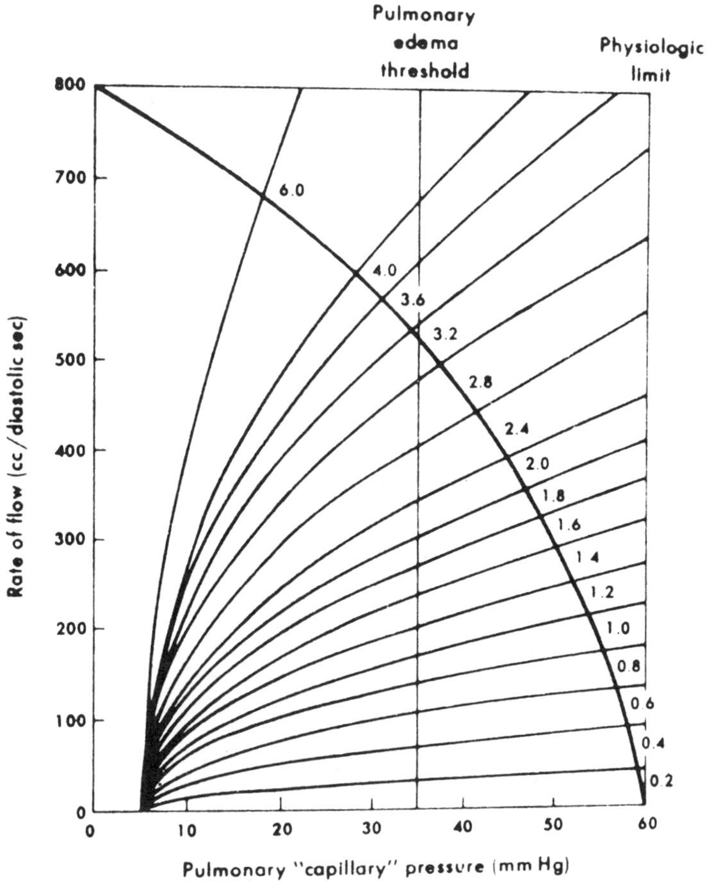

Figure 14-1 This "three-dimensional" plot demonstrates the interrelationship between transmitral flow, mitral orifice size, and pulmonary capillary wedge pressure. At low flow rates, even patients with severe stenoses may have relatively normal left atrial pressures. (Reproduced with permission from Grossman W: *Cardiac Catheterization and Angiography*, ed 2. Philadelphia, Lea & Febiger, p 127).

assessment of cardiac disability to hemodynamic measurements, it is particularly noteworthy that the closest relationship was present in mitral stenoses.[12] Exercise pulmonary capillary wedge pressure, in particular, was useful in distinguishing New York Heart Association functional class I, II, and III patients. Thus, these measurements can be very helpful in evaluating the significance of lesions in mitral stenosis patients who are otherwise difficult to assess.

Aortic Stenosis

Hemodynamic measurements during exercise are not commonly employed in the evaluation of aortic stenosis. In part, this reflects the risks of syncope and ventricular arrythmias incurred by exercising these patients. Perhaps more importantly, the appropriate management of aortic stenosis can generally be determined by the history, clinical findings, and resting hemodynamics. Unlike the situation with mitral stenosis, transvalvular gradients in aortic stenosis are large enough to be measured reliably. Nonetheless, it is of interest to review the published findings.

A number of articles have evaluated the hemodynamic response to supine bicycle exercise in isolated aortic stenosis.[13–16] The cardiac output rises in most subjects, but less than normally for the increase in oxygen consumption. As a result of the increase in systolic flow the transaortic valvular gradient often rises, potentially to high levels. Many cases in which left ventricular systolic pressure during exercise exceeds

250 mmHg have been reported. However, increases in aortic valve gradient are not a uniform finding, since the relative duration of systole may increase proportionally to flow, and their magnitude is not predictable from the resting measurements. The gradient change is proportionately small compared to the changes between rest and exercise in mitral stenosis. As with mitral stenosis, with exercise there may be a modest increase in the calculated aortic valve area, suggesting the presence of a dynamic component to the obstruction.[16,17]

The increased load encountered by the left ventricular myocardium makes the response of left ventricular end-diastolic pressure noteworthy. In children with congenital aortic stenosis, end-diastolic pressure remains unchanged during supine exercise,[18] but most studies in adults report increases. Bache et al found a significant correlation between the rise in end-diastolic pressure and age, but not with the severity of stenosis, suggesting that it may reflect the chronicity of the pressure overload.[16]

The mechanism of exertional syncope in aortic stenosis has been investigated by exercise hemodynamic studies. While some patients probably develop ventricular arrythmias, possibly secondary to imbalances between myocardial oxygen supply and demand, abrupt hypotension due to peripheral vasodilation or acute left ventricular failure has been documented in others.[19] An elegant study by Mark et al demonstrated inappropriate exercise-induced peripheral vasodilation in nonworking tissue in patients with aortic stenosis and a history of syncope.[20] Their findings suggest that the exertional hypotension may in part reflect autonomic dysfunction.

Mitral Regurgitation

Patients with mitral regurgitation are, perhaps, the most heterogeneous group with valvular heart disease. In adults, regurgitation often results from abnormalities of the subvalvular apparatus, including the chordae tendineae, the papillary muscles, and the myocardium adjacent to the papillary muscles. The most common causes of subvalvular dysfunction are coronary artery disease and cardiomyopathies. Thus, the major determinant of the hemodynamic response to exercise in mitral insufficiency is often not the severity of the regurgitation but the nature of the underlying cause and the status of the myocardium. Another important factor is the compliance of the left atrium. A small left atrium may yield high pressures with relatively modest mitral regurgitation, but patients with very dilated atria may maintain normal pressures at rest with severe regurgitation. In the latter, an additional volume load during exercise may cause marked pressure elevations. Thus, while hemodynamic measurements may deteriorate markedly during exercise, it may be difficult to determine whether this reflects a poorly compensated volume overload, myocardial abnormalities, or the underlying condition. Since the optimal timing of valve replacement in mitral regurgitation is often problematic and may be affected by many of these factors, the exercise hemodynamic findings can be helpful in establishing the need or the potential value of valve surgery, although they have not been as popular in this lesion as with mitral stenosis.

Published studies confirm the heterogeneous response to exercise in mitral regurgitation, but the general trend is toward deterioration.[21,22] In general, pulmonary artery and pulmonary capillary wedge pressures increase. The magnitude of increase reflects in large part the status of the myocardium. The rise in forward cardiac output is usually subnormal for the level of exercise, though it may be substantial. Despite the decrease in peripheral vascular resistance during exercise, the one study which evaluated the severity of regurgitation during exercise showed no change from rest.[21] There are no longitudinal exercise hemodynamic data available, but because of the role of the myocardium, it is certain that these changes with exercise do not indicate the severity of regurgitation and are not necessarily reversible.

The most valuable applications of exercise hemodynamics in mitral regurgitation are to provide objective measurements in symptomatic patients in whom the significance of the valvular abnormality is unclear. There are two situations in which this information may be most useful. One is the patient with episodic papillary muscle dysfunction due to ischemia, in whom the dramatic appearance of regurgitant "v" waves and pulmonary hypertension during exercise may clarify the etiology of exertional dyspnea. The second is in patients with normal resting pressures and moderate mitral insufficiency, in whom exercise-induced pulmonary hypertension may be the single indicator that the regurgitation is severe or poorly tolerated.

Aortic Regurgitation

The determination of the optimal time for surgical intervention in patients with aortic regurgitation is one of the most difficult and controversial problems in cardiology.[23] There is general agreement that patients with more than minimal symptoms should undergo valve replacement. Unfortunately, in some of these patients preoperative left ventricular dysfunction has been found to persist or even worsen postoperatively and morbidity and mortality are increased when left ventricular dysfunction is present.[24,25] Therefore, consideration is often given to early intervention in patients with severe aortic insufficiency with mild symptoms or who are asymptomatic. However, the generally long natural history of aortic insufficiency, which often includes a prolonged asymptomatic period, and the not infrequent complications of valve replacement create a difficult dilemma as to when to intervene.

The possibility that exercise hemodynamics might delineate groups of patients who might benefit from early surgical intervention has generated considerable interest in these measurements. Hemodynamic studies have shown heterogeneous responses. The decrease in peripheral resistance coupled with the increase in heart rate almost invariably result in a reduction in regurgitant fraction.[21,26,27] This permits aortic insufficiency patients to increase their cardiac output significantly, and many have a normal cardiac output response to exercise.[21,26–29] The responses of left ventricular end-diastolic and left atrial pressures are more variable, with some symptomatic patients exhibiting little or no increases and some asymptomatic individuals displaying marked rises. In fact, the exercise hemodynamics do not correlate well with the severity of regurgitation or the associated symptoms,[12] although the measured exercise capacity has correlated with the postoperative prognosis and left ventricular function.[30]

Because of the lack of a close relationship between these invasive exercise hemodynamic measurements and symptoms or severity of regurgitation, they are not often employed in the evaluation of patients. However, noninvasive exercise radionuclide angiography remains popular in aortic regurgitation, and this will be discussed further below.

Exercise Hemodynamics for Evaluating Surgical and Medical Therapy

Valve replacement may be the most critical event in the clinical course of a patient with valvular disease, but it often does not render the patient permanently asymptomatic. Among the multiple factors which can continue to produce symptoms are residual (or even resultant) left ventricular dysfunction, pulmonary vascular disease, and residual stenosis or insufficiency due either to inadequate commisurotomy, inadequate prosthesis orifice size, or prosthetic valve dysfunction. As a result, considerable attention has been devoted to the measurement of exercise hemodynamics postoperatively.

Exercise hemodynamics were found to be a valuable aid in assessing the outcome of mitral commisurotomy.[31] In a group of 35 patients undergoing the procedure, resting hemodynamics improved in most but often larger changes were apparent in the exercise measurements. The most dramatic changes were reductions in exercise mean left atrial pressure from 30 to 17 mmHg, with individual reductions being as great as 40 mmHg, and a mean decrease in exercise pulmonary vascular resistance from 4.2 to 2.6 units. Of note is that though maximal cardiac index did not change much (a mean increase of 0.3 L/min/m^2), the mean transvalvular gradient during exercise fell from 20 to 9 mmHg, compared to a decrease from 14 to 6 mmHg at rest. The improvements tended to be better in the group with the largest postoperative valve area, but generally correlations between the hemodynamic measurements and postoperative valve area were poor, suggesting that other factors such as myocardial function may have affected the results. Similar findings were reported in patients undergoing mitral valve replacement for either stenosis or regurgitation.[32–34] The most striking improvements are in exercise left atrial or pulmonary capillary wedge pressures, although these still rise to a mean of 20 mmHg, and in pulmonary artery pressure. The change in exercise cardiac index was variable and the exercise transvalvular gradient averaged 10 mmHg. These findings indicate that after mitral valve surgery, modest transvalvular gradients develop during exercise and that hemodynamic abnormalities persist, probably reflecting residual myocardial abnormalities.

Exercise hemodynamics have also been reported in patients undergoing aortic valve replacement.[35,36] In general, these have been relatively normal in patients who had normal left ventricular function preoperatively. Transvalvular gradients were noted in most patients, but were generally 30 mmHg or less, yielding calculated valve areas of 1.0 to 2.0 cm.

Since gradients have almost invariably been found across prosthetic valves and the physiologic significance of these can often be better assessed during exercise when flow is increased, exercise hemodynamics have been measured to evaluate the degree of stenosis imparted by several types of prostheses. The greatest concern has been with the bioprostheses, since the effective orifice in bioprostheses is smaller than that of many mechanical valves. Indeed, large gradients have been noted in two series in which mean transaortic gradients of 70 mmHg and 51 mmHg during exercise were reported.[37,38] Usually, smaller gradients have been present with the low-profile Bjork-Shiley valves[39] and with more recent bioprostheses, such as the Carpentier-Edwards.[40] Nonetheless, the obstructive properties of all valves must be considered when determining the need for valve replacement.

Exercise hemodynamics have also been employed to confirm the value of vasodilator therapy in regurgitant valvular lesions. In both aortic and mitral disease, Greenberg et al demonstrated that hydralazine hydrochloride increased exercise cardiac output and decreased pulmonary capillary wedge pressure.[22,41] These beneficial effects were present in patients with both normal and impaired left ventricular function, and presumably reflect a reduction in regurgitant fraction as well as unloading of the left ventricle.

NONINVASIVE EXERCISE MEASUREMENTS

Exercise Radionuclide Angiography

Because of the limitations of invasive exercise hemodynamic measurements discussed above and the difficulty in performing serial studies, attention has shifted to noninvasive measurements of left ventricular performance in valvular heart disease. The most successful of these techniques has been exercise radionuclide angiography, which permits serial measurements of left ventricular ejection fraction during supine, and in some laboratories, upright bicycle exercise. Techniques are also available to measure left ventricular end-diastolic and end-systolic volume and to estimate the severity of regurgitation, though these are less widely utilized.

The greatest interest has been in evaluating patients with aortic regurgitation, since this is the lesion which presents the most difficulty relative to the timing of surgical intervention and because the status of the left ventricle is the major determinant of therapy. Borer et al first performed radionuclide measurements in patients with aortic insufficiency.[42] They detected a deterioration in left ventricular function during exercise, irrespective of the resting ejection fraction, in nearly all symptomatic patients, but a variable response in asymptomatic subjects. Only six of 22 asymptomatic patients showed an increment in ejection fraction of the order usually seen in normal subjects. This finding raised the exciting possibility that a subset of asymptomatic patients might have reduced myocardial reserve and therefore be candidates for early surgical intervention in order to preserve myocardial function. In symptomatic patients undergoing valve replacement, the exercise ejection fraction response was noted to improve postoperatively, but not always to totally normalize.[43]

Other workers have subsequently confirmed the observation of variable exercise ejection fraction responses in asymptomatic aortic regurgitation.[44–49] These studies have shown a consistent decrease in regurgitant fraction and little change or a tendency toward a decrease in end-diastolic volume when these were measured. Thus, it is the variable change in end-systolic volume which determines the ejection fraction response. However, the effects of exercise on the heart in aortic regurgitation are complex. The tachycardia and peripheral vasodilation tend to reduce the proportion, and possibly even the total amount of regurgitation.[50] Left ventricular afterload may be reduced by both the declining systemic vascular resistance and, if end-diastolic volume falls, reduced wall tension. On the other hand, systolic blood pressure may rise significantly during exercise in patients with regurgitation and, if they have dilated hearts with relatively thin walls, systolic wall stress may be elevated. In fact, echocardiographic-radionuclide correlative studies suggest that the subjects whose systolic wall stress is increased at rest are those who exhibit the most abnormal ejection fraction response during exercise.[51,52]

As a result of all these factors, the exercise ejection fraction response in aortic regurgitation cannot be considered to reflect myocardial function alone. Nonetheless, two studies in which both invasive exercise hemodynamics and scintigraphy have been performed in the same patients confirm the value of the noninvasive measurements.[27,29] We noted that patients whose ejection fraction rose or remained essentially

Table 14-2
Hemodynamic Correlates of the Exercise Ejection Fraction (EF) Response in Aortic Regurgitation

	Response of EF During Exercise		
	EF Unchanged or Increased	EF Decreased	*P*
Δ* Cardiac index (L/min/m^2)	+6.1	+4.2	<.001
Δ Stroke index (mL/beats/m^2)	+30	+10	<.01
Δ Pulmonary capillary wedge pressure (mmHg)	+11	+22	<.05
Δ End-diastolic volume index (mL/m^2)	−34	+3	<.05
Δ End-systolic volume index (mL/m^2)	−12	+40	<.05

*Change from rest to maximum exercise measurements.

constant during exercise showed marked differences from those whose ejection fraction fell by more than 0.05 (Table 14-2). The former showed greater increases in cardiac index and stroke index and a smaller rise in pulmonary capillary wedge pressure. The correlation between the change in ejection fraction and the rise in cardiac index was highly significant ($r = 0.81$, $P < .001$). An important study by Bonow et al in which 88 initially asymptomatic patients with aortic regurgitation were followed for a mean of 4 years further demonstrates the value of the exercise ejection fraction response.[53] The ten patients who required valve replacement all exhibited a fall in ejection fraction during exercise, and these ten represented 25% to 30% of patients with an abnormal exercise response (Figure 14-2) Thus, exercise radionuclide angiography appears to provide a useful indication of the patients who require the most careful follow-up.

Studies employing exercise radionuclide angiography in patients with other valve lesions are much more limited. In significant aortic stenosis, ejection fraction consistently falls or fails to rise normally with exercise.[54] After valve replacement, a normal exercise response is restored. However, there appears to be no useful correlation between the change in ventricular function from rest to exercise and the severity of aortic stenosis, so the clinical role of such measurements is limited. Newman evaluated nine patients with mitral stenosis.[55] As might be expected, end-diastolic volume remained constant or fell and though left ventricular ejection fraction tended to rise, stroke volume was unchanged. Thus, these patients increased their cardiac output during exercise only by virtue of a rise in heart rate. Postcommissurotomy, stroke volume rose significantly during stress. However, since left atrial or pulmonary artery pressure, which are the most important measurements in mitral stenosis, cannot be determined noninvasively, the technique is of limited value.

Few data are available in mitral regurgitation, probably as a result of the high prevalence of atrial fibrillation, which interferes with scintigraphic evaluation, and of accompanying coronary disease. If the latter patients are excluded, the ejection fraction response was usually normal in one study.[32] This finding was somewhat surprising in view of the expected presence of associated left ventricular dysfunction. It is noteworthy, however, that the outcome of surgery in the patients with abnormal ejection fraction responses was poor.

Measurements of Exercise Capacity

A great deal of clinically useful information can also be obtained by objective measurements of exercise capacity, particularly in patients whose symptoms do not correspond with other assessments of the severity of valvular disease. Since exercise is usually limited by the patients' ability to increase their forward cardiac output, such measurements can reveal a great deal about cardiac function, although they do not determine whether the limitation is from valve disease or associated myocardial involvement. Indeed, Bonow et al have reported that preoperative exercise capacity is a good indicator of postoperative prognosis, even though it does not correlate well with resting measurements of left ventricular function.[30] Interestingly, a second group of investigators has found a close relation between the measured exercise capacity and the exercise ejection fraction response in aortic regurgitation.[56] However, more data are needed in both aortic regurgitation and other valvular diseases to determine the value of exercise testing in determining prognosis and the need for thereapeutic interventions.

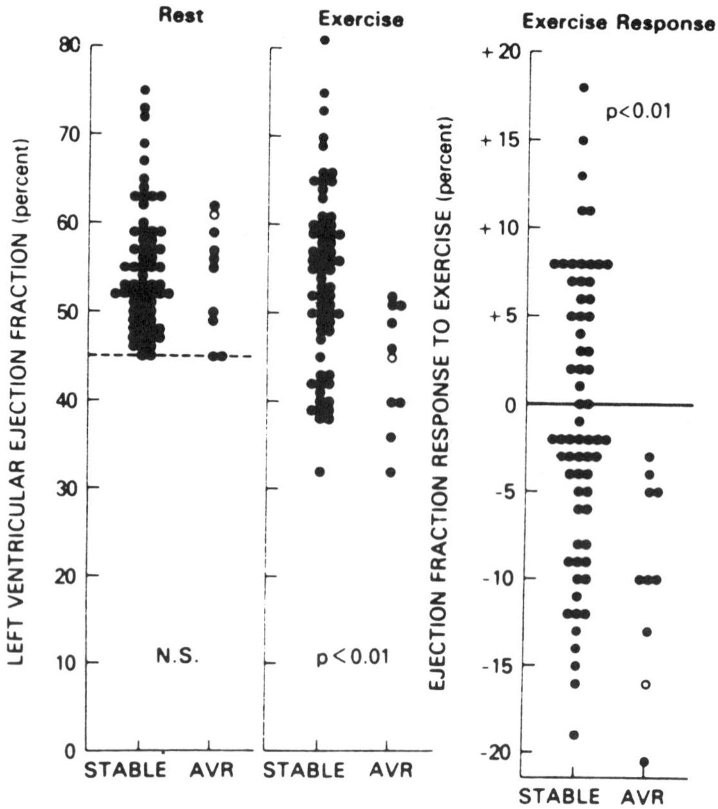

Figure 14-2 These plots show the baseline measurements of left ventricular ejection fraction at rest and during exercise, as well as the rest-to-exercise changes, in a group of asymptomatic patients with aortic regurgitation. They are divided into those who remained asymptomatic and those who subsequently required aortic valve replacement (AVR) because of symptoms. All patients who subsequently deteriorated were among those whose ejection fraction fell during exercise. (Reproduced with permission from Bonow et al[53] and the American Heart Association).

The capability for on-line measurements of respiratory gas exchange is becoming more widespread, permitting objective and reproducible measurements of exercise capacity, anaerobic threshold, and some indication of cardiac output. The added value of these indices over the determination of exercise duration on a standard protocol is unclear, but all of these techniques permit careful observation of patients to determine the degree and nature of their limitation — findings that can be of enormous clinical value.

SUMMARY

The hemodynamic response to exercise in patients with valvular heart disease has been studied since the availability of cardiac catheterization, and much of the current knowledge dates back to these early studies. The clinical role of these measurements has declined somewhat, and they are no longer routinely made in most laboratories. Nonetheless, they may be helpful in evaluating selected patients. The most appropriate candidates are patients with borderline mitral stenosis, patients with mitral insufficiency in whom the resting hemodynamics are normal, and patients with any valve lesion in whom there is a discrepancy between the resting hemodynamics and clinical presentation. In addition, exercise hemodynamics are sometimes useful in evaluating patients with postoperative symptoms of uncertain etiology.

Noninvasive evaluation of the left ventricular response to exercise by scintigraphic techniques has become increasingly popular. This is particularly useful in aortic regurgitation, where the noninvasive findings correlate significantly with invasive measurements but may be of even greater clinical utility. Objective assessment of exercise capacity can also be helpful clinically, but its role in the management of valvular heart disease remains to be defined.

REFERENCES

1. Smith EE, Guyton AC, Manning RD, et al: Integrated mechanisms of cardiovascular response and control during exercise in the normal human. *Prog Cardiovasc Dis* 1976;18:42–444.
2. Vatner SF, Pagani M: Cardiovascular adjustments to exercise: Hemodynamics and mechanisms. *Prog Cardiovasc Dis* 1976;19:91–108.
3. Clement DL, Shepard JT: Regulation of peripheral circulation during muscular exercise. *Prog Cardiovasc Dis* 1976;19:23–31.
4. Epstein SE, Beiser GD, Stampfer M, et al: Characterization of the circulatory response to maximal upright exercise in normal subjects and patients with heart disease. *Circulation* 1967; 35:1049–1062.
5. Epstein SE, Beiser GD, Stampfer M, et al: Exercise in patients with heart disease: Effects of body position and type and intensity of exercise. *Am J Cardiol* 1969;23:572–576.
6. Thadani U, Parker JO: Hemodynamics at rest and during supine and upright exercise in normal subjects. *Am J Cardiol* 1978;41:52–59.
7. Kramer B, Massie B, Topic N: Hemodynamic differences between supine and upright exercise in patients with congestive heart failure. *Circulation* 1982;66:820–825.
8. Poliner LR, Dehmer GJ, Lewis SE, et al: Left ventricular performance in normal subjects: A comparison of the responses to exercise in the upright and supine positions. *Circulation* 1980; 62:528–534.
9. Gorlin R, Sawyer CG, Haynes FW, et al: Effects of exercise on circulatory dynamics in mitral stenosis. III. *Am Heart J* 1951;41:192–203.
10. Ross J Jr, Gault JH, Mason DT, et al: Left ventricular performance during muscular exercise in patients with and without cardiac dysfunction. *Circulation* 1966;34:597–608.
11. Kasalicky J, Hurych J, Widimsky J, et al: Left heart haemodynamics at rest and during exercise in patients with mitral stenosis. *Br Heart J* 1968; 30:188–195.
12. Tsagaris T, Samuelson C, McDonnell M, et al: Comparison of clinical and hemodynamic assessment of cardiac disability. *Cardiology* 1975;60: 50–61.
13. Gorlin R, McMillan IKR, Medd WE, et al: Dynamics of the circulation in aortic valvular disease. *Am J Med* 1955;18:855–870.
14. Anderson FL, Tsagaris TJ, Tikoff G, et al: Hemodynamic effects of exercise in patients with aortic stenosis. *Am J Med* 1964;46:872–885.
15. Lee SJK, Johnson B, Bevegard S, et al: Hemodynamic changes at rest and during exercise in patients with aortic stenosis of varying severity. *Am Heart J* 1970;79:318–331.
16. Bache RJ, Wang Y, Jorgensen CR: Hemodynamic effects of exercise in isolated valvular aortic stenosis. *Circulation* 1971;44:1003–1013.
17. Richardson JW, Anderson FL, Tsagaris TJ: Rest and exercise hemodynamic studies in patients with isolated aortic stenosis. *Cardiology* 1979;64:1–11.
18. Cueto L, Moller JH: Haemodynamics of exercise in children with isolated aortic valvular disease. *Br Heart J* 1973;35:93–98.
19. Flamm MD, Branniff BA, Kimball R, et al: Mechanism of effort syncope in aortic stenosis. *Circulation* 1967;35(suppl 2):II–109.
20. Mark AL, Kioschos JM, Abboud FM, et al: Abnormal vascular responses to exercise in patients with aortic stenosis. *J Clin Invest* 1973;52: 1138–1146.
21. Levinson GE, Grank MJ, Schwartz CJ: The effect of rest and physical effort on the left ventricular burden in mitral and aortic regurgitation. *Am Heart J* 1970;80:791–801.
22. Greenberg BH, DeMots H, Murphy E, et al: Arterial dilators in mitral regurgitation: Effects on rest and exercise hemodynamics and long-term clinical follow-up. *Circulation* 1982;65:181–187.
23. Bonow RO, Rosing DR, Kent KM, et al: Timing of operation for chronic aortic regurgitation. *Am J Cardiol* 1982;50:325–336.
24. Gault JH, Covell JW, Braunwald E, et al: Left ventricular performance following correction of free aortic regurgitation. *Circulation* 1970;42: 773–780.
25. Forman R, Firth BG, Barnard MS: Prognostic significance of pre-operative left ventricular ejection fraction and valve lesion in patients with aortic valve replacement. *Am J Cardiol* 1980; 45:1120–1125.
26. Lewis RP, Bristow JD, Griswald HE: Exercise hemodynamics in aortic regurgitation. *Am Heart J* 1970;80:171–176.
27. Massie BM, Kramer BL, Loge D, et al: Ejection fraction response to supine exercise in asymptomatic aortic regurgitation: Relation to simultaneous hemodynamic measurements. *J Am Coll Cardiol* 1985;5:847–855.
28. Goldberg HA, Bakst AA, Bailey CP: The dynamics of aortic valvular disease. *Am Heart J* 1959;47:527–559.
29. Boucher CA, Wilson RA, Kanarek DJ, et al: Exercise testing in asymptomatic or minimally symptomatic aortic regurgitation: relationship of left ventricular ejection fraction to left ventricular filling pressure during exercise. *Circulation* 1983; 67:1091–1100.
30. Bonow RO, Borer JS, Rosing DL, et al: Preoperative exercise capacity in symptomatic patients with aortic regurgitation as a predictor of postoperative left ventricular function and long-term prognosis. *Circulation* 1980;62:1280–1290.
31. Feigenbaum H, Linback RE, Nasser WK: Hemodynamic studies before and after instrumental mitral commissurotomy. *Circulation* 1968; 38:261–276.
32. Peter CA, Austin EH, Jones RH: Effect of valve

replacement for chronic mitral insufficiency on left ventricular function during rest and exercise. *J Thorac Cardiovasc Surg* 1981;82:127–135.

33. Morrow AG, Oldham HM, Elkins RC, et al: Prosthetic replacement of the mitral valve. Preoperative and postoperative clinical and hemodynamic assessments in 100 patients. *Circulation* 1967;35:962–979.
34. Hultgren H, Hubis H, Shumway H: Cardiac function following mitral valve replacement. *Am Heart J* 1968;75:302–312.
35. Bristow JD, McCord CW, Starr A, et al: Clinical and hemodynamic results of aortic valvular replacement with a ball-valve prosthesis. *Circulation* 1964;29 (suppl 1):36–46.
36. Ross J, Morrow AG, Mason DT, et al: Left ventricular function following replacement of the aortic valve. Hemodynamic responses to muscular exercise. *Circulation* 1966;33:507–516.
37. Hamner H, Reis RL: Current status of porcine heterograft prostheses. *Circulation* 1976;54 (suppl 3):27–31.
38. Johnson H, Thompson S, Vieney WVR, et al: Evaluation of the in vivo function of the Hancock porcine xenograft in the aortic position. *J Thorac Cardiovasc Surg* 1978;75:599–605.
39. Bjork VO, Henze A, Holmgren A: Central haemodynamics at rest and during exercise before and after aortic valve replacement with the Bjork-Shiley tilting disc valve in patients with isolated aortic stenosis. *Scand J Thor Cardiovasc Surg* 1973;7:111–130.
40. Dyrda I, Grondin CM: Hemodynamic evaluation of the Carpentier-Edwards porcine xenograft. *Circulation* 1979;60:1170–1182.
41. Greenberg BH, DeMots H, Murphy E, et al: Beneficial effects of hydralazine on rest and exercise hemodynamics in patients with chronic severe aortic insufficiency. *Circulation* 1980;62: 49–55.
42. Borer JS, Bacharach SL, Kent KM, et al: Exercise-induced left ventricular dysfunction in symptomatic and asymptomatic patients with aortic regurgitation: Assessment with radionuclide cineangiography. *Am J Cardiol* 1978;42:351–357.
43. Borer JS, Rosing DR, Kent KM, et al: Left ventricular function at rest and during exercise after aortic valve replacement in patients with aortic regurgitation. *Am J Cardiol* 1979;44: 1297–1305.
44. Dehmer CJ, Firth BG, Hillis LO, et al: Alterations in left ventricular volumes and ejection fraction at rest and during exercise in patients with aortic regurgitation. *Am J Cardiol* 1981;48:17–27.
45. Steingart RM, Yee C, Weinstein L, Scheuer J: Radionuclide ventriculographic study of adaptations to exercise in aortic regurgitation. *Am J Cardiol* 1983;51:483–488.
46. Huxley RL, Gaffney A, Corbett JR, et al: Early detection of left ventricular dysfunction in chronic aortic regurgitation as assessed by contrast angiography, echocardiography, and rest and exercise scintigraphy. *Am J Cardiol* 1983;51:1542–1550.
47. Iskandrian AS, Hakki A, Manno B, et al: Left ventricular function in chronic aortic regurgitation. *J Am Coll Cardiol* 1983;1:1374–1380.
48. Johnson LL, Powers ER, Tzall WR, et al: Left ventricular volume and ejection fraction response to exercise in aortic regurgitation. *Am J Cardiol* 1983;51:1379–1385.
49. Massie B, Kramer B, Topic N, et al: Exercise hemodynamic responses in asymptomatic aortic regurgitation. *J Am Coll Cardiol* 1984;3:534.
50. Judge TP, Kennedy JW, Bennett LJ, et al: Quantitative hemodynamic effects of heart rate in aortic regurgitation. *Circulation* 1971;44:355–367.
51. Lewis SM, Riba AL, Berger HJ, et al: Radionuclide angiographic exercise left ventricular performance in chronic aortic regurgitation: Relationship to resting echographic ventricular dimensions and systolic wall stress index. *Am Heart J* 1982;103:498–594.
52. Greenberg B, Massie B, Thomas D, et al: Association between exercise, ejection fraction response and systolic wall stress in patients with chronic aortic insufficiency. *Circulation* 1985;71:458–465.
53. Bonow RO, Rosing DR, McIntosh CL, et al: The natural history of asymptomatic patients with aortic regurgitation and normal left ventricular function. *Circulation* 1983;68:509–517.
54. Borer JS, Bacharach SL, Green MV, et al: Left ventricular function in aortic stenosis: Response to exercise and effects of operation. *Am J Cardiol* 1978;41:382.
55. Newman GE, Rerych SK, Bounous PE, et al: Noninvasive assessment of hemodynamic effects of mitral valve commissurotomy during rest and exercise in patients with mitral stenosis. *J Thorac Cardiovasc Surg* 1979;78:750–756.
56. Boucher CA, Kanarek DJ, Okada RD, et al: Exercise testing in aortic regurgitation: Comparison of radionuclide left ventricular ejection fraction with exercise performance at the anaerobic threshold and peak exercise. *Am J Cardiol* 1983; 52:801–808.

CHAPTER 15
Emergencies in Valvular Heart Disease

Dean J. Kereiakes
Thomas A. Ports

Emergent situations may complicate the course of established valvular heart disease, or may be the initial manifestation of valvular dysfunction. Valves on the left side of the heart are particularly vulnerable and their dysfunction may produce life-threatening hemodynamic alterations. Familiarity with the clinical presentation, and appropriate diagnostic evaluation and therapeutic approach to emergencies in valvular heart disease will facilitate the care of these critically ill patients, and can be life-saving. For the sake of convenience in the discussion to follow, emergencies involving the mitral and aortic valves will be grouped into stenotic and regurgitant categories. Emergencies complicating the use of valvular prosthetic devices will be dealt with separately.

ACUTE AORTIC REGURGITATION

The clinical significance of aortic insufficiency depends on the volume of regurgitation, the time course over which it occurs, and the underlying state of the left ventricular myocardium. Severe aortic regurgitation may be well tolerated when it develops insidiously, allowing time for adaptation to the volume load.

Acute severe aortic regurgitation (AAR) precludes the time necessary for compensatory adaptation.[1,2] Left ventricular end-diastolic pressure rises abruptly with little increase in end-diastolic fiber length or volume. Thus, forward stroke volume cannot increase adequately to compensate for a large regurgitant volume and forward cardiac output falls. Reflex sympathetic activation causes heart rate and peripheral vascular resistance to rise. Without augmentation in left ventricular end-diastolic fiber length, the velocity of left ventricular contraction, left ventricular stroke volume, and, consequently, aortic systolic pressure, cannot increase. The fall in aortic diastolic pressure, which is so prominent in chronic aortic regurgitation, is limited by marked elevation in left ventricular end-diastolic pressure and the attenuation of peripheral run-off by an increased vascular resistance. Pulse pressure, therefore, may rise little, if at all, in AAR. In mid- to-late diastole, rapidly rising left ventricular pressure may exceed left atrial pressure, causing premature closure of the mitral valve. Mitral "preclosure" may protect the pulmonary circulation from the linear transmission of left ventricular pressure which continues to rise and may equilibrate with aortic pressure by end diastole. Prolongation of ventricular systolic ejection by the acutely imposed volume load and abbreviation of diastole by tachycardia and mitral preclosure combine to increase the duration of systole relative to diastole, and limit the duration of mitral valve opening. Acute severe aortic regurgitation (AAR) may be more poorly tolerated when regurgitant flow enters a left ventricle which is less than normally compliant because of pre-existent hypertrophy or hemopericardium.

Clinical Manifestations

Although the etiology of AAR may vary, the hemodynamic sequelae and clinical manifestations are remarkably constant. The patient appears acutely and seriously ill. Symptoms of pulmonary congestion predominate, and if not present at rest, will occur with minimal exertion.

The rapid progression of AAR seldom allows time for secondary renal salt and water retention, therefore, edema or weight gain are infrequently found. The extremities may be cool and mottled, reflecting diminished peripheral perfusion. Tachycardia is invariable and its absence cautions against the diagnosis of AAR. The pulse pressure, for reasons noted previously, is normal or only slightly increased. The carotid upstroke is not brisk and the contour, which may occasionally be bisferiens, is usually monophasic. Pulsus alternans, reflecting left ventricular dysfunction, is common and is best appreciated in the femoral arteries. In contrast to findings in chronic aortic regurgitation, prominent pulsations in the neck are usually venous, not arterial, and reflect secondary right ventricular dysfunction. The apex impulse is not laterally displaced or hyperdynamic, and a double impulse in diastole may be found on inspection or palpation. The initial outward diastolic movement of the apex reflects rapid ventricular filling and is the mechanical correlate of a third heart sound. This is followed by an inward movement which coincides with mitral valve preclosure and a second outward movement reflecting continued aortic insufficiency.[2] On auscultation, the first heart sound may be diminished by early mitral closure. The intensity of the aortic component of the second heart sound may be decreased or absent if the valve leaflets are damaged. Thus, diminution in the intensity of the first and second heart sounds combined, with an increase in the duration of systole relative to diastole, obscures the timing of systole and diastole on auscultation. Simultaneous palpation of the carotid upstroke during auscultation is, therefore, frequently required to distinguish systole from diastole.

The murmur of AAR begins with the aortic second sound and is of medium frequency. The murmur may be deceptively soft and brief, as rapid equilibrium of aortic and left ventricular pressure occurs. This is in stark contrast to the pure, high frequency and long blowing diastolic murmur characteristic of chronic aortic regurgitation. Occasionally, a fenestrated or flail cusp may produce a loud, musical diastolic murmur or more rarely, a coarse, sawing sound simulating the murmur of aortic stenosis (Key-Hodgkin murmur).[3] A third heart sound is common, but a fourth sound is not, because early mitral closure prevents presystolic filling of the ventricle. The Austin-Flint murmur, a mid- to-late diastolic rumble, is frequently heard between the apex and left sternal border.[4,5]

Etiology

The major etiologies of AAR are as follows:

1. Infective endocarditis
2. Aortic dissection
3. Trauma
4. Spontaneous rupture of normal or myxomatous valve
5. Rheumatologic disorders (ankylosing spondylitis, rheumatoid arthritis, etc)
6. Surgical valvotomy

Infective endocarditis often involving a functionally normal, previously unrecognized bicuspid valve is the most common etiology.

Aortic insufficiency may complicate over half of proximal aortic dissections and is poorly tolerated in the presence of hypertensive left ventricular hypertrophy.[6] The patient should be evaluated for associated coarctation, signs of Marfan's syndrome, bicuspid aortic valve, or aortic stenosis. Dissection may produce aortic insufficiency through annular dilatation, annular disruption, or downward displacement of one or more cusps.[7]

Aortic insufficiency is the most common valvular lesion in patients surviving blunt chest trauma.[8–10] Valvular damage may be found in 9% of postmortem examinations in subjects dying from blunt chest damage, and is almost always (96%) associated with other cardiac injuries.[8] The nature and severity of cardiac damage resulting from blunt chest trauma depends on the direction and velocity of compression, the phase of the cardiac cycle at impact, and the level of intracardiac pressure produced. The aortic valve is most vulnerable in early diastole when a sudden impact may tear an aortic leaflet, avulse a commissural attachment, or create an aortic intimal tear with subsequent leaflet prolapse into the left ventricular outflow tract.[11,12] The regurgitant murmur may not become evident for some time following the trauma and may have an unusual musical quality. The prognosis depends both on the severity of regurgitation and associated cardiac and noncardiac injuries.

Severe AAR may result from spontaneous rupture or prolapse of a myxomatous, or, more rarely, normal aortic valve.[13] Valve incompetence may result from fenestrations, from valve rupture or perforation, or from prolapse of one or more cusps. Spontaneous rupture may also involve the bicuspid aortic valve. Significant aortic insufficiency following surgical aortic valvotomy for congenital aortic stenosis has become extremely uncommon in modern surgical practice.

Laboratory Features

The ECG in severe AAR shows sinus tachycardia with nonspecific ST segment and T wave abnormalities. The presence of left ventricular hypertrophy implies preexistent cardiovascular disease, particularly hypertension or aortic stenosis. Intraventricular or atrioventricular conduction abnormalities may indicate extravalvular extension of infection in patients suspected of having endocarditis.[14] The chest film usually shows pulmonary edema and relatively normal cardiac chamber sizes. The presence of a widened mediastinum or irregularities in aortic contour, often best seen in a left anterior oblique view, may suggest aortic dissection. Separation of intimal calcium from the outer border of the aortic wall by 6 mm or more may reflect intramural hematoma.[15]

Echocardiographic Findings

The noninvasive assessment of AAR has been facilitated by echocardiography. Two-dimensional echocardiography is superior to M-mode echocardiography for delineating aortic root and valvular pathology and thus identifying the etiology of AAR.[16,17] The ascending aorta is best imaged using the parasternal long and short axis views. The retrocardiac descending aorta can be visualized using the same transducer position or by moving the transducer laterally in the third or fourth intercostal space.[18] Suprasternal views, obtained with the transducer in the suprasternal notch directed inferoposteriorly and leftward (parallel to the long axis of the aorta) may detect abnormalities of the aortic arch or great vessels. Dilatation of the root (> 42 mm), thickening of the anterior (> 16 mm) or posterior (> 10 mm) aortic walls, or separation of the single dominant echo of a wall into two discreet echoes moving in unison, suggest the diagnosis of aortic dissection.[19] Oscillation of an intimal flap may be seen.[20,21] A flail aortic leaflet from endocarditis, trauma, or spontaneous rupture may exhibit diastolic flutter and wide systolic excursion.[22,23] Valvular vegetations of 2 mm in diameter or greater, and occasionally annular abscesses may be visualized in infective endocarditis.[24–26] Dilatation of the aortic valve ring, sinuses of Valsalva, and ascending aorta may occur in Marfan's syndrome and should prompt further evaluation for an associated aortic dissection or ruptured myxomatous valve.

Associated echocardiographic findings following blunt cardiac trauma include global and segmental abnormalities in ventricular function, ventricular mural thrombi, and pericardial effusion.[27] Echocardiographic abnormalities of the mitral valve in AAR may provide both qualitative and quantitative information. Delayed opening, decreased amplitude of excursion, reduction in the e-f slope, and fluttering in diastole may be present in echoes of the anterior mitral leaflet. Premature mitral valve closure (before inscription of the QRS complex on a simultaneously recorded ECG) in the presence of sinus rhythm and a normal P-R interval usually denotes severe acute aortic regurgitation with marked elevation of left ventricular diastolic pressures (Figure 15-1).[28] Occasionally, the diastolic pressure may be so high that the aortic valve opens prematurely.[29] By evaluating the direction and velocity of blood flow, continuous-wave Doppler echocar-

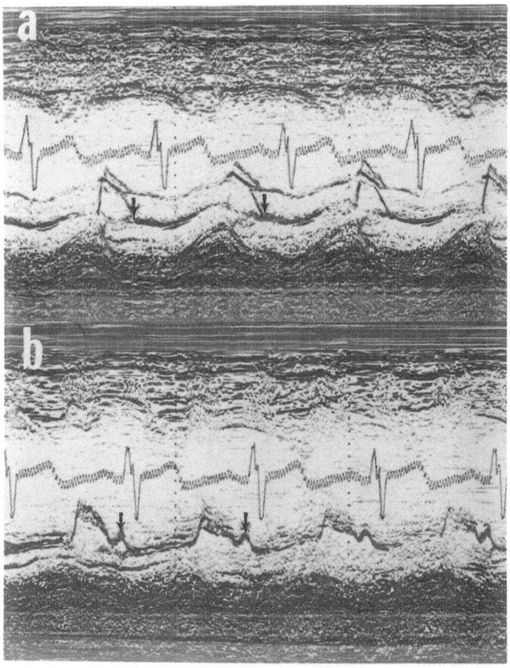

Figure 15-1a and b (a) M-mode echocardiogram of the left ventricle at the level of the mitral valve demonstrating early mitral valve closure. The arrow indicates closure of the mitral valve prior to the Q wave of the simultaneous ECG. (b) M-mode echocardiogram obtained in the same patient following reduction in the left ventricular end-diastolic pressure from 36 mmHg. to 18 mmHg with intravenous nitroprusside therapy. The mitral valve now opens with atrial contraction (arrow) and early closure is no longer present.

diography can detect the reversal and exaggeration of diastolic aortic flow indicative of aortic regurgitation.[30] Intravenous (IV) digital subtraction angiography has also been used to visualize abnormalities of the aorta.[31] Contrast-enhanced computed tomography (CT) may be particularly suited for the evaluation of an aortic dissection because of its tomographic format and ability to differentiate hematoma from vessel wall.[32]

Cardiac Catheterization

When the diagnosis of severe AAR is made clinically and is substantiated by noninvasive techniques, cardiac catheterization may not be necessary and indeed may carry a significant risk. The decision to perform cardiac catheterization must be made on an individual basis after weighing the risk of subjecting a critically ill patient to contrast angiography with its attendent volume load and obligatory delay in surgery against the anticipated benefit of obtaining information with differential diagnostic or therapeutic utility. If the diagnosis or severity of the lesion is in question, catheterization should be performed. Catheterization may also identify and quantitate the severity of associated abnormalities, such as an unsuspected valve ring abscess, ruptured sinus of Valsalva aneurysm, or multiple valve involvement in patients with infective endocarditis.[33] In patients with aortic dissection, angiographic evaluation with cut film or cineangiography may demonstrate the false lumen, intimal flap, or true lumen compression by hematoma. Knowledge of aortic arch and coronary anatomy may aid surgical repair.

Therapy

Severe AAR is best treated by aortic valve replacement. Medical therapy directed at reducing pulmonary congestion and improving forward output by lowering impedance to left ventricular ejection may be instituted under close hemoydnamic monitoring while awaiting operation. Reduction in systemic vascular resistance, regurgitant fraction, left ventricular end-diastolic volume, and pressure can be achieved with nitroprusside.[34] Hydralazine hydrochloride will also lower impendance to left ventricular ejection, thus reducing regurgitant volume and improving forward output.[35] Hydralazine, however, is not as effective as nitroprusside in lowering pulmonary capillary wedge pressure and relieving pulmonary congestion. Further improvement in forward output can be obtained with an inotropic agent, particularly dobutamine. Dopamine hydrochloride may be used, but has the potential through α-adrenergic stimulation to increase vascular resistance and regurgitant fraction. Further preload reduction and relief of pulmonary congestion may accompany the use of a loop diuretic. Digoxin, which has a more delayed onset and lower magnitude of effect than dobutamine, is less useful in the patient with severe AAR. Rapid administration of digoxin may increase vascular resistance through a direct arteriolar constricting effect and worsen the severity of regurgitation. A slower infusion given over 20 to 30 minutes will minimize this effect on vascular resistance and may be used in patients with mild symptomsy. Although the use of the intra-aortic balloon pump in aortic insufficiency is contraindicated because the augmentation of aortic diastolic pressure will aggravate regurgitation, a reduction in regurgitant volume has been achieved experimentally with an inflatable, spherical balloon "valve."[36] This valve, which is inserted in the same manner as an intra-aortic balloon pump and positioned above the aortic anulus, can be operated by commerically available balloon pump consols.

Definitive therapy of AAR is valve replacement. In patients with infective endocarditis, the risk of aortic valve replacement is proportional to the degree of preoperative hemodynamic compromise. The decision for operation must be based on the hemodynamic status of the patient and not the duration of preoperative antibiotic therapy. In the patient with severe AAR, the risk of waiting exceeds that of operation and blood cultures should be obtained, broad-spectrum antibiotics begun and valve replacement performed immediately. Overall mortality for the procedure is 7% to 20%, and in patients matched for New York Heart Association congestive heart failure functional class, early surgical results are comparable to these of aortic valve replacement in noninfected patients.[37–42] Postoperative periprosthetic leaks have been reported in 15% of patients,but recrudescence of infection is rare.[43] Aorto-left ventricular discontinuity caused by annular erosion or abscess may require primary closure with horizontal pledget support mattress sultures or use of a Teflon patch graft.[44,45] Although congestive heart failure is the major indication for aortic valve replacement in infective endocarditis, other indications include infection with certain gram-negative or fungal organisms, recurrent systemic emboli, persistent sepsis, and evidence of extravalvular extension of infection.

The risk of aortic valve replacement is greatest in patients with AAR secondary to aortic dissection. Operative mortality approaches 30% and is greatest in patients with shock from tamponade.[6] Native valve reconstruction can be performed in the majority of patients, although valve replacement is required in those with annular disruption.[46–48] This is accomplished by utilizing a composite prosthetic valve – Dacron tube conduit.[49] Reanastamosis of the coronary arteries to the conduit or saphenous vein bypass may be necessary to preserve the coronary circulation. The majority of patients with traumatic aortic valve disruption will require valve replacement.[11] Surgical outcome in these patients is influenced by concomitant cardiac and noncardiac injuries.

ACUTE MITRAL REGURGITATION

Acute mitral regurgitation (AMR) delivers a volume load into a relatively noncompliant, normal-sized left atrium. Left atrial pressure rises rapidly and is freely transmitted in the form of a regurgitant wave to the pulmonary venous and arterial systems. Acute mitral regurgitation of moderate severity increases left atrial dimension and is associated with enhanced left atrial transport function as reflected by an increased amplitude of diastolic fractional shortening.[50] More severe degrees of regurgitation further increase left atrial dimension and impair left atrial function as the length-function curve of atrial myocardium is exhausted and left atrial afterload (left ventricular diastolic pressure) rises.[51] In mitral regurgitation, the left atrium provides a low impedance outlet to the left ventricle in systole, and left ventricular end-systolic pressure and volume diminish. Total stroke volume and ejection fraction are increased, although net forward flow is reduced.[52] Tachycardia and increased systemic vascular resistance accompany the decline in forward cardiac output seen in AMR. The acute mitral regurgitant volume returns to augment left ventricular filling in diastole, causing elevation in left ventricular diastolic pressures and small increments in end-diastolic volume. Thus, enhanced preload (end-diastolic fiber length) and diminished outflow impedance combine to increase the velocity and extent of left ventricular contraction in AMR.

Clinical Signs

Acute mitral regurgitation, unlike acute aortic insufficiency, may follow a more protracted course, with signs and symptoms being dependent on the volume of regurgitation, the rapidity with which it develops, and the presence of associated myocardial disease. Certain clinical characteristics of AMR differentiate it from chronic regurgition. The onset of dyspnea, fatigue, and muscle weakness, reflecting both pulmonary congestion and low forward output, may be well localized in time by the patient. Tachycardia is invariable, and the precordium is frequently hyperdynamic, reflecting the increased force and velocity of left ventricular contraction. A palpable presystolic distention at the cardiac apex is common and occasionally an apical thrill is present. A fourth heart sound is characteristic of AMR and helps differentiate it from chronic regurgitation. The second sound may have wide splitting with accentuation of the pulmonic component. The murmur of AMR, most frequently detected at the cardiac apex, is often not pansystolic in duration, but may have a descrescendo or diamond-shaped configuration. Early termination of the murmur occurs as left atrial pressure rises, and the gradient for flow from the left ventricle to the left atrium declines. An apical third heart sound or diastolic rumble may reflect a large regurgitant volume and augmentation of left ventricular filling in diastole.

Etiology

Papillary muscle disorders Acute mitral regurgitation may be classified according to the part of the mitral apparatus involved and the etiology of the involvement (Table 15-1). Although papillary muscle dysfunction may arise from abscess, vasculitis, amyloidosis, or other infiltrative diseases and trauma, the most frequent cause is ischemia from coronary artery disease.[53,54] Ischemia may impair systolic papillary muscle contraction or cause regional left ventricular free wall dysfunction at the base of a papillary muscle with subsequent failure of mitral leaflet coaptation. Ischemia causing necrosis may result in papilary muscle rupture, which has been found in 1% to 5% of patients dying of infarction.[55] Papillary muscle dysfunction (PMD) may be clinically detected in over half of patients with acute myocardial infarction.[56] The murmur of PMD is highly variable in onset, duration, and configuration. Although classically described as an ejection type (crescendo-decrescendo) murmur occurring in mid- to late systole, the murmur is frequently pansystolic. The intensity bears little relationship to the severity of regurgitation and may be deceptively soft or absent when left

Table 15-1
Etiologies of Acute Mitral Regurgitation

I. Disorders of papillary muscles
  A. Papillary muscle dysfunction or rupture
    1. Ischemia, acute myocardial infarction
    2. Infiltrative disease (amyloidosis, sarcoidosis, etc)
    3. Infectious disease (endocarditis, syphilis, etc)
    4. Vasculitis
    5. Blunt chest trauma
  B. Altered geometric relationship of papillary muscle to mitral anulus and leaflets (left ventricular dilatation)

II. Ruptured chordae tendineae
  A. Idiopathic
  B. Infectious endocarditis
  C. Rheumatic heart disease
  D. Mitral valve prolapse (myxomatous degeneration)
  E. Blunt chest trauma
  F. Disorders of collagen production (Ehlers-Danlos syndrome, osteogenesis imperfecta, Marfan's syndrome, etc)

III. Disorders of mitral leaflets
  A. Perforation due to infective endocarditis
  B. Fenestration or rupture due to blunt chest trauma

ventricular dysfunction is present. Systolic clicks with or without a murmur may also reflect papillary muscle dysfunction. Although rarely silent, papillary muscle rupture is usually accompanied by a pansystolic murmur at the cardiac apex radiating to the axilla and at times associated with a thrill. This murmur may be confused with the pansystolic murmur of ventricular septal rupture (VSR), which is usually loudest at the left sternal edge and more frequently associated with a thrill. Differentiation may require bedside hemodynamic monitoring with a flow-directed pulmonary artery catheter. Oxygen saturations must be determined at the right atrium, right ventricle, and pulmonary artery. The presence of a step-up in excess of 5% oxygen saturation between right atrium and pulmonary artery or a recirculation peak on the thermodilution cardiac output curve reflects the left-to-right shunt of VSR.[57] Large "v" or regurgitant waves in the wedge pressure tracing may reflect AMR. The normal "v" waves reflects the passive component of left atrial filling. Its magnitude depends on left atrial filling volume and compliance and may be increased in a variety of disorders.[58,59] The augmented left atrial filling from increased pulmonary venous inflow of an acute left-to-right shunt accompanying VSR may be asociated with an exaggerated "v" wave in the wedge pressure tracing, stimulating AMR.[60] The onset of this "v" wave is normal with respect to the QRS complex of a simultaneously recorded ECG and its peak rarely, if ever, exceeds the systolic pressure in the pulmonary arterial tracing. In AMR, the "v" wave is, in truth, a "c-v" or regurgitant wave having earlier onset in reference to the QRS and obscuring the x-descent of the left atrial pressure tracing. The presence of normal pulmonary vascular resistance in AMR facilitates retrograde transmission of this regurgitant "v" wave, which not infrequently exceeds peak systolic pressure in the pulmonary artery.[61]

Two-dimensional echocardiography may aid in the detection of papillary muscle dysfunction or rupture.[62] Parasternal and apical long axis views may demonstrate failure of one or both mitral leaflets to reach their normal systolic position in the plane of the mitral anulus ("incomplete leaflet closure"[63]) with associated left ventricular free wall dysfunction at the base of a papillary muscle. Anterior leaflet involvement is universal, regardless of which papillary muscle is invovled, with posterior leaflet dysfunction occurring in a smaller percentage of cases. Papillary muscle rupture is suggested by the presence of a flail mitral leaflet with systolic prolapse into the left atrium. A mass of tissue representing the ruptured papillary muscle head may accompany the flail leaflet.[62] The major differential diagnostic consideration in papillary muscle rupture, ventricular septal rupture, may be visualized with apical or subxyphoid four-chamber or parasternal short axis views. Intravenous saline contrast injection may demonstrate the intraventricular communication by showing a negative contrast effect in the right ventricle or contast entering the left ventricle.[64] Doppler ultrasound may be useful to detect and help quantify both AMR and the shunt of VSR.[65,66] Radionuclide angiography can be used to demonstrate, help quantify, and differentiate AMR from the left-to-right shunt of ventricular septal rupture.[67] Cardiac catheterization may be done to confirm the diagnosis, assess hemodynamic severity, and evaluate associated coronary artery disease.

Chordal Rupture Although rupture of chordae tendinae may occur on the basis of infection, trauma, rheumatic heart disease, angina or infarction, underlying collagen disorders, or mitral valve prolapse syndrome, the majority of episodes occur spontaneously with grossly normal valves.[68] Spontaneous rupture occurs most frequently in males aged 40 to 60 years and involves the posterior mitral leaflet nine times more frequently than the anterior leaflet. Other etiologies do not have this characteristic age and sex distribution or proclivity for posterior leaflet involvement. The murmur of spontaneous chordal rupture frequently radiates to the base or left ventricular outflow tract and may be accompanied by a palpable thrill at the apex or, less commonly, the primary aortic area. This characteristic radiation results from rupture of chordae from the anterolateral papillary muscle to the lateral aspect of the posterior mitral leaflet with a resultant anterosuperiorly directed jet stream causing vibration of the intra-atrial septum and adjacent posterior aortic wall.[69,70] Thus, the murmur of posterior leaflet chordal rupture may be confused with aortic stenosis. Important findings favoring chordal rupture are a brisk carotid upstroke and wide splitting of the second heart sound with an early aortic component.

The chest film in chordal rupture reveals relatively normal left atrial and ventricular sizes, with pulmonary vascular congestion. The ECG shows normal sinus rhythm and may demonstrate a negative terminal P wave in lead V_1 attributed to left atrial pressure overload.[71] The two-dimensional echocardiogram is the most sensitive and specific noninvasive evaluation for the detection of chordal rupture.[72] Parasternal long axis or apical four-chamber views will show loss of systolic leaflet coaptation, systolic leaflet prolapse, and leaflet flutter throughout the cardiac cycle. The tip of the flail leaflet points toward the left atrium at end systole and toward the left ventricle at end diastole (Figure 15-2). Systolic vibration of the intra-atrial septum and posterior aortic wall may occur in spontaneous chordal rupture. Cardiac catheterization may be performed if the severity of the mitral regurgitant lesion is in question or associated vallvular abnormalities are suspected, and for the evaluation of coexistent coronary artery disease.

Therapy

The medical therapy of acute severe mitral

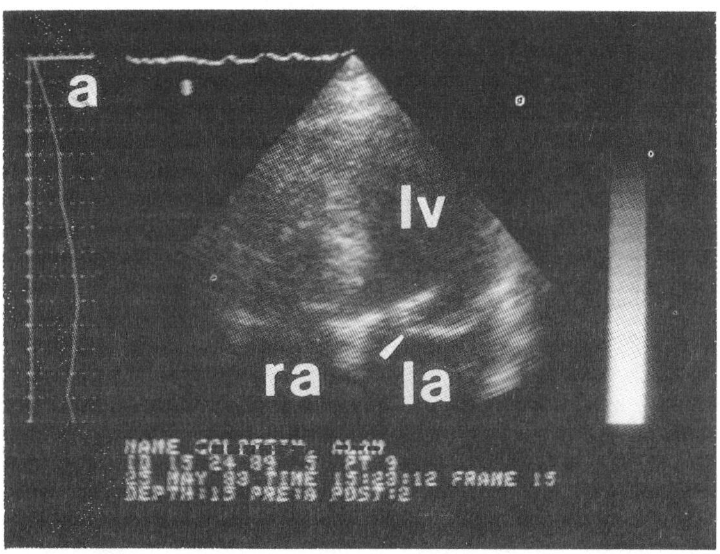

Figure 15-2 Two-dimensional echocardiogram, apical four-chamber view and systolic frame in a patient with flail posterior mitral leaflet. Flail posterior leaflet (arrow) is seen prolapsing in systole into the left atrium. RA = right atrium, LA = left atrium, LV = left ventricle.

regurgitation is directed toward reducing impedance to forward left ventricular outflow and toward lowering elevated left ventricular pressure and volume. Bedside hemodynamic monitoring should be performed with a balloon-tipped, flow-directed catheter. The magnitude of regurgitant volume is dependent on mitral regurgitant orifice size, systolic pressure gradient from left ventricle to left atrium, and the duration of left ventricular systole. Recent data suggest that mitral regurgitant orifice size is not static in disorders of the subvalve apparatus, but varies directly with left ventricular volume.[73] The relative importance of regurgitant orifice size can be demonstrated through an adaptation of the Gorlin formula: mitral regurgitant flow equals mitral regurgitant orifice size times the square root of the systolic pressure gradient across the valve (left ventricle to left atrium). Viewed in this context, one can appreciate the importance of even minor changes in orifice size relative to similar changes in the pressure gradient. A reduction in left ventricular volume will reduce regurgitant orifice size and thus the severity of mitral regurgitation.

Nitroprusside is particularly useful therapeutic agent because of its ability to both lower systemic impedance and reduce left ventricular volume and, therefore, mitral regurgitant orifice size. Experimental observations suggest the latter mechanism to be the predominant beneficial influence of nitroprusside in acute mitral regurgitation.[74] Hydralazine may also be used to reduce systemic vascular resistance, but lacks the effect on left ventricular volume and mitral regurgitant orifice size seen with nitroprusside.[75] Further reductions in outflow impedance can be obtained with intra-aortic balloon counterpulsation.[76] The augmentation of aortic diastolic pressure with balloon pumping may improve coronary artery perfusion and allow more aggressive use of vasodilators such as nitroprusside. Further improvement in left ventricular function can be achieved by the addition of an inotropic agent, particularly dobutamine. Dobutamine is preferred over dopamine because the α-adrenergic agonist properties of the latter are at least of theoretical disadvantage with respect to left ventricular outflow impedance. Digoxin, with its delayed onset, difficult titration, and relatively low magnitude of inotropic effect is not recommended for therapy of acute severe mitral regurgitation. Rapid IV infusion of digoxin may increase systemic vascular resistance through a direct arteriolar constricting effect and exacerbate mitral regurgitation. Furosemide and nitrates may be useful in manipulating left atrial pressure to meet the desired response.

Mitral regurgitation from papillary muscle dysfunction or chordal rupture may markedly improve with institution of the above measures. Residual regurgitation may be managed with an oral regimen of digitalis, diuretics and hydralazine, if necessary. These patients may be treated medically until symptoms of mitral regurgitation become refractory to such treatment and consideration of surgical correction is necessary. Acute mitral regurgitation refractory to medical therapy may require early surgical intervention. The decision to intervene surgically should not be made without knowledge of the level of left ventricular function as both operative and alte postoperative survival is directly influenced by the preoperative left ventricular ejection fraction.[77,78] The choice of surgical procedure depends on the mechanism of AMR and the personal experience and preference of the surgeon. Many patients with chordal rupture are candidates for valve repair. Normal left ventricular geometry and papillary muscle function may be maintained with valve repair and long-term anticoagulation has not been necessary.[79–81] Mitral valve repair may also be used in patients with papillary muscle rupture by reattachment of the ruptured muscle head to the left ventricular wall or adjacent papillary muscle with Teflon felt reinforced mattress sutures.[82,83] Both operative and long-term mortality following mitral valve replacement for papillary muscle rupture are dependent on left ventricular function and are inversely related to the preoperative ejection fraction.[83,84] Although concomitant coronary bypass grafting does not appear to influence acute surgical mortality, improvement in long-term survival may accompany coronary revascularization.[83,84]

AORTIC STENOSIS

Aortic stenosis usually develops gradually, imposing an incremental pressure load on the left ventricle which is hemodynamically significant when aortic valve surface area reaches 0.75 cm^2 or less and the peak transvalvular pressure gradient in systole is 50 mmHg or greater in the presence of a normal cardiac output. Concentric left ventricular hypertrophy develops in an attempt to normalize systolic wall stress and preserve left ventricular stroke volume. Although myocardial hypertrophy is a key compensatory mechanism in preserving systolic ventricular function, the consequent increase in ventricular wall thickness and reduction in compliance results in elevation of left ventricular diastolic pressures. In patients with severe aortic stenosis, atrial contraction serves a particularly important "booster pump" function by augmenting left ventricular end-diastolic pressure and contributing substantially to left ventricular stroke volume.[85] The loss of appropriately timed, vigorous atrial contractions may precipitate clinical deterioration.

Any event causing cardiovascular decompensation in the patient with significant aortic stenosis presents an emergent situation. Excessive reduction in preload accompanying the osmotic diuresis following contrast angiography, vigorous diuretic therapy, the use of vasodilators, or gastrointestinal (GI) hemorrhage may precipitate a fall in cardiac output and systemic hypotension. The increase in myocardial oxygen consumption and reduction in diastolic coronary perfusion time and pressure accompanying reflex tachycardia are poorly tolerated by the hypertrophied left ventricle. In patients with significant aortic stenosis, the capacity of the coronary arteries to increase flow above resting levels (coronary vascular reserve) to meet an increase in myocardial oxygen demand may be reduced in rough proportion to the degree of left ventricular hypertrophy.[86] This limited coronary reserve may further compromise oxygen supply and may contribute to the development of ischemia, even in the absence of significant coronary obstructions. The loss of atrial transport function accompanying atrial fibrillation or atrioventricular dissociation, as noted above, may also precipitate clinical deterioration.

Clinical Features

In previously unsuspected cases, the diagnosis of critical aortic stenosis must be arrived at quickly. The cardinal symptoms of aortic stenosis, including angina, syncope, and congestive heart failure, should be sought. Palpation of the carotid artery reveals a slowly rising, low-amplitude impulse frequently with an anacrotic shoulder or transmitted shudder. A bisferiens impulse suggests significant valvular insufficiency. Although narrowing of the systemic arterial pulse pressure may accompany severe aortic stenosis, older patients with arterial inelasticity and consequent elevation in systolic blood pressure may have a wide pulse pressure in the presence of severe valvular obstruction.[87] The apical impulse is widened, sustained, and nondisplaced in the absence of ventricular dilatation and a prominent presystolic impulse is frequently present. A palpable lag time between the onset of apical and carotid impulses may be appreciated on simultaneous palpation.[88] A fourth heart sound is almost always present and the first heart sound is diminished in intensity. the aortic component of the second heart sound is delayed in occurrence and diminished in intensity. Marked prolongation of left ventricular systole may result in reversed splitting of the second sound. The systolic ejection murmur of aortic stenosis has an intensity and duration that bears a rough relationship to the severity of stenosis in the absence of valvular insufficiency or congestive heart failure. A reduction in gradient and therefore the intensity of the murmur will accompany a fall in cardiac output, but the murmur remains audible even in the moribund patient.

The ECG may provide supportive evidence of the diagnosis and will show typical changes of left ventricular hypertrophy in 85% of cases where significant valvular obstruction exists.[89] Abnormalities in intraventricular and atrioventricular conduction are more common with aortic stenosis than with other valvular lesions.[90] These include varying degrees of atrioventricular block, left anterior hemiblock, bundle-branch block, and intraventricular conduction defect. The rhythm is usually sinus and the occurrence of atrial fibrillation suggests left ventricular failure or associated coronary or mitral valve disease.[91]

The chest film will demonstrate poststenotic dilatation of the ascending aorta in 80% or more of patients with significant aortic stenosis, but the degree of dilatation bears no relationship to the severity of the stenosis. The aortic valve should be assessed for the presence of calcium on the routine chest roentgenogram, as well as by fluoroscopy. The absence of calcium in subjects over the age of 40 years virtually excludes the presence of significant valvular aortic stenosis.[92] However, marked calcification can be present in the absence of significant obstruction. Fluoroscopy done at the bedside with a portable unit can provide valuable information in the acute assessment of previously undiagnosed aortic stenosis.

Two-dimensional echocardiography, quickly and conveniently done at the bedside, can both detect and estimate the severity of aortic stenosis. Leaflet thickening and impaired mobility is universally present in severe cases. By measuring the maximum aortic cusp separation in the long axis or the valve surface area directly in the short axis, a rough approximation of the severity of obstruction can be obtained. In combined series, all patients with critical aortic valve stenosis (valve surface area $\leqslant 0.75\ cm^2$) have had a maximal cusp separation or 11 mm or less.[93] Cusp separation of 13 mm or more has high predictive accuracy for mild stenosis. Direct assessment of aortic valve surface area in adults with calcific aortic stenosis may be extremely difficult as the orifice is often small, irregular, and densely calcified. In those patients in whom a well-defined orifice can be recorded, however, there is a reasonable correlation between the echocardiographic and hemodynamic estimation of orifice size.[94] Qualitative evaluation of aortic leaflet motion helps to identify those patients in whom maximal cusp separation alone may overestimate the severity of stenosis. Indirect estimation of the severity of aortic stenosis can be obtained by assessing left ventricular wall thickness or left atrial size.[95] Pulsed and continuous-wave Doppler techniques combined with echocardiography can demonstrate the level of obstruction. The peak pressure drop across the orifice can be calculated from the maximum velocity recorded and has relatively good correlation with catheterization data.[96,97]

Once the diagnosis of critical aortic stenosis has been established, valve replacement can be performed electively in the stable patient. If the severity of stenosis has not been determined, cardiac catheterization with direct determination of the transvalvular gradient should be performed, if the clinical situation permits. As this gradient is flow-dependent, it must be interpreted in the context of a simultaneously obtained cardiac output. Aortic valve surface area can then be calculated from these data.

Coronary angiography should be performed, if possible, so that saphenous vein bypass of significant stenoses can be done at the time of valve replacement. In the moribund patient, catheterization imposes added risk and delays urgent valve replacement. Reliance on clinical examination and noninvasive evaluation must suffice in this situation. Medical treatment of acute decompensation in the patient with critical aortic stenosis should be directed toward the precipitating event when one can be identified. Electrical cardioversion of atrial fibrillation or flutter should be attempted promptly. Subsequent treatment with digoxin and a type 1 antiarrhythmic agent may prevent recurrence or better control the ventricular response, if atrial fibrillation should recur prior to valve replacement. High-degree atrioventricular block should be treated by insertion of a temporary pacemaker, to be replaced by a permanent pacemaker at the time of valve surgery. Hypotension may be corrected by volume replacement if pulmonary congestion is not present. Since vigorous volume infusion in the face of diminished left ventricular compliance can precipitate pulmonary edema, close hemodynamic monitoring with a flow-directed, balloon-tipped catheter is often necessary.

Hypotension not rapidly responsive to volume infusion requires hemodynamic evaluation and treatment with inotropic and/or pressor agents. Dobutamine, by improving the force of left ventricular contraction, may increase forward output and lower the pulmonary capillary wedge pressure. Although some improvement in arterial pressure may accompany the increase in cardiac output from dobutamine, the α-adrenergic stimulation of dopamine will be more effective in raising arterial pressure directly. A combination of these agents may be useful for maintaining arterial pressure and improving forward output.[98] Relief of pulmonary congestion is best accomplished with a loop diuretic. Attempts at pharmacologic afterload reduction are not advised. Such attempts are unlikely to alter the fixed obstruction to left ventricular outflow imposed by a stenotic valve and may have the detrimental effect of lowering coronary perfusion pressure. For similar reasons, effective afterload reduction cannot be expected to accompany intra-aortic balloon counterpulsation. However, augmentation of diastolic blood pressure may improve ischemic left ventricular dysfunction, particularly if maximum coronary autoregulation has already occurred. Flow to ischemic myocardium in situations of limited coronary vascular reserve may be highly pressure-dependent, and thus improved by the diastolic pressure augmentation achieved with balloon counterpulsation. Such measures are only temporal and valve replacement on an emergent basis should be performed on patients with clinical deterioration.

Critical aortic stenosis is most effectively treated by surgical valve replacement. Improvement in left ventricular function with regression of left ventricular hypertrophy, and improved long-term survival, will follow valve replacement in the vast majority of patients.[99,100] While elective aortic valve replacement can be accomplished with less than 5% operative mortality, replacement on an emergency basis has approximately a 10% mortality in combined series.[101,102]

Operative mortality is greatest in those patients suffering preoperative cardiac arrest, shock, or renal failure, and valve replacement should be performed, if at all possible, prior to the occurrence of these events.

MITRAL STENOSIS

Although the natural history of mitral stenosis (MS) is one of gradual progression following the onset of symptoms, certain clinical situations may be associated with abrupt hemodynamic deterioration requiring emergent treatment. The most common event precipitating clinical deterioration in mitral stenosis is atrial fibrillation, which will occur in 30% to 50% of patients with symptomatic MS. Atrial fibrillation may be transient, associated only with palpitations, or sustained, causing pulmonary venous hypertension. The clinical impact of atrial fibrillation on the patient with MS is determined by the resultant ventricular rate much more so than the loss of atrial contraction per se.[103,104] With a rapid ventricular response, left atrial pressure rises abruptly, causing pulmonary congestion or frank pulmonary edema. Pulmonary venous and arterial pressure rise passively with little or no change in pulmonary vascular resistance. Left ventricular stroke volume and forward cardiac output fall from the loss of atrial contribution and the abbreviation of diastolic filling time, causing varying degrees of systemic hypoperfusion. Although these changes are most frequently seen in association with atrial fibrillation, they may accompany any supraventricular tachyarrhythmia with a rapid ventricular response.[105,106]

Clinical Features

Dyspnea, orthopnea, and cough, the symptoms of pulmonary congestion, predominate. When congestion is severe, frothy pink or blood-tinged sputum may be expectorated. Bronchial edema may precipitate wheezing (cardiac asthma) causing confusion with primary airway hyperactivity. On examination of the precordium, a palpable pulmonary arterial pulsation or pulmonic valve closure in the second left intercostal space denotes pulmonary hypertension. An accentuated first heart sound may be felt at the lower left sternal border or apex and may be accompanied by a palpable diastolic thrill. The ausculatory hallmarks of mitral stenosis include accentuation of the first heart sound, a low frequency diastolic rumble at the apex, and a mitral valve opening snap characteristically following aortic valve closure by 60 to 80 ms. The interval between aortic valve closure and mitral opening snap is inversely proportional to the level of left atrial pressure in normal sinus rhythm. This interval will vary directly with R-R cycle length in atrial fibrillation.

Laboratory Findings

When atrial fibrillation precipitates clinical deterioration, the ventricular response is usually in excess of 130 beats/min. Rightward deviation of the frontal plane QRS axis is common and evidence of right ventricular hypertrophy may be found. The chest film will show evidence of an enlarged left atrium causing straightening of the left heart border. Posterior and rightward displacement of the esophagus, elevation of the left main bronchus, or a double-density at the right heart border. Redistribution of pulmonary venous and arterial flow to upper lung zones is characteristic of mitral stenosis and may be associated with varying degrees of interstitial and alveolar pulmonary edema. The presence of Kerley B lines caused by thickened interlobular septae has been correlated with mean left atrial pressures in excess of 20 mmHg.[107]

The noninvasive diagnosis of mitral stenosis can be made echocardiographically by finding thickened mitral valve leaflets, a reduction in mitral diastolic closing velocity, or e-f slope and an abnormal pattern of anterior movement of the posterior mitral leaflet in diastole. Two-dimensional echocardiography will demonstrate doming of the mitral valve in diastole and the mitral orifice size can be determined in the parasternal short axis view.[108,109] The left atrium should be evaluated for the presence of thrombus.[110] Echocardiography, combined with Doppler techniques, is helpful in both the qualitative and quantitative assessment of mitral stenosis.[97] Doppler recording can be used to obtain an estimate of transmitral gradient and, thus, calculated mitral valve surface area.[111]

The therapeutic approach to tachyarrhythmias in patients with mitral stenosis is determined by the severity of hemodynamic compromise. Frank pulmonary edema associated with systemic hypoperfusion is most effectively treated with prompt electrical cardioversion using an energy level of at lealst 100 watt-seconds. Immediately following cardioversion the patient should receive a loading dose of 1.0 to 1.5 mg of digoxin in divided doses over 24 hours, followed by a daily maintenance dose adjusted for renal function, so that ventricular rate will be better controlled should atrial fibrillation recur. The addition of quinidine or procainamide hydrochloride may help prevent recurrence. Less severe degrees of pulmonary congestion in the presence of adequate systemic perfusion can be managed pharmacologically with a diuretic to help reduce left atrial pressure, as well as with agents directed at slowing the heart rate. Although digoxin is most frequently used, propranolol hydrochloride, verapamil, or diltiazem hydrochloride may also be effective. These agents may be given orally or IV, depending on the urgency of the situation, to bring the heart rate to 100 beats-min or less. When given IV, verapamil is the most rapidly acting, having a peak effect on the ventricular response within five minuts of an IV dose.[112] An initial dose of 5 mg IV may be followed in ten minutes by a 10-mg dose, if heart rate does not slow appropriately. Verapamil is the pharmacologic treatment of choice for supraventricular tachycardia from atrioventricular nodal reentry. In the patient who has already received digoxin, the addition of small doses of propranolol may be effective in further slowing the ventricular rate in atrial fibrillation.

Other etiologies pertinent to the differential diagnosis of mitral stenosis include left atrial ball valve thrombus, large endocarditic vegetations, and left atrial tumors. Obstruction by thrombus or vegetation most frequently complicates underlying rheumatic mitral stenosis. Treatment centers on surgical excision of the obstructing mass. There are no available data on the use of fibrinolytic agents in the treatment of mitral valve obstruction from left atrial thrombus.

PROSTHETIC HEART VALVES

The development of prosthetic heart valves has been a major advance in cardiovascular medicine. However, significant complications, at times life-threatening, may accompany the use of these devices.[113] All prostheses currently in use are intrinsically stenotic, resulting in a small pressure gradient at rest. Severe prosthetic stenosis may arise from intrinsic valve dysfunction, prosthesis chamber disproportion, valve thrombosis, and the vegetations of infective endocarditis. Extrinsic obstruction of the valve orifice may result from pannus ingrowth or extension of left atrial thrombus.[114,115]

Silicon ball swelling (ball variance) in the early model Starr-Edwards ball-in-cage prostheses occasionally caused trapping of the ball in the closed position, but this does not occur in newer models. Interference with tilting disc or ball motion may occur when the valve is too large for the chamber in which it rests (prosthesis chamber disproportion).[116] This is a particular problem with ball-in-cage prostheses in the mitral position, but may also occur with lower profile tilting disc designs.

The clinical findings accompanying prosthetic valve thrombosis are those of pulmonary edema, low cardiac output, and occasionally syncope. Prosthetic valve sounds may be changed in intensity and timing or absent. Murmurs consistent with valve stenosis are usually present. With the Bjork-Shiley prosthesis, thrombosis usually obliterates the smaller valve aperture causing fixation of the disc, which normally opens 60° in the direction of flow at a 45° to 60° angle.[117] This results in both stenosis and insufficiency and the vast majority of these patients will have both systolic and diastolic murmurs on examination.

Interference with tilting disc motion causing valve stenosis has also resulted from tissue overgrowth around the sewing ring, migration of suture material, or trapped residue of chordal tissue.[118] Left atrial thrombus or vegetations from infective endocarditis may cause severe obstruction of a mitral prosthesis. Fibrosis and calcification of xenograft prostheses may hinder leaflet motion and result in progressive stenosis. This occurs more frequently in young persons and in the presence of abnormalities in calcium metabolism.[119,120]

Normal mechanical prostheses may be associated with some degree of closure backflow or regurgitation, particularly under conditions of low cardiac output and tachycardia.[121] Significant prosthetic insufficiency results most commonly from disruption of the sutures between the sewing ring and valve annulus. Spontaneous suture dehiscence is more frequently found in the presence of heavy calcification of the mitral annulus or aortic root and in patients with myxomatous degeneration. Dehiscence may also result from prosthetic valve infective endocarditis. Prosthetic thrombosis may interfere with disc or poppet motion and result in regurgitation as noted previously. Xenograft prostheses, particularly in the mitral position, are subject to mechanical damage, calcification, and immunologically mediated host rejection, which may culminate in leaflet tear or rupture.[122,123]

Although regurgitant murmurs usually accompany valve dehiscence, clinical examination may be difficult, especially in the postoperative period. Prosthesis dehiscence should be suspected in any patient with postoperative hemodynamic deterioration, even when a murmur is absent. The noninvasive evaluation of prosthetic dysfunction may utilize the phonocardiogram, fluoroscopy, echocardiogram, Doppler ultrasound, or spectral analysis. Phonocardiographic analysis of the presence and timing of prosthetic sounds is particularly useful if baseline postoperative studies are available.[124,125] Lengthening of the second heart sound to mitral valve opening may indicate sticking or immobility of the tilting disc or ball. Shortening of this interval may accompany an increased left atrial pressure resulting from valvular obstruction or paravalvular leak. Valve opening sounds appear to occur more frequently with Ionescu-Shiley prostheses than with porcine valves and have acoustic qualities similar to those of mechanical prostheses.[126] Fluoroscopic evaluation of the prosthetic valve ring may detect excessive movement or rocking consistent with dehiscence. This should be considered in Bjork-Shiley prostheses when the angle of tilt exceeds 6° in the aortic and 10° in the mitral position.[127] The movement of a poppet or disc occulder may be evaluated as well.

Two-dimensional and M-mode echocardiography may provide complementary information in the evaluation of prosthetic valves. Two-dimensional echocardiography is superior to M-mode technique in detecting primary failure of bioprosthetic valves,[128] but mechanical prostheses may be difficult to evaluate due to the highly reflective nature of their inert components, requiring lower gain settings for better visualization. Combined M-mode echocardiography and phonocardiography are particularly useful in relating auscultatory events to valve motion. A rounded upstroke in opening and down stroke in closing may accompany the reduced velocity of disc movement with thrombosis of the Bjork-Shiley valve.[129] Normal displacement of the tilting disc in this prosthesis averages 1.4 cm.[130] An early "diastolic hump" on the M-mode echocardiogram has been seen with valve dehiscence and exaggerted movement of the annulus.[131] Motion of an aortic prosthesis which is not concordant with that of the adjacent root, annulus, and upper interventricular septum suggests valvular dehiscence of between 40% to 95% of the annular circumference.[132] The normal porcine xenograft has three smooth contoured leaflets, 3 mm or less in thickness, attached to a sewing ring that moves in concert with the native valve anulus.[133,134] Leaflet thickening alone does not distinguish between leaflet changes due to degeneration and those due to growth of vegetations.[132] Prolapse of leaflet-associated echoes below the level of the prosthetic ring may be observed both with torn leaflets and leaflet vegetations. Although infrequently observed, the antegrade extension of leaflet-associated echoes to above the level of the prosthetic stents appears to be highly specific for the presence of vegetations.[132] The Ionescu-Shiley pericardial xenograft has a normal cusp excursion by M-mode echocardiogram of 19 mm in the aortic and 21 mm in the mitral position.[135] Echocardiography also gives valuable information about left ventricular function.

Pulsed wave or continuous Doppler ultrasound may detect and help quantify gradients across prosthetic valves.[136,137] An estimate of the peak gradient across a stenotic prosthesis can be obtained by placing the Doppler sample downstream from the valve and measuring the velocity of flow. The velocity across a stenotic valve can be directly related to the transvalvular pressure gradient by the Bernoulli equation:

$$\triangle P = \tfrac{1}{2}p \triangle V^2 - R$$

where P = pressure drop across the stenosis, p = density of the fluid, V = change in velocity, and R = viscus loss. This can be converted to pressure in mmHg and simplified so that the following relation exists

$$\triangle P = 4V^2$$

where P = transvalvular pressure gradient in mmHg and V = maximal velocity recorded in m/s. This latter equation can be readily used to calculate pressure gradients from the Doppler measured peak velocities, as illustrated in Figure 15-3. An approximation of valve surface can be derived for the mitral valve by first determining the mitral pressure half-time (time required for the transvalvular gradient to fall to half its initial value). As pressure can be determined from velocity (as noted above) pressure half-time ($P_{t\frac{1}{2}}$) can be expressed as the time required for initial velocity (V_0) to fall to a value equal to v_0 divided by the square root of 2 ($P_{t\frac{1}{2}} = v_0/\sqrt{2}$). An estimate of mitral valve area is obtained by dividing 220 by the pressure half-time expressed in milliseconds.[97]

Cardiac catheterization should be performed if there is a question in the diagnosis or if clinical and noninvasive evaluations are discrepant.[138] Catheterization may also be performed to evalu-

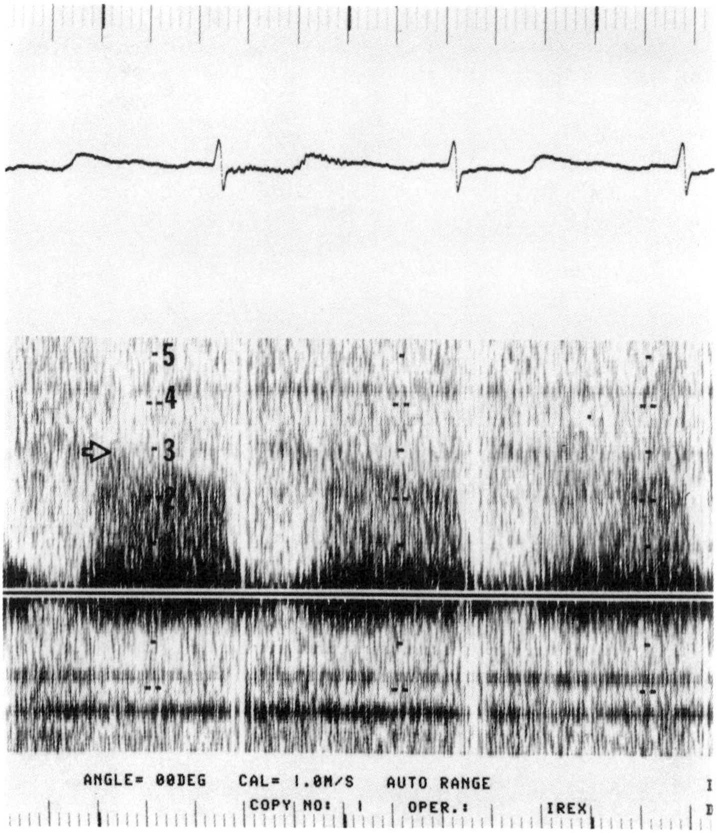

Figure 15-3 Continuous mode Doppler ultrasound record with the sample directed across the partially thrombosed Bjork-Shiley mitral prosthesis. Simultaneous ECG is shown above. The peak gradient across the valve can be determined from the peak velocity of the jet (arrow) which, in this example, is 3 m/s. This velocity corresponds with a peak gradient of 36 mmHg and a calculated valve orifice area of 0.6 cm^2.

ate associated disease of the coronary arteries or great vessels. When clinical findings consistent with severe valve dysfunction are corroborated by noninvasive techniques, catheterization entails an unnecessary risk and delays surgical correction.

The medical management of hemodynamic abnormalities accompanying prosthetic valve dysfunction parallels that of similar lesions affecting native valves. For pulmonary edema caused by stenotic left heart lesions, reduction in left atrial presure and improved forward output may be achieved by the judicious use of furosemide and dobutamine, as arterial pressure permits. Hypotension may require the addition of dopamine or other pressors. Regurgitant lesions can be managed with vasodilators and inotropic agents, as noted previously.

Thrombolytic agents (streptokinase, urokinase) have been used in the medical treatment of prosthetic valve thrombosis.[139–142] These may be particularly useful for thrombolysis of tricuspid valve prosthesis, where hemodynamic deterioration usually follows a subacute course. Resolution of presumed thrombotic mitral or aortic prosthetic dysfunction has been reported following IV infusion of a thrombolytic agent. Use of these agents for left-sided prosthetic thrombosis is at this time experimental and should not delay surgery in the critically ill patient.

Prosthetic valve replacement can be accomplished with a mortality between 5% and 15%.[143,144] Mortality is proportional to the severity of preoperative hemodynamic compromise; therefore, surgery must be performed early, before significant deterioration occurs. In cases of prosthetic valve thrombosis, thrombectomy without valve replacement may be performed, and appears more easily achieved with aortic than with mitral prostheses.[145]

REFERENCES

1. Morganroth J, Perloff JK, Zeldis Sm, et al: Acute severe aortic regurgitation, pathophysiology, clinical recognition and management. *Ann Intern Med* 1977;87:233–232.
2. Wigle ED, Labrosse CJ: Sudden, severe aortic insufficiency. *Circulation* 1965;32:708–20.
3. Hodgkin T: On retroversion of the valves of the aorta. *London Medical Gazette* 1829;(March 7): 433–443.
4. Flint A: On cardiac murmurs. *Am J Med Sci* 1862;44:29–54.
5. Laniado S, Yellin EL, Yoran C, et al: Physiologic mechanisms in aortic insufficiency. I. The effect of changing heart rate on flow dynamics. II. Determinants of Austin-Flint murmur. *Circulation* 1982;66:226–235.
6. Dalen JE, Pape LA, Conn LH, et al: Dissection of the aorta: pathogenesis, diagnosis and treatment. *Prog Cardiovasc Dis* 1980;23:237–245.
7. Slater EE, DeSanctis RW: The clinical recognition of dissecting aortic aneurysm. *Am J Med* 1976;60:625–633.
8. Parmley LF, Manion WC, Mattingly TW: Nonpenetrating traumatic injury of the heart. *Circulation* 1958;18:371–396.
9. Payne DD, Deweese JA, Mahoney EB, et al: Surgical treatment and traumatic rupture of the normal aortic valve. *Ann Thorac Surg* 1974;17: 223–229.
10. McIlduff JB, Foster ED: Disruption of a normal aortic valve as a result of blunt chest trauma. *J Trauma* 1978;18:373–375.
11. Jackson DH, Murphy GW: Nonpenetrating cardiac trauma. *Mod Concepts Cardiovasc Dis* 1976; 45:123–128.
12. Symbas PN: Traumatic heart disease. *Cur Probl Cardiol* 1982;7:1–35.
13. Najafi H, Dye WS, Javia H, et al: Rupture of an otherwise normal aortic valve. Report of two cases and review of the literature. *J Thorac Cardiovasc Surg* 1968;56:57–62.
14. Arnett EN, Roberts WC: Valve ring abscess in active infective endocarditis: frequency, location and clues to clinical diagnosis from the study of 95 necropsy patients. *Circulation* 1976;54: 140–145.
15. Baron MG: Dissecting aneurysm of the aorta. *Circulation* 1971;43:933–943.
16. Imaizumi T, Orita Y, Koiwaya Y, et al: Utility of two-dimensional echocardiography in the differential diagnosis of the etiology of aortic regurgitation. *Am Heart J* 1982;103:887–896.
17. Smuckler AL, Nomeir AM, Watts E, et al: Echocardiographic diagnosis of aortic root dissection by M-mode and two-dimensional techniques. *Am Heart J* 1982;103:897–904.
18. Come PC: Improved cross-sectional echocardiographic technique for visualization of the retrocardiac descending aorta in its long axis. *Am J Cardiol* 1983;51:1029–1033.
19. Brown OR, Popp RL, Kloster FE: Echocardiographic criteria for aortic root dissection. *Am J Cardiol* 1975;36:17–21.
20. Victor MF, Mintz GS, Kotler MN, et al: Two-dimensional echocardiographic diagnosis of aortic dissection. *Am J Cardiol* 1981;48:1155–1160.
21. Rubenson DS, Fowles RE, Miller DC, et al: Spontaneous dissection of the ascending aorta diagnosed by two-dimensional echocardiography. *Chest* 1981;8:587–591.
22. Gay JA, Gottdiener JS, Gomes MN, et al: Echocardiographic features of traumatic disruption of the aortic valve. *Chest* 1983;83:150–151.
23. Strom J, Becker R, Davis R, et al: Echocardiographic and surgical correlations in bacterial endocarditis. Circulation 1980;62(suppl 1): 164–167.
24. Wann LS, Dillon JC, Weyman AE, et al: Echocardiography in bacterial endocarditis. *N Engl J Med* 1976;295:135–139.
25. Stewart JA, Silimperi D, Harris P, et al: Echocardiographic documentation of vegetative lesions in infective endocarditis: clinical implications. *Circulation* 1980;61:374–380.
26. Griffiths BE, Petch MC, English TAH: Echocardiographic detection of subvalvular aortic root aneurysm extending to mitral valve annulus as complication of aortic valve endocarditis. *Br Heart J* 1982;47:392–396.
27. Miller FA, Seward JB, Gersh BT, et al: Two-dimensional echocardiographic findings in cardiac trauma. *Am J Cardiol* 1982;50:1022–1027.
28. Botvinick EH, Schiller NB, Wickramasekaran R, et al: Echocardiographic demonstration of early mitral valve closure in severe aortic insufficiency. It clinical implications. *Circulation* 1975; 51:836–847.
29. Weaver WF, Wilson CS, Rourke T, et al: Mid-diastolic aortic valve opening in severe acute aortic regurgitation. *Circulation* 1977; 55: 145–148.
30. Boughner DR. Assessment of arotic insufficiency by transcutaneous doppler ultrasound. *Circulation* 1975;52:874–879.
31. Myerowitz PD, Turnipseed ND, Shaw CG, et al: Computerized fluoroscopy. New technique for the noninvasive evaluation of the aorta, coronary artery bypass grafts and left ventricular function. *J Thorac Cardiovasc Surg* 1982;83:65–73.
32. Brundage BH, Lipton MJ: The emergence of computed tomography as a cardiovascular diagnostic technique. *Am Heart J* 1982;103:313–316.
33. Mills J, Abbott J, Utley JR, et al: Role of cardiac catherization in infective endocarditis. *Chest* 1977;72:576–581.
34. Miller RR, Vismara LA, DeMaria AN, et al: Afterload reduction therapy with nitroprusside in severe aortic regurgitation: Improved cardiac performance and reduced regurgitant volume. *Am J Cardiol* 1976;38:564–567.
35. Greenberg BH, DeMots H, Murphy E, et al: Mechanism for improved cardiac performance with arteriolar dilators in aortic insufficiency. *Circulation* 1981;63:263–268.
36. Moulopoulos SD, Anthopoulos LP, Antonatos PG, et al: Intra-aortic balloon pump for relief of aortic regurgitation. Experimental study. *J Thorac*

Cardiovasc Surg 1980;80:38–44.
37. Griffin FM, Jones G, Cobbs CG: Aortic insufficiency in bacterial endocarditis. *Ann Intern Med* 1972;76:23–29.
38. Young JB, Welton DE, Raizner AE, Surgery in active infective endocarditis. *Circulation* 1979; 60(suppl 1):77–81.
39. Croft CH, Woodward W, Elliot A, et al: Analysis of surgical versus medical therapy in active complicated native valve infective endocarditis. *Am J Cardiol* 1983;51:1650–1655.
40. Cukingnan RA, Carey JS, Wittig JH, et al: Early valve replacement in active infective endocarditis. Results and late survival. *J Thorac Cardiovasc Surg* 1983;85:163–173.
41. Parrott JCW, Hill JD, Kerth WJ, et al: The surgical management of bacterial endocarditis. A review. *Ann Surg* 1976;183:289–292.
42. Stinson EB: Surgical treatment of infective endocarditis. *Prog Cardiovasc Dis* 1979;22:145–148.
43. Dinubile MJ: Surgery in active endocarditis. *Ann Intern Med* 1982;96:650–659.
44. Symbas PN, Vlasis SE, Zacharopoulos L, et al: Acute endocarditis: surgical treatment of aortic regurgitation and aortico-left ventricular discontinuity. *J Thorac Cardiovasc Surg* 1982;84: 291–296.
45. Bailey WW, Ivey TD, Miller DW: Dacron patch closure of aortic annulus mycotic aneurysms. *Circulation* 1982;66(suppl 1);127–130.
46. Meng RL, Natafi H, Jauid H, et al: Acute ascending aortic dissection: surgical management. *Circulation* 1981;64(suppl 1):231–234.
47. Miller DC, Stinson EB, Oyer PE, et al: Operative treatment of aortic dissections, experience with 125 patients over a sixteen year period. *J Thorac Cardiovasc Surg* 1979;78:365–382.
48. Cachera JP, Vouche PR, Loisance DY, et al: Surgical management of acute dissections involving the ascending aorta. *J Thorac Cardiovasc Surg* 1981;82:576–584.
49. Kouchoukos NT, Kard RB, Leil WA: Replacement of the ascending aorta and aortic valve with a composite graft: results in 25 patients. *Ann Thorac Surg* 1977;24:140–148.
50. Sasayama S, Takahashi M, Osakada G, et al: Dynamic geometry of the left atrium and left ventricle in acute mitral regurgitation. *Circulation* 1979;60:177–186.
51. Sasayama S, Takahashi M, Kawai C: Left atrial function in acute mitral regurgitation. *Herz* 1981; 6:156–165.
52. Linhart JW, Hildner FJ, Barold SS, et al: A hemodynamic study of acute mitral valvar regurgitation in man. *Chest* 1970;57:22–27.
53. Sanders CA, Armstrong PW, Willerson JT, et al: Etiology and differential diagnosis of acute mitral regurgitation. *Prog Cardiovasc Dis* 1971;14: 129–150.
54. DeBusk RF, Harrison DC: The clinical spectrum of papillary muscle disease. *N Engl J Med* 1969; 281:1458–1467.
55. Wei JY, Hutchins GM, Bulkley BH: Papillary muscle rupture in fatal acute myocardial infarction. *Ann Intern Med* 1979;90:149–152.
56. Heikkila J: Mitral incompetence as a complication of acute myocardial infarction. *Acta Med Scand Suppl* 1967;475:7–149.
57. Meister SG, Helfant RH: Rapid bedside differentiation of ruptured interventricular septum from acute mitral insufficiency. *N Engl J Med* 1972;287:1024–1025.
58. Fuchs RM, Heuser RR, Yin FP, et al: Limitations of pulmonary wedge V waves in diagnosing mitral regurgitation. *Am J Cardiol* 1982;49: 849–854.
59. Pichard AD, Kay R, Smith H, et al: Large V waves in the pulmonary wedge tracing in the absence of mitral regurgitation. *Am J Cardiol* 1982;50:1044–1050.
60. Bethea CF, Peter RH, Behar VS, et al: The hemodynamic simulation of mitral regurgitation in ventricular septal defect after myocardial infarction. *Cathet Cardiovasc Diagn* 1976;2: 97–104.
61. Carley JE, Wong BYS, Pugh DM, et al: Clinical significance of the V wave in the main pulmonary artery. *Am J Cardiol* 1977;39:982–985.
62. Mintz GS, Victor MF, Kotler MN, et al: Two-dimensional echocardiographic identification of surgically correctable complications of acute myocardial infarction. *Circulation* 1981;64: 91–96.
63. Godley RW, Wann LS, Rogers EW, et al: Incomplete mitral leaflet closure in patients with papillary muscle dysfunction. *Circulation* 1981; 63:565–572.
64. Drobac M, Gilbert B, Howard R, et al: Ventricular septal defect after myocardial infarction: diagnosis by two-dimensional contrast echocardiography. *Circulation* 1983;67:335–341.
65. Stevenson JG, Kawabori I, Dooley TK, et al: Diagnosis of ventricular septal defect by pulsed Doppler echocardiography — sensitivity, specificity, limitations. *Circulation* 1978;58:322–329.
66. Abbasi AS, Allen MW, DeCristofaro D, et al: Detection and estimation of the degree of mitral regurgitation by range-gated pulsed Doppler echocardiography. *Circulation* 1980;61:143–147.
67. Hecht HJS, Zibelli LR: First pass radionuclide angiography in visualization of acute myocardial infarction, ventricular septal defect and assessment of ventricular function. *Am Heart J* 1982; 103:436–438.
68. Selzer A, Kelley JJ, Vannitamby M, et al: The syncrome of mitral insufficiency due to isolated rupture of the chordae tendineae. *Am J Med* 1967;43:822–836.
69. Antman EM, Angoff GH, Sloss LT: Demonstration of the mechanism by which mitral regurgitation mimics aortic stenosis. *Am J Cardiol* 1978; 42:1044–1048.
70. Tei C, Tanaka H, Nakao S, et al: Motion of the interatrial septum in acute mitral regurgitation. *Circulation* 1980;62:1080–1088.
71. Cooksey J, Parker BM, Aker U, et al: Mitral regurgitation secondary to ruptured chordae tendinease: Clinical, hymodynamic and electrocardiographic findings. *South Med J* 1976;69: 864–867.
72. Mintz GS, Kotler MN, Parry WR, et al: Statistical comparison of M-mode and two-dimensional echocardiographic diagnosis of flail mitral leaflets. *Am J Cardiol* 1980;45:253–259.

73. Yoran C, Yellin EL, Becker RM, et al: Dynamic aspects of acute mitral regurgitation: effects of ventricular volume, pressure and contractility on the effective reguritant orifice area. *Circulation* 1979;60:170–176.
74. Yoran C, Yellin EL, Becker RM, et al: Mechanism of reduction of mitral regurgitation with vasodilator therapy. *Am J Cardiol* 1979;43: 773–777.
75. Greenberg BH, Massie BM, Brundage BH, et al: Beneficial effects of hydralazine in severe mitral regurgitation. *Circulation* 1978;58:273–279.
76. Gold HK, Leinbach RC, Sanders CA, et al: Intra-aortic balloon pumping for ventricular septal defect or mitral regurgitation complicating acute myocardial infarction. *Circulation* 1973;47: 1191–1196.
77. Phillips HR, Levine FH, Carter J, et al: Mitral valve replacement for isolated mitral regurgitation: Analysis of clinical course and late postoperative left ventricular ejection fraction. *Am J Cardiol* 1981;48:647–654.
78. Kennedy JW, Doces JG, Stewart DK: Left ventricular function before and following surgical treatment of mitral valve disease. *Am Heart J* 1979;97:592–598.
79. Bonchek LI: Correction of mitral valve disease without valve replacement. *Am Heart J* 1982; 104:865–868.
80. Kay JH, Zubiate P, Mendex MA, et al: Surgical treatment of mitral insufficiency secondary to coronary artery disease. *J Thorac Cardiovasc Surg* 1980;79:12–18.
81. David TE, Uden DE, Strauss HD: The importance of the mitral apparatus in left ventricular function after correction of mitral regurgitation. *Circulation* 1983;68(suppl 2):76–82.
82. Gula G, Yacoub MH: Surgical correction of complete rupture of the anterior papillary muscle. *Ann Thorac Surg* 1981;32:88–91.
83. Merin G, Giuliani ER, Pluth JR, et al: Surgery for mitral valve incompetence after myocardial infarction. *Am J Cardiol* 1973;32:322–324.
84. Cohn LH: Surgical management of acute and chronic cardiac mechanical complications due to myocardial infarction. *Am Heart J* 1981;102: 1049–1060.
85. Stott DK, Marpole DGF, Bristow JD, et al: The role of left atrial transport in aortic and mitral stenosis. *Circulation* 1970;41:1031–1041.
86. Marcus ML, Doty DB, Hiratzka LF, et al: Decreased coronary reserve. A mechanism for angina pectoris in patients with aortic stenosis and normal coronary arteries. *N Engl J Med* 1982;307:1362–1366.
87. Andersen JA, Hansen BF, Lungborg K: Isolated valvular aortic stenosis. Clinicopathological findings in an autopsy material of elderly patients. *Acta Med Scand* 1975;197:61–64.
88. Chun PKC, Dunn BE: Clinical clue of severe aortic stenosis. Simultaneous palpation of the carotid and apical impulses. *Arch Intern Med* 1982;142:2284–2288.
89. Wood P: Aortic stenosis. *Am J Cardiol* 1958;1: 553–571.
90. Ohingra RC, Amat-Y-Leon F, Pietras R, et al: Sites of conduction disease in aortic stenosis. Significance of valve gradient and calcification. *Ann Intern Med* 1977;87:275–280.
91. Myler RK, Sanders CA: Aortic valve disease and atrial fibrillation. *Arch Intern Med* 1968;121: 530–533.
92. Glancy DL, Freed TA, O'Brien KP, et al: Calcium in the aortic valve; Roentgenologic and hemodynamic correlations in 148 patients. *Ann Intern Med* 1969;71:245–250.
93. Weyman AE: *Cross-Sectional Echocardiography*, Philadelphia, Lea & Febiger, 1982, pp 219–221.
94. Demaria AN, Bommer W, Joye J, et al: Value and limitations of cross-sectional echocardiography of the aortic valve in the diagnosis and quantification of valvular aortic stenosis. *Circulation* 1980;62:304–312.
95. Schwartz A, Vignola PA, Walker HJ, et al: Echocardiographic estimation of aortic valve gradient in aortic stenosis. *Ann Intern Med* 1978;89:329–335.
96. Hattle L: Non-invasive assessment and differentiation of left ventricular outflow obstruction with Doppler ultrasound. *Circulation* 1981;64: 381–387.
97. Stamm RB, Martin RP: Quantification of pressure gradients across stenotic valves by Doppler ultrasound. *J Am Coll Cardiol* 1983;2:707–718.
98. Richard C, Ricome JL, Rimailho A, et al: Combined hemodynamic effects of dopamine and dobutamine in cardiogenic shock. *Circulation* 1983;67:620–626.
99. Ross J: Left ventricular function and the timing of surgical treatment in valvular heart disease. *Ann Intern Med* 1981;94:498–504.
100. Schwarz F, Baumann P, Manthey J, et al: The effects of aortic valve replacement on survival. *Circulation* 1982;66:1105–1110.
101. Sanders JH, Cohn LH, Dalen JE, et al: Emergency aortic valve replacement. *Am J Surg* 1976;131:495–498.
102. Louw JWK, Kinsley RH, Dion RAE, et al: Emergency heart valve replacement: An analysis of 170 patients. *Ann Thorac Surg* 1980;29: 415–422.
103. Carleton RA, Graettinger JS: The hemodynamic role of the atria with and without mitral stenosis. *Am J Med* 1967;42:532–538.
104. Selzer A: Effects of atrial fibrillation upon the circulation in patients with mitral stenosis. *Am Heart J* 1960;59:518–526.
105. Thompson ME, Shaver JA, Leon DF: Effect of tachycardia on atrial transport in mitral stenosis. *Am Heart J* 1977;94:297–306.
106. Arani DT, Carleton RA: The deleterious role of tachycardia in mitral stenosis. *Circulation* 1967; 36:511–516.
107. Chen JTT, Behar VS, Morris JJ, et al: Correlation of roentgen findings with hemodynamic data in pure mitral stenosis. *Radiology* 1968;102: 280–292.
108. Nichol PM, Gilbert BW, Kisslo JA: Two-dimensional echocardiographic assessment of mitral stenosis. *Circulation* 1977;55:120–133.
109. Martin RP, Rakowski H, Cleinman JH, et al: Reliability and reproducibility of two-dimensional echocardiographic measurement of the stenotic mitral valve orifice area. *Am J Cardiol*

1979;43:560–568.

110. Shrestha NK, Moreno FL, Narciso FU, et al: Two-dimensional echocardiographic diagnosis of left atrial thrombus in rheumatic heart disease. A clinicopathologic study. *Circulation* 1983;67: 341–347.

111. Holen J, Simonsen S: Determination of pressure gradient in mitral stenosis with Doppler echocardiography. *Br Heart J* 1979;41:529–536.

112. Talano JV, Tommaso C: Slow channel calcium antagonists in the treatment of supraventricular tachycardia. *Prog Cardiovasc Dis* 1982;25: 141–156.

113. Kloster FE: Diagnosis and management of complications of prosthetic heart valves. *Am J Cardiol* 1975;35:872–885.

114. Braunwald NS, Morrow AG: Tissue ingrowth and the rigid heart valve. *J Thorac Cardiovasc Surg* 1968;56:307–322.

115. Shachar G, Vlodaver Z, Joyce LD, et al: Mural thrombosis of the left atrium following replacement of the mitral valve. *J Thorac Cardiovasc Surg* 1981;82:595–600.

116. Roberts WC. Complications of cardiac valve replacement: Characteristic abnormalities of prostheses pertaining to any or specific site. *Am Heart J* 1982;103:113–122.

117. Wright JO, Hiratzka LF, Grandt B, et al: Thrombosis of the Bjork-Shiley prosthesis. Illustrative cases and review of the literature. *J Thorac Cardiovasc Surg* 1982;84:138–144.

118. Williams DB, Pluth JR, Orszulak TA: Extrinsic obstruction of the Bjork-Shiley valve in the mitral position. *Ann Thorac Surg* 1981;32:58–62.

119. Hetzer R, Hill JD, Kerth WJ, et al: Thrombosis and degeneration of Hancock valves: Clinical and pathological findings. *Ann Thorac Surg* 1978;26: 317–322.

120. Schoen FJ, Collins JJ, Cohn LH: Long term failure rate and morphologic correlations in porcine bioprosthetic heart valves. *Am J Cardiol* 1983;51:957–964.

121. Dellsperger KC, Wieting DW, Baehr DA, et al: Regurgitation of prosthetic heart valves: dependence on heart rate and cardiac output. *Am J Cardiol* 1983;51:321–328.

122. Warnes CA, Scott ML, Silver GM, et al: Comparison of late degenerative changes in procine bioprostheses in the mitral and aortic valve position in the same patient. *Am J Cardiol* 1983; 51:965–968.

123. Rocchini AP, Weesner KM, Heidelberger K, et al: Porcine xenograft failure in children: An immunologic response. *Circulation* 1981;64 (suppl 2):162–171.

124. Brodie BR, Grossman W, McLaurin L, et al: Diagnosis of prosthetic mitral valve malfunction with combined echo-phonocardiography. *Circulation* 1976;53:93–100.

125. Cunha CLP, Giuliani ER, Callahan JA, et al: Echocardiographic findings in patients with prosthetic heart valve malfunction. *Mayo Clin Proc* 1980;55:231–242.

126. Szkopiec RL, Desser KB, Benchimol A, et al: Phonocardiographic findings in patients with normally functioning Ionescu-Shiley prostheses. *Am J Cardiol* 1983;51:969–972.

127. Heystraten FMJ, Paplman H: Cineradiographic evaluation of Bjork-Shiley mitral and aortic valves. A study of sixty cases. *Ann Radiol* 1981;24:346–348.

128. Kotler MN, Mintz GS, Panidis I, et al: Noninvasive evaluation of normal and abnormal prosthetic valve function. *J Am Coll Cardiol* 1983;2:151–173.

129. Bernal-Ramirez JA, Phillips J: Echocardiography study of malfunction of the Bjork-Shiley prosthetic heart valve in the mitral position. *Am J Cardiol* 1977;40:449–453.

130. Chandraratna PAN, Lopez JM, Hildner FJ, et al: Diagnosis of Bjork-Shiley aortic valve dysfunction by echocardiography. *Am Heart J* 1976;91: 318–324.

131. Jacovella G, Giampaolo P, Gabelli G, et al: Echocardiographic patterns of prosthetic valve malfunction. *Am J Cardiol* 1978;42:876.

132. Effron MK, Popp RL: Two-dimensional echocardiographic assessment of bioprosthetic valve dysfunction and infective endocarditis. *J Am Coll Cardiol* 1983;2:597–606.

133. Schapira JN, Martin RP, Fowles RE, et al: Two-dimensional echocardiographic assessment in patients with bioprosthetic valves. *Am J Cardiol* 1979;43:510–519.

134. Alam M, Madrazo AC, Magilligan DJ, et al: M-mode and two-dimensional echocardiographic features of porcine valve dysfunction. *Am J Cardiol* 1979;43:502–509.

135. Szkopiec RL, Torstveit J, Desser KB, et al: M-mode and two-dimensional echocardiographic characteristics of Ionescu-Shiley valve in the mitral and aortic positions. *Am J Cardiol* 1983; 51:973–980.

136. Hatle E: Pulsed and continuous wave Doppler in diagnosis and assessment of various heart lesions, in Gatle E, Angelsen B (eds): *Doppler Ultrasound in Cardiology*, ed 2. Philadelphia, Lea & Febiger, 1985, pp 121–126.

137. Wilkes HS, Berger M, Gallerstein PE, et al: Left ventricular outflow obstruction after aortic valve replacement: Detection with continuous wave doppler ultrasound recording. *J Am Coll Cardiol* 1983:1:550–553.

138. Morton MJ, McAnulty JH, Rahimtoola SH, et al: Risks and benefits of post-operative cardiac catheterization in patients with ball valve prostheses. *Am J Cardiol* 1977;40:870–875.

139. Witchitz S, Yeyrat C, Moisson P, et al: Fibrolytic treatment of thrombus and prosthetic heart valves. *Br Heart J* 1980;44:545–554.

140. Luluaga IT, Carrera D, d'Oliviera J: Successful thrombolytic therapy after acute tricuspid valve obstruction. Lancet 1971;1:1067–1068.

141. Inberg MV, Havia T, Arstila M: Thrombolytic treatment for thrombotic complication of valve prosthesis after tricuspid valve replacement. *Scand J Thorac Cardiovasc Surg* 1977;11: 195–198.

142. Witchitz S, Veyrat C, Moisson P, et al: Thromboses tardives des prostheses valvulaires mitrales et tricuspidiennes. Diagnostic phonomecanographique et traitement. *Ann Cardiol Angeiol* 1974;23:399–409.

143. Wideman FE, Blackstone EH, Kirklin JW, et al:

Hospital mortality of re-replacement of the aortic valve. *J Thorac Cardiovasc Surg* 1981;82: 692–698.

144. Cohn LH, Koster JK, Vandervanter S, et al: The in-hospital risk of re-replacement of dysfunctional mitral and aortic valves. *Circulation* 1982; 66(suppl 1):153–156.

145. Ayuso LA, Joffe A, Rufilanchas JJ, et al: Thrombectomy: Surgical treatment for the thrombosed Bjork-Shiley prosthesis. *J Thorac Cardiovasc Surg* 1982;84:906–910.

CHAPTER 16
Endocarditis

Randolph C. Byrd
Melvin D. Cheitlin

Endocarditis, more than most diseases, involves a diverse group of specialists in its treatment and prevention. The diagnosis is suspected by the primary care physician, the internist, or cardiologist, The treatment of the acute problem is the responsibility of the internist, the cardiologist, and the thoracic surgeon. In those patients who survive, there is frequently limitation in cardiac function due to valvular insufficiency and in those who have had surgery, there remains the problems related to the postoperative state — the patient with a prosthetic valve. Every effort is made to prevent infective endocarditis by health professionals involved in dentistry, gynecology, pediatrics, internal medicine, surgery and geriatrics. It is obvious that the problem of infection endocarditis is important to a wide variety of physicians.

DEFINITION

Endocarditis is commonly used to include any inflammatory or noninflammatory disease involving the endocardial lining of the heart or as endarteritis, the endothelial lining of the ascending aorta and pulmonary artery. It can be subdivided into infective and noninfective endocarditis. Pathologically, this disease is characterized grossly by a vegetation, primarily occuring on the cardiac valves but also on the endocardium of the ventricle, atrium, or in the large arteries. The vegetation consists of a collection of platelets and fibrin with or without bacterial organisms. This vegetation may occur at the attachment of foreign bodies placed in the heart as a result of operation including prosthetic or bioprosthetic valves, conduits, patches, baffles, sutures, and pacemaker leads. Infections involving pre-existing endocardial clots or myocardial tumors also come under the head of endocarditis.

Classically, infective endocarditis has been categorized as subacute and acute. This terminology, referring to the clinical status of the patient, has become less important as the picture of endocarditis changes with the advent of modern medicine and its numerous invasive procedures as well as the greater and earlier availability of medical treatment. With the decline in the frequency of chronic rheumatic heart disease and the rise in the frequency of intravenous (IV) drug abuse and prosthetic valve implants, a more useful classification of endocarditis is based on whether the involved valve is native or prosthetic, right- or left-sided, the type of organism involved, and whether the patient is or is not an IV drug abuser. In addition, the importance of thrombotic noninfective endocarditis is rising as the average age of the general population increases. Any proposed classification of endocarditis therefore should include the following descriptors: (1) infective or noninfective endocarditis, (2) valve or site involved, (3) causative organism(s), (4) whether the valve or site is native or prosthetic, and (5) whether the patient is an IV drug abuser.

PATHOGENESIS

Pre-existing cardiac disease increases the risk of infective endocarditis by causing injury to the endocardium of the heart and the endothelium of the great arteries. Intimal and endothelial injury results from jets of blood striking the walls, valves, and supporting structures in the heart.[1] Injury may also occur on the endocardium near an orifice from a Venturi effect.[2] Vegetations always occur on the low pressure side of the jet. Therefore the lesion occurs on the atrial surface of the mitral valve, or the endocardium of the atrium, in mitral insufficiency; and on the ventricular surface of the aortic valve, septum, or anterior leaflet of the mitral valve where the jet of aortic insufficiency strikes. The lesion occurs on the right ventricular endocardium in the patient with a small ventricular septal defect or on the crista supraventricularis or the septal leaflet of the tricuspid valve, and less frequently on the pulmonic valve. This also explains why it is more common to see endocarditis with small ventricular septal defects with high-velocity jets than with large ventricular septal defects with high pulmonary vascular resistance where there is no high-velocity jet.

When endocardial injury occurs, the underlying collagen matrix is exposed to a precipitating deposition of platelets and, subsequently, fibrin, which form a sterile platelet-fibrin micro-thrombus. Healing usually occurs without infection, even when bacteremia is present. Implantation does not occur due to the low invasive capability of the organisms or as a result of low numbers of circulating organisms as may occur with the simple act of brushing the teeth. Endocarditis may be more likely to occur when the number of circulating organisms is high as occurs after dental manipulation. Circulating antibodies may increase the adherence of the organism by clumping and holding larger numbers of organisms on the platelet-fibrin clot in the subacute form. Bacterial endocarditis can occur on apparently previously normal valves; thus the presence of previous valvular pathology is not essential. The organisms' inherent invasiveness and ability to adhere to the endocardial surface is much more important. Adherence is highest with *Staphylococcus aureus* and enterococci, lower with *Streptococcus viridans*, *S epidermidis*, and *Pseudomonas aeruginosa*, and least with *Escherichia coli*.[3,4] *S aureus* and *S viridans* have been shown to preferentially adhere to endothelial cells of the heart as a result of certain endothelial cell characteristics and surface glycoproteins such as fibronectin.[5] Certainly, other as yet unknown factors are operative since among immunosuppressed hosts, either from disease or from therapy, the incidence of endocarditis is rather low. This is surprising when one considers the frequency of bacteremias with high circulating numbers of organisms in these patients.

PREDISPOSING FACTORS

Before infection can occur on either normal or abnormal cardiac valves or endocardial surfaces, infecting organisms must be present in the bloodstream. Until recently bacteremia or fungemia generally came from the oral cavity or from skin infections. Transient bacteremias are known to occur with dental procedures, and even from minimal trauma such as brushing and cleaning of the teeth. These organisms are primarily streptococci but on occasion are enterococci. Recently, with the numerous types of diagnostic and therapeutic procedures such as bronchoscopy, sigmoidoscopy, and colonoscopy, involving structures normally inhabited by organisms, more unusual types of bacteria are seen causing infective endocarditis.[6,7] Fortunately this is still uncommon. Genitourinary procedures may produce bacteremias with a wide variety of organisms in 31% of patients when there is pre-existing urinary tract infection. Vaginal deliveries, abortions, and dilatation and curettage frequently produce bacteremias whereas cesarian section does not. Hemodialysis has rarely been associated with *S aureas* endocarditis. Indwelling catheters, especially Swan-Ganz catheters and hyperalimention lines, have been reported to cause a secondary valve infection.[8] Morgan et al[9] reported a 1% incidence of septicemia associated with over 1000 consecutive patients with permanent pacemakers. With *S aureas* present in 83% of these cases, treatment was generally ineffective when the pacing system was retained, whereas in those patients in whom the line was promptly removed, survival was 100%. Other sources of bacteremia which have been reported to occasionally lead to endocarditis include active infections in other major organ systems, ie, osteomylitis, usually with *S aureus* with *Hemophilus influenzae* pneumonia, and pyelonephritis with *E coli* and other Gram-negative organisms. Cirrhosis has also been associated with a slight increase in the risk of endocarditis as has chronic alcoholism.[10]

PRE-EXISTING HEART DISEASE

Rheumatic Heart Disease

Chronic rheumatic valvular disease has long

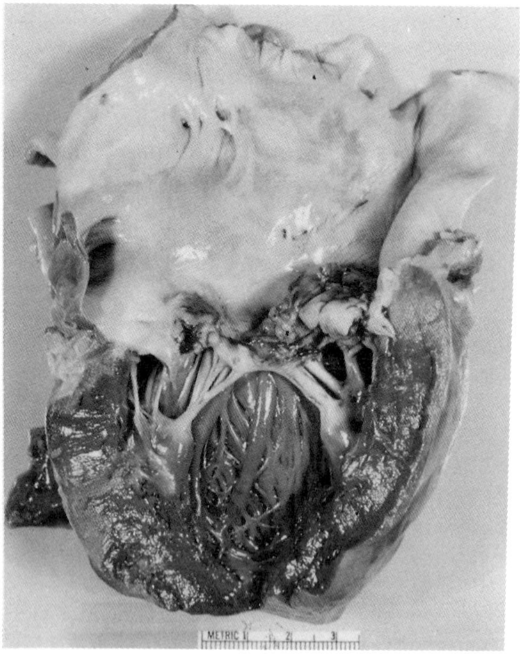

Figure 16-1 A mitral valve damaged by rheumatic fever. The chordae tendineae are fused and thickened, and the leaflets are thickened and rolled. The patient died from an embolic complication caused by endocarditis.

been recognized as the major underlying heart disease in patients who develop endocarditis (Figure 16-1). The overall incidence of underlying rheumatic heart disease in all cases of bacterial endocarditis has declined from 80% to 90% incidence in the preantibiotic era to a 40% to 60% incidence reported by Lerner and Weinstein in 1966[11] to a 30% incidence reported by Pelletier and Petersdorf[12] in a report from the decade 1963–1972. This incidence is echoed in a report of 30% by Leitersdorf et al in 92 patients with native and prosthetic valve endocarditis in Jerusalem[13] between 1970 and 1980, even though these patients come from an area of the world where rheumatic fever is still prevalent. In a 40-year review of bacterial endocarditis in infancy and childhood from 1933 to 1972, Johnson et al[14] reported a decline in the frequency of associated rheumatic heart disease from 21% to 5%. Although it is true that most murmurs in the past where attributed to rheumatic heart disease, this apparent decrease in the percentage of rheumatic valvular disease as predisposing factor in endocarditis is also due to present recognition that rheumatic heart disease was overdiagnosed, the emergence of prosthetic valve endocarditis, the increase in recognized lesions of congenital heart disease, and an increase in endocarditis in the elderly.

Congenital Heart Disease

Some authors have suggested that the incidence of endocarditis in the general nonaddict population is declining. However, the incidence in infancy and childhood may be rising as reported by Johnson et al.[14] They ascribed the increased incidence of endocarditis to the rising age and number of older patients with congenital heart disease who are still at an increased risk of endocarditis compared to the general population. They reported 149 episodes in 141 patients under age 25. Thirty-two episodes were associated with some identifiable predisposing factor accounting for the source of bacteremia (22%), ie, secondary to surgical procedures including open heart surgery, dental procedures, and infections such as urinary tract infections, meningitis, and osteomyelitis. Only rarely was preceding cardiac catheterization cited as a predisposing factor. They noted that tetralogy of Fallot, small ventricular septal defects, and aortic stenosis had a significantly increased risk of endocarditis. Most cases of bacterial endocarditis were caused by α-streptococcal species with *S aureas* being the second most common organism.[14] Survival rates in this group of patients have improved from 0% in the preantibiotic era to 81% in the 1960s. The increase in survival is due to earlier and more aggressive therapy with antibiotics and surgical correction of the congenital defect.

Cardiac Surgery

Cardiac surgery has emerged over the past 10 years as a major predisposing factor to endocarditis second only to IV drug abuse. Infections are more common when valvular prostheses are implanted and less frequent in other open heart procedures.[15] In a report by Rositer et al[16] a 1% per year infection rate was seen with mitral prosthesis and a 2.2% per year incidence with aortic prosthesis. Clearly with 10,000 valves being placed annually in the United States, cardiac surgery has an impressive impact on the incidence of bacterial endocarditis.

Intravenous Drug Abuse

The exact pathophysiologic mechanism by which IV drug abusers have an increased susceptibility to develop infective endocarditis is at present still unknown, though bacteremias are certainly common either from the injection of bacteria directly into the bloodstream[17] or as a result of hematologic seeding in association with skin and intramuscular abscesses, suppurative thrombophlebitis, or as a result of contamination of the needle from the skin flora.

In addicts only 26%[18] may have underlying heart disease as compared to 60% in nonaddicts.[19] The size of the inoculum may be important. Those patients who have pre-existing heart disease may be infected even if a small inoculum is introduced whereas laboratory studies have demonstrated, that in the absence of a damaged endothelial lining, even a large inoculum will not result in implantation of infecting organisms in large enough quantity to establish growth and resultant vegetation formation. One proposed theory suggests that some component of the injectate such as talc causes endothelial damage to the tricuspid valve thus resulting in the deposition of a fibrin platelet clot leading to eventual colonization by circulating bacteria. However, examination at our institution of the hearts of IV drug abusers who died from noncardiac causes have failed to demonstrate any loss of integrity of the endothelial surface of the tricuspid valve. Furthermore, this theory would not explain infections on the left side of the heart. The possibility of immunologic compromise in drug abusers as a predisposing factor has not been ruled out. It is interesting to note that there have been cases in our institution where the initial episode of endocarditis occurred in addicts after 35 years of abuse as well as in those who reported having had only a single injection.

Other Heart Conditions

Other valvular lesions have become recognized as predisposing factors in infective endocarditis. In their review of idiopathic hypertrophic subaortic stenosis, Wang et al[20] found a 4% to 9% incidence of endocarditis usually with α-streptococci.

Another predisposing disease which has had recent notoriety is mitral valve prolapse.[21] *S aureus* and *S albus* as well as α-streptococci have been reported. Many authorities recommend prophylaxis in any patient, even those with only a nonejection click, and others believe it to be necessary only when a mitral systolic murmur is present.[22] This is still an area of some controversy. Prophylaxis probably is not necessary in patients without auscultatory findings where mitral valve prolapse is diagnosed only by echocardiography.

Endocarditis may also develop in mural thrombi which have formed at the site of a myocardial infarct or in the infarcted muscle. False aneurysms of the myocardium have also been reported to have become infected. False aneurysms may actually be caused by endocarditis when abscess formation burrows through the necrotic myocardium.[23] These superinfections generally occur in the first week after infarction (or later in the case of false aneurysm infection) possibly with septicemia related to instrumentation. A case has also been reported in which endocarditis complicated a ventricular septal defect secondary to myocardial infarct.

Endocarditis has also been reported in association with left atrial myxoma,[24] in heart transplant recipients, and in calcification of the mitral anulus fibrosus. Endarteritis occurs at the low pressure side of arteriovenous fistulas, the patent ductus arteriosus, and in the mural thrombi of aortic aneurysms.

DIAGNOSIS

When presenting with the classic picture of fever, malaise, new murmur, peripheral emboli, petechiae, and sublingual and subungual hemorrhases, bacterial endocarditis is not difficult to diagnose. However, in many cases the diagnosis may be subtle, especially in the elderly, and may be masked due to prior inappropriate antibiotic treatment administered by patients themselves or by well-meaning physicians treating "flu-like" symptoms. Establishing the diagnosis in patients with an extracardiac source of infection such as osteomyelitis or subcutaneous abscess will present a challenge even to the most knowledgeable of physicians, and the diagnosis of culture-negative endocarditis is generally made by exclusion in a patient with an otherwise typical clinical picture. In the literature the following diagnostic criteria have been proposed:[13,24–32]

1. A definite diagnosis of infective endocarditis can only be made on the basis of a histopathologic examination of material obtained at autopsy, during open heart surgery, or from embolectomy.

2. A probable diagnosis of infective endocarditis can be made when two or more positive blood cultures are present with one or more organisms, and if one or more of the following conditions are present:

a. A new regurgitant murmur is present, or an old regurgitant murmur increases by two grades. The presence of an old regurgitant murmur is used by some authors. One must use caution in accepting these criteria in the presence of conditions which could cause valvular regurgitation such as acute rheumatic fever, severe hypertension, type I dissecting aneurysm, chronic aortic valve disease of various types, acute myocardial infarction, congestive cardiomyopathy, mitral valve prolapse, chronic rheumatic heart disease, and pulmonary hypertension, either acute or chronic.

b. Emboli, either systemic or pulmonary, have occurred. The presentation of an IV drug abuser with often multiple bilateral lung infiltrates, fever, positive blood cultures, and absence of an extracardiac source of infection has become almost pathognomonic for tricuspid valve endocarditis even in the absence of a typical regurgitant murmur or any murmur at all. However, addicts with sepsis and suppurative skin infections can present with this picture without endocarditis. When systemic embolism has occurred in the presence of sepsis, endocarditis is certainly the most likely diagnosis, but the presence of alternate possible sources of emboli reduce the certainty in making this diagnosis. These include carotid artery disease, old myocardial infarction, cardiomyopathy, left heart failure, aortic and mitral valve disease, and atrial fibrillation.

c. Peripheral stigmata of endocarditis have occurred such as Osler's nodes, Janeway lesions, Roth's spots, splinter hemorrhages, and petechiae.[12]

d. Observation by M-mode (Figure 16-2) or two-dimensional echocardiography of a mass compatible with a vegetation which has newly appeared or one that has increased in reflectance. The myxomatous valve of mitral valve prolapse, torn chordae tendineae, old healed endocarditis, rheumatic heart disease, and calcific aortic valve disease can produce similar echo patterns to those of vegetations, and may result in a false-positive diagnosis.

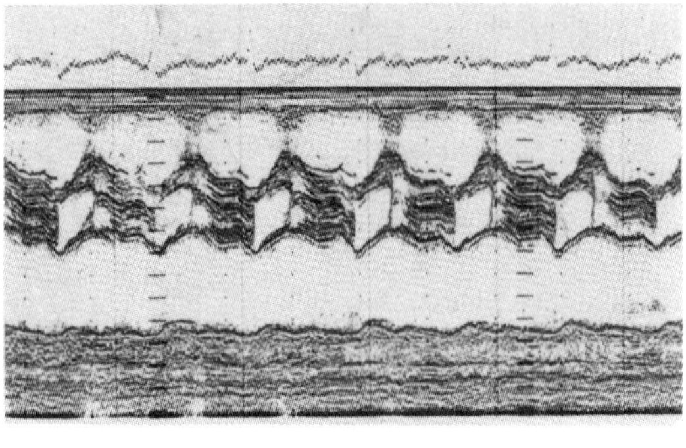

Figure 16-2 M-mode echocardiogram showing a large vegetation on the aortic valve due to enterococcal infection in a 33-year-old male drug addict.

3. A diagnosis of possible infective endocarditis can be made when two or more blood cultures are positive with the same organism and an extracardiac source of sepsis is not apparent in the presence of one or more of the following: (*a*) recurrence of bacteremia after cessation of therapy or (*b*) known underlying valvular heart disease or other disease predisposing to endocarditis (eg, arteriovenous fistula).

4. A probable diagnosis of culture-negative infective endocarditis can be made if a patient has a persistent fever (>38°C), a new regurgitant murmur or an old regurgitant murmur which increased by two grades, and an embolic event. A possible diagnosis is tenable in a patient with fever, known underlying cardiac disease, and embolic events.

5. Infective endocarditis is highly likely in any patient with a prosthetic valve and unexplained sepsis with positive blood culture, even in the absence of paravalvular leak, dehiscence, or emboli.

CLINICAL PRESENTATION

Infection endocarditis results in pathophysiologic derangements causing signs and symptoms by four mechanisms:

1. Infection and sepsis: This results in fever, malaise, leukocytosis, and elevation in nonspecific inflamatory serum reactants such as ESR and C-reactive protein. Also, metastatic infection occurs resulting in visceral abscesses, osteomyelitis, annular and myocardial abscesses, meningitis, and pericarditis.

2. Embolization: Vegetations result in embolization causing acute ischemia, infarction, and infection distal to the embolized artery. Clinically this causes strokes, pulmonary infarction, splenic, renal, and myocardial infarction, and peripheral arterial occlusion. Osler nodes, Janeway lesions, and Roth's spots probably result from microemboli.[33]

3. Immune complex disease: This results from the constant antigenemia and antibody formation fixing complement which deposits on basement membranes causing glomerulonephritis, petechiae, and arthritis. Roth's spots and Janeway lesions[34] may occur by an immunologic mechanism but probably are microemboli.

4. Valvular destruction: The valvular infection weakens and destroys the valve leaflets and/or

Table 16-1
Clinical Manifestations of Endocarditis

	Intravenous drug abuse (%)	Native Valve (%)	Infants and Children (%)	Age > 60 (%)	Early Prosthetic Valve (%)	Late Prosthetic Valve (%)	Culture-Negative (%)	Gram-Negative (%)
Fever	95–100	84–100	90–95	55–93	93–96	96–100	90	100
Never or changing murmur	55–85	80–95	21–98	66–68	60–70	37–60	100	83
Sepsis or shock	...	20–60	...	27	33–35	<5	<5	...
CNS manifestations	5–10	10–30	21–25	35	30–40	30	...	35
Peripheral emboli	15–25	5–30	30	...	7–13	7–26	30–40	50
Splenomegaly	...	30–60	65	10–15	20–30	18–45	29	20–50
Leukocytosis	...	40–60	...	62	40–60	28–50	...	...
References	13,18 25,26 39,40	6,11 13,41	14	42,43	44–46	34, 44–46	27,47	28

Ellipses indicate no or questionable data.

supporting structures resulting in valvular insufficiency.

Infective endocarditis presents a clinical continuum ranging from the chronic, nonspecific to the acute, fulminant, and obvious.[13,14,25,35–37] Over the past 40 years, since the introduction of penicillin, the literature suggests that the characteristics of this continuum may be changing with the introduction of indwelling catheters, increasing numbers of IV drug abusers, cardiac surgery with patch grafts and prosthetic valves, extracorporeal renal dialysis, the increasing number of people over the age of 60, and the increasing average age of the population with congenital heart disease.

Native valve endocarditis from streptococcal and staphylococcal species continue to present in much the same way as it did in the preantibiotic era. The subacute presentation so common with streptococci (though staphylococcal infections can present in a similar fashion) is one of a flu-like syndrome of chronic duration, a month to even 1 year,[35] with symptoms of malaise, anorexia, fatigue, and weakness with weight loss in most patients.[37] Nonspecific musculoskeletal complaints of chest pain, back pain, myalgias and arthralgias are also seen frequently.[38] In the early antibiotic era and especially in the preantibiotic era, petechiae, Roth's spots, Osler's nodes, Janeway lesions and subungual and sublingual hemorrhages were classic peripheral stigmata of subacute bacterial endocarditis. Now, the reported incidence of these peripheral manifestations have fallen dramtically, in part due to early recognition and institution of effective antibiotics.[11,13,31,35,36] The findings of splenomegaly as well as clubbing of the fingers have likewise decreased in frequency.

In our experience patients with acute bacterial endocarditis generally present to hospital within a week of the onset of symptoms. Most cases are caused by *S aureus* but the acute picture can also be seen in infection by Gram-negative organisms, *Streptococcus pyogenes*, and *Streptococcus pneumoniae*.[37] The clinical picture is one of an acutely septic course with fever of 39 to 40°C with rigors and prostration. Nonspecific complaints of chest and back pain with myalgia and arthralgia are common. A new pathologic murmur is usually heard at presentation or within a week of hospitalization. Unfortunately, many patients also have one or more of the many complications discussed below on initial presentation. Some of the symptoms and signs present with endocarditis in various groups are summarized in Table 16-1.*

LABORATORY FINDINGS

Laboratory tests, with the exception of the blood culture, are of little help in the diagnosis of

*References 6, 11, 13, 14, 18, 25–28, 34, 39–47

endocarditis because of their nonspecific nature. Of the various blood tests, the ESR is elevated in almost all patients with infective endocarditis. Without this finding the diagnosis should be seriously questioned. The WBC reflects any chronic or acute infection. Leukocytosis is variable, even occasionally normal with the subacute form, but may be marked in the acute form or with prosthetic valve endocarditis. The degree of leukocytosis depends most especially on the infecting organism. A shift to the left is found in most cases. Toxic granulation and bacteria in the buffy coat are seen primarily in only the minority of staphylococcal cases.[48]

Blood Cultures

In evaluating any patient with fever, sepsis, or suspected endocarditis, bacteriologic culture of the blood is necessary and should be obtained in the most optimal fashion.

Studies done in the early and midantibiotic era confirmed that three separate cultures in a 24-hour period would be adequate to confirm 98% to 100% of streptococcal and staphylococcal infections in patients who had not taken antibiotics in the prior 14 days.[49,50] Werner et al[50] reported that 100% of cases due to organisms other than the above were positive from one of the first two cultures. Of course these reports excluded cases of culture-negative endocarditis. It is with the latter that improved microbiological techniques have increased our diagnostic abilities.

The number of patients with negative cultures may be minimized by continued incubation for up to 4 weeks in order to grow fungi, some slow-growing Gram-negative bacilli, and microaerophilic streptococci. At present the incidence of culture-negative endocarditis is in the range of 3%. In our population of IV drug abusers, over 90% of all blood cultures drawn on entry into the hospital grew organisms. In cases when the diagnosis is in doubt, antibiotics should be withheld and cultures redrawn startings from two to seven days after cessation of antibiotic therapy. Special microbacteriologic techniques are required to grow some of the more fastidious organisms such as providing CO_2 atmosphere and special media for *Neisseria* and *Brucella* species. Slow-growing organisms such as microaerophilic streptococci, *Eikenella*, *Haemophilus*, *Actinobacillus*, and *Aspergillus* may require 2 weeks or longer to produce positive cultures. It may be very difficult to culture organisms such as *Rickettsia*, *Chlamydia*, *Brucella*, and fungi, in which case serologic testing may lead to the diagnosis.

GENERAL PRINCIPLES OF MANAGEMENT

Acute bacterial endocarditis must be treated with high doses of IV bactericidal antibiotics as soon as cultures on the patient have been obtained. A minimum of three blood cultures should be obtained five minutes apart from different sites. A urine culture should always be obtained as well as sputum and skin cultures. Antibiotics should then be started immediately after obtaining the cultures and definitely before other routine diagnostic tests are performed because of the rapidly destructive course of the acute variety of endocarditis where a few hours may possibly mean the difference between medical therapy alone vs surgical therapy. When symptoms are mild and the course seems subacute, then antibiotics may be given on a less emergent basis but should be given as soon as practical after appropriate cultures. Therapy should not be withheld for 24 to 48 hours pending identification of the causative organism as some authors have suggested. Though they are probably correct in stating the safety of such action, the cost of the additional day in the hospital is much greater than 24 to 48 hours of parenteral antibiotics.

Empirical therapy started in the absence of knowledge of the causative organism in the septic patient should include broad coverage against penicillinase-producing staphylococci, enterococci, and penicillin-sensitive streptococci. Nafcillin sodium 2 g IV every four hours, tobramycin 1 mg/kg intramuscularly (IM) or IV every eight hours, and penicillin G 4 million units IV every four hours will provide this coverage. Vancomycin hydrochloride 7.5 mg/kg every six hours plus tobramycin 1 mg/kg IM. or IV every eight hours may be substituted for those patients with an allergy to penicillin. If prosthetic valve endocarditis is suspected, a combination of vancomycin hydrochloride 7.5 mg/kg IV every six hours, rifampin 300 mg orally every 12 hours, and tobramycin 1 mg/kg IM or IV every eight hours should prove adequate to cover methicillin sodium–resistant *S epidermidis*, *S aureus*, streptococci (*viridans*, non-enterococcal group D, and enterococcal), diphtheroids, and some Gram-negative bacilli. For subacute native valve endocarditis penicillin G plus streptomycin will provide adequate initial coverage.

Invariably, initial empirical regimens require modification after the results of microbiologic studies. Antibiotics should then be adjusted based on sensitivity testing, initial minimal inhibitory concentration (MIC), minimal bactericidal concentration (MBC), and synersisms. After 48 hours of this new regimen, blood cultures are repeated and peak serum antibiotic levels are measured. The MIC and MBC are determined with the patient's serum. Dosages should be increased or new antibiotics selected to provide a peak bactericidal titer in a dilution of 1:8 or greater. Antibiotics should be administered parenterally except in unusual cases (ie, rifampin) and continued for a minimum of 4 weeks in most cases. Penicillin-sensitive *S viridans* streptococci and *Streptococcus bovis* may be cured after only 2 weeks when combination therapy of penicillin G and streptomycin is given. Enterococal infections may require 8 weeks of therapy with resistant strains.

During therapy a daily or, better, twice daily physical examination should be performed. A cardiology consultation should be requested along with an echocardiogram. If acute left-sided infection is present or if a prosthetic valve is involved, then consultation with a cardiac surgeon is manditory. A rapid improvement in the patient's feelings of well-being should occur within 48 to 72 hours of effective antibiotic therapy. This findings often precedes the drop in temperature followed by the normalization of the laboratory values. Barring complications, patients usually feel quite recovered for most of the time of treatment.

During the course of therapy, a portal of entry should be sought. Abscesses should be treated and any required dental work be performed during antibiotic treatment. If *S bovis* was causative, colonoscopy should be performed since infection with this organism is frequently associated with colonic carcinoma.

After discharge repeat blood cultures are performed at 30 and 60 days. This will find the majority of relapses. Education on prophylaxis must be given prior to discharge and reinforced at each outpatient visit.

ECHOCARDIOGRAPHY

In our experience at a general hospital treating primarily addict-associated endocarditis, the enchocardiogram has had little impact on the management of patients. This is true in both left-sided as well as right-sided infections. Though echocardiography has greatly added to our understanding of this disease and its natural history, its actual day-to-day usefulness is limited to a few situations which are discussed below.

Dillon et al,[51] reporting on eight patients with surgically proven endocarditis, concluded that a vegetation of 2 mm or greater could be identified with M-mode echocardiography. Using the two-dimensional technique, however, Berger et al[52] could not reliably detect a vegetation of 3 mm or less on the aortic valve.

Several attempts have been reported to determine the sensitivity, specificity, and diagnostic accuracy of echocardiographic endocarditis.[53–61] Autopsy studies and surgery provide the only source of study material and these are biased as at present they are primarily associated with acute septic cases, and with moderate-size vegetative lesions involving staphylococcus and streptococcus, whereas subacute cases typically have smaller vegetations.[55,58,59] Nevertheless, echocardiography can identify the involved valve and especially with Doppler techniques can diagnose significant valvular dysfunction in 80% to 90% of cases. Sensitivity is improved by two-dimensional echocardiographic studies and is best when these are combined with the M-mode technique.[56,57,59] Left-sided lesions are detected more reliably,[61] and vegetations in younger patients are detected more frequently due to the increased number of technically adequate studies. No reliable method has been found to distinguish vegetation on previously abnormal valves or in cases where a prosthesis is in place. The echocardiogram may be helpful in confirming the diagnosis when culture-negative endocarditis is suspected[62] or when slow-growing organisms are present.[63]

Patients with detectable vegetation have a worse prognosis, higher complication rate, higher mortality, and increased requirement for surgery.[55,64–66] Larger vegetations are more likely to embolize. However, the echocardiogram has been of no significant value over clinical evaluation in directing the course of therapy or in determining immediate prognosis. After embolization has occurred the degree of reflectance may be notably reduced; however, the risk of a subsequent embolus is still higher. This observation has given rise to the suggestion that surgical intervention be instituted in those patients because of the generally catastrophic consequences

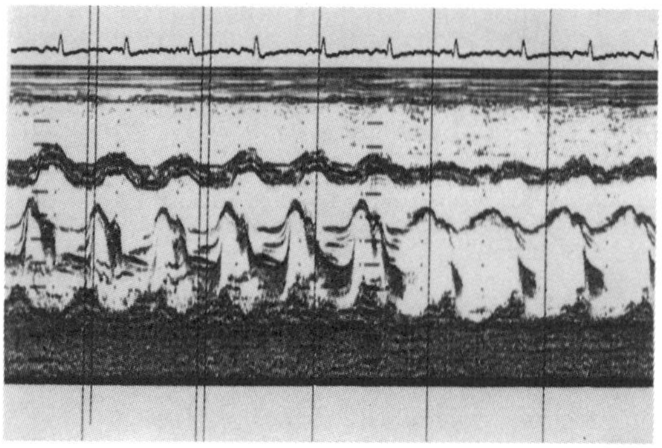

Figure 16-3 M-mode echocardiogram. Sweep of the left ventricle and aorta revealing a highly reflectant mass on the anterior and posterior mitral leaflets. The vegetation appears to protrude into the left atrium during systole. Mitral insufficiency was present in this patient.

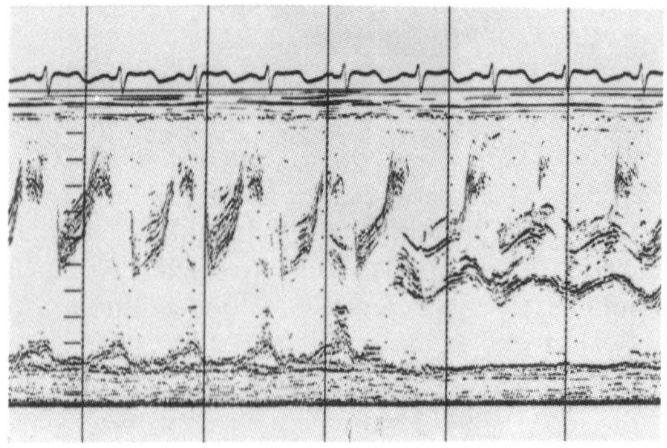

Figure 16-4 M-mode echocardiogram. Sweep of the tricuspid valve and aorta demonstrating moderate reflectance of a vegetation on the tricuspid valve caused by *S aureus* infection in a drug addict.

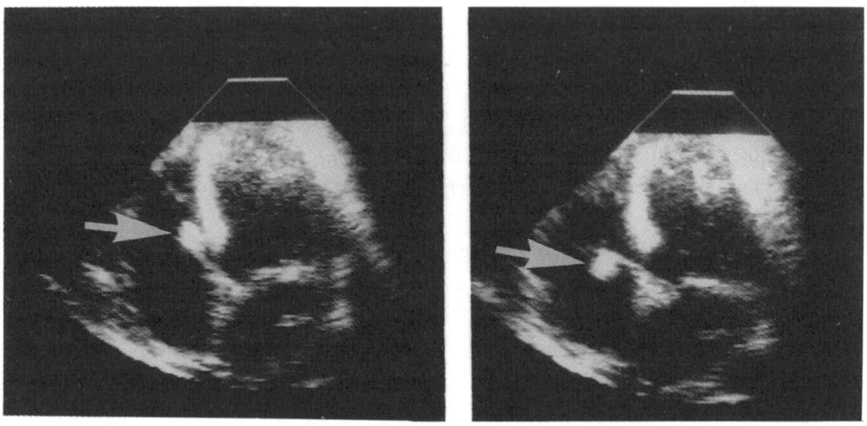

Figure 16-5 Two-dimensional echocardiogram. Apical four-chamber view showing a large vegetation (arrow) on the tricuspid valve. Left panel in diastole, right panel in systole.

of large vessel emboli. Figures 16-3 and 16-4 show the echocardiographic pattern of vegetation of the mitral and tricuspid valves respectively. Figure 16-5 illustrates the appearance of a vegetation on the tricuspid valve in the apical four-chambered view obtained by two-dimensional echocardiography.

Formation of myocardial abscess has in the past been generally undetectable except at post mortem or at surgery. The overall incidence of abscesses is unknown, as is their role in the pathogenesis of myocardial failure, though present in 20% to 30% of patients at autopsy.[67,68] Two-dimensional echocardiographic techniques have proved useful in detecting this condition[69] but the sensitivity is unknown and the number of false-positives may be high.[57] Gallium scanning and thallium perfusion techniques may also be useful as a means of detecting myocardial abscess.

Uses and Limitations of Echocardiography

Our cardiac consultation service is frequently asked to "rule out" endocarditis using echocardiography but we are infrequently asked to "rule in" endocarditis. On the one hand, we may be able to support the clinical diagnosis if echocardiographic features compatible with endocarditis are found; however, we cannot exclude the presence of endocarditis if none are found. Though few false-positive studies have been reported the risk is certainly present, especially in the older age group where fibrotic, calcific or myxomatous changes in the valve may be present, or when other pathology is present such as rheumatic heart disease, calcific aortic stenosis, congenital heart disease, or valvular prosthesis[59,70,71] all of which obscure the echographic picture.

Situations in which echocardiography is helpful include patients with: (1) peripheral emboli, (2) multiple pulmonary emboli, (3) congestive heart failure, (4) preoperative evaluation, (5) suspected culture-negative endocarditis, (6) sepsis when the diagnosis of endocarditis is not clear, (7) suspected marantic endocarditis, (8) Löeffler's endocarditis, and (9) prosthetic valve endocarditis. Furthermore, echocardiography, especially in association with Doppler techniques, is valuable in assessing the significance of the valvular insufficiency and the functional state of the ventricle.

CATHETERIZATION

The role of cardiac catheterization in the management and preoperative evaluation of the endocarditis patient is in the process of being reassessed.[72-73] It is important to know whether to perform catheterization, especially when the diagnosis seems apparent on clinical grounds and by noninvasive tests, or whether it is even safe to perform because of the risk of dislodging a vegetation or because it may delay surgery, albeit for only a few hours.

Mills, et al[73] reported the experience at San Francisco General Hospital in 19 patients who were catheterized prior to surgery. The clinical diagnosis was proved correct in 74% of patients in regard to valvular involvement and the presence of heart failure. Three of the patients required catherization to determine the degree of aortic insufficiency and mitral insufficiency when both were present in the same patient. Four of seven aortic ring abscesses were detected by angiocardiography, all of which were "missed" clinically. There were two patients with severe aortic insufficiency who clinically worsened after study and one died.

Welton et al[74] found slightly different results in 35 patients studied. They reported 66% of the clinical diagnosis to either be incorrect or incomplete. They noted that catheterization was helpful in evaluating multivalvular involvement.[74] Hosenpud and Greenberg[72] found the clinical diagnosis to be 95% sensitive and 89% correct. Only one of 19 study patients developed a nonfatal complication from catheterization. The 19 patients in their study all had clinical criteria for early surgical intervention; congestive heart failure, systemic emboli, persistent infection, or new conduction abnormalities. Of these, one patient was found not to have congestive heart failure by hemodynamic measurement and was spared surgery. In this case the clinical picture was confusing.

These studies support the conclusion that angiocardiography and catheterization should be performed preoperatively in patients in whom (1) multiple valve involvement is suspected, (2) the clinical diagnosis of congestive failure or the site of infection is confusing or ambiguous, or (3) coronary bypass surgery is also a consideration. Catheterization does not appear to be needed in patients with severe mitral insufficiency when the diagnosis is certain clinically and the echocardiogram is consistent.[75] Catheterization probably should not be done in patients with rapidly progressive heart failure due to wide open aortic insufficiency because any delay in the definitive therapy of valve replacement may prove detrimental. Its place in evaluating patients with prosthetic valve endocarditis has not been defined as yet.

COMPLICATIONS

All too often, patients seek medical care initially for treatment of one of the many complications of endocarditis. These complications can generally be divided into cardiac and extracardiac, and may be present when the diagnosis is first made, or occur during the course of the illness and treatment of endocarditis.

Congestive Heart Failure

Congestive heart failure, primarily due to aortic insufficiency (Figure 16-6) or mitral insufficiency (Figure 16-7) from perforation or destruction of the valve, continues to be the leading cause of death from endocarditis, although on occasion myocarditis, myocardial abscess, or acute myocardial infarction from emboli can be responsible for congestive heart failure.[13,24,76] When congestive heart failure occurs in the course of infective endocarditis, valvular insufficiency with few exceptions has proved to be the cause. Heart failure is usually sudden and may be devastating in patients with acute aortic regurgitation or may be slowly progressive over weeks or months. Mixed valvular lesions with congestive heart failure carry the highest mortality rate.[12] The reported incidence of congestive

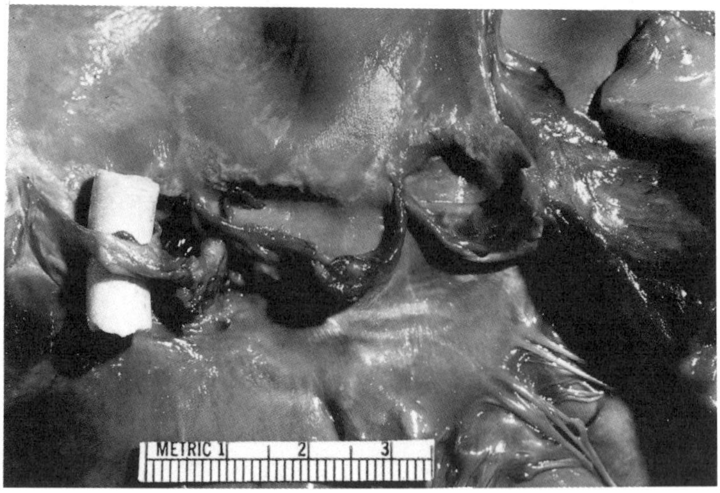

Figure 16-6 Perforation of the right coronary cusp in a 55-year-old women who died from pneumococcal aortic valve endocarditis (nonaddict).

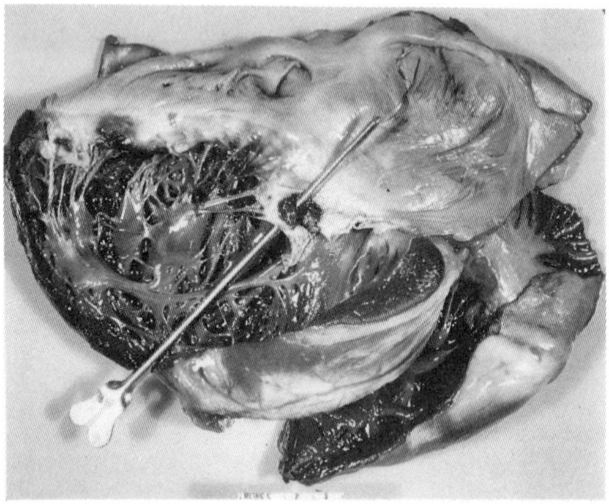

Figure 16-7 The probe is in a perforation of the anterior leaflet of the mitral valve from a 60-year-old white male who died from acute endocarditis caused by *S aureau* and α-hemolytic streptococci.

heart failure ranges between 25%[77] to 67%[12] depending on the criteria of congestive heart failure used and the population under study.

Hubbel et al[25] in reporting our experience in a group of 97 IV drug abusers with infective endocarditis, found 57% of aortic valve infections and 38% of mitral valve infections to present with evidence of heart failure. In this series 100% of mixed aortic and mitral valve infections presented with congestive heart failure. Of the entire 97 patients a total of 37 (38%) had congestive heart failure of whom 35 (95%) had involvement of one or more left-sided valves. The lower incidence of congestive heart failure in this group was in part related to the lower incidence of congestive heart failure associated with tricuspid valve infection common in IV drug abusers. Pulmonary emboli from the tricuspid valve, however, can lead to pulmonary hypertension, which intensifies the degree of tricuspid insufficiency and may lead to the development of right heart failure.

Valvular Obstruction

Both aortic stenosis and mitral stenosis have been reported secondary to infective endocarditis associated with large vegetative lesions often seen in fungal infections. The mitral stenosis may be associated with a valve vegetation originating from the endocardium of the left atrium behaving much the same as the ball valve mass often present with left atrial myxoma.[78,79] Myxomas themselves may become infected and present not only with obstruction to flow but also with multiple embolic events.

Myocardial and Ring Absceses

The development of myocardial abcess is a serious cardiac complication of endocarditis and carries a grave prognosis. Abscesses associated with endocarditis may be the result of direct spread of the infection, hematologic spread via the bloodstream, or due to an infected embolus. Abscess formation is usually associated with aortic and mitral valve infection and rarely with tricuspid valve infection. The abscesses are most commonly found in the perivalvular areas.[80,81] They are more commonly seen in patients with prosthetic valve endocarditis, especially in the aortic position.[82] Myocardial abscesses are present in approximately 20% of patients dying from endocarditis seen at autopsy.

Abscesses may be multiple and widespread throughout the myocardium and occasionally be associated with pericarditis. An unusual complication of myocardial abscess is rupture of the wall of the myocardium, causing tamponade and death. Septal abscesses may rupture creating an intraventricular septal defect which if unrecognized and not promptly treated by surgical placement of a patch, will result in the death of the patient. A report of 95 necropsy patients with native valve endocarditis found 27 (28%) patients with ring abscesses involving 30 valves.[68] The aortic valve ring was affected in 24 patients, the mitral valve in two and the tricuspid valve in one patient. *S aureus*, pneumococcus, and non-α-streptococci were the most frequently observed infecting organisms. Because most of the abscesses are located in the upper septum or in the right fibrous trigone near the atrioventricular (A-V) node and bundle of His, varying degrees of heart block and infra-His bundle block can occur. Electrocardiographic abnormalities are usually present consisting of first degree A-V block, Mobitz II heart block, or third degree heart block. Left bundle-branch block is more commonly seen than right bundle-branch block and may signal the imminent occurrence of third degree heart block. Paravalvular abscesses can sometimes be detected by a gallium scan, thallium 201 myocardial perfusion study, or two-dimensional echocardiogram when suspicion is raised by the presence of new right or left bundle-branch block and/or any A-V block. Surgical drainage is usually necessary, although there are case reports of medical cures with antibiotics alone.

When rapidly progressive, unremittant heart failure is present, and patients are taken to surgery for valve replacement before antibiotic therapy can be completed. If a prosthetic valve has to be replaced in the presence of a valve ring abscess, the prospect for survival is poor in spite of surgical débridement and attempts to obliterate the abscess cavity and close the septal defect. However, in cases of aortic valve endocarditis associated with severe congestive heart failure, the high surgical mortality is acceptable as medical management is attended with almost 100% fatality.[24]

Any degree of A-V block or infra-His bundle block should alert the clinician to the possibility of myocardial abscess, particularly when the infection is associated with the aortic valve. Among 142 cases of bacterial endocarditis, Wang et al[83] reported a 4% incidence of complete heart block and a 10% incidence of either first or second degree A-V block. The aortic valve was involved in 90% of cases with A-V conduction disturbances including all six patients with third degree A-V block. Five of the six patients with complete heart block died suddenly and one patient survived with temporary pacing, finishing antibiotic treatment to receive a prosthetic aortic valve. In view of the serious prognosis of this findings and the usual progression of conduction defect, any degree of new A-V block or the appearance of right or left bundle-branch block should be an indication for temporary tranvenous pacing.

Embolization

Whereas emboli, either microscopic or macroscopic, occur in almost all patients with endocarditis, emboli have been reported in earlier studies to be clinically manifest in only 15% to 35% of nonaddicts.[19,41] However, the incidence of clinically apparent systemic embolic phenomena in more recent reports ranges between 5% and 10% for a mixed addict and nonaddict population[26,84]; systemic emboli are distributed randomly through the body, being clinically manifest most commonly when involving the brain (Figure 16-8), coronary vessels, spleen, kidney (Figure 16-9), and peripheral circulation. Patients dying from overwhelming sepsis invariably have embolic phenomena with microscopic abscesses involving all major organ systems. This may help explain the somewhat higher figures

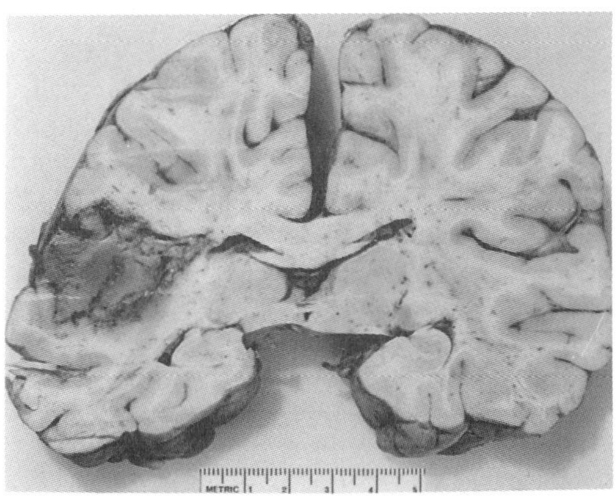

Figure 16-8 Left hemispheric embolic infarct in a patient with *S aureus* aortic valve infection.

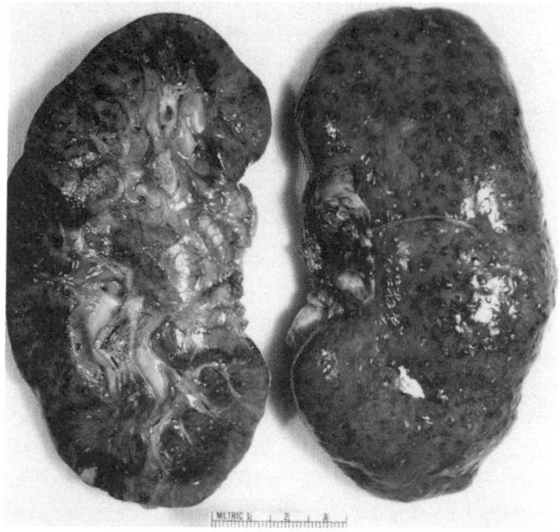

Figure 16-9 Multiple small macroabscesses in the kidney of a patient with acute *S aureus* endocarditis.

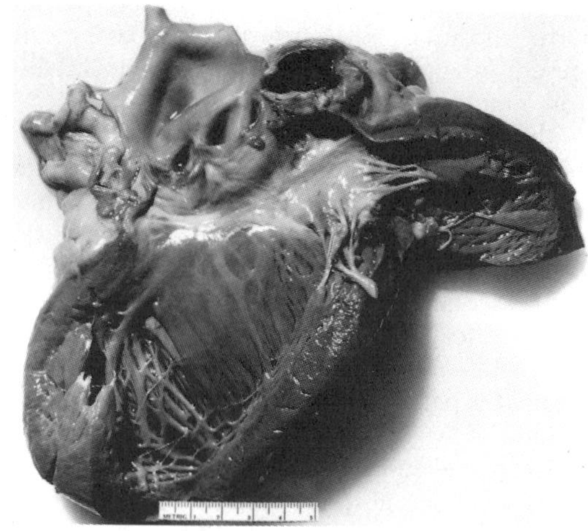

Figure 16-10 Sinus of Valsalva aneurysm (topcenter) was found at autopsy, complicating the course in a drug addict with enterococcal aortic valve infection.

reported in autopsy reports. Major emboli generally occur early, mostly at presentation or in the first week of therapy. Thereafter, major embolic phenomena are more unusual but have been reported to occur months after completion of therapy. In endocarditis involving the right side of the heart (mostly the tricuspid valve, less commonly the pulmonary valve and right ventricular endocarditis from an intraventricular septal defect) the usual clue is the radiographic appearance of multiple infiltrates in one or both lungs consistent with multiple septic pulmonary emboli.

Other Cardiac Complications

Other unusual cardiac complications include: aneurysms of the aortic sinus of Valsava (Figure 16-10) which may or may not rupture into the atrium, pericardial space, right ventricle, or myocardium. False aneurysm of the left ventricle due to perforation of the mitral aortic intravalvular fibrosa has also been reported.[85] Although pericardial effusion is not uncommon, clinical pericarditis is rarely seen with infective endocarditis and is probably the result of a local reaction to the deposition of immune complexes. Pericarditis associated with abscess formation may herald the rupture of a myocardial abscess into the pericardial sac causing purulent pericarditis. Pericarditis also may be a secondary phenomonen related to uremia, pneumonia, or as a result of penetrating injury to the heart which resulted in the initial infection. Purulent pericarditis necessitates urgent surgical drainage with continued antimicrobial therapy.

The presence of myocarditis as part of the infective picture received some discussion in the past. Whether the histologic findings represent ischemic damage, direct myocardial invasion by bacteria, or deposition of immune complexes has not been adequately evaluated. A deposition of immune complexes may be the most likely etiology of myocarditis and might be similar to the microvasculitis producing the patterns characteristic in the flea-bitten kidney and glomerulonephritis.

Noncardiac Complications

Noncardiac complications of endocarditis are caused by three mechanisms: embolic phenomena, hematalogic spread of the infecting agent, and deposition of immune complexes. The most devastating noncardiac complications include nephritis, neurologic abnormalities, and mycotic aneurysms as well as acute vasculitis of the skin.

Microscopic hematuria probably is a result of the deposition of immune complexes in the glomeruli and not due to emboli to the kidney. Gross hematuria, on the other hand, probably does result from macroemboli to the kidney.

Mycotic aneurysms (Figure 16-11) (probably as a result of septic emboli to the small arteries or to the vasa vasorum of the large arteries) are becoming less frequent with endocarditis probably due to earlier recognition of the disease and more aggressive therapy. However, aneurysms are reported in up to 2.5% of patients today,[86] with the majority of mycotic aneurysms involving the aorta or its major branches. When present in

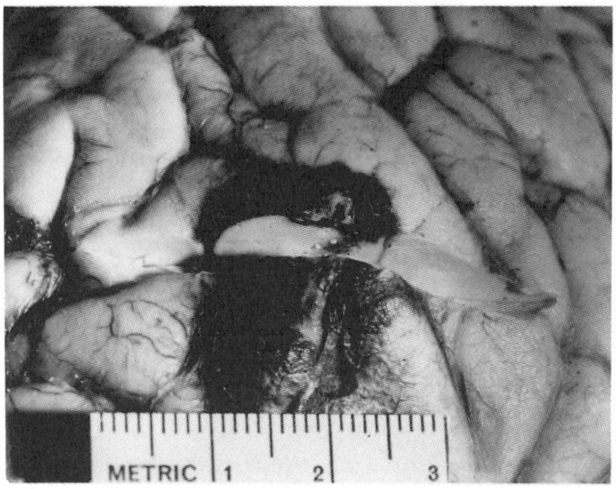

Figure 16-11 Ruptured mycotic aneurysm of the left superior cerebral artery in a 26-year-old female drug addict with rheumatic heart disease and enterococcal endocarditis of the aortic and mitralvalves.

the cerebrovascular arteries they may remain silent until they rupture producing catastrophic hemorrhage into the brain tissue. The diagnosis should be suspected and angiography or computed tomography (CT) with contrast enhancement performed whenever focal neurologic findings are present. Surgical therapy is the treatment of choice although at times mycotic aneurysms seen on angiography have later been shown to resolve spontaneously.

Metastatic infections due to infected emboli are not uncommon and are often associated with *S aureus* infections. Whereas embolic phenomena are seen frequently in streptococcal infections, metastatic infections are unusual with this organism, probably due to its relatively slow rate of growth and low virulence. Staphloccocal infections on the other hand, invariably produce an infection at most sites of embolization. Metastatic infections found in the lung are generally from right-sided involvement but may also be seen with left-sided infections.

PROSTHETIC VALVE ENDOCARDITIS

Studies reporting results of follow-up in cardiac surgical patients have subdivided their results into early (within 2 months of surgery) and late (after 2 months) infections.[34,44,45,87] Infections generally occur at the site of attachment of the prosthetic valve in both early and late infections, probably as a result of suture material providing a nidus for circulating bacteria to attach and invade the tissues contiguous with the sewing ring. This is especially common in patients with active endocarditis under treatment who, due to devastating congestive heart failure from valvular incompetence, require emergency valve replacement. Not only are the technical results suboptimal in these cases, prognosis is also poor and recurrence of infection somewhat higher.[88] Infection may also occur on the bioprosthetic valve leaflets themselves, usually resulting in acute valvular degeneration. Ring abscesses are much more frequently seen in infections with prosthetic valves as compared to native valves, and may result in valve dehiscence and catastrophic paravalvular insufficiency.

Clinically, patients with prosthetic valve endocarditis usually present much the same as do patients with native valve endocarditis (Table 16-1). However, patients may not present with an insufficiency murmur in spite of the extensive involvement of the sewing ring of the valve in abscess formation. This is seen in the case of the aortic valve when it has lost much of its attachment and is tilting off its attachments during systole but occludes the aortic orifice with diastole. When paraprosthetic valvular insufficiency is present, the leak may be along a large percentage of the circumference of the valve, creating a fanlike jet which may not result in a murmur audible at the chest surface. These silent perivalvular leaks occur more frequently in the mitral position than in the aortic position. Risk factors for developing early prosthetic valve endocarditis include valve replacement for native valve endocarditis, mechanical prothesis *v* bioprosthesis, black race, and longer cardiopulmonary bypass time. Early endocarditis usually results from some predisposing extracardiac infection such as skin abscesses, sternal wound infections, mediastinal infections, and urinary tract infections, usually with a predominance of infections with *S* aureus, *S epidermidis*, and Gram-negative bacilli. Late infections account for approximately 50% to 80% of all prosthetic valve infections. Most are caused by streptococci but staphlococci and Gram-negative organisms are also seen. Late infections are frequently associated with some predisposing factor producing bacteremia.

Antibiotics alone do not cure the majority of cases of prosthetic valve endocarditis and valve replacement is required. Surgery should not be delayed, even one day, in an attempt at an antibiotic cure in patients whose valves have become severely insufficient or are in the process of detaching. Unfortunately, repeat operation carries a much higher morbidity and mortality, especially in the acutely ill individual. Furthermore, in our experience replacement of an artificial valve in IV drug abusers carries with it a 70% to 80% 2- to 3- year mortality (unpublished data) due to reinfection and heart failure.

ENDOCARDITIS IN INTRAVENOUS DRUG ABUSERS

Endocarditis among IV drug abusers differs in several respects from endocarditis in nondrug abusers. Addicts tend to be younger than nonaddicts with a higher male-to-female ratio (31 *v* 21), and pre-existing or prior heart disease, including congenital heart disease and rheumatic heart disease, tends to be less likely. In addicts the tricuspid valve is involved much more frequently than in nonaddicts and the staphylococcus is the predominant organism; therefore, presentation is generally more acute but survival with the first infection is higher due to the predominance of right-sided infections. In addition, recurrences are higher on both native valves as well as prosthetic valves.

Intravenous drug abusers not only include those patients who inject heroin, reported in the early 1970s by Tuazon to be as many as 650,000 in the United States,[17] but also includes patients who inject a variety of other drugs including methylphenidate hydrochloride, amphetamines, cocaine, and barbituates. It is estimated that one out of ten people in San Francisco have injected IV drugs at some time in their life, which amounts to a potential population at risk of 90,000 people. The risk of developing endocarditis has been estimated to be between one and two cases per 1000 drug abusers.[89] However, the relative risk may vary from region to region and may fluctuate from year to year due to the nature of the drug, the source of the drug, the adulterants, the habits of the community of IV drug abusers, and the techniques of injection.[40]

The disease generally presents clinically with an acute course reflecting the high frequency of *S aureus* infection. Ninety-five to 100% of patients either have had a history of fever or on admission have a temperature greater than 38°C. Other presenting complaints include respiratory problems in 50% to 60% of cases, gastrointestinal (GI) symptoms in 10% to 20%, arthritis in 10% to 15%, extremity pain in 10% to 15%, various neurologic complaints in 5% to 10% and renal problems in less than 5% of patients.[13,25,26,39,40,90]

Anterior chest pain and back pain is another common complaint in our patients. In *S aureus* infection involving the tricuspid valve, over three fourths of the patients will have either multiple infiltrates or abscess formation in the lung. With right-sided infection in this group a murmur of tricuspid insufficiency may be present in only one third of cases, though when looked for carefully, a systolic murmur along the lower left sternal border compatible with tricuspid insufficiency is present at some time during hospitalization in nearly one half of the patients.

In our experience the tricuspid valve is involved 52% of the time, the aortic valve 17%, the mitral valve 14%, and the pulmonic valve 1%. Staphylococci are involved in 80% of cases of tricuspid infection but in only 27% of left-sided infections. Enterococci produce 27% of left-sided infections and *S viridans* 19% of left-sided infections. Both Gram-negative organisms and fungal species are more common in this group than in the nonaddict population.[18]

ENDOCARDITIS IN THE ELDERLY

The average age of the population with endocarditis has increased compared to earlier studies. Endocarditis is recognized in the younger population of adults more frequently ante mortem due to a higher index of suspicion and more obvious presenting symptoms than in the older population. This is reflected in the higher mortality of endocarditis in the elderly.[12]

Two reviews, by Thell et al[42] and Applefeld and Hornick,[43] address this problem specifically. Both studies stress the problems in making the diagnosis of endocarditis. Not surprisingly 60% to 70% of patients who came to autopsy had underlying valvular disease, consisting primarily of aortic valve disease with calcification or rheumatic mitral valve disease. The aortic valve was most commonly involved (40% to 50%), the mitral valve next (30% to 40%) and the tricuspid valve least with 10% to 20% of the cases. This distribution is quite similar to that reported in the younger nonaddict population. Clinically, patients presented much the same as their younger cohorts; however, the degree of change in the clinical laboratory findings were not as marked. Fever and leukocytosis were present in most patients, petechiae were seen in approximately 30% of cases and splenomegaly in 10% to 15% of cases. Generally an equal number of cases are caused by staphylococci and streptococci which make up over 80% of infecting agents. Bacterial endocarditis was suspected ante mortem in only 40% of cases reported by Thell, in spite of a murmur being present in 68% and a fever in 93%, often with a septic pattern.[42] Endocarditis was suspected in only 38% of patients who presented with fever, while 54% of cases were suspected when a murmur was present. Applefeld and Hornick reported that 48% of their patients received inappropriate antibiotics and had a 72% overall mortality.[43]

Frequently, endocarditis in older patients can present without fever and with only an unexplained change in mental status, anemia, or uremia. In the presence of an organic heart murmur, endocarditis should be suspected in these clinical situations and blood cultures obtained.

CULTURE-NEGATIVE ENDOCARDITIS

Patients who present with fever, a new valvular insufficiency murmur, embolic phenomena either to the peripheral circulation or to the lungs, with or without splenomegaly or the peripheral stigmata of endocarditis, where no obvious source of infection is found, and whose blood cultures are sterile, are said to have culture-negative endocarditis. This definition includes patients who have noninfective thrombotic endocarditis as well as patients with culture-negative infective endocarditis.

In the preantibiotic era the mortality of both culture-negative and culture-positive endocarditis was essentially 100%.[91] Now, in the decades since the introduction of penicillin, the mortality in culture-negative endocarditis has decreased to around 40% and a similar decrease has been observed in culture-positive endocarditis. With the advance of medical knowledge and microbiological techniques, the percentage of all endocarditis diagnosed as culture-negative endocarditis has decreased from a high of 50% to the 5% to 10% range reported by most competent laboratories.

At the Mayo Clinic the percentage of culture-negative endocarditis is 3%. In a review Pesanti and Smith[27] studied the clinical records of 52 patients diagnosed as having endocarditis with negative blood cultures. They found these patients to have more frequently received antibiotics prior to the cultures in comparison to a similar culture-positive cohort. Twice as many patients had a history of rheumatic heart disease and congenital heart disease, whereas fewer patients had a prosthetic valve in place. Both major emboli and congestive heart failure were twice as frequent, as was splenomegaly. Petechiae, hematuria, and Osler's nodes were likewise more frequently seen in this group. The distribution of the involved valves paralleled that found in the culture-positive cohort.[27]

Empirical therapy produces a high survival rate in patients who become afebrile in the first week of therapy. But half of those who do not respond in this first week will die.[27]

Possible etiologies include *Eikenella*, Brucella, *Neisseria*, Q fever, fungi, acid-fast organisms, *Chlamydia*, nutritionally deficient forms of streptococci, and possibly right-sided infective endocarditis where the infective organism is filtered by the lung so that culturing of the systemic circulation alone will fail to yield organisms.[31] This latter situation probably occurs only rarely since the lung may filter and reduce the concentration of bacteria, but never removes all the organisms. Diseases which resemble infective endocarditis and must be distinguished from it include myxoma, rheumatic fever, systemic lupus enythematosus, marantic endocarditis, endocardial fibroelastosis, Löffler's myocarditis, and carcinoid.

RELAPSE AND RECURRENT ENDOCARDITIS

The return of signs and symptoms of endocarditis after completion of medical therapy is termed a "relapse" if it occurs within 6 months and a "recurrence" when it occurs after 6 months. When the illness recurs and involves the same organism it is usually believed to be a relapse and when it involves a different organism, a recurrence. It is obvious that recurrences can occur with a similar organism but it is not possible to prove this.

A definite exception to this involves a primary infection with fungi or yeast which commonly relapses in spite of vigorous therapy. This recurrence most likely is a result of failure of the antifungal agent to penetrate into the bulky vegetatons common to these organisms in sufficient concentrations to sterilize them. Because of this experience, surgical débridement of the valve with removal of the infected tissue is almost always required to provide a "medical" cure and is the treatment of choice in the majority of these patients.

The frequency of reinfection varies widely in the literature. In early reports involving primarily nondrug abusers with congenital and rheumatic heart disease, the incidence was as low as 2% to 4% to as high as 22%.[43] In more recent reports the percentage of recurrence in native valve endocarditis is as high as 30% to 40% in IV drug abusers mostly due to *S aureus*.[92]

Relapse and recurrence were seen in less than 10% of nondrug abusers.[93] Among nondrug abusers recurrence is associated with a higher frequency of α-streptococcal species and occurs more frequently in younger patients with congenital heart disease. Cure rate and mortality figures were equal in the first and second episodes with this group. Among patients with valvular prostheses, drug abusers had a much higher recurrence rate approaching 90% to 100%[92] and had a lower cure rate and higher mortality.

In our own experience, M-mode echocardiography has been helpful as a predictor of those, primarily IV drug abusers, who were at risk of subsequent relapses. Among patients with a normal M-mode echocardiogram, there was only a 5% recurrence rate, whereas in patients with either an echocardiogram suggestive of valvular vegetation or other abnormality including torn chordae tendineae, right ventricular enlargement, left ventricular enlargement, or aortic insufficiency a 50% to 60% recurrence rate was noted with long-term follow-up (unpublished data).

MARANTIC ENDOCARDITIS

Marantic endocarditis is a primary form of nonbacterial vegetative endocarditis. The disease is characterized by vegetative lesions occurring on the contact surfaces predominantly of the mitral and aortic valves usually occurring in association with chronic illnesses, notably malignant tumors (60% of cases) (Figure 16-12) Involvement of the contact surfaces of the leaflets is characteristic in this disorder and other cardiac structures are typically spared. The valve leaflets appear swollen and marked destruction may be present.

The patient's primary clinical presentation is generally that of an older patient with chronic disease, usually a malignancy, and the marantic endocarditis is either silent and found incidentally at postmortem examination or is suspected as a result of one or more embolic episodes frequently to the brain, occurring in 14% to 33%.[94] Noncancerous diseases associated with marantic endocarditis include hepatic cirrhosis, diabetes, tuberculosis, pneumonia, and chronic obstructive pulmonary disease.[95] Occasionally, patients have a clinical course typical of endocarditis associated with congestive heart failure and embolic phenomena.

Because the endocarditis is noninfectious the diagnosis is difficult to make in the living patient in the absence of new valvular insufficiency murmur or clinically manifest emboli. However, congestive heart failure in association with aortic or mitral insufficiency murmur, or a peripheral embolus or acute myocardial infarction in asso-

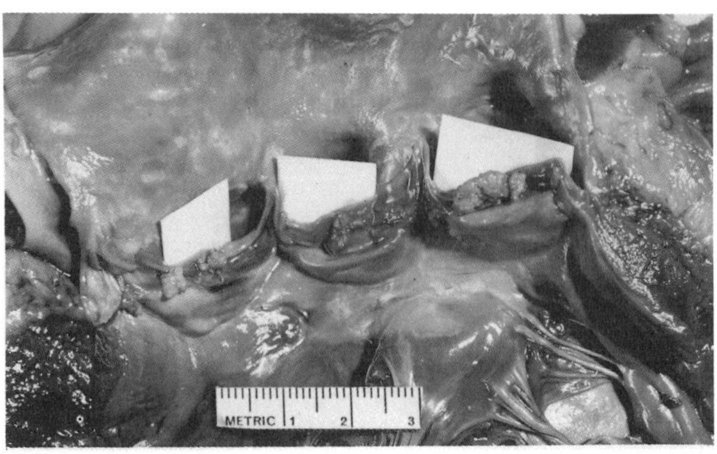

Figure 16-12 Veruccal vegetation on the contact surfaces of the aortic valve in marantic endocarditis. The patient was a 60-year-old male who died from mucinous adenocarcinoma of the lung.

ciation with a chronic disease, especially malignancy, should alert the clinician to the possibility of the presence of marantic endocarditis. In these cases echocardiography may be helpful in establishing the diagnosis.

Once the diagnosis is made, careful consideration should be given to valvular replacement in patients with left-sided involvement when the ultimate prognosis appears to be more related to the valvular insufficiency than to the underlying disease.

LÖFFLER'S ENDOCARDITIS

Löffler's endocarditis is the result of systemic hypereosinophilia which involves the myocardium in 95% of cases. The final stages of this disease are characterized by endocardial fibrosis with superimposed thrombus with congestive heart failure and cardiac enlargement. Etiologies for the hypereosinophilia include leukemia, profound parasitic infection, drug reaction, polyarteritis nodosa, Hodgkin's disease, tumors, and idiopathic causes.[96,97]

The disease occurs predominantly in white men and half of the patients present with cardiomegaly, frequently a murmur of mitral regurgitation and congestive heart failure, poorly responsive to therapy.[98,99] Major systemic emboli are the rule, at times leading to serious neurologic complications including stroke. Due to extensive fibrosis the heart failure has a restrictive pathophysiology. Primary destruction of the right ventricle may lead to a clinical picture of right heart failure with tricuspid valve insufficiency. Death occurs within months of the development of congestive failure. The major pathologic findings of thickened endocardium, mitral, or tricuspid valve can easily be demonstrated on two-dimensional echocardiography.

Surgical removal of endocardial clots with some successful resolution of the restrictive pathophysiologic picture has been reported.

SURGICAL THERAPY

When congestive heart failure occurs surgery continues to be life-saving. The timing and indications for surgical intervention may change, perhaps dramatically, in the next few years with our increasing ability to manage moderate to severe congestive heart failure with more powerful inotropic agents and afterload reducing agents. Also, the rapid proliferation of new antibiotics may prove very effective in controlling infection before valve destruction has occurred or where previously uncontrollable abscesses and resistant bacteria made surgical intervention necessary. Also, as the reliability and long-term effectiveness and safety of prosthetic valves increase, indications for valve replacement may become more liberal.

At the present time indications for surgical intervention are:

1. Moderate to severe congestive heart failure due to aortic and/or mitral insufficiency[70,100–104]
2. Aortic valve endocarditis with acute, severe aortic insufficiency[70,100,103]
3. Fungal endocarditis[70,71,100,103]
4. Left-sided infection with Gram-negative organism (possible exception of *Haemophilus* sp)[70,100,103,105–107]
5. Left ventricular and/or aortic aneurysm[105]
6. Myocardial abscess with heart block or resistant to therapy (except sensitive streptococci)[70,100]
7. Prosthetic valve endocarditis (except sensitive streptococcus species)[70,100,104]
8. Recurrent endocarditis (with resistant organisms or after repeated failure of a trial of medical treatment with sensitive organisms[70,100]
9. Massive pulmonary emboli with right-sided endocarditis and vegetations (unpublished data)
10. Clinical nonresponders with culture-negative endocarditis (controversial)[42]
11. Recurrent systemic emboli[70,100,102]
12. Large left-sided vegetation on echocardiogram (controversial)[55,65,66]

Congestive Heart Failure

Numerous studies have demonstrated the life-saving effect of surgical intervention in patients with moderate to severe congestive heart failure when due to valvular insufficiency.[70,100–104] This is most clearly the case in patients who develop rapidly progressive aortic insufficiency characterized by unremittant congestive heart failure. In these patients, unless surgical intervention is performed, mortality may approach 100% from heart failure or due to a sudden, arrhythmic death. Surgical survival may be as high as 70%.

The benefits of immediate mitral valve replacement in congestive heart failure due to acute mitral insufficiency has not been so clearly demonstrated, although in those patients with uncontrollable congestive heart failure due to mitral insufficiency, urgent valve replacement remains the treatment of choice.[73] However, in moderate congestive heart failure which is controllable with inotropic support and diuretics with or without afterload reduction, the patient may not require urgent valvular replacement because the incidence of sudden death is much lower in this group. A more conservative approach — initial medical management with subsequent elective surgical corrective procedure if failure continues — may be more desirable here. In our experience with proper medical treatment, patients with mitral insufficiency may be controlled allowing for completion of antibiotic therapy with the conversion of the patient from acute mitral insufficiency to a stable patient with chronic mitral insufficiency who may be managed for several years medically without valve replacement. In addition, those patients who develop either mitral insufficiency or aortic insufficiency slowly, ie, over a period of 2 to 3 weeks, may respond well to medical management and not require any surgical intervention.

Those patients, predominantly IV drug abusers, who develop tricuspid or pulmonary valvular insufficiency, seldom require surgical intervention. Diuretics and digitalis may be of some use in controlling mild to moderate right-sided congestive heart failure. Severe right ventricular failure is seen rarely, most often in association with left ventricular failure or, in the case of IV drug abusers, with mild to moderate pulmonary hypertension as a consequence of increased pulmonary vascular resistance secondary to pulmonary vascular disease due to their addiction. In our experience tricuspid valve replacement has been necessary on three occasions in the past 10 years for unremittant right ventricular failure in the face of chronic pulmonary hypertension. All three cases came to operation after completion of antibiotic therapy but subsequently died within 6 weeks to 1 year as a result of pulmonary complications of their primary disease.

Not all infective left-sided valves that come to surgery require prosthetic replacement. We have had on occasion patients with severe intractable failure who at operation had a perforation of the aortic or mitral valve leaflet amenable to valvuloplasty. In the future this may be even more frequent as mitral valvular reconstructive techniques continue to improve. Figure 16-3 is a flow chart which summarizes the management of patients with valvular insufficiency.

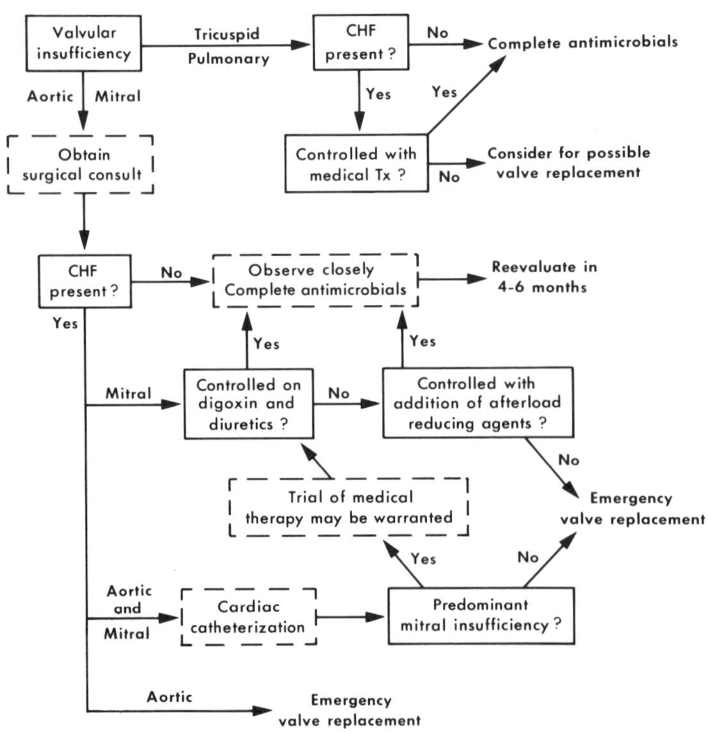

Figure 16-13 A useful flow chart for the management of patients with valvular insufficiency due to endocarditis.

Fungal Infections

Medical treatment alone of fungal endocarditis without surgery should not be attempted unless there is a clear contraindication to surgery. This is even more important when fungal endocarditis occurs on prosthetic valves.[71] With right-sided native valve fungal endocarditis in drug addicts, the general tendency is to attempt a medical cure. Although there have been isolated reports of medical cure, the chance of this occurring is remote and a high rate of subsequent relapse has been reported.

It is generally recommended that surgical intervention be done after seven to ten days of antifungal therapy; however, the benefit of any such delay has not been demonstrated. Early in the growth of the fungal vegetation the bulk of the growth protrudes freely into the bloodstream with only minimal damage to the underlying valve tissue allowing the removal of the infected mass and the preservation of the valve. This is especially true with infections of the tricuspid valve but also has been possible occasionally with mitral and aortic valves.

Left-sided infections are characterized by large vegetations on the mitral and/or aortic valve with a high tendency to embolization. Unfortunately, embolization may occur prior to the growth of this organism in culture. For this reason, in patients whose initial blood cultures have failed to culture organisms within 72 hours, the findings of a large vegetation by two-dimensional echocardiography in a patient with the clinical features of endocarditis may provide enough information to bring the patient urgently to surgery, thus preventing a catastrophic outcome.

Gram-Negative Infections

Medical thereapy alone has generally been unsuccessful in valvular endocarditis due to Gram-negative organisms[71,103,105] with the possible exception of infection with *Hemophilus* species.[28,107]

It has been reported that addicts have a higher incidence of right-sided *Pseudomonas* infection as compared to nonaddicts and 50% or more of these right-sided infections in addicts can be cured medically.[89] In general, combined medical-surgical therapy should be used in most if not all cases of left-sided Gram-negative infection with the possible exception of those with *Hemophilus* species, where a trial of medical therapy should be given. In IV drug abusers with right-sided *Pseudomonas* infections, medical therapy should be first attempted but surgical therapy should be considered rapidly in those patients who show persistance of their infection due either to recurrent episodes of sepsis, persistant fever, pulmonary emboli, or right ventricular failure. Arbulu and Asfaw recommend removal of the infected tricuspid valve without prosthetic valve replacement in those with normal pulmonary vascular resistance.[108]

Aneurysm and Abscess

All patients with aneurysms involving the heart or aorta should probably be treated surgically. This includes free wall aneurysms of the left ventricle from abscess formation or secondary to septic emboli to the coronary arteries with myocardial infarction,[109] sinus of Valsalva aneurysms, and false aneuryms of the left ventricle due to perforation of mitral/aortic intervalvular fibrosa.[105] When these diagnoses are suspected, although echocardiography can frequently demonstrate the presence of these problems, cardiac catheterization and angiocardiography and/or coronary arteriography should be done to definitely delineate the extent of the problem.

Prosthetic Valve Endocarditis

The need for valve replacement is primarily related to the inability of antibiotics to eradicate the infection in the presence of the prosthetic valve and in the presence of complications of the infection. Generally accepted indications for valve replacement include most *S aureus* infections, all fungal infections, recurrent macroemboli, myocardial abscess formation, severe valve dysfunction, persistently positive blood cultures, and relapse of infection.* Patients with very sensitive streptococcal infections, which excludes enterococcus, can be cured medically without valve replacement and an attempt at medical sterilization should be made in these cases.[46] With failure on one attempt, the patient should be treated surgically with antibiotics administered for 4 weeks after surgery.

All patients with prosthetic valve endocarditis should be followed closely since emergency surgery might be needed at any time as a result of destruction of the bioprosthetic leaflets, dehiscence, or obstruction of the valve by large clots. In addition, the paravalvular leak may be so severe as to result in congestive heart failure, which may be uncontrollable by medical management. All patients with prosthetic endocarditis should have repeated cardiac fluoroscopy in

*References 16, 44–46, 70, 74, 82, 104, 110

order to detect the dehiscence of the prosthesis. This may be entirely inapparent clinically even with the presence by fluoroscopy or two-dimensional echocardiography of violent rocking of the valve due to detachment of most of the circumference of the suture line.

Recurrent Endocarditis

Recurrence or relapse of endocarditis has been suggested as an indication for surgical intervention especially in light of the report by Welton et al[92] who noted an increased mortality among their patients with recurrence. This finding is supported by our own experience (unpublished data). In the case of IV drug abusers, however, the placement of a prosthetic valve for recurrence of endocarditis alone is not warranted due to the high recurrence rate after surgery, and morbidity and mortality in this group of patients with a prosthetic valve.[25,92] If the patient is hemodynamically stable, a repeat trial of antibiotics should be instituted.

In nonaddicts valve replacement should not be done for recurrence alone without other complicating factors such as severe valve insufficiency with heart failure or significant recurrent systemic emboli. Surgery must be weighed against the risk associated with the placement and presence of a prosthetic valve, ie surgical mortality and morbidity, risk of emboli from a prosthetic valve, and risk of anticoagulation.

Pulmonary Emboli

Right-sided infection may cause emboli large enough to produce one or more large pulmonary infarctions. In unusual patients with either staphylococcal or streptococcal tricuspid valve endocarditis, emboli may be large enough to acutely compromise the patient, thus prompting the addition of anticoagulant therapy, though, it is not clear that anticoagulation is useful.

In our experience in a large population of IV drug abusers, 1% to 2% of patients with tricuspid valve endocarditis had recurrence of massive multiple pulmonary emboli in spite of anticoagulation therapy and required surgical débridement of the vegetation or even excision of the tricuspid valve with or without placement of a bioprosthesis. On several occasions pulmonary embolectomy has been attempted with uniformly poor results. These patients generally have some degree of pulmonary hypertension as a result of emboli and IV drug abuse, and may not be appropriate candidates for tricuspid valve excision alone without valve replacement.

Culture-Negative Endocarditis

Studies have demonstrated that patients with culture-negative endocarditis who respond clinically within the first week of antibiotic therapy generally have a good prognosis whereas those who do not respond during the first week have a poor prognosis.[27] Possibly, surgical intervention in these nonresponders in which an etiologic agent has not been determined may be beneficial both by reducing the infecting mass and by allowing direct examination and culture of the vegetation in an attempt to determine the cause.

Recurrent Systemic Emboli

Our present approach to the problem of recurrent systemi emboli in IV drug abusers is to not replace a valve for recurrent emboli alone because of the high subsequent reinfection rate and high mortality rate. In nonaddicts valve replacement is indicated if an embolus affects the CNS and leaves the patient with relatively good residual function, if the event occurred in the early part of treatment, and if the echocardiogram continues to show large vegetations. If the first embolus was not to the brain or if it occurred late in the course of treatment or if there are no large vegetations (>1.0 cm) by echocardiography, then surgery is not recommended unless a second event occurs. Figure 16-14 outlines our approach to this problem.

Left-sided Vegetation on Echocardiogram

A prospective multicenter study must be performed to determine the predictability of embolization by echocardiography. To date no clear criteria exist which would allow the prediction of an embolus with sufficient certainty to warrant prophylactic valve replacement. However bulky vegetations demonstrated by echocardiography have been noted to embolize frequently,[111] often with catastrophic results — thus the controversy exists.[55,65,66] At present we do not, as yet, operate on this indication alone.

PROPHYLAXIS

Though no prophylactic regimen provides complete protection against all possible bacteria, studies have shown the effectiveness in animal models of several regimens against the more common strains of streptococci, staphylococci, and enterococci which cause the vast majority of procedure-related episodes of endocarditis. Table

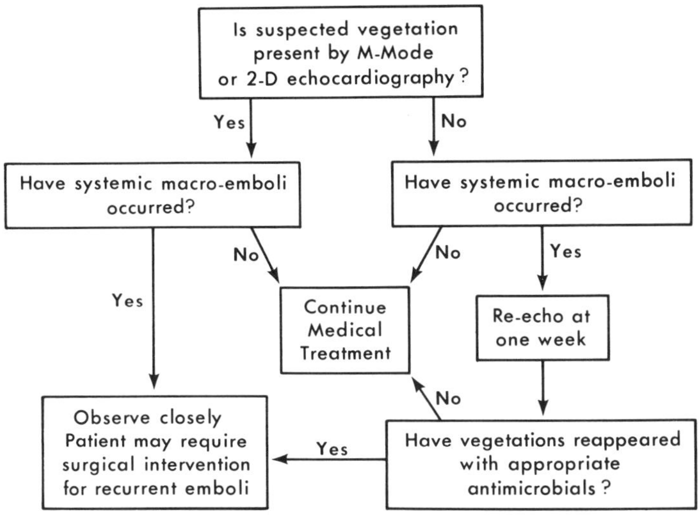

Figure 16-14 A decision tree presenting the authors' recommendations for managing systemic macroemboli resulting from left-sided *bacterial* endocarditis. Fungal endocarditis typically has a large vegetation on the echocardiogram. These patients, however will require surgical therapy.

Table 16-2
Cardiovascular Conditions for Which Bacterial Endocarditis Prophylaxis is Given

Conditions with highest risk
Prosthetic heart valves
Previous episode of infectious endocarditis within 6 months*
Conditions with medium risk
Acquired valvular disease (eg, rheumatic, calcific [aorta and mitral anulus], syphilitic, atherosclerotic, idiopathic)
History of rheumatic fever
Congenital heart disease (excluding uncomplicated secundum atrial septal defect and ligated and divided patent ductus arteriosus)
Intravenous drug abusers*
Idiopathic hypertrophic subaortic stenosis
Previous episode of infective endocarditis >6 months*
Mitral valve prolapse with mitral regurgitation
Conditions with lowest risk†
Transvenous pacemakers
Mitral valve prolapse without mitral regurgitation
Tricuspid valve prolapse (isolated)*
Indwelling catheters, arteriovenous shunts, and ventriculoatrial shunts

*Authors' opinion.
†Questionable need for prophylaxis.

16-2 lists the cardiovascular conditions considered to increase the risk for endocarditis related to the procedures listed in Table 16-3.[122]

The general principles which guide the administration of antibiotics are provided by animal research and common sense. Of primary importance is the selection of an antibiotic regimen which is highly bactericidal against the expected organism. The identity of the organism may be known from prior cultures or may be a highly likely offenders such as streptococci from the upper respiratory tract, enterococci from the genitourinary tract, or staphylococci from abscesses in the skin and subcutaneous tissues. The drugs should be given to provide the highest blood levels at the time of the expected bacteremia. In the case of surgical operation, the bacteremia is biphasic, corresponding to opening

Table 16-3
Procedures That may Cause Transient Bacteremia

Streptococci — necessity for prophylaxis is certain in:
- Dental care where bleeding may be produced
- Surgery, procedures or instrumentation on the lower and upper respiratory tract, and maxillofacial region
- Upper gastrointestinal (GI) endoscopy with biopsy
- Bronchoscopy
- Nasotracheal intubation

Streptococci — necessity for prophylaxis is uncertain in*:
- Liver biopsy
- Upper GI endoscopy without biopsy
- Orotracheal intubation

Enterococci — necessity for prophylaxis is certain in:
- Surgery, procedures, or instrumentation on the genitourinary tract, biliary system, and lower GI tract
- Septic abortion or peripartum infection
- Sigmoidoscopy or colonoscopy with biopsy
- Rectal biopsy

Enterococci — necessity for prophylaxis is uncertain in*:
- Sigmoidoscopy or colonoscopy without biopsy
- Barium enema
- Normal vaginal delivery
- Uncomplicated insertion or removal of intrauterine device
- Dilatation and curettage of the uterus
- Proctoscopy
- Pelvic examination

Staphylococci — necessity for prophylaxis is certain in:
- Manipulation or drainage of abscesses
- Débridement of burns

*Recommended by authors for highest risk group only (see Table 16-2)

and closing the skin, and antibiotics should be repeated prior to skin closure if the operation is longer than 4 hours. The need to continue antibiotic prophylaxis after surgery for 24 to 48 hours has not been proved. Since timing is of critical importance when the patient is at high risk and when the oral route is not an option, then a parenteral route is preferred. In general, prophylaxis is not indicated when surgery is done through an incision where sterilization of the skin is possible and there is no opening of a organ normally inhabited by bacteria.

Allergic sensitivities will influence the choice of antibiotic. The risk to the patient of any drug and its route of administration should be carefully weighed against the benefit desired ie, the reduction of the risk of endocarditis. For instance, it has been noted that the incidence of penicillin anaphylaxis is similar in magnitude to the incidence of endocarditis following tooth extractions.[113,114]

In 1977 a committee of the American Heart Association presented recommendations for antimicrobial prophylaxis in patients with underlying cardiac disease.[115] These recommendations have since been criticized on various grounds: (1) Their recommendations are based primarily on animal studies and not on human clinical trials. (2) The regimens suggested may be excessive in the amount of drug and in the duration of therapy. (3) The routine regimen is generally uncomfortable, painful, and unacceptable to the patient. (4) The risk benefit ratio is low with some indications. (5) The recommendations are not being used in actual practice. Not only is the oral route preferred by dentists over the recommended parenteral route for most dental procedures; it is not even given in the regimen suggested by the American Heart Association committee. (6) The development of new-generation antibiotics may be more effective. These criticisms are, in our own experience, for the most part valid. Thus we support the modifications of Oakley and Somerville and Keys with our own adjustments as presented in Table 16-4.[116–118]

We believe that these recommendations incorporate recent clinical work, are acceptable to the usual patient, and are easily applied by the practicing dentist and clinician.

Table 16-4
Recommended Antibiotic Regimens for Antimicrobial Prophylaxis

Streptococci	
Nonpenicillin-allergic	Amoxicillin 3.0 g orally 1h before procedure or when NPO
	Amoxicillin 1.0 g IM 30 min before procedure
Penicillin-allergic	Erythromycin 2.0 g orally 1h before procedure or when NPO
	Vancomycin hydrochloride 1.0 g IV 1h before procedure
Enterococci	
Nonpenicillin-allergic	Amoxicillin 1.0 g IM or IV plus tobramycin 1.0 mg/kg IM or IV 1h before and 12 h after procedure
Penicillin-allergic	Vancomycin 1.0 g IV plus tobramycin 1.0 mg/kg IM or IV 1h before and 12 h after procedure
Staphylococci Penicillin-allergic	Vancomycin 1.0 g IV plus tobramycin 1.0 mg/kg IM or IV 1h before and 12h after procedure

Adult doses with normal renal function. Patients with impaired renal function may not require repeat dose depending on degree of dysfunction.
Pediatric doses: amoxicillin 50 mg/kg, erythromycin 40 mg/kg, vancomycin 20 mg/kg (not to exceed maximum adult dose).

REFERENCES

1. Lepeschkin E: On the relation between the site of valvular involvement in endocarditis and the blood pressure resting on the valve. *Am J Med Sci* 1952;224:318–319.
2. Rodbard S: Blood velocity and endocarditis. *Circulation* 1963;27:18–28.
3. Holmes RK, Ramirez-Ronda CH: *Adherence of Bacteria to the Endothelium of Heart Valves. Infective Endocarditis.* American Heart Association, monograph No. 52, 1977, pp 12–13.
4. Gould K, Ramirez-Ronda CH, Holmes Rk, et al: Adherence of bacteria to heart valves in vitro. *J Clin Invest* 1975;56:1364–1370.
5. McCarthy JB, Jacob HS, Moldow CF: Bacteral adherence to fibronectin and endothelial cells: a possible mechanism for bacterial tissue tropism. *J Lab Clin Med* 1984;103:34–43.
6. Le Frock JL, Ellis CA, Klainer A, Weinstein L: Transient bacteremia associated with barium enema. *Arch Intern Med* 1975;135:835–840.
7. Le Frock JL, Ellis CA, Turchick JB, et al: Transient bacteremia associated with sigmoidoscopy. *N Engl J Med* 1973;289:467–469.
8. Ehrie M Morgan AP, Moore FD, et al: Predisposing causes of bacterial endocarditis. *J Trauma* 1978;18:664–666.
9. Morgan G, Ginks W, Siddons H, et al: Septicemia in patients with an endocardial pacemaker. *Am J Cardiol* 1979;44:221–224.
10. Buchbinder NA, Roberts WC: Alcoholism. An important but unemphasized factor predisposing to infective endocarditis. *Arch Intern Med* 1973; 132:689–692.
11. Lerner PE, Weinstein L: Infective endocarditis in the antiobiotic era. *N Engl J Med* 1966;274: 259–266.
12. Pelletier LL Jr, Petersdorf RG: Infective endocarditis: A review of 125 cases from the University of Washington Hospitals, 1963–72. *Medicine* 1977;4:287–313.
13. Leitersdorf E, Friedman G, Gozal D, et al: Infective endocarditis in Jerusalem. A comparative analysis of native and prosthetic valve endocarditis. *Isr J Med Sci* 1983;19:491–494.
14. Johnson DH, Rosenthal A, Nadas A: A forty-year review of bacterial endocarditis in infancy and childhood. *Circulation* 1975;51:581–588.
15. Stein PD, Harken DE, Dexter L: The nature and prevention of prosthetic valve endocarditis. *Am Heart J* 1966;71:393–407.
16. Rossiter SJ et al: Prosthetic valve endocarditis. *J Thorac Cardiovasc Surg* 1978;76:795–803.
17. Tuazon CV, Hill R, Sheagren JN: Microbiologic study of street heroin and injection paraphernalia. *J Infect Dis* 1974;29:327–329.
18. Reisberg BE: Infective endocarditis in the narcotic addict. *Prog Cardiovasc Dis* 1979;22: 193–204.
19. Lerner PI, Weinstein L: Infective endocarditis in the antibiotic era. *N Engl J Med* 1966;274: 199–206.
20. Wang K, Gobel F, Geason DF: Bacterial endocarditis in idiopathic hypertrophic subaortic stenosis. *Am Heart J* 1975;89:359–365.
21. Lachman AS, Bramwell-Jones DM, Lakier JB, et al: Infective endocarditis in the billowing mitral leaflet syndrome. *Br Heart J* 1975;37: 326–330.
22. Weinstein AJ, McHenry M: Bacterial endocarditis in a patient with mitral valve prolapse. *Arch Intern Med* 1979;139:1191–1192.
23. Kuhn C, Weber N: Mural bacterial endocarditis of a ventricular friction lesion. *Arch Pathol* 1973;95:92–93.
24. Quinn TJ, Codini MA, Harris AA: Infected cardiac myxoma. *Am J Cardiol* 1984;53:381–382.
25. Hubbell GM, Cheitlin MD, Rapaport E: Presentation, management, and follow-up evaluation of infective endocarditis in drug addicts. *Am Heart J* 1981;102:85–94.
26. Chambers HF, Korzeniowski OM, Sande MA, et al: *Staphylococcus aureus* endocarditis: clinical

manifestations in addicts and nonaddicts. *Medicine* 1983;62:170–177.
27. Pesanti EL, Smith IM: Infective endocarditis with negative blood cultures. *Am J Med* 1979;66: 43–50.
28. Cohen PS, Maguire JH, Weinstein L: Infective endocarditis caused by gram-negative bacteria: a review of the literature, 1945–1977. *Prog Cardiovasc Dis* 1980;23:205–242.
29. Sklaver AR, Hoffman TA, Greenman RL: Staphylococcal endocarditis in addicts. *South Med J* 1978;71:638:643.
30. Wilson WR, Giuliani ER, Danielson GK, et al: General considerations in the diagnosis and treatment of infective endocarditis. *Mayo Clin Proc* 1982;57:81–85.
31. Brandenburg RO, Giuliani ER, Wilson WR, et al: Infective endocarditis — a 25 year overview of diagnosis and therapy. *J Am Coll Cardiol* 1983;1: 280–291.
32. Von Reyn CF, Levey BS, Arbeit R, et al: Infective endocarditis. An analysis based on strict case definitions. *Ann Intern Med* 1981;94:505–518.
33. Alpert JS, Kraus HF, Dalen JE, et al: Pathogenesis of Osler's nodes. *Ann Intern Med* 1976; 85:471–473.
34. Karchmer AW, Dismukes WE, Buckley MJ, et al: Late prosthetic valve endocarditis. *Am J Med* 1978;64:199–206.
35. Kerr A Jr,: *Subacute Bacterial Endocarditis*. Springfield, Ill, Charles C Thomas Publisher, 1955.
36. Weinstein L: Modern infective endocarditis. *JAMA* 1975;233:260–265.
37. Hermans PE: The clinical manifestations of infective endocarditis. *Mayo Clin Proc* 1982;57: 15–21.
38. Churchill MA Jr, Geraci JE, Hunder GG: Musculoskeletel manifestations of bacterial endocarditis. *Ann Intern Med* 1977;87:754–759.
39. Mills J, Drew D: *Serratia marcescens* endocarditis: a regional illness associated with intravenous drug abuse. *Ann Intern Med* 1976;84: 29–35.
40. Lange M, Salaki JS, Middleton JR, et al: Infective endocarditis in heroin addicts: epidemiological observations and some unusual cases. *Am Heart J* 1978;96:144–152.
41. Linde LM, Rao PS: A modern view of infective endocarditis. *Cardiology* 1973;2:15–34.
42. Thell R, Martin FH, Edwards JE: Clinicopathologic correlations — bacterial endocarditis in subjects 60 years of age and older. *Circulation* 1975; 51:174–182.
43. Applefeld MM, Hornick RB: Infective endocarditis in patients over age 60. *Am Heart J* 1974;88: 90–94.
44. Wilson WR, Jaumun Pm, Danielson GK, et al: Prosthetic valve endocarditis. *Ann Intern Med* 1975;82:751–756.
45. Watanakunakorn C: Prosthetic valve infective endocarditis. *Prog Cardiovasc Dis* 1979;22: 181–192.
46. Masur H, Johnson WD: Prosthetic valve endocarditis. *J Thorac Cardiovasc Surg* 1980;80: 31–37.
47. Van Scoy RE: Culture negative endocarditis. *Mayo Clin Proc* 1982;57:149–154.
48. Powers DL, Mandel GL: Intraleukocytic bacterial in endocarditis patients. *JAMA* 1974;227: 312–313.
49. Beli J, Waisbren BA: The numbers of blood cultures necessary to diagnose most cases of bacterial endocarditis. *Am J Med Sci* 1956;232: 284–288.
50. Werner AS, Cobbs CG, Kaye D, et al: Studies on the bacteremia of bacterial endocarditis. *JAMA* 1967;202:199–203.
51. Dillon JC, Feigenbaum H, Konecke LL, et al: Echocardiographic manifestations of valvular vegetations. *Am Heart J* 1973;86:698–704.
52. Berger M, Gallinstein PE, Benhuri P, et al: Evaluation of aortic valve endocarditis by two-dimensional echocardiography. *Chest* 1981;80: 61–64.
53. Thomson KR, Nanda NC, Gramiak R: The reliability of echocardiography in the diagnosis of infective endocarditis. *Radiology* 1977;125: 473–476.
54. Come PC, Isaacs RE, Riley MF: Diagnostic accuracy of M-mode echocardiography in active infective endocarditis and prognostic implications of ultrasound-detectable vegetations. *Am Heart J* 1982;103:839–847.
55. Wann LS, Dillon JC, Weyman AE, et al: Echocardiography in bacterial endocarditis. *N Engl J Med* 1976;295:135–139.
56. Mintz GS, Kotler MN, Segal BL, et al: Comparison of two-dimensional and M-mode echocardiography in the evaluation of patients with infective endocarditis. *Am J Cardiol* 1979;43:738–744.
57. Wann S, Hallam C, Dillon JC, et al: Comparison of M-mode and cross-sectional echocardiography in infective endocarditis. *Circulation* 1979;60: 728–733.
58. Roy P, Tajik AJ, Giuliani ER, et al: Spectrum of echocardiographic findings in bacterial endocarditis. *Circulation* 1976;53:474–482.
59. Strom J, Becker R, Davis R, et al: Echocardiographic and surgical correlations in bacterial endocarditis. *Circulation* 1980;62:I-164–I-166.
60. Ginzton LE, Siegel RJ, Criley JM: Natural history of tricuspid valve endocarditis: a two dimensional echocardiographic study. *Am J Cardiol* 1982;49:1853–1860.
61. Andy JJ, Sheikh MU, Ali N, et al: Echocardiographic observations in opiate addicts with active infective endocarditis. Frequency of involvement of the various valves and comparison of echocardiographic features of right- and left-sided cardiac valve endocarditis. *Am J Cardiol* 1977;40: 17–23.
62. Rubenson DS, Tucker CR, Stinson EB, et al: The use of echocardiography in diagnosing culture-negative endocarditis. *Circulation* 1981;64: 641–646.
63. Gottlieb S, Khuddus SA, Balooki H, et al: Echocardiographic diagnosis of aortic valve vegetations in candida endocarditis. *Circulation* 1974; 50:826–830.
64. Mintz GS, Kotler MN, Segal BL, et al: Survival of patients with aortic valve endocarditis. The prognostic implications of the echocardiogram. *Arch Intern Med* 1979;139:862–866.

65. Davis RS, Strom JA, Frishman W, et al: The demonstration of vegetations by echocardiography in bacterial endocarditis. An indication for early surgical intervention. *Am J Med* 1980; 69:57–63.
66. Stewart JA, Silimperi D, Harris P, et al: Echocardiographic documentation of vegetative lesions in infective endocarditis: clinical implications. *Circulation* 1980;61:374–379.
67. Buchbinder NA, Roberts WC: Left-sided valvular active infective endocarditis. *Am J Med* 1972;53:20–35.
68. Arnett EN, Roberts WC: Valve rings abscess in active infective endocarditis. *Circulation* 1976; 54:140–145.
69. Scanlan JG, Seward JB, Tajik AJ: Valve ring abscess in infective endocarditis: visualization with wide angle two dimensional echocardiography. *Am J Cardiol* 1982;49:1794–1800.
70. Dinubile MJ: Surgery in active endocarditis. *Ann Intern Med* 1982;96:650–659.
71. Utley JR, Mills J, Roe BB: The role of valve replacement in the treatment of fungal endocarditis. *J Thorac Cardiovasc Surg* 1975;69:255–258.
72. Hosenpud JD, Greenberg BH: The preoperative evaluation in patients with endocarditis. Is cardiac catheterization necessary? *Chest* 1983;84: 690–694.
73. Mills J, Abbott J, Utley JR, et al: Role of cardiac catheterization in infective endocarditis. *Chest* 1977;72:576–582.
74. Welton DE, Young JB, Raizner AE, et al: Value and safety of cardiac catheterization during active infective endocarditis. *Am J Cardiol* 1979;44: 1306–1310.
75. Cheitlin MD, Mills J: Infective endocarditis: is cardiac catheterization usually needed before cardiac surgery? *Chest* 1984;86:4–6.
76. Mills J, Utley J, Abbott J: Heart failure in infective endocarditis: predisposing factors, course, and treatment. *Chest* 1974;66:151–157.
77. Lerner PI, Weinstein L: Infective endocarditis in the antibiotic era. *N Engl J Med* 1966;274: 388–393.
78. Roberts WC, Ewy GA, Glancy DL, et al: Valvular stenosis produced by active infective endocarditis. *Circulation* 1967;36:449–451.
79. Sacks PV, Lakier JB, Barlow JB: Severe aortic insufficiency in the same patient caused by bacterial endocarditis. *Br Med J* 1969;3:97–98.
80. Ryan DS, Pastor BH, Meyerson RM: Abscess of the myocardium. *Am J Med Sci* 1966;251: 698–705.
81. Sanson J, Sladki S, Gouhn JG: Myocardial abscesses. *Am Heart J* 1963;66:301–308.
82. Wilson WR, Danielson GK, Siuliani ER, et al: Prosthetic valve endocarditis. *Mayo Clin Proc* 1982;57:155–161.
83. Wang K, Gobel F, Gleason DF, et al: Complete heart block complicating bacterial endocarditis. *Circulation* 1972;46:939–946.
84. Wilson WR, Giuhani ER, Danielson GK, et al: Management of complications of infective endocarditis, *Mayo Clin Proc* 1982;57:162–170.
85. Qizilbaxh AH, Schwartz CJ: False aneurysm of left ventricle due to perforation of mitral-aortic intervalvular fibrosa with rupture and cardiac tamponade. *Am J Cardiol* 1973;32:110–112.
86. Roach MR, Drake CG: Ruptured cerebral aneurysms caused by microorganisms. *N Engl J Med* 1965;273:240–244.
87. Kaplan EL, Rich H, Gersony W, et al: A collaborative study of infective endocarditis in the 1970's. *Circulation* 1979;59:327–339.
88. Ivert TSA, Dismukes WE, Cobbs CG, et al: Prosthetic valve endocarditis. *Circulation* 1984; 69:223–232.
89. Banks T, Fletcher R, Ali N: Infective endocarditis in heroin addicts. *Am J Med* 1973;55: 444–451.
90. Stimmel B, Donoso E, Dack S: Comparison of infective endocarditis in drug addicts and nondrug users. *Am J Cardiol* 1973;32:924–928.
91. Keefer CS: Subacute bacterial endocarditis: active cases without bacteremia. *Ann Intern Med* 1937;11:714–720.
92. Welton DE, Young JB, Gentry WO, et al: Recurring infective endocarditis: analysis of predisposing factors and clinical features. *Am J Med* 1979;66:932–938.
93. Levison ME, Kaye D, Mandell GL, et al: Characteristics of patients multiple episodes of bacterial endocarditis. *JAMA* 1970;211:1355–1357.
94. Waller BF, Knapp WS, Edwards JE: Clincopathologic correlations. *Circulation* 1973;48: 644–650.
95. Chino F, Kodama A, Otake M, et al: Nonbacterialthrombotic endocarditis in a Japanese autopsy sample. A review of eighty cases. *Am Heart J* 1975;90:190–198.
96. Olsen EG: Endomyocardial fibrosis and Löffler's endocarditis parietalis fibroplastica. *Postgrade Med J* 1977;53:538–540.
97. Brockinston IF, Olsen EGJ: Löffler's endocarditis and Davies endomyocardial fibrosis. *Am Heart J* 1973;85:308–322.
98. Chusid MJ, Dale DC, West BC, et al: The hypereosinophilic syndrome analysis of fourteen cases with review of the literature. *Medicine* 1975;54:1–27.
99. Scott ME, Bruce JH: Löffler's endocarditis. *Br Heart J* 1975;37:534–538.
100. Karp RB: Role of surgery in infective endocarditis, in Brest AN (ed): *Cardiovascular Clinics*. Philadelphia, FA Davis Co, 1982, pp 157–175.
101. Wilson WR, Danielson GK, Giuliani ER, et al: Cardiac valve replacement in congestive heart failure due to infective endocarditis. *Mayo Clin Proc* 1979;54:223–226.
102. Jung JY, Saab SB, Almond CH: The case for early surgical treatment of left-sided primary infective endocarditis. *J Thorac Cardiovasc Surg* 1975;70:509–518.
103. Boyd AD, Spencer FC, Isom OW, et al: Infective endocarditis. An analysis of 54 surgically treated patients. *J Thorac Cardiovasc Surg* 1977;73: 23–30.
104. Richardson JV, Karp RB, Kirklin JW, et al: Treatment of infective endocarditis: a 10-year comparative analysis. *Circulation* 1978;58: 589–597.
105. Saksena FB, Kramer NE, Towne WD, et al: Infective aneurysm of the left ventricle: angiographic and echocardiographic features. *Am*

Heart J 1978;96:384–388.
106. Levitsky S, Mammana RB, Silverman NA, et al: Acute endocarditis in drug addicts: surgical treatment for gram-negative sepsis. *Circulation* 1982; 66:I-135–I-138.
107. Geraci JE, Wilson WR: Endocarditis due to gram-negative bacteria. *Mayo Clin Proc* 1982;57: 145–148.
108. Arbulu A, Asfaw I: Tricuspid valvulectomy without prosthetic replacement. *J. Thorac Cardiovasc Surg* 1981;82:684–691.
109. Mildvan D, Goldberg E, Berger M, et al: Diagnosis and management of septal myocardial abscess: a complication of bacterial endocarditis. *Am J Med Sci* 1977;274:311–316.
110. Sandza JG, Clark RE, Ferguson TB, et al: Replacement of prosthetic heart valves. *J Thorac Cardiovasc Surg* 1977;74:864–874.
111. Wann LS, Dillon JC, Weyman AE, et al: Echocardiography in bacterial endocarditis. *N Engl J Med* 1976;295:135–139.
112. Lowy L, Steigbigel NH: Infective endocarditis. Part III. Prevention of bacterial endocarditis. *Am Heart J* 1978;96:689–695.
113. Rudolph AH, Price EV: Penicillin reactions among patients in venereal disease clinic patiens. *JAMA* 1973;223:499–501.
114. Brown WJ, Simpson WG, Price EV: Reevaluation of reactions to penicillin in venereal disease clinic patients. *Public Health Rep* 1961;76: 189–198.
115. American Heart Association Committee: Prevention of bacterial endocarditis. *Circulation* 1977;56:139A–143A.
116. Oakley C, Somerville W: Prevention of infective endocarditis. *Br Heart J* 1981;45:233–235.
117. Keys TF: Antimicrobial prophylaxis for patients with congenital or valvular heart disease. *Mayo Clin Proc* 1982;57:171–175.
118. Shonson DC, Ashford RFU, Singh J: High-dose amoxycillin for preventing endocarditis. *Br Med J* 1980;280:446.

CHAPTER 17
Prosthetic Cardiac Valves

Edward S. Murphy

The development of prosthetic cardiac valves has been a major advance in the management of patients with valvular heart disease. Undoubtedly, many patients' lives have been prolonged by valve replacement surgery and many more have been allowed to lead more active and useful lives. However, valve replacement is a palliative and not a curative procedure. Patients with artificial heart valves continue to face a substantial risk of death or serious complication during their cardiac surgery and continuously thereafter. Initial and continued symptomatic improvement is not insured.

In making the decision for cardiac valve replacement, the physician must balance the risk of the procedure and subsequent complications of prosthetic valves against the natural history of the valvular heart disease. For the clinician to make an informed decision as to the timing of cardiac valve replacement and selection of prosthesis, it is important that he have an understanding of the types of valves, the functional and hemodynamic results of valve surgery, as well as the prognosis and complications of prosthetic valves.

The ideal valve substitute, ie, one having excellent hemodynamic performance, resistance to thrombogenesis and thromboemboli, and absence of degeneration throughout the human lifespan, is not available. Any selection of a valve prosthesis is a compromise. There are four functional categories of prosthetic valves: (1) caged ball, (2) caged disc, (3) tilting disc, and (4) tissue valve. (Figures 17-1–17-5).

The ball valve has been in continuous use for the longest time with the Starr-Edwards and Smeloff-Cutter prostheses the most commonly used.[1] The ball-valve prosthesis has remained in

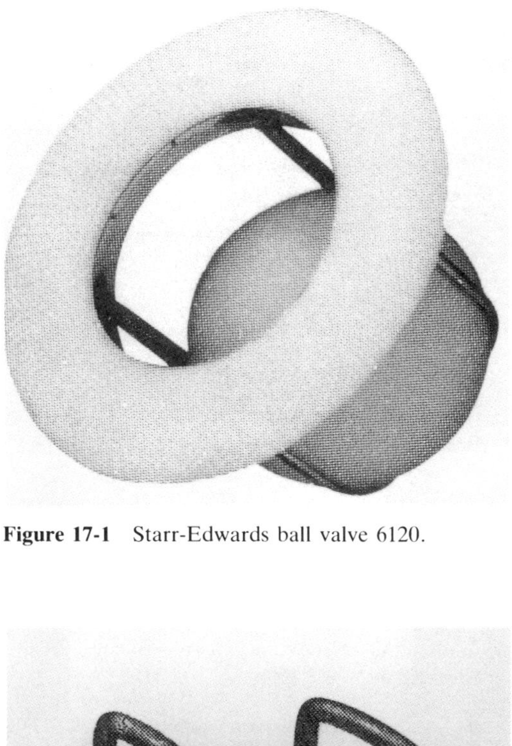

Figure 17-1 Starr-Edwards ball valve 6120.

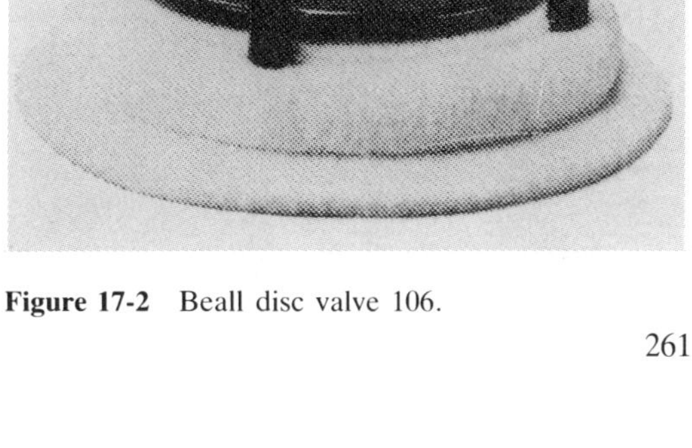

Figure 17-2 Beall disc valve 106.

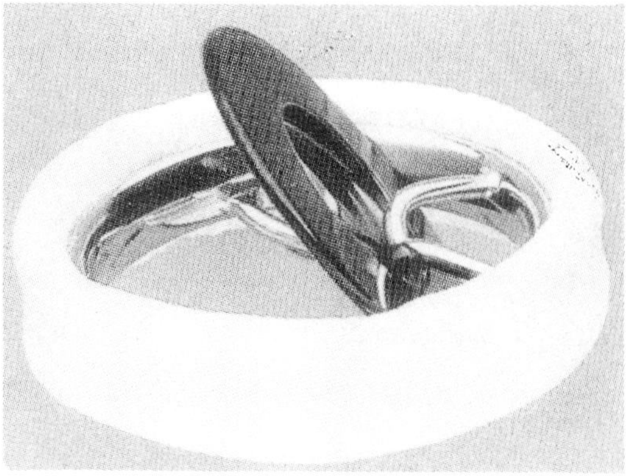

Figure 17-3 Björk-Shiley tilting-disc valve.

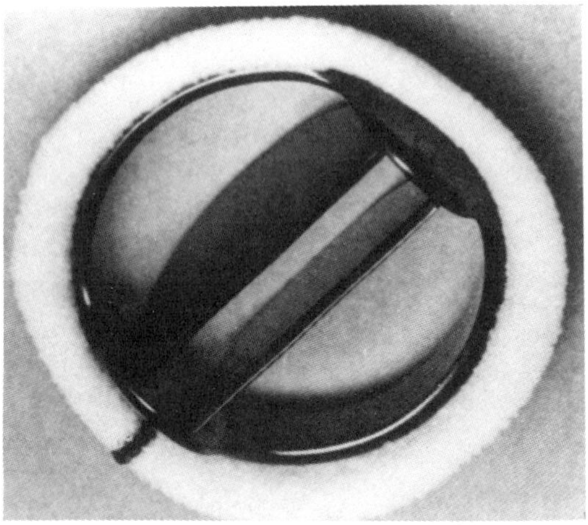

Figure 17-4 St. Jude tilting-disc valve.

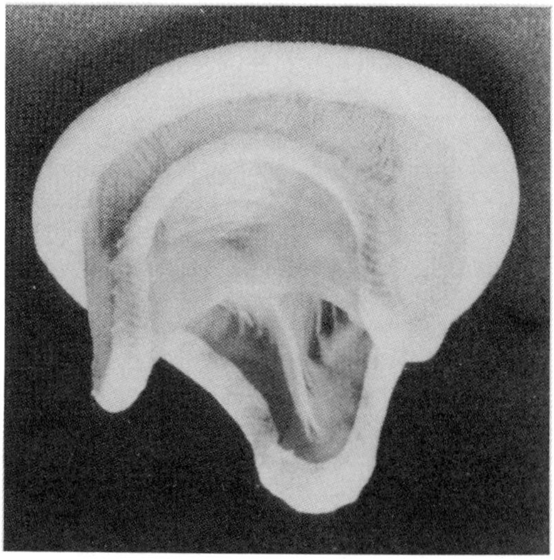

Figure 17-5 Carpentier-Edwards porcine valve.

use because of its generally satisfactory hemodynamic function and proven durability.[2] A major problem associated with the ball valve and other mechanical prostheses has been systemic thromboembolism, even with chronic anticoagulation therapy. For example, approximately 45% of the 10- to 15-year survivors of Starr-Edwards prostheses will have suffered a systemic embolus.[3]

Cloth-covered prostheses were developed in an attempt to reduce the incidence of thromboembolism by encouraging the ingrowth of neointima into the fabric.[4] Although there was some encouraging initial evidence of improvement in diminished thromboembolism rate, most of this improvement has subsequently been attributed to generally lower thromboemboli rates in patients currently undergoing valve replacement.[5] The cloth-covered valve is troubled with an increased rate of thrombosis and hemolysis.[6]

Ball variance due to absorption of lipid into the silastic poppet with swelling and fracture of the ball was an important early problem with ball-valve prostheses. Modifications in 1965 essentially eliminated the development of ball variance.[7]

Caged disc valves were developed because of concern about accommodation of the cage and poppet of the ball valve in the left ventricle.[8] The major problem with the disc valves is that of disc and strut wear with an incidence of thromboembolism and hemoydnamics similar to or worse than the ball valves.[9] Caged disc valves are not commonly used currently.

A variation of the original disc valves was the evolution of the tilting-disc valve originally introduced as the Björk-Shiley valve and Lillehei-Kaster valves in the late 1960s.[10,11] The central flow design was proposed in an attempt to improve hemoydnamics compared with the lateral flow of the ball-valve prosthesis. Newer variations of the tilting-disc valve include the MedTronic-Hall, Omniscience, and St. Jude bileaflet. Hemodynamics are generally satisfactory with thromboemboli comparable to ball-valve prostheses but with the persistent requirement of chronic anticoagulation.[12]

Tissue valves have been developed in an attempt to diminish the thromboembolic rate and minimize the requirement for anticoagulation.[13] Initially, several sterilization and preservation techniques as well as sources of valves were used including use of aortic homografts, porcine aortic valve, or bovine pericardium prepared with antibiotics, freezing, or gluteraldehyde. At present the most widely used tissue valves are the Hancock and Carpentier-Edwards. Both use the porcine aortic valve but differ in the stent composition and concentration of gluteraldehyde used in the tanning process. The major advantage of tissue valves is the relatively low incidence of thromboembolism, diminishing the necessity for long-term anticoagulation therapy.[12] Hemodynamic function is similar to that in the ball-valve and other mechanical prostheses (the newer mechanical tilting-disc prostheses appear to have better hemodynamics than the tissue valves.)[14] The major disadvantage of tissue valves has been the degeneration of the leaflets with resultant valve failure. The durability of tissue valves in the early years after implantation has been satisfactory but with evidence accomulating that their 8-year valve failure rate approaches 20% to 30%.[15,16]

At present, several different types of prosthetic valves are being used, each with its own advantages and disadvantages. Continuing analysis of long-term durability of the gluteraldehyde-preserved porcine valve and detailed comparison with mechanical valves should allow an informed selection of the most satisfactory cardiac valve substitute device.

AORTIC VALVE REPLACEMENT

The operative mortality of aortic valve replacement is currently 4% to 8%.[17,18] Perioperative myocardial infarction, which can contribute to poor late results, was 15% in early series but has been reduced to about 5% with current techniques of operative myocardial preservation.[19] Lesser degrees of myocardial damage related to operation are likely to be more prevalant. Current studies report 5-year survival of 70% to 75% for all patients undergoing aortic valve replacement, 10-year survival of 55%, and 15-year survival of 50%.[20–22] Selected subsets can be identified which have even better survival. The major cause of early deaths are cardiac failure, intraoperative deaths, embolic events, infection, hemorrhage, or sudden arrhythmic death. Of all late deaths 80% to 90% will be cardiac-related with myocardial infarction (0.3% per year), cardiac failure (0.7% to 1.0% per year), and sudden or arrhythmic death (1.5% per year) accounting for almost half the late deaths. Embolic events, prosthetic valve complications, infection, or hemorrhage constitute the remainder of the cardiac deaths. After recovery from the operation, the yearly mortality with prosthetic valves ranges from 2.0% to 4.7% per year.[20,21] The prosthesis may contribute directly to the cause of death in 20% to 30% of patients by precipitating endocarditis (<1% per year), thromboembolism (1% to 4% per year), prosthesis failure, or hemorrhage secondary to anticoagulation.[20–22] (Table 17-1). In addition, complications related to the prosthetic valve can contribute to late congestive heart failure, myocardial infarction, and unexplained sudden death. The mechanism of late sudden death is not firmly established but is associated with patients who are in New York Heart Association functional class III or IV postoperatively and have more frequent ventricular rhythm disturbances.[23]

The major variables influencing long-term prognosis in aortic valve replacement also tend to increase operative mortality. Advanced age, severe functional impairment (functional class IV), evidence of prior myocardial infarction in a severely damaged left ventricle, prior cardiac surgery, and concomitant operative interventions, as well as the operative factors of method and duration of myocardial preservation, all contribute both to operative mortality and diminished long-term survival.[17,24] The type of valve lesion has little effect on late survival. The adverse impact of coronary disease on late survival has been diminished by recent surgical techniques.[25] However, even in the elderly or in

Table 17-1
Complications of Prosthetic Valves

	Total	Fatal
Prosthetic valve failure	1.0%–4%/yr	0.1%–1.2%/yr
Endocarditis	0.8%/yr	0.4%/yr
Reoperation	1.0%–2.0%/yr	
Heart failure		0.7%/yr
Sudden death		0.8%/yr
Anticoagulation-related hemorrhage	3.5%/yr	0.1%–1%/yr
Emboli		
Aortic	0.5%–4%/yr	0.1%/yr
Mitral	1.0%–5.0%/yr	0.5%/yr

patients with severe left ventricular dysfunction, aortic valve replacement for aortic stenosis, functional improvement, and survival can be very encouraging.[26]

Despite limitations in the measurement of functional classification, this can be a useful guide. Of operative survivors of aortic valve replacement, between 70% and 90% will be functional class I or II with many asymptomatic during normal or strenuous activity, with this improvement sustained for 5 and even 10 years.[20] The social and economic impact of this improvement varies greatly with as few as 20% of patients reported to have resumed household duties or gainful employment after aortic valve replacement.[27] Clearly, factors other than functional class enter into rehabilitation and employability of patients with prosthetic heart valves.

More detailed discussion of the hemodynamic performance of prosthetic valves will be taken up below but after prosthetic replacement of the aortic valve, the average left ventricle-to-aorta peak systolic pressure gradient varies from 7 to 19 mmHg with most normally functioning prostheses, depending upon valve size, type of prosthesis, and stroke volume[12] (Table 17-2). Many patients will have no detectable gradient at rest. The average calculated valve area ranges from 1.3 to 2.0 cm^2. With exercise, the peak transvalvular gradient usually does not become significiantly higher, except for the occasional patient with a small aortic root who requires a prosthesis that is disproportionately small for his/her body size or in subsets of patients who achieve high levels of cardiac output. In these patients, serious outflow obstruction may persist in the presence of "normal" prosthesis function. The likelihood of this developing appears to be less with the Bjork-Shiley valve and St. Jude valve which may be particularly useful when smaller valve sizes are required.

After successful aortic valve replacement, cardiovascular performance generally improves although it is usually not normal. Cardiac output may increase normally with a return toward normal of left ventricular ejection fraction with a decrease in left ventricular mass and increase in mean velocity of circumferential fiber shortening.[28] Left ventricular end-diastolic pressure often stays the same with biopsy evidence showing continuing evidence of myocardial fibrosis.[29]

In patients undergoing aortic valve replacement for aortic regurgitation, left ventricular mass and end-diastolic volume index can decrease, although less consistently than in those patients with aortic stenosis.[28] Left ventricular ejection fraction and mean velocity of circumferential fiber shortening may change little, although marked improvement has been observed in 50% of patients with preoperative left ventricular dysfunction.[29] In some individuals, particularly in those with chronic marked aortic regurgitation, left ventricular dilatation, and severe impairment of function preoperatively, the clinical result is disappointing and impaired left ventricular function persists.[30]

MITRAL VALVE REPLACEMENT

The operative mortality of mitral valve replacement is 4% to 10% currently.[18,31,32] The 5-year survival of all patients varies between 60% and 77% 10-year survival of all patients is approximately 55%, and 15-year survival is 40% to 45%.[20,22] Congestive heart failure and unexplained sudden death remain the most common cause of late death as in aortic valve replacement but thromboembolism is more common with mitral prostheses accounting for 20% or more of all late deaths of patients. Newer types of valves, earlier operation, and meticulous anticoagulation regimens may diminish that figure. Prostheses-related problems (prosthesis failure, emboli, thrombosis, endocarditis, and

Table 17-2
Aortic Valve Gradients and Area

Model	Average Resting Gradient (range) (mmHg)	Exercise Gradient (mmHg) (range)	Average area (cm^2)
Starr-Edwards 1260	7 (0–15)	14 (6–37)	1.6
Smeloff-Cutter	14 (0–34)	29 (8–38)	
Lillehei-Kaster	19		2.0
Björk-Shiley	14 (0–37)	17 (0–59)	2.0–3.5
St. Jude	3	7	1.6–3.3
Porcine xenograft	18 (5–32)	(20–125)	1.3–2.5

anticoagulant-related hemorrhage) account for 10% to 20% of late deaths.[20,33]

Of patients surviving mitral valve replacement, 80% to 90% will be improved one or more functional classes from their preoperative status and this improvement will be maintained for several years. Of operative survivors 30% to 40% will be reported to be in functional class I. Unfortunately, there is sometimes marked discrepancies between excellent symptomatic improvement with disappointingly poor hemodynamic results. Treadmill exercise tests or hemodynamic evaluation can more objectively evaluate functional state.

Hemodynamic improvement results from successful mitral valve replacement with a fall in the left atrial pressure and reduction in pulmonary vascular resistance, often to normal. Mean diastolic pressure gradients across normally functioning prosthetic mitral valves average 4 mmHg, and calculated valve areas average between 1.6 and 2.7 cm^2[12] (Table 17-3). As with aortic prostheses, the hydraulic function varies, depending upon prosthesis, type of valve, size, and stroke volume, but is especially sensitive to diastolic filling time as reflected in heart rate because of the lower opening and closing pressures, and shortening of diastolic flow period associated with tachycardia. For this reason, the gradient can become severely elevated with exercise, particularly in patients with smaller-size prostheses. At least half of all patients with mitral prostheses will have abnormal responses in cardiac output or left atrial pressures during exercise.[34] Unfortunately, there is often little change of left ventricular pump function after mitral valve replacement, although left ventricular size can diminish after successful mitral valve replacement for mitral regurgitation, but ejection fraction may deteriorate postoperatively.[35] After the initial operative and first-year period (10% mortality the first postoperative year), yearly mortality is 2.5% to 5.0% per year.[20]

Long-term survival is diminished in patients with associated severe right heart failure, advanced preoperative functional class, and severe left ventricular dysfunction.[36,37] Also, preoperative duration of symptoms and response to medication may be a factor as unsatisfactory results are common in patients who are allowed to deteriorate over long periods and become refractory to medical management before undergoing surgery. Patients whose predominant valve lesion is mitral stenosis have a better long-term prognosis while those with mitral regurgitation due to ischemic disease have the poorest prognosis.[36,38] Other associated cardiac diseases contribute to late mortality as well. The major long-term complications of prosthetic mitral valve replacement include embolic events (2.5% per year), endocarditis (0.5 to 1.0% per year) hemorrhagic complications in patients on anticoagulation (2.0% to 4.5% per year), sudden death (approximately 0.8% per year)[20,33] (Table 17-1).

MULTIPLE VALVE REPLACEMENT

The operative mortality of double-valve replacement currently is in the range of 10% with hospital mortality of triple-valve replacement approximately 20% (see chapter 11). The 5-year survival of all patients undergoing double-valve replacement is approximately 60% with significant clinical improvement in about 80%.[39] Hemodynamic improvement can be striking with increased cardiac output, regression of severe pulmonary hypertension, and lowering of right heart pressures. Generally, however, a persistently abnormal response to exercise remains. Ten-year survival of double-valve replacement is reported to be 45% with triple-valve replacement

Table 17-3
Mitral Valve Gradients and Area

Model	Average Resting Gradient (mmHg) (range)	Exercise Gradient (mmHg) (range)	Average area (cm^2)
Starr-Edwards 6120	4.2	9	2.4
Smeloff-Cutter	5.2	4–15	
Lillehei-Kaster	6	14	1.8–2.4
Björk-Shiley	5	(8–12)	2.6
St. Jude	2	4	2.5
Porcine xenograft	6 (2–8)	(7–18)	2.0–2.9

slightly less.[40] Preoperative functional class is again an important factor in long-term survival with 70% of those in functional class III preoperatively alive in 3 years compared with only 30% of functional class IV patients, congestive heart failure and sudden death being the most common causes of late deaths in patients with multiple valve replacements.[39]

Only small numbers of patients with isolated tricuspid valve replacement are reported and series include patients with congenital heart disease, as well as traumatic and acquired inflammatory valvular lesions.[41] Generally, the overall survival is similar to that among patients undergoing multiple valve replacement. Of particular concern has been the late malfunction of mechanical tricuspid prostheses due to restriction of poppet or leaflet excursion by subvalvular muscle tissue.[42] Currently, tissue valves are preferred in the tricuspid position (see chapter 5).

CARDIAC VALVES IN CHILDREN

Children who require cardiac valve replacement represent a special problem. These special problems include the variety of etiologies of heart disease requiring valve replacement in children including complex congenital diseases, as well as rheumatic disease. Other special problems include hemodynamic function of smaller valve sizes, growth and development of the child, the control and risks of anticoagulant therapy in patients receiving mechanical prostheses, and the increased risk of earlier bioprosthetic degeneration noted in children. In a recent study, close to 40% of the bioprostheses placed in children had evidence of failure by 5 years.[43] The selection of prostheses centers on the trade-off between control and risks of anticoagulant therapy for a mechanical prostheses versus the risk of reoperation for the biologic prostheses (approximately 7% per year in children). Children's growth has not necessarily necessitated frequent reoperation to insert larger prosthesis, particularly if the child is over 5 years of age when receiving the initial prosthesis.[44] Careful clinical evaluations, frequently requiring hemodynamic studies, are required to allow appropriate timing of second operations. Currently, many clinics are favoring mechanical valves, either the tilting-disc type (either Björk or St. Jude) or ball cage (Starr-Edwards) for valve replacement in children.[45–47] Although there are suggestions of diminished risk of thromboembolic phenomena in children with mechanical valves and antiplatelet agents alone have been recommended, anticoagulation with warfarin sodium is probably safest until more information is available.

EVALUATION OF THE PATIENT WITH A PROSTHETIC VALVE

The length and quality of life after valve replacement are determined by preoperative clinical and hemodynamic status of the patient, operative morbidity and mortality, hemodynamic function of the substituted valve, postoperative cardiac performance, and adverse effects of the prosthetic valve.

Despite continuing advances in surgical techniques, postoperative care, and improvements in design of prosthetic heart valves, complications after valve replacement remain a substantial source of morbidity and mortality[16,19–21,32,48–52] (Table 17-1). The risk of a specific complication in a given patient may vary depending on the underlying heart disease and the prosthetic device use, but the major complications are common to all prostheses.

In the evaluation of a patient after he/she has received a prosthetic valve, several items in the patient's history are particularly important. The current clinical status of the patient must be evaluated and compared to the preoperative clinical status and early phases of the postoperative period. Recent or rapid clinical deterioration requires more intense and speedy evaluation.

The preoperative hemodynamics (left ventricular function and associated cardiac lesions), etiology of valve disease, operative findings, duration and type of myocardial preservation, size of valve, and perioperative course all have a bearing on evaluation of clinical findings after valve replacement. For example, the evaluation of breathlessness in a patient with a mitral valve who had had severe mitral regurgitation due to coronary disease with left ventricular dysfunction as opposed to the patient with mitral valve regurgitation due to acute chord rupture and normal left ventricle should be different. An understanding of the natural history of the specific type of prostheses the patient has received and its requirement for anticoagulation can also help direct the evaluation. The physician must then probe for anticipated complications, ie, thromboembolism, thrombosis, prosthesis failure, hemorrhage, endocarditis.

When comparing current clinical status and

symptom limitation with the preoperative status, as well as the peak performance in the postoperative period, it is valuable to quantitate the level of exercise. Additional historical details to elicit are evidence of infections or related organ dysfunction that might predispose to increased risk of infection, ie, dental or urologic problems. In addition, evaluation for hemorrhagic complications in patients on anticoagulation or factors that might accentuate hemorrhagic problems, especially peptic disease, should be explored.

The physical examination of a patient with a prosthetic valve can be complex and it is best not to rely on any single finding, but rather on a constellation of findings to assist in the evaluation of a patient. Evidence of pulmonary or systemic congestion or ventricular overload has similar clinical importance in the postoperative state, as it has preoperatively, but auscultation can represent particular problems. Analysis of carotid upstroke in the postoperative state is not sufficiently precise to include or exclude the diagnosis of aortic prosthesis obstruction.

Auscultatory examination can be confusing.[53] All prosthetic valves produce alterations in the normal laminar pattern of blood flow and all have a significantly smaller orifice than normal native valves. These valves are implanted in patients with abnormal cardiovascular systems which often possess residual abnormalities. The prosthesis sounds themselves may camouflage the appreciation of normal acoustic events, and significant valvular dysfunction may occur without audible changes.

Seven percent to 15% of prosthetic valves have paravalvular regurgitation, although only half of this will be audible.[54] Occasionally, patients have severe paravalvular leak that is not detected by clinical examination due to radiation of murmur, masking by other heart sounds, or associated low-output states. Diastolic rumbles are detected in one third of biologic prostheses in the mitral position and may be a "normal" finding, ie, not associated with severe valvular stenosis, although only half of severe valvular stenoses of biologic mitral prostheses have diastolic rumbles; thus, the sensitivity and specificity of diastolic rumbles in mitral biologic prostheses is low.[54,55] Diastolic flow sounds tend to be uncommon with mechanical mitral valves and if detected point toward a severe valvular obstruction. It can be very difficult to reliably distinguish a paravalvular mitral regurgitant murmur from aortic stenosis murmur or an outflow murmur due to turbulence within the left ventricular outflow tract.

Despite these limitations, the examiner should focus on the opening and closing sounds of the prosthesis. This is especially important in mechanical prostheses as diminished opening or closing sounds have been associated with valve dysfunction which can be precipitous and catastrophic. Also, an attempt should be made to carefully evaluate for the presence of valve regurgitation. The development of new prosthetic regurgitation can be associated with endocarditis or valve dysfunction. A comparison of previous ascultatory findings and evidence of associated cardiac disease (tricuspid regurgitation, S_3 of left ventricular dysfunction, etc) can help to interpret the clinical observations.

In addition to providing evidence of cardiac enlargement, change in cardiac chamber size, and pulmonary venus congestion, the chest roengenogram can also be used to establish the type of prosthesis. Atlases are available that identify specific model types of valves based upon radiographic appearance, although it should be noted that both the St. Jude and the Angell-Shiley valve are not usually visible on routine chest films.[56–58]

Gated blood pool scans can demonstrate left ventricular size and ejection fraction. Severely impaired left ventricular performance, ie, ejection fractions below .30 in the presence of mitral valve replacement, indicate severe left ventricular dysfunction as likely to be the dominant etiology of cardic failure. However, with an aortic prosthetic valve, the presence of aortic prosthesis stenosis could contribute to a decline in ejection fraction that could be reversible with replacement of an obstructed prosthesis.

Other laboratory tests can occasionally give clues to malfunction. Significant intravascular hemolysis with lactic dehydrogenase (LDH) values over 600 IU are virtually never seen in a modern, normally functioning prosthesis. The presence of moderate or severe hemolysis makes paravalvular leak and/or prosthetic malfunction likely. An exception are the cloth-covered Starr-Edwards prostheses (2300-2400, 6300-6400) which may develop severe hemolysis secondary to cloth tear and not imply hemodynamic deterioration.

Other noninvasive tests that have been utilized to analyze prosthetic function include phonocardiography, echocardiography, cinefluoroscopy, and Doppler analysis of the flow characteristics of the prostheses.[59]

Analysis of phonocardiographic time intervals and altered, typically diminished valve opening or closing sounds can provide supportive evidence of prosthetic malfunction, although these intervals are particularly prone to patient-to-patient variation, and changes in rhythm and hemodynamic status. A shortened A_2-mitral valve opening suggests mitral obstruction or severe mitral regurgitation. Delayed aortic and mitral valve opening has been associated with impaired poppet motion as occurs with tissue ingrowth or left ventricular dysfunction. Similarly, reduction or alteration of tricuspid valve opening implies impairment of poppet motion. Delayed and/or diminished aortic valve opening can indicate obstruction with poppet or leaflet problems. However, because of marked individual variations and alterations in hemodynamic states, it is unusual for any specific phonocardiographic finding to provide sufficient information for optimal management for the patient. In the severely ill patient, the absence of a poppet-opening sound in a mechanical prosthesis implies thrombotic obstruction, and emergency surgery may be necessary. In most circumstances, fluoroscopy, echocardiography, or hemodynamic studies will be required to characterize the status of the prosthesis.

Cinefluoroscopy can be used to evaluate prostheses for poppet or disc motion when they are radiopaque.[59] The opening is related to orientation of the valve and to the instantaneous aortic flow rate and is reduced when there are low levels of cardiac output and aortic flow. Cinefluoroscopy is most useful for disc-type prostheses to evaluate completeness of opening and closing of the disc. For example, the Björk-Shiley valve opens to 60° and closes at 0°. Failure of complete opening or closing implies thrombotic obstruction. Cinefluoroscopy is less useful for ball valves as even thrombotic obstruction may not impair poppet motion.

Valve dehiscence may be identified by cinefluoroscopy by noting the angle of tilting of the base of the prosthesis. Ordinarily the aortic valves tilt 8° to 10° and mitral valves 9° to 12°. Excessive tilting of the prostheses can suggest extensive valvular disruption, but high-output states can also exaggerate tilting motion.

The value of M-mode echocardiography in detecting mechanical prosthetic valve malfunction is limited because of extensive echoes and reverberations from the ball and disc. Unfortunately, even two-dimensional echocardiography does not appear to completely solve these problems. Characterization of the motion of the poppet or leaflet may provide some guidance. Measuring poppet or leaflet excursion and opening and closing velocities have been suggested as valuable tools to evaluate mechanical prostheses as diminished rates of opening, incomplete opening, or impaired poppet or leaflet motion can occasionally identify malfunctions. Echoproducing masses in the vicinity of the prosthetic valve with total absence of disc-ball motion can indicate thrombus or vegetation, but false-positive responses may be observed. Early diastolic rounding of initial diastolic or systolic motion also has been described with malfunctioning disc or leaflet poppet motion. The sensitivity, specificity, and acuracy of these findings, however, are not established.

Echocardiography, especially two-dimensional has been evaluated in biologic valves in attempt to identify findings of degeneration, endocarditis, and regurgitation.[59–61] Prolapse of leaflets, extension of the leaflet echo beyond the plane of strut, a large leaflet image (greater than 3 mm), fluttering of the leaflets while the valve is in a closed position indicating severe valve regurgitation, and discordant motion of the valve are the most useful findings of leaflet dysfunction. Many of these findings may be associated with either primary leaflet degeneration or endocarditis, and two-dimensional echocardiograph is not able to make that distinction. The diagnosis depends upon associated clinical findings. Unfortunately there can be technical problems in analyzing leaflet motion and size, which are affected by focal deposition of calcium (radiographically present in virtually all valves implanted for more than 5 years).[55] Cusp motion is difficult to analyze because all portions of the cusp may not be well visualized with echocardiography. Thus the identification of bioprosthetic valve stenosis by leaflet motion alone is poor.

Doppler echocardiography studies, which identify the direction and velocity of flow, and indirectly the pressure gradient have shown evidence of assisting in the evaluation of prosthetic valves.[62] The Doppler technique is capable of identifying prosthetic valve regurgitation, and giving information about the velocity and pattern of flow across the prostheses, ie, pandiastolic flow across the mitral valve would tend to be asociated with more severe obstruction while intermittent biphasic diastolic flow with rapid diminution of flow in early diastole would support little important porsthetic valve stenosis.[63] However, the Doppler flow patterns will be importantly affected by the direction of flow, the type of prosthesis, the rhythm, and hemodynamic status of the patients.[64] There has been encouraging initial work reporting correlations of Doppler-determined gradients, and the technique shows promise of aiding the hemodynamic evaluation of prostheses.[65]

HEMODYNAMICS OF PROSTHESES

Since the primary indication for cardiac valve surgery is for a hemodynamic disturbance with symptomatic consequences, success must be defined by both a symptomatic and hemodynamic reponse. From the Gorlin formula the relationship of valve area to gradient is such that the gradient is related to the inverse of the square of the area of the orifice[66]:

$$\text{gradient } \delta \ 1/(\text{area})^2$$

Thus, after a 50% reduction in area, for each additional increment in reduction of area, there is a marked increase in gradient. When the orifice size of a native valve is reduced to less than 25% of normal, the gradient rises precipitously. Conversely, small increases of valve area of severely narrow valve will result in large reduction of gradient. Thus, if valve area is increased only from severe to a moderately stenotic range, a large reduction in gradient will occur. Current prostheses have an in vitro effective orifice area that is smaller than that of the normal human valve, and in fact, most prosthetic valves are the in the area where slight reductions in area produce a large increase in gradient.[67] (Figure 17-6). Thus a prosthetic valve converts a severe hemodynamic burden into a mild or moderate one. Despite successful surgery, every patient with a prosthetic valve has a residual obstruction to ventricular inflow or outflow. The clinical significance of this residual obstruction will vary from patient to patient depending upon the type and size of prosthesis placed, the size of the patient, the exercise and/or flow states that the patient will be subjected. In addition, approximately 10% to 20% of prostheses placed will have a degree of regurgitation, some of which may be clinically important in the presence of a relatively stenotic device.[68] The addition of even mild to moderate amounts of additional hemodynamic burden due to regurgitation can be clinically devastating.

Also, the hemodynamics of the prosthesis may change over time. For example, Lipson noted that a third of biologic prostheses placed for 5 or more years had a reduction in calculated valve area.[68] Over time, there may be an additional

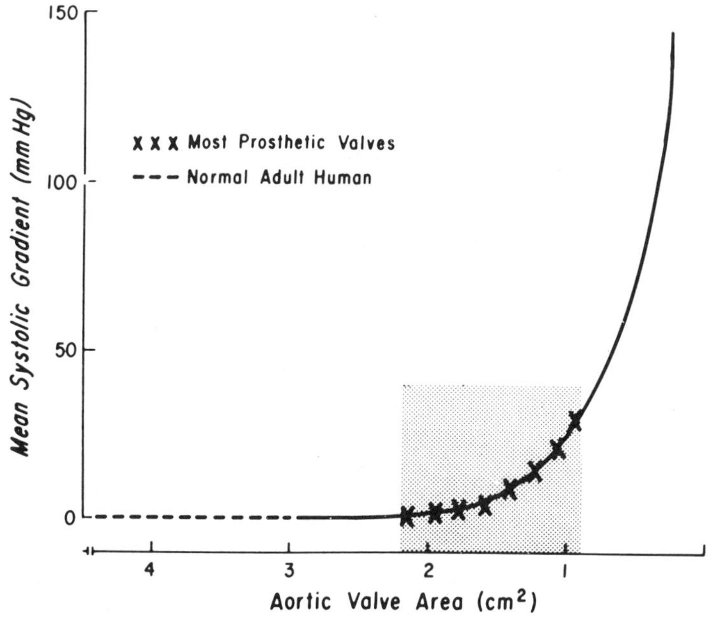

Figure 17-6 Diagrammatic representation of the relationship of systolic gradient to the aortic valve area. The curve and approximate zone of a prosthetic valve area are based upon a constant cardiac output and velocity of flow and published data. (Reproduced with permission from Rahimtoola[67] and the American Heart Association.)

small amount of tissue ingrowth, thrombus, or stiffening of the valve leaflets which may produce critical stenosis that can place patients at risk for a sudden deterioration of cardiac function. This may account for some instances of late unexplained sudden death.

Hemodynamics of prostheses are usually described in terms of gradient and valve area. It is more precise to think of prosthetic valve hemodynamics in terms of the relationship of flow to gradient to orifice size in a prosthesis. The Gorlin formula for valve area presupposes a constant flow rate throughout systole (or diastole) and can only be utilized as an approximation of effective orifice size.

Recently, several authors have presented the hemodynamics of a prosthesis by plotting the change in gradient as the flow changes for each type and size of prosthesis.[14,70,71] (Figure 17-7) Hemodynamically, the best prosthesis would be one with the lowest gradient at both high and low flow states, no changeover time, and the least amount of regurgitation. These principles are important when interpreting hemodynamic data. Because of intrinsic impedance problems with prostheses at low flow, even as the flow becomes lower, the gradient has a tendency to remain the same. Thus, calculated orifice areas can be small in low flow states especially in biologic prostheses (Figure 17–8). This by itself may not indicate prosthesis malfunction, but it may be a consequence of the low flow state, and when the patient then exercises, the actual gradient stays the same and occasionally even falls, indicating relatively "normal" prosthesis function.[70,72]

The optimal hemodynamic evaluation of a prosthesis is performed invasively with pressures measured in the chamber immediately on either side of the prosthesis with simultaneous flow studies (cardiac output). Two flow states are often preferred (rest and exercise), as well as angiographic evaluation for the presence of any valvular regurgitation. Clinical circumstances can modify this approach and useful data can be obtained by more indirect means utilizing wedge pressures instead of left atrial pressures, although this could potenitally lead to inacurrate pressure analyses and result in an erroneous conclusion.[73]

THROMBOEMBOLISM

Thromboembolic complications have been a continuing and distressing problem with prosthetic valves.[74,75] Even with improved valve design, increased awareness of the importance of effect-

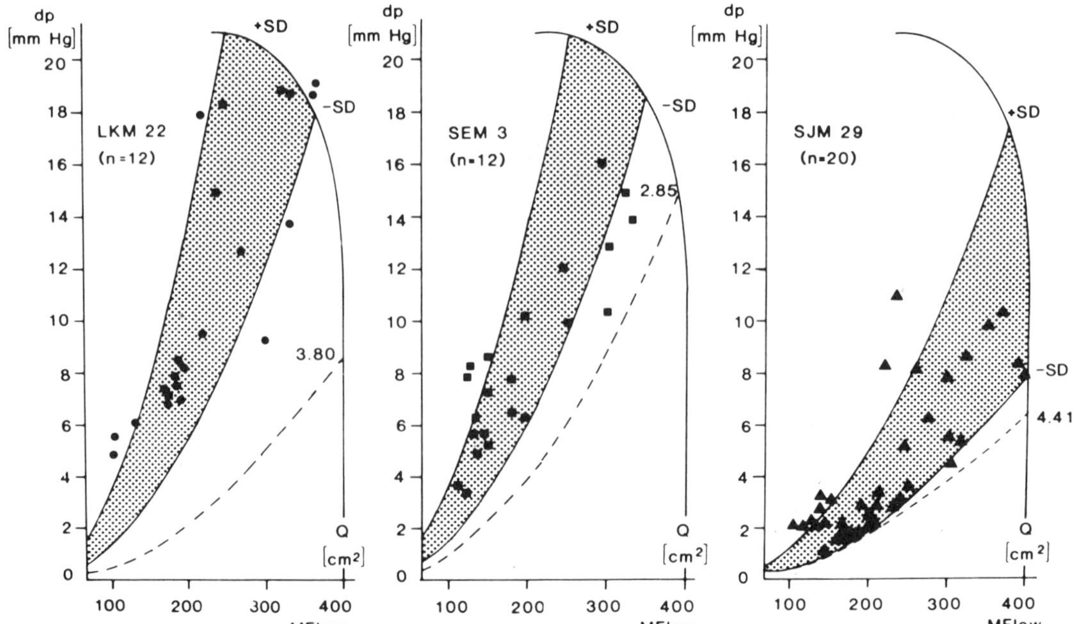

Figure 17-7 Relationship between pressure gradient (δp), diastolic mitral flow (M flow), and geometric orifice area in Lillehei-Kaster (LKM), Starr-Edwards (SEM), and St. Jude Medical (SJM) mitral valve prostheses (Reproduced with permission from Horstkotte et al[14] and the American Heart Association.)

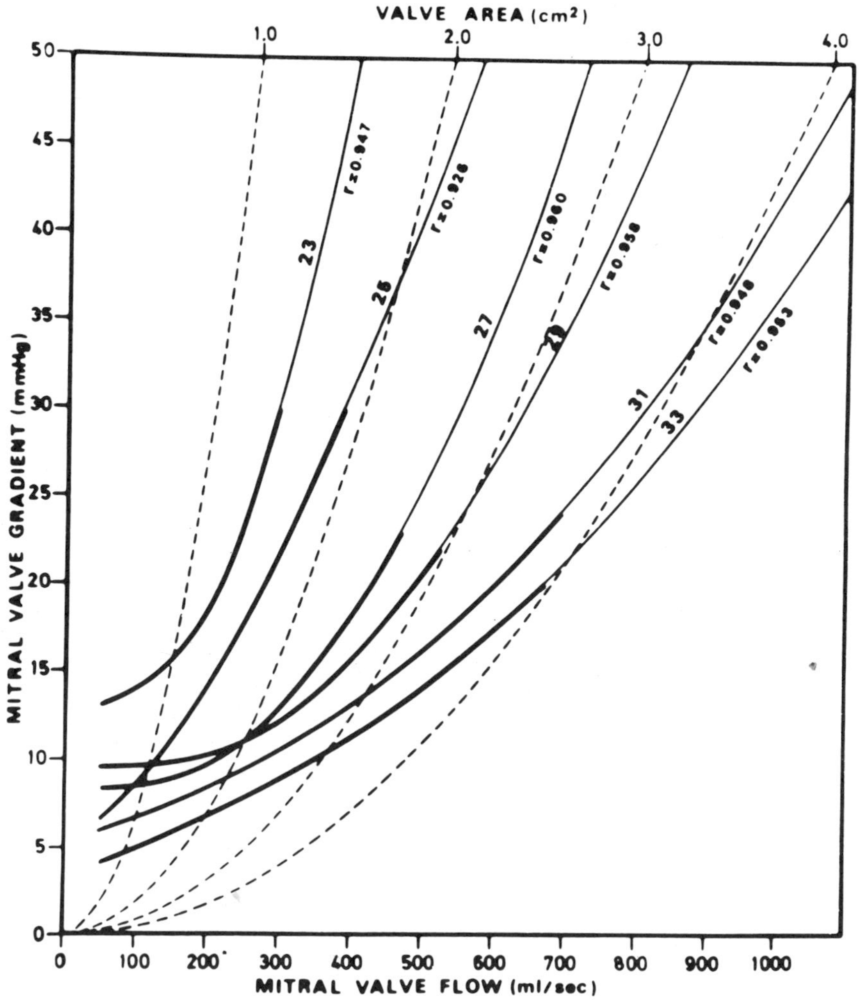

Figure 17-8 Flow-gradient relationship for each Hancock porcine xenograft valve size. Dotted lines show Gorlin flow-pressure curves for different orifice areas. Thick lines correspond to observed data. Figures on each curve indicate the Hancock valve size and correlation. *Note*: At low flows (< 200 mL/s) the gradient remains the same and the calculated valve area becomes markedly reduced. (Reproduced with permission from Ubago et al[70] and the American Heart Association.)

ive anticoagulation in mechanical valves and awareness of subsets at increased risk, it remains a substantial problem. In the earliest model Starr-Edwards prostheses, thromboembolism was found to be a major continuing complication in spite of anticoagulation, with only 55% of the surviving patients free of thromboembolic complications at 15 years.[22] Up to 80% of the clinically evident emboli leave a residual neurologic defect, and approximately 10% lead to death.

The incidence of embolism from Starr-Edwards valves implanted in the 1960s is higher than from identical valves implanted in more recent years, and the rate of embolism associated with these latter valves may be equivalent to that associated with other valve types currently available.[5] This may be due to early operative intervention in the natural history of the disease with fewer patients in atrial fibrillation and very large left atrium, and perhaps some improvement in anticoagulation. Current thromboembolic rates from Starr-Edwards prostheses range from two to four events per 100 patient-years in the aortic position and two to five in the mitral position.[20] The rate of embolic events of the Björk-Shiley tilting-disc valve of one to three events per 100 patient-years in the aortic position and one to four in the mitral position is not very different from that of the Starr-Edwards valve.[12,50,51,52] The Björk-Shiley tilting-disc valve is susceptible to the development of sudden thrombosis leading to rapid deterioration of valve function due to clot interfering with disc movement, and is a continuing risk that may be as high as 8% or more per year in the poorly anticoagulated patient.[12,76] The newer Björk models may be less susceptible to this complication although recent reports of strut fracture of the Björk-Shiley convex-concave model are alarming.[77]

Biologic valves tend to have a slightly lower incidence of emboli even when most of the patients are not anticoagulated.[12] However, even when up to one third of the patients are being anticoagulated, the overall rate of three to four events per 100 patient-years from the mitral valve, and 0.5 to 2.0 events from the aortic valve have been reported.[74] Many of these emboli in biologic valves, up to 40%, occur within the first month of placement.[78] Most of the emboli occur in the patients with atrial fibrillation or large left atrium.

The most important risk factor for systemic embolism in mechanical valves is the presence of inadequate anticoagulation.[3] The mitral prosthetic mechanical valves, especially Björk-Shiley valves, are particularly susceptible to the development of thrombosis in the presence of poor anticoagulation with incidences up to 8% to 10% per year.[12] Atrial fibrillation, perhaps enlarged left atrium, the early postoperative period of biologic valves and poor cardiac output, also appear to be risk factors for the development of systemic embolism in the mitral position.

Several studies indicated that the addition of aspirin or dipyridamole to warfarin anticoagulation for mechanical valves effected a significant further reduction in embolic events.[79,80] Unfortunately, antiplatelet agents alone have not proved to be successful in diminishing the risk of embolic episodes in mechanical valves.[81] A recent prospective study from the Mayo Clinic of the addition of dipyridamole 400 mg daily or aspirin 500 mg daily to warfarin sodium demonstrated excessive bleeding with the aspirin combination with a trend toward diminished thrombolic complications with the dipyridamole.[79]

Every patient with a mechanical prosthetic valve should be placed on long-term anticoagulation with warfarin. The addition of dipyridamole appears safe and is likely to achieve a slight additional reduction in thromboembolic complications. Aspirin, although it may reduce the incidence of thromboembolic complication, tends to be associated with excessive bleeding, and should not be routinely utilized. Biologic valves should be anticoagulated with warfarin for 3 months, and longer if the patient is at high risk for emboli, ie, atrial fibrillation, large left atrium, and the risk of anticoagulation is acceptable. Antiplatelet agents may have a role in biologic valves alone, but there is not enough evidence to be certain.[82]

Chronic warfarin anticoagulation is associated with a significant risk of bleeding complications, some of which can be fatal. Only half of the patients will have their warfarin anticoagulation within therapeutic range 70% or more of the time.[79] In patients with poorer control, the risk of hemorrhagic or thromboembolic complications is increased. The risk of hemorrhagic complication in patients on warfarin is between 3% and 6% per year with the incidence of serious hemorraghic complications requiring transfusion or serious morbidity or mortality approximately half of that.[20,21,33,83] Cerebral hemorrhage is the major fatal hemorrhagic complication.

SPECIAL PROBLEMS WITH ANTICOAGULATION

The development of cerebral embolization during anticoagulation therapy is a difficult clinical problem. The clinician is concerned about development of hemorrhagic infarct with the continuation of anticoagulation versus the risk of a recurrent embolic rate.[84] Although there are no definitive data, evidence suggests that the recurrence rate of a thromboembolic episode is likely to be greater than a provocation of a hemorrhagic infarct. A reasonable recommendation is to withhold anticoagulation and allow the prothrombin time to drift lower until a computed tomographic (CT) scan can be obtained to confirm that there is no bleeding within the CNS. At that time full anticoagulation is reinstituted with careful control keeping the prothrombin time about one and a half times normal with careful clinical follow-up. If the patient is lethargic or has a very large defect on CT scan, the risk of hemorrhage may be great and anticoagulation probably should be delayed. If signs of intracranial hemorrhage develop, neurosurgical evacuation of the hematoma can be lifesaving.[85] Similar considerations enter the decision in the management of anticoagulants in the presence of infective endocarditis of prosthetic valves.[86] If no cerebral embolism has occurred, and the prosthesis is a mechanical one that requires anticoagulation, anticoagulants should be continued because the risk of embolism is probably greater than the risk of bleeding from a mycotic aneurysm. If the prosthesis is a biological prosthesis, and chronic anticoagulation is not required, the anticoagulation probably should be withheld. If embolism does occur and the risk from hemorrhagic complication may be increased, anticoagulants probably should be temporarily withheld. Certainly meticulous control of anticoagulation (probably in the low therapeutic range), coupled with careful clinical follow-up, is essential in an attempt to chart the safest course.

Warfarin had been associated with teratogenic effects which justifies switching to subcutaneously administered heparin during the first 3 months of pregnancy and then continuing with heparin sodium or warfarin for the balance.[87] Heparin may also be given during the last month of pregnancy to avoid perinatal hemorrhage in the event of premature labor (see chapter 12).

Ordinarily withholding anticoagulation temporarily for noncardiac surgery and reinstitution immediately postoperatively is safe, but in individuals who are believed to be at increased risk of thromboembolic complications, ie, history of prior emboli, mitral mechanical valves, tilting-disc type valves, or atrial fibrillation, converting to intravenous (IV) heparin until shortly preoperatively and then reinstituting heparin 12 to 24 hours postoperatively until the prothrombin time returns to normal seems to provide the additional protection of emboli in the high-risk patient, but has been associated with delayed hemorrhage from the operative site.[88–90] Some authorities have advised empirical substitution of dipyridamole 400 mg daily during the time that warfarin is withheld.[75]

THROMBOTIC OBSTRUCTION

Thrombotic obstruction of a prosthetic mechanical valve is a serious and potentially catastrophic complication.[12] Occasionally even with tissue valves thrombosis can occur.[91] Although chronic anticoagulation diminishes the risk of latent thrombosis, there is a small but potentially catastrophic risk of acute or chronic thrombotic obstruction of all mechanical valves even when the patient is on effective anticoagulation.[12] Poor anticoagulation increases the risk at least tenfold. Unfortunately aspirin or dipyridamole does not protect mechanical prostheses from this complication.[81] Detection of thrombosis on a prothesis depends primarily on demonstration of prosthetic valve dysfunction due to impaired poppet or leaflet motion or a decreased area of the valve orifice. Clinical examination may reveal no abnormal function or may clearly identify evidence of thrombus on the prosthesis. Common ausculatory findings include variation in intensity and diminution or loss of prosthetic valve opening sounds due to the thrombus interrupting poppet or leaflet motion.[92] New murmurs of valvular regurgitation due to incomplete closure of the prosthesis or murmurs of mitral or tricuspid stenoses are particularly important observations. Isolated diastolic mitral murmurs, or aortic regurgitant murmurs by themselves, may not be clinically important; however, the presence of a diastolic murmur in any patient should be compared with the clinical presentation of the patient, and as discussed above phono- and echocardiography can supply valuable corroborative information.

Cardiac fluoroscopy is occasionally helpful in demonstrating impaired poppet or leaflet motion prostheses with poppets or discs of radiopaque materials.[93] However, the fluoroscopic appearance may be entirely normal in patients with a ball-type prosthesis with severe stenosis of a prosthesis caused by thrombus occluding the valve orifice, but not impeding poppet motion. Cardiac catheterization and angiography may not be necessary when a patient has clear clinical evidence of prosthetic valve dysfunction and there are strong supporting data from noninvasive studies. This most often occurs when the need for reoperation appears urgent, as in an obstruction of a tricuspid prosthesis, or in the patient who is severely ill with acute thrombotic dysfunction of a Björk-Shiley valve with sudden onset of severe aortic regurgitation or stenosis due to thrombotic restriction of the movement of the occluder. Often the clinical and laboratory findings are less convincing, and a comprehensive evaluation is desired before therapeutic decisions are made that might include a reoperation.

Cardiac catheterization studies are usually not productive in demonstrating abnormal prosthesis function in patients with isolated embolic phenomena unless there are other clinical findings that point to protheses dysfunction, such as evidence of infection, obstruction, regurgitation, or hemodynamic deterioration.[94] To detect prosthesis dysfunction the hemodynamic evaluation should include measurement of the pressure gradient across the prosthesis in question with simultaneous cardiac output determinations to permit calculation of the effect orifice area. It is also important to evaluate for the presence of regurgitation across the prosthesis even in the absence of a regurgitant murmur since serious paravalvular mitral regurgitation has been reported without a significant murmur. The highest incidence of abnormal hemodynamic and angiocardiographic findings in patients with prosthetic valves is in those with late clinical deterioration of failure to improve after an operation.[94]

When significant prosthetic valve dysfunction due to thrombus is present, prompt reoperation is usually necessary. The urgency of reoperation is obvious in patients with clinical difficulty with heart failure, low cardiac output, hypotension, or arrhythmias. Even patients in whom the need for operation appears less urgent may be at risk for precipitous deterioration in some circumstances and early reoperation is encouraged. When clinical and laboratory findings are equivocal and hemodynamic data are borderline, patients may be observed for a time, but must be followed closely with clear instructions to return promptly if they experience any change in symptoms.

The risk of elective reoperation in experienced hands is similar to the risk of the original operation.[95] With urgent reoperation of the desperately ill patient the risk is substantially increased (25% to 50%).[95,96] Although complete valve replacement is often required, in experienced hands thrombotic débridement can be satisfactory and there have even been reports of streptokinase infusions to remove thrombus from obstructive prostheses.[97]

EMBOLI

Systemic emboli are a continuing problem with all prostheses and occur at a rate of 2% to 5% per year.[12,74–75] In the clinical evaluation of an individual who has had an embolic episode or when there is consideration of thrombotic complications, the physician should evaluate the anticoagulant history of the patient, the complications of anticoagulation, the limitations of more effective anticoagulation, the type of prosthesis and its requirement for anticoagulation, and the possibility of other precipitants of embolic or thrombotic episodes such as endocarditis or change of rhythm. An embolic episode justifies a search for endocarditis. After endocarditis has been excluded and the clinical and historical data are such that the patient is unlikely to have prosthesis dysfunction, the clinician can manage the patient by attempting to improve anticoagulation control by more meticulous follow-up, often with the addition of an antiplatelet agent (dipryidamole 400 mg daily), and with more frequent clinical evaluation for reassurance as to the continuing hemodynamic stability of the prosthesis. If the patient has clinical evidence of hemodynamic deterioration, more detailed investigations will be necessary to determine if prosthetic valve replacement is required.

Recurrent thromboembolic episodes can occur in a few patients, despite optimal anticoagulant and antiplatelet therapy. Reoperation to replace a mechanical prosthesis with a biologic prosthesis has been reported and may be justified in selected circumstances.[98]

INFECTIOUS ENDOCARDITIS

The presence of a prosthesis both increases the vulnerability of the patient to endocarditis and makes eradication of the infection more difficult. The incidence of late endocarditis in patients with prosthetic valves is between 0.5% and 1.0% per year and is a continuous risk throughout the life of the patient with a prosthesis.[20,21,33,48]

Prosthetic valve endocarditis occurring early after operation (within 60 days) is usually due to contamination during the surgical procedure or to obvious infections in noncardiac areas during the immediate postoperative period.[99] The infecting organisms are staphylococci in about half the cases, and fungal or Gram-negative organisms in the remainder. The response to therapy is poor, reoperation is usually required, and the mortality high at 70% to 90%. In contrast, prosthetic valve endocarditis developing late after operation is more similar to classic subacute bacterial endocarditis. The infecting organisms are more like those seen with infections of natural valves with stretococcal species most common, staphylococcus less common, and Gram-negative bacilli or fungal infections rare. The mortality rate is 35% to 45%. The clinical presentation of prosthetic valve endocarditis is related to the time of onset after operation. The clinical course is more often insidious and prolonged in late onset infection, but may be acute and rapidly progressive with either late or early onset. Fever is present in virtually all patients with fatigue, malaise, lethargy, and anorexia as well as sweating and chills are usually present although occasionally patients will feel quite well.

New murmurs of regurgitation may appear, usually indicating late disruption of the prosthetic suture line, but may also appear as a result of vegetations on the prosthetic valve preventing complete opening or closure of the poppet. Sytemic arterial embolism occurs in 30% to 40% of patients with endocarditis and may be the presenting symptom.[100] A systemic embolic episode should always suggests the possible presence of endocarditis. The importance of immediately suspecting infectious endocarditis in any patient with a prosthetic valve who has intermittent or persistent fever, a new murmur, embolic phenomena, or development of clinical deterioration cannot be overemphasized.

The diagnosis is usally established by demonstration of bacteremia in the appropriate clinical setting. Occasionally a patient with cardiac valve prosthesis is febrile with clinical findings consistent with infectious endocarditis, but negative blood cultures despite repeated attempts and careful search for unsual organisms including anaerobes. Other clinical data may provide supporting evidence including echocardiographic evidence of vegetation. The success of treatment of prosthetic valve endocarditis with antibiotics alone depends upon the type of organism. Medical therapy is more likely to be successful when the organism is streptococcal, there is no new valvular regurgitation, and no congestive heart failure.[101] The principles of antibiotic selection and management are similar for endocarditis whether or not a prosthesis is present and includes use of bactericidal drugs, and confirmation of adequate drug effect against the organism with careful clinical and laboratory follow-up to insure elimination of infection.[102]

Failure of medical management is indicated by uncontrolled infection, large or multiple systemic emboli, valve disruption, valve obstruction, or progressive congestive heart failure. Failure of medical therapy must be indentified promptly and reoperation considered without delay.[103] Hesitation can commonly lead to progressive cardiac deterioration and increasing morbidity and mortality.

If the infected prosthesis is a mechanical prosthesis, continuing anticoagulation is required with careful control of the prothrombin time at one and a half to two times normal.[86]

The importance of prevention is obvious in a disease as potentially catastrophic and difficult to treat as prosthetic valve endocarditis. Adequate coverage with antibiotic prophylaxis during procedures or illnesses with a potential for bacteremia is imperative in an attempt to prevent late prosthetic valve endocarditis. Although there has been continuing debate about the optimal antibiotic regimen, the American Heart Association recommendation is the most intensive and wisest choice[105] (see Chapter 16, Table 4). The requirement for prophylaxis is well recognized for dental or genitourinary procedures in which a high incidence of bacteremia has been demonstrated, but should include other procedures as well[104] (see Chapter 16, Table 3). In addition, any infection in a patient with a prosthetic valve should receive prompt and vigorous treatment. The selection of a drug should be individualized on the basis of expected bacterial flora or culture material from the patient, and the elimination of infection should be confirmed. Prompt control of infections and the requirement for good dental and urologic care makes the patient an important partner for protection from endocarditis.

PROSTHESIS DYSFUNCTION

Acute valve dysfunction can present without warning and may be life-threatening or fatal (see chapter 15). Modes of valve failure vary widely with different prostheses and include development of serious valvular regurgitation due to disruption of a tissue leaflet, thrombotic obstruction of mechanical or tissue valves, or wear with sticking or even dislodgment of occluders as well as strut fractures.[12,77] The valve failure rate for currently available mechanic prostheses is probably less than 1% per year, but unfortunately follow-up of earlier prostheses demonstrated that valve failure may only become apparent or may precipitously increase several years after implant.[12]

With biologic valves pathologic and radiographic evidence of wear appears in virtually every prostheses after 5 years.[62] Late calcification with gradual stenosis and obstruction of the prosthesis appears to be the most common mode of late biologic prosthetic dysfunction although leaflet dysfunction with rent and tear along the insertion sites, commissures, or in the middle of the leaflets are also frequent[105,106] (Figures 17-9 and 17-10). The estimated failure rate of biological prostheses is 20% to 30% at 8 years.[15,16,107] The degeneration of biological prostheses is fastest in patients under 35 years of age and greatest in adolescents.[108]

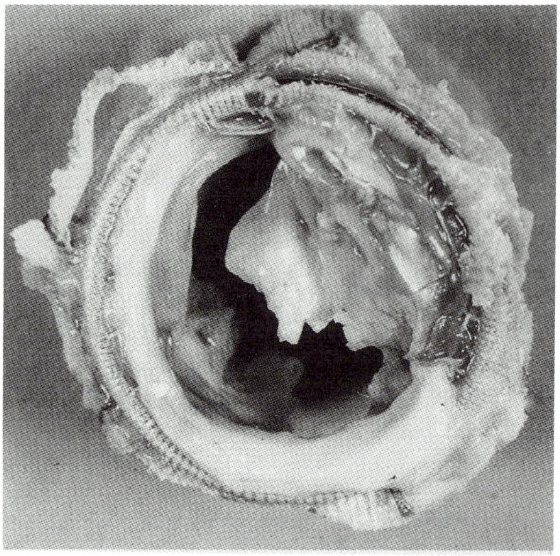

Figure 17-9 Degenerated biologic prosthesis which had been in the aortic position for 5 years, with cusp tear disintegration.

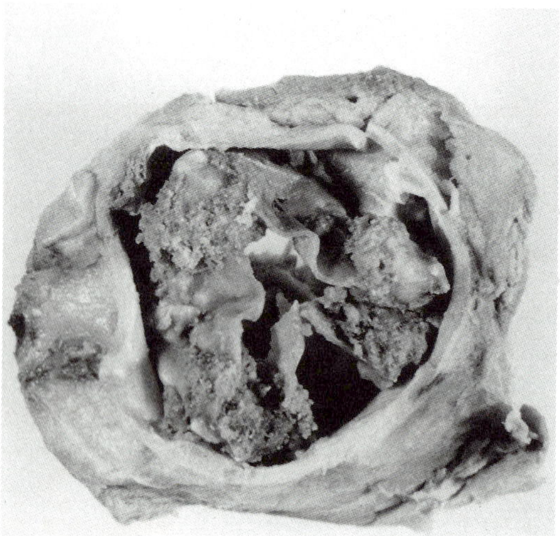

Figure 17-10 Calcified biologic prosthesis which had been in the aortic position for 18 months in a 54-year-old man with renal failure. (Valve courtesy of Dr W. Mayer.)

In any patient with a prosthetic valve, the development of new or increased angina, episodes of faintness, diaphoresis, shortness of breath, accelerating hemolysis, or cardiac failure should be regarded as possible signs of impending valve failure, and prompt evaluation is warranted. Careful clinical examinations, roentgenography, ECG, and occasionally echocardiography can help, but hemodynamic and angiographic studies are often necessary to critically evaluate the function of a prosthesis. Elective reoperation can generally be done reasonably safely except in the most urgent situation where operative mortality approaches 40%.[95,96]

HEMOLYTIC ANEMIA

Intravascular hemolysis is generally a trivial problem with current heart prostheses although in older type prostheses it was a more significant problem. In the Braunwald-Cutter or Beall prostheses the development of hemolysis was associated with severe occluded wear problems and a sign of impending valve failure.[109,110] Starr-Edwards cloth-covered prostheses had a tendency for the cloth to wear and to develop severe hemolysis (LDH greater than 1000), which alone did not imply hemodynamic deterioration and could often be controlled with oral iron therapy.[111] Nevertheless, the development of hemolysis in a patient with prosthetic valves should make the clinician highly suspicious of prostheses dysfunction or paraprosthetic valve regurgitation. There is virtually never severe hemolysis of a prosthesis in the mitral position unless there is valve dysfunction or regurgitation. Occasionally the regurgitation may produce severe hemolysis through a small slitlike defect in the sewing ring even though the degree of regurgitation is not hemodynamically significant.

Evaluation should demonstrate the presence of anemia, the presence and severity of the hemolysis, and any deficiency state secondary to iron loss, or accelerated hematopoiesis, ie, folate deficiency. Special attention should be given to factors contributing to increased hemolysis, particularly dysfunction of the prosthesis, paravalvular regurgitation, or high transvalvular pressure gradient. Management consists of replacing a seriously defective prosthesis. If the prosthesis is not seriously defective (ie, small amount of regurgitation or cloth tear), oral iron and folate therapy usually control the anemia. Occasionally transfusions and reoperation are required.

UNSATSIFACTORY LATE RESULTS

Although symptomatic improvement after valve replacement is generally gratifying, 10% or more of patients may fail to improve, develop recurrent cardiac symptoms, or even worsen. The differential diagnosis and approach to the patient depends upon the timing after operation, the underlying cardiac disease, as well as the specific cardiac prosthesis. The most common recurrent or new cardiac symptoms are angina or congestive heart failure.

If angina develops or presents early after replacement, the physician should consider the presence or progression of previously overlooked disease (eg, idiopathic hypertrophic subaortic stenosis, coronary atherosclerosis, as well as perioperative injury to the coronary ostia or coronary vessels.) Mechanical dysfunction or hemodynamically unsatisfactory prostheses are important problems that should be considered if angina develops after cardiac valve replacement. An embolus to a coronary artery can present as unstable angina or myocardial infarction after valve replacement. Late after valve replacement, development of coronary artery disease or prosthetic dysfunction may be the more likely causes of new angina.

Congestive heart failure after cardiac valve replacement may be due to residual uncorrected valve disease, pre-existing or perioperative myocardial dysfunction, prosthetic valve malfunction, or prosthesis/patient mismatch. The term "prosthetic valve mismatch" has been used to describe the situation where a relatively stenotic valve must be placed in a large or active patient and moderate valve stenosis persists.[67] High flow states over a prolonged period can then result in marked cardiac enlargement and hemodynamic burden despite a "normal" prosthesis. Other valve disease or coronary disease can develop late after valve surgery and may present with new clinical symptoms. Unusual problems that cause hemodynamic deterioration include pericardial restriction, new shunts, or regurgitant lesions related to the cardiac operation. It can be very difficult to establish by noninvasive means the precise cause and relation of clinical and hemodynamic deterioration in many of these patients, especially when there is a combination of aortic disease, left ventricular dysfunction, and mitral disease. Detailed evaluation including hemodynamic and angiographic studies produces a high yield in terms of identifying the specific reason for deterioration. Seventy-five percent of patients with clinical deterioration will have significant abnormalities discovered by postoperative hemodynamic studies.[94] Frequently, these lesions are correctable by reoperation.

SPECIAL PROBLEMS

Additional problems which may arise in the management of patients with prosthetic valves include pregnancy (discussed in chapter 12) and management during general surgery.

In the management of patients with prosthetic valves undergoing general surgery, attention should be directed to management of anticoagulation as well as bacterial endocarditis prophylaxis. Ordinarily if anticoagulation is stopped one to three days before the surgical procedure and restarted one to two days after, the risk of hemorrhage and thromboembolic phenomena is extremely low.[88] Dipyridamole 400 mg daily, while the warfarin is withheld, has been advised empirically by some to help minimize the risk.[75] Special circumstances might arise in which the complication of a hemorrhage may be very serious and anticoagulation would have to be withheld for a longer time (eg, neurosurgical procedures). Because of recorded cases of acute massive thrombosis of the Björk-Shiley valve after anticoagulation was stopped for only a short period of time, Björk and Henge recommended that anticoagulation be maintained with only temporary reduction to subtherapeutic levels.[112] Alternatively, a recent study indicated that preoperative anticoagulation with heparin after the warfarin has been withheld for a series of days and then reheparinization during the time before the warfarin has had an opportunity to be effective diminishes the embolic and hermorrhagic complications, and may have an advantage in the tilting-disc type prosthesis, especially in the mitral position or in patients who are believed to be at particularly high risk for thromboembolic complications.[89] Infective bacterial endocarditis prophylaxis should be given to patients undergoing general surgical procedures, particularly dental and urologic procedures.[104]

CONCLUSION

Cardiac valve replacement has been a substantial advance in the management of patients with valvular heart disease. However, a patient with a prosthesis has a new disease, "prosthetic valve disease," of which we have a reasonable assessment of the ten-year mortality and morbidity. The durability of currently used prostheses and the steps taken to diminish cardiac and prosthesis-related morbidity and mortality continue to be areas of active investigation and research.

REFERENCES

1. Starr A, Edwards ML: Mitral valve replacement: Clinical experience with a ball-valve prosthesis.

Ann Surg 1961;154:726–740.
2. McClung JA, Stein JH, Ambrose JA, et al: Prosthetic heart valves: A review. *Prog Cardiovasc Dis* 1983;26:237–270.
3. Fuster V, Pumphrey CW, McGoon MD, et al: Systemic thromboembolism in mitral and aortic Starr-Edwards prostheses: A 10–19 year followup. *Circulation* 1982;66:(suppl 1):157–161.
4. Starr A, Grunkemeier G, Lambert L, et al: Mitral valve replacement: A 10-year followup of non-cloth-covered vs. cloth-covered caged ball prosthesis. *Circulation* 1976;54(suppl 3):47–56.
5. Macmanus Q, Grunkemeier GL, Lambert LE, et al: Year of operation as a risk factor in the late result of valve replacement. *J Thorac Cardiovasc Surg* 1980;80:834–841.
6. Bonchek LI, Starr A: Ball valve prosthesis: Current appraisal of late results. *Am J Cardiol* 1975;843–854.
7. Hylen JC, Kloster FE, Starr A, et al: Aortic ball variance: Diagnosis and treatment. *Ann Intern Med* 1970;72:1–8.
8. Beall AC, Bloodwell RD, Liotta D, et al: Clinical experience with a Dacron velour-covered Teflon-disc mitral valve prosthesis. *Ann Thorac Surg* 1968;5:402–407.
9. Roberts WC, Fishbein MC, Golden A: Cardiac pathology after valve replacement by disc prostheses: A study of 61 necropsy patients. *Am J Cardiol* 1975;35:740–760.
10. Björk VO: The development of the Björk-Shiley artificial heart valve. *Clin Cardiol* 1984;7:3–5.
11. Lillehei CW, Koster RL, Coleman M, et al: Heart valve replacement with Lillehei-Koster pivoting disc prosthesis. *NY State J Med* 1974;74: 1426–1441.
12. Starr A, Greenkemeier GL: Selection of a prosthetic heart valve. *JAMA* 1984;251:1739–1742.
13. Angell WW, Angell JD: Porcine valves. *Prog Cardiovasc Dis* 1980;23:141–166.
14. Horstkotte D, Haerten K, Seipel L, et al: Central hemodynamics at rest and during exercise after mitral valve replacement with different prostheses. *Circulation* 1983;68(suppl 2):161–168.
15. Gallo, I, Ruiz B, Nistol F, et al: Degeneration in porcine bioprosthetic cardiac valves: Incidence of primary tissue failures among 938 bioprostheses at risk. *Am J Cardiol* 1984;53:1061–1065.
16. Cohn LH, Mudge GH, Pratter F, et al: Five to eight-year followup of patients undergoing porcine heart valve replacement. *N Engl J Med* 1981; 304:258–262.
17. Cohn LH, Allred EN, DiSesor VJ, et al: Early and late risk of aortic valve replacement. *J Thorac Cardiovasc Surg* 1984;88:695–705.
18. Marshall WG, Kouchoukos NT, Pollock SB, et al: Early results of valve replacement with the Björk-Shiley convexo-concave prosthesis. *Ann Thorac Surg* 1984;37:398–403.
19. Kirklin JW, Conti VR, Blackstone FH: Prevention of myocardial damage during cardiac operations. *N Engl J Med* 1979;301:135–141.
20. Teply JF, Grunkemeier GL, Sutherland D, et al: The ultimate prognosis after valve replacement: An assessment at twenty years. *Ann Thorac Surg* 1981;32:112–118.
21. Miller DC, Oyer PE, Mitchell RS, et al: Performance characteristics of the Starr-Edwards 1260 aortic valve prosthesis beyond ten years. *J Thorac Cardiovasc Surg* 1984;88:193–207.
22. McGoon MD, Fuster V, McGoon DC, et al: Aortic and mitral valve incompetence: Long-term followup (10 to 19 years) of patients treated with the Starr-Edwards prosthesis. *J Am Coll Cardiol* 1984;3:930–938.
23. Santinga JT, Kirsh MM, Flora JD, et al: Factors relating to late sudden death in patients having aortic valve replacement. *Ann Thorac Surg* 1980; 29:249–253.
24. Copeland JG, Griepp RB, Stinson EB, et al: Long-term followup after isolated aortic valve replacement. *J Thorac Cardiovasc Surg* 1977;74: 875–889.
25. Nunley DL, Grunkemeier GL, Starr A: Aortic valve replacement with coronary bypass grafting. *J Thorac Cardiovasc Surg* 1983;85:705–711.
26. Murphy ES, Lawson RM, Starr A, et al: Severe aortic stenosis in patients 60 years of age and older: Left ventricular function and 10-year survival after valve replacement. *Circulation* 1981;64(suppl 2):184–188.
27. Carey JS, Hughs RK, Plested WG, et al: Functional rehabilitation after cardiac valve surgery. *Ann Thorac Surg* 1973;16:492–504.
28. Pantely G, Morton M, Rahimtoola SH: Effects of successful uncomplicated valve replacement on ventricular hypertrophy, volume, and performance in aortic stenosis and in aortic incompetence. *J Thorac Cardiovasc Surg* 1978;75: 383–391.
29. Hess OM, Ritter M, Schneider J, et al: Diastolic stiffness and myocardial structure in aortic valve disease before and after valve replacement. *Circulation* 1984;69:855–865.
30. Clark DG, McAnulty JH, Rahimtoola SH: Valve replacement in aortic insufficiency with left ventricular dysfunction. *Circulation* 1980;61: 411–421.
31. Starr A, Grunkemeier, Lambert L, et al: Mitral valve replacement. *Circulation* 1976;54(suppl 3): 47–56.
32. Chaux A, Czer LSC, Matleff JM, et al: The St. Jude medical bileaflet valve prosthesis. *J Thorac Cardiovasc Surg* 1984;88:706–717.
33. Miller DC, Oyer PE, Stinson EB, et al: Ten to fifteen year reassessment of the performance characteristics of the Starr-Edwards Model 6120 mitral valve prosthesis. *J Thorac Cardiovasc Surg* 1983;85:1–20.
34. Bristow JD, Kremkau EL: Hemodynamic changes after valve replacement with Starr-Edwards prosthesis. *Am J Cardiol* 1975;35:716–724.
35. Schuler G, Peterson K, Johnson A, et al: Temporal response of left ventricular performance to mitral valve surgery. *Circulation* 1979;59: 1218–1231.
36. Solomon NW, Stinson EB, Griepp RB, et al: Patient-related risk factors as predictors of results following mitral valve replacement. *Ann Thorac Surg* 1977;24:519–530.
37. Dalby AJ, Firth BG, Forman R: Preoperative factors affecting the outcome of isolated mitral valve replacement: A 10 year review. *Am J Cardiol* 1981;47:826–833.

38. Pinson CW, Cobanoglu A, Metzdorff MT, et al: Late surgical results for ischemic mitral regurgitation: Role of wall motion score and severity of regurgitation. *J Thorac Cardiovasc Surg* 1984;88: 663–672.
39. Stephenson LW, Edie RN, Harken AH, et al: Combined aortic and mitral valve replacement: Changes in practice and prognosis. *Circulation* 1984;69:640–644.
40. Macmanus Q, Grunkemeier G, Starr A: Late results of triple valve replacement: A 14-year review. *Ann Thorac Surg* 1978;25:402–406.
41. Sanfelippo PM, Giuliani ER, Danielson GK, et al: Tricuspid valve prosthetic replacement. Early and late results with the Starr-Edwards prosthesis. *J Thorac Cardiovasc Surg* 1976;71: 441–445.
42. Vander Veer JB, Rhyneer GS, Hodam RP, et al: Obstruction of tricuspid ball-valve prosthesis. *Circulation* 1971;43(suppl 1):62–67.
43. Williams DB, Danielson GK, McGoon DC, et al: Porcine heterograft valve replacement in children. *J Thorac Cardiovasc Surg* 1982;84:446–450.
44. Friedman S, Edmunds LH, Cuaso CC: Long-term mitral valve replacement in young children: Influence of somatic growth on prosthetic valve adequacy. *Circulation* 1978;57:981–986.
45. Schaff HV, Danielson GK, DiDonato RM, et al: Late results after Starr-Edwards valve replacement in children. *J Thorac Cardiovasc Surg* 1984; 88:583–589.
46. Iyer KS, Reddy KS, Rao IM, et al: Valve replacement in children under twenty years of age: Experience with the Björk-Shiley prosthesis. *J Thorac Cardiovasc Surg* 1984;88:217–224.
47. Pass HI, Sade RM, Crawford FA, et al: Cardiac valve prostheses in children without anticoagulation. *J Thorac Cardiovasc Surg* 1984;87: 832–835.
48. Marshall WG, Kouchoukos NT, Karp RB, et al: Late results after mitral valve replacement with the Björk-Shiley and porcine prostheses. *J Thorac Cardiovasc Surg* 1983;85:902–910.
49. Murphy DA, Levine FH, Buckley MJ, et al: Mechanical valves: A comparative analysis of the Starr-Edwards and Björk-Shiley prostheses. *J Thorac Cardiovasc Surg* 1983;86:746–752.
50. Perier P, Deloche A, Chauvaud S, et al: Comparative evaluation of mitral valve repair and replacement with Starr, Björk, and porcine valve prosthesis. *Circulation* 1984;70(suppl 1):187–192.
51. Cheung D, Flemma RJ, Mullen DC, et al: Ten-year follow-up in aortic valve replacement using the Björk-Shiley Prosthesis. *Ann Thorac Surg* 1981;32:138–145.
52. Lepley D, Flemma RJ, Mullen DC, et al: Long-term follow-up of the Björk-Shiley prosthetic valve used in the mitral position. *Ann Thorac Surg* 1980;30:164–172.
53. Smith ND, Raizada V, Abrams J: Auscultation of the normally functioning prosthetic valve. *Ann Intern Med* 1981;95:594–598.
54. Björk VO, Holmgren A, Olin C, et al: Clinical and hemodynamic results of aortic valve replacement with the Björk-Shiley tilting disc valve prosthesis. *Scand J Thorac Cardiovasc Surg* 1971; 5:177–191.
55. Schapira JN, Martin RP, Fowles RE, et al: Two dimensional echocardiographic assessment of patients with bioprosthetic valves. *Am J Cardiol* 1979;43:510–519.
56. Chun PKC, Nelson WP: Common cardiac prosthetic valves: Radiologic identification and associated complications. *JAMA* 1977;238:401–403.
57. Mehlman DJ, Resnekov L: A guide to the radiographic identification of prosthetic heart valves. *Circulation* 1978;57:613–623.
58. Mehlman DJ: A guide to the radiographic identification of prosthetic heart valves: An addendum. *Circulation* 1984;69:102–105.
59. Kotler MN, Mintz GS, Panidis I, et al: Noninvasive evaluation of normal and abnormal prosthetic valve function. *J Am Coll Cardiol* 1983;2:151–173.
60. Effron MK, Popp RL: Two-dimensional echocardiographic assessment of bioprosthetic valve dysfunction and infective endocarditis. *J Am Coll Cardiol* 1983;4:597–606.
61. Grenadier E, Sahn DJ, Roche AH, et al: Detection of deterioration or infection of homograft and porcine xenograft bioprosthetic valves in mitral and aortic positions by two-dimensional echocardiographic examination. *J Am Coll Cardiol* 1983;3:452–459.
62. Cipriano PR, Billingham ME, Oyer PE, et al: Calcification of porcine prosthetic heart valves: a radiographic and light microscopic study. *Circulation* 1982;66:1100–1104.
63. Quinones MA, Young JB, Waggoner AD, et al: Assessment of pulsed Doppler echocardiography in detection and quantification of aortic and mitral regurgitation. *Br Heart J* 1980;44:612–620.
64. Stamm RB, Martin RP: Quantification of pressure gradients across stenotic valves by Doppler ultrasound. *J Am Coll Cardiol* 1983;4:707–718.
65. Gross CM, Wann LS: Doppler echocardiographic diagnosis of porcine bioprosthetic cardiac valve malfunction. *Am J Cardiol* 1984;53: 1203–1205.
66. Herman MV, Cohn PF, Gorlin R: Resistance to blood flow by stenotic valves: Calculation of orifice area, in Grossman W (ed): *Cardiac Catheterization and Angiography*. Philadelphia, Lea & Febiger, 1980, pp 124–130.
67. Rahimtoola SH: The problem of valve prosthesis-patient mismatch. *Circulation* 1978;58:20–24.
68. Miller HC, Gibson DG, Stephens JD: Role of echocardiography and phonocardiography in diagnosis of mitral paraprosthetic regurgitation with Starr-Edwards prosthesis. *Br Heart J* 1973; 35:1217–1225.
69. Lipson LC, Kent KM, Rosing DR, et al: Long-term hemodynamic assessment of the mitral position: Late development of valvular stenosis. *Circulation* 1981;64:397–401.
70. Ubago JL, Figueroa A, Colman T, et al: Hemodynamic factors that affect calculated orifice areas in the mitral Hancock xenograft valve. *Circulation* 1980;61:388–394.
71. Gray RJ, Chaux A, Matloff JM, et al: Bileaflet, tilting disc and porcine aortic valve substitutes: In vivo hydrodynamic characteristics. *J Am Coll Cardiol* 1984;3:321–327.
72. Chaitman BR, Bonan R, LePage G, et al:

Hemodynamic evaluation of the Carpentier-Edwards porcine xenograft. *Circulation* 1979;60: 1170–1182.

73. Hosenpud JD, McAnulty JH, Morton MJ: Overestimation of mitral valve gradients obtained by phasic pulmonary capillary wedge pressure. *Cathet Cardiovasc Diagn* 1983;9:283–290.
74. Edmunds LH: Thromboembolic complications of current cardiac valvular prostheses. *Ann Thorac Surg* 1982;34:96–106.
75. Pumphrey CW, Fuster V, Chesebro JH: Systemic thromboembolism in valvular heart disease and prosthetic heart valves. Mod Concepts Cardiovasc Dis 1982;51:131–136.
76. Björk VO, Henze A: Ten years' experience with the Björk-Shiley tilting disc valve. *J Thorac Cardiovasc Surg* 1979;78:331–342.
77. Complications of convexo-concave heart valves. *FDA Drug Bull* 1984;14:22.
78. Chesebro JH, Fuster V, Fisher L, et al: Thromboembolism after biologic prosthetic heart valve replacement. *J Am Coll Cardiol* 1985;5:459.
79. Chesebro JH, Fuster V, Elveback LR, et al: Trial of combined warfarin plus dipyridamole or aspirin therapy in prosthetic heart valve replacement. Danger of aspirin compared with dipyridamole. *Am J Cardiol* 1983;51:1537–1541.
80. Dale J, Myhre E, Storstein O, et al: Prevention of arterial thromboembolism with acetylsalicylic acid: A controlled clinical study in patients with aortic ball valves. *Am Heart J* 1977;94:101–111.
81. Brott WH, Zajtchuk R, Bowen TE, et al: Dipyridamole-aspirin as thromboembolic prophylaxis in patients with aortic valve prosthesis: Prospective study with the Model 2320 Starr-Edwards prosthesis. *J Thorac Cardiovasc Surg* 1981;81:632–635.
82. Muñez L, Aguado MG, Celemín, et al: Aspirin or coumadin as the drug of choice for valve replacement with porcine bioprosthesis. *Ann Thorac Surg* 1982;33:354–358.
83. Forfar JC: A 7-year analysis of haemorrhage in patients on long-term anticoagulant treatment. *Br Heart J* 1979;42:128–132.
84. Lieberman A, Hass WK, Pinto R, et al: Intracranial hemorrhage and infarction in anticoagulated patients with prosthetic heart valves. *Stroke* 1978;9:18–24.
85. Yatsu FM, Mohr JP: Anticoagulation therapy for cardiogenic emboli to brain. *Neurology* 1982;32: 274–275.
86. Wilson WR, Geraci JE, Danielson GK, et al: Anticoagulant therapy and central nervous system complications in patients with prosthetic valve endocarditis. *Circulation* 1978;57:1004–1007.
87. Salazar E, Zajarias A, Gutierrez N, et al: The problem of cardiac valve prostheses, anticoagulants, and pregnancy. *Circulation* 1984;70 (suppl 1):169–177.
88. Tinker, JH, Tarhan S: Discontinuing anticoagulant therapy in surgical patients with cardiac valve prostheses: Observations in 180 operations. *JAMA* 1978;239:738–739.
89. Katholi RE, Nolan SP, McGuire LB: The management of anticoagulation during noncardiac operations in patients with prosthetic heart valves: A prospective study. *Am Heart J* 1978;96:163–165.
90. Bristow JD, Seaman AJ, Kloster FE, et al: Late, heparin-induced bleeding after retrograde arterial catheterization. *Circulation* 1968;37:393–396.
91. Cohen DJ, Kishel J, Likoff M, et al: Risk of prosthetic thrombosis with a porcine heterograft valve in the aortic position: Case reports. *Milit Med* 1982;147:1056–1058.
92. Copans H, Lakier JB, Kinsley RH, et al: Thrombosed Björk-Shiley mitral prostheses. *Circulation* 1980;61:169–174.
93. Björk VO, Henze A, Hindmarsh T: Radiopaque marker in the tilting disc of the Björk-Shiley heart valve. *J Thorac Cardiovasc Surg* 1977;73: 563–569.
94. Morton MJ, McAnulty JH, Rahimtoola SH, et al: Risks and benefits of postoperative cardiac catheterization in patients with ball valve prostheses. *Am J Cardiol* 1977;40:870–875.
95. Husebye DG, Pluth JR, Piehler JM, et al: Reoperation on prosthetic heart valves: An analysis of risk factors in 552 patients. *J Thorac Cardiovasc Surg* 1983;86:543–552.
96. Cohn LH, Koster JK, Van de Vanter S, et al: The in-hospital risk of re-replacement of dysfunctional mitral and aortic valves. *Circulation* 1982; 66(suppl 1):153–156.
97. Moulton AL: Thrombectomy for clotted Björk-Shiley prostheses: Is it really a proven procedure? *J Thorac Cardiovasc Surg* 1984;87: 147–148.
98. Reitz BA, Stinson EB, Griepp RB, et al: Tissue valve replacement of prosthetic heart valves for thromboembolism. *Am J Cardiol* 1978;41: 512–515.
99. Wilson WR, Danielson GK, Giuliani ER, et al: Prosthetic valve endocarditis. *Mayo Clinic Proc* 1982;57:155–161.
100. Kloster FE: Infective prosthetic valve endocarditis, in Rahimtoola SH (ed): *Infective Endocarditis*. New York, Grune & Stratton Inc, 1978, pp 291–305.
101. Karchmer AW, Dismukes WE, Buckley MJ, et al: Late prosthetic valve endocarditis: Clinical features influencing therapy. *Am J Med* 1978;64: 199–206.
102. Wilson WR, Giuliani ER, Danielson GK, et al: General considerations in the diagnosis and treatment of infective endocarditis. *Mayo Clin Proc* 1982;57:81–85.
103. Richardson JV, Karp RB, Kirklin JW, et al: Treatment of infective endocarditis: A 10-year comparative analysis. *Circulation* 1978;58: 589–598.
104. Shulman ST, Amren D, Biono A, et al: Prevention of bacterial endocarditis. *Circulation* 1984; 70:1123A–1127A.
105. Milano A, Bortolotti U, Talenti E, et al: Calcific degeneration as the main cause of porcine bioprosthetic valve failure. *Am J Cardiol* 1983;53: 1066–1070.
106. Ishihara T, Ferrans VJ, Boyce SW, et al: Structure and classification of cuspal tears and perforations in porcine bioprosthetic cardiac valves implanted in patients. *Am J Cardiol* 1981;48: 665–678.
107. Schoen FJ, Collins JJ, Cohn LH: Long-term

failure rate and morphologic correlations in porcine bioprosthetic heart valves. *Am J Cardiol* 1983;51:957–964.

108. Magilligan DJ, Lewis JW, Jara FM, et al: Spontaneous degeneration of porcine bioprosthetic valves. *Ann Thorac Surg* 1980;30:259–265.

109. Blackstone EH, Kirklin JW, Pluth JR, et al: The performance of the Braunwald-Cutter aortic prosthetic valve. *Ann Thorac Surg* 1977;23: 302–318.

110. Clark RE, Pavlovic TA, Knight BE, et al: Quantification of wear, hemoloysis and coagulation deficits in patients with Beall mitral valves. *Circulation* 1977;56(suppl 2):139–143.

111. Kloster FE: Diagnosis and management of complications of prosthetic heart valves. *Am J Cardiol* 1975;35:872–885.

112. Björk VO, Henge A: Management of thromboembolism after aortic valve replacement with the Björk-Shiley tilting disc valve. *Scand J Thorac Cardiovasc Surg* 1975;9:183–191.

Index

Adenosine diphosphate (ADP), in aortic stenosis, 139
Adenosine triphosphatase (ATPase), with cardiac muscle hypertrophy, 4
Adolescence, aortic stenosis in, 133–139, 143
Amyloidosis, 219
Angell-Shiley prosthesis, 267
Angina pectoris
  aortic regurgitation and, 197, 198–199, 200
  aortic stenosis and, 149, 156, 195, 196–197, 200, 223
  management of, 199–200
  medical therapy for, 200
  mitral regurgitation and, 221
  prosthetic valves and, 276, 277
  surgical therapy for, 200
Angiography
  aneurysmal dilatation of sinus of Valsalva on, 127
  aortic insufficiency on, 162–163, 210
  aortic stenosis with, 71, 179, 210, 224
  aortic valve congenital anomalies with, 132
  cleft mitral leaflet on, 88
  Ebstein's anomaly with, 41–43
  endocarditis and, 243
  evaluation in valvular heart disease with, 29, 30
  mitral insufficiency with, 114–115
  mitral regurgitation on, 221
  multivalvular heart disease with, 179
  pregnancy and use of, 184
  prosthetic valves and, 273
  pulmonic stenosis on, 70–71
  tricuspid atresia on, 36
  tricuspid regurgitation on, 54
Ankylosing spondylitis, 157, 161
Antibiotics
  endocarditis management with, 240–241, 247, 275
  endocarditis prophylaxis with, 254–257
  pregnancy and use of, 186
Anticoagulation therapy, 25
  mitral stenosis and, 105
  mitral valve disease surgery with, 84
  pregnancy and use of, 185
  prosthetic valves and, 263, 266, 271, 272–273
Aortic coarctation, 148
  bicuspid aortic valve with, 125, 131
  mitral regurgitation with, 78, 83, 85–86
Aortic insufficiency, 26, 157–168
  aortic regurgitation with, 216, 218
  asymptomatic, 164–165, 166
  bicuspid valve and, 148
  chest roentgenogram in, 160–161
  child and adolescent, 137
  echocardiography in, 162
  electrocardiography (ECG) in, 161
  endocarditis and, 235, 250
  etiology and pathology of, 157–158
  evaluation of, 159–165
  exercise measurement in, 205, 209, 210
  history in, 159
  left ventricular dysfunction, 166–167
  management of, 165–167
  mitral stenosis and, 98, 104
  murmur in, 160
  natural history of, 163–165
  pathophysiology of, 158–159
  physical examination in, 151, 159–160
  radionuclide angiography in, 162–163, 210
  rheumatic carditis with, 97
  valve replacement in, 165, 166–167
  vasodilator therapy in, 167–168
Aortic regurgitation
  acute (AAR), 215–219
  aneurysmal dilatation of sinus of Valsalva in, 127
  angina in, 197, 198–199, 200
  aortic insufficiency and, 159, 163
  aortic stenosis with, 137, 141, 145
  bisferiens pulse in, 26
  cardiac catheterization in, 218
  causes of, 24
  chamber stiffness in, 21
  clinical manifestations of, 215–216
  clinical significance of, 215
  congenital anomaly and, 143–145
  coronary flow in, 197–199
  echocardiography in, 144, 217–218
  electrocardiography in, 217
  etiology of, 216–217
  exercise measurement in, 208–209, 210–211
  heart sounds in, 27
  laboratory features in, 217
  left ventricular function and, 15, 178
  mitral stenosis with, 177–178
  multivalvular heart disease with, 175–176, 177–178, 179
  murmur in, 144, 179, 216
  myocardial contractility and, 15, 16
  palpation of precordium in, 27
  pregnancy and, 189–190
  quadricuspid aortic valve with, 126
  radionuclide angiography in, 28, 210
  rheumatic fever and, 143–144
  therapy in, 218–219
  valve replacement in, 218–219, 264
  vasodilator therapy in, 181, 210
  volume overload and, 12, 13, 15, 21
Aortic root pathology
  chest roentgenography in, 161
  echocardiography in, 28

Aortic sinus of Valsalva — right ventricular fistula, 12
Aortic stenosis, 147–157
angina in, 149, 156, 195, 196–197, 200
angiography of, 71, 179, 224
aortic regurgitation with, 137, 141, 145, 216
asymptomatic, 156
atrial transport function in, 7–8
biscuspid valve with, 125, 129, 147–148, 152
bisferiens pulse in, 26
cardiac catheterization in, 138–139, 154, 156
cardiac muscle contractility in, 6, 7
causes of, 24
chamber stiffness in, 20–21
chest roentgenogram in, 133, 134, 152, 223
child and adolescent, 133–139, 140, 143
clinical features of, 223–225
coronary bypass surgery with surgery for, 157
coronary flow in, 195–197
diagnosis of, 149–154
Doppler ultrasound in, 28, 136, 154, 224
echocardiography in, 133, 136, 152–154, 223–224
elderly patients and surgery in, 156–157
electrocardiography (ECG) in, 28, 133, 134–135, 138, 223
emergency with, 222–225
endocarditis and, 236
estimating severity of, 224
etiology and pathology of, 147–148
exercise measurement in, 135–136, 204, 205, 207–208, 211
heart sounds in, 27, 223
idiopathic hypertrophic subaortic (IHSS), 151, 152, 237, 277
infant, 132–133, 142–143
left outflow tract anomalies differentiated from, 129
left ventricular-aortic pressure gradient in, 141
left ventricular hypertrophy in, 5, 149, 150
long-term follow-up after surgery for, 143
management of, 155–157, 189, 224–225
mitral regurgitation with, 78, 176
mitral stenosis and, 177
multivariate analysis in, 135
murmur in, 123, 151–152, 223
natural course of, 136–141, 147, 149, 154–155
oxygen consumption in, 195
palpation of precordium in, 27
parachute mitral valve with, 83
pathogenesis of progression of severity of, 139
pathophysiology of, 129, 148–149
peripheral pulse contour and blood pressure in, 134
physical activity and sports in, 134, 141
physical examination in, 150–152
pregnancy and, 189
prophylactic surgery in, 156
pulmonary hypertension and, 140–141
quadricuspid aortic valve with, 126
reoperation in, 143
subvalvular, 128
sudden death and, 139–141, 155
supravalvular, 128, 129
surgical treatment of, 141–143, 155–157
symptoms in, 149–150
tricuspid aortic valve with cusps of unequal size in, 125
valve replacement in, 224–225, 264
vasodilator therapy in, 181
Aortic valve
bicuspid, 124–125, 128–129, 130–131
bicuspid, with cystic medial necrosis of aorta and dissecting aneurysm, 127–128
calcification of, 150, 152, 154, 155
fungal endocarditis and, 253
intravenous drug abuse and, 248
normal morphology of, 123–124
prolapse of, 158
prosthetic valve replacement of, 263–264
quadricuspid, 125–127
tricuspid, with cusps of unequal size, 125
unicommissural, 125
Aortic valve congenital anomalies, 123–145
aneurysmal dilatation of sinus of Valsalva in, 127
aortic regurgitation due to, 143–145
clinical features and diagnosis of, 129–136
echocardiography in, 131–132
incidence of, 123
left outflow tract anomalies in, 124–128, 130
morphology/pathology of, 123–128
pathophysiology of, 128–129
physical signs in, 129–130
see also specific conditions
Aortic valve disease
electrocardiography (ECG) in, 28
heart sounds in, 27
triscuspid stenosis with, 56
Aortic valve prostheses, 228, 229
Aortocaval fistula, and volume overload, 15
Aortoinferior vena cava, and volume overload, 12, 15, 20
Arrhythmias
aortic insufficiency and, 159
aortic stenosis and, 150, 207, 208
bicuspid aortic valve with, 131
history in evaluation of valvular heart disease and, 25
mitral insufficiency and, 109
mitral stenosis with, 225–226
prosthetic valves and, 263, 274
pulmonic stenosis with, 64
see also specific arrhythmias
Arterial pulses, in physical examination, 26
Arteriosclerotic heart disease, and mitral insufficiency, 106–107, 110, 117
Arteriovenous fistula
endocarditis and, 237
volume overload and, 12, 20
Arthritis, 25
Aspirin, 185, 272

Atherosclerosis
aortic stenosis and, 147
prosthetic valves and, 277
Atria, *see* Left atrium; Right atrium
Atrial fibrillation
aortic stenosis and, 150, 154, 224
mitral regurgitation with, 55
mitral stenosis and, 98, 99, 105, 225
prosthetic valves and, 272
treatment of, 105
tricuspid regurgitation with, 55
Atrial septal defect
Ebstein's anomaly associated with, 38
Noonan's syndrome with, 62
mitral valve disease with, 77, 78–79, 80
pulmonic stenosis with, 72
treatment of, 72
volume overload and, 12, 15
Atrioventricular valve, and volume overload, 12
Auscultation of heart
aortic regurgitation with, 216
Ebstein's anomaly with, 38
mitral stenosis and, 225
multiple positions used in, 27
physical examination in valvular heart disease with, 27
prosthetic valves and, 267
pulmonic stenosis with, 63
tricuspid atresia with, 34
tricuspid regurgitation with, 50
see also specific heart sounds
Austin-Flint murmur, 144, 160, 179, 216

Back pain, 25
Bacteremia
antibiotic prophylaxis in, 255–256
endocarditis and, 235, 236
pregnancy and, 186
procedures that may cause, 255, 256
Bacterial endocarditis
pathogenesis of, 235
pregnancy and, 188, 190
pulmonic stenosis with, 60, 73
Ball prosthetic valves, 261–262
Beall prosthesis, 276
Bernoulli principle, 102, 154, 227
Bicuspid aortic valve
aortic regurgitation with, 144, 216
aortic stenosis with, 125, 129, 147–148, 152
clinical features and diagnosis of, 130–131
cystic medial necrosis of aorta and dissecting aneurysm with, 127–128
echocardiography in, 131–132, 158
incidence of, 123
pathogenesis of progression of severity of, 139
pathology of, 124–125
pathophysiology of, 128–129
Billowing mitral leaflet syndrome, 109
Bisferiens pulse, 26
aortic insufficiency with, 159
aortic regurgitation with, 216
aortic stenosis and, 223
Björk-Shiley prosthesis, 226, 227, 262, 266, 268, 271–272, 273, 277
Blalock-Taussig shunt, and tricuspid atresia, 34
Blood cultures, in endocarditis, 240
Brain embolization, with endocarditis, 245
Braumwald-Cutter prosthesis, 276

Caged disc valves, 262
Calcium-channel blockers, 185
Carcinoid syndrome
pulmonic stenosis with, 60
tricuspid regurgitation and, 48
Cardiac catheterization
aortic stenosis with, 133, 137, 138–139, 141, 154, 156
as baseline for later evaluation, 30
Ebstein's anomaly with, 41–43
endocarditis and, 243
evaluation in valvular heart disease with, 29–30
mitral insufficiency with, 114–115
mitral regurgitation with, 221
mitral stenosis with, 103–104
mitral valve disease with, 79–80
multivalvular heart disease with, 179
pregnancy and use of, 184
presurgical use of, 29–30
prosthetic valves and, 227–228, 273–274
pulmonic stenosis with, 68–71
tricuspid atresia with, 36
tricuspid stenosis with, 53–54
Cardiac chamber
pressure overload and, 2–3
prosthetic valves and size of, 267
volume overload and, 12–15
Cardiac muscle contractility
aortic regurgitation and, 15, 16
aortic stenosis and, 6, 7
determining, 7
diastolic function in, 1, 2–3
end-systolic stress-volume relation (ESSVR) in, 16–19
exercise and, 205
mitral insufficiency and, 116–117
mitral regurgitation and, 15–16
pressure overload and, 1–3, 7
pressure-volume loop in, 3
systolic function in, 1–2, 3, 6
volume overload and hypertrophy and, 15–19, 21–22
Cardiac muscle hypertrophy
aortic stenosis and, 222–223
concentric, 13
myocardial constituents in, 4–5
pressure overload and, 3–5
regression of, 9–10
stimulus for, 4

volume overload and, 13, 15–19, 22
see also Left ventricular hypertrophy
Cardiac muscle mass
pressure overload and, 3
volume overload and, 21, 22
Cardiomegaly, with tricuspid atresia, 33
Cardiomyopathy, with mitral valve disease, 93
Carotid pulse
aortic insufficiency with, 159–160
aortic regurgitation with, 216
aortic stenosis with, 151
physical examination in valvular heart disease with, 26–27
Carpentier–Edwards valve, 262
Carvallo's sign, 50
Catheterization, *see* Cardiac catheterization
Chest pain
aortic insufficiency and, 159
aortic stenosis and, 149
endocarditis and, 248
history in evaluation of valvular heart disease and, 25
pulmonic stenosis with, 61
Chest radiography
aortic insufficiency on, 160–161
aortic regurgitation on, 217
aortic stenosis on, 133, 152, 223
Ebstein's anomaly on, 39–40
evaluation in valvular heart disease with, 28
mitral insufficiency on, 110, 113
mitral regurgitation on, 221
mitral valve disease on, 79
mitral stenosis on, 99–100
multivalvular heart disease with, 178
pregnancy and radiation exposure in, 183–184
prosthetic valves on, 267
pulmonic stenosis on, 65–66
tricuspid atresia on, 35–36
tricuspid valve disease on, 51
Children
aortic stenosis in, 133–139, 140, 143, 208
exercise measurement in, 208
prosthetic valves and, 266
Chordae tendinae
endocarditis and, 238, 250
mitral valve disease and, 78, 80, 83, 85
mitral valve function and, 92–93
Chordae tendinae rupture
heart sounds in, 27
mitral insufficiency and, 107, 110, 111, 112
mitral regurgitation and, 221, 222
Cineangiography
Ebstein's anomaly on, 42
pulmonic stenosis on, 70
Cleft mitral leaflet, 87–88
Cloth-covered valve, 262
Collagen disease
endocarditis and, 235
mitral insufficiency and, 107
pressure overload and, 1, 4–5
Computed tomography (CT)
aortic insufficiency on, 158, 160
aortic regurgitation on, 218
tricuspid regurgitation on, 54–55
radioisotope evaluation in, 54
Concentric hypertrophy, 13
Congenital heart disease, 190
aortic stenosis and, 147
aortic regurgitation and, 218
endocarditis and, 236, 243, 249, 250
mitral valve disease with, 82, 83, 93–94, 107
multivalvular heart disease and, 174
pulmonic stenosis with, 58
tricuspid valve anomalies in, 32
Congestive heart failure
aortic stenosis and, 138, 149, 150, 156, 223
endocarditis and, 243–244, 250, 251–252
physical examination in valvular heart disease with, 26, 27
prosthetic valves and, 263, 264, 277
pulmonic stenosis with, 60
tricuspid atresia with, 33
Connective tissue disorders, 78
Constrictive pericarditis, 48, 49
Contractility of muscle, *see* Cardiac muscle contractility
Cortriatriatum, 80–81, 94
Coronary arteriography
exercise measurement and, 205
mitral stenosis on, 104
Coronary artery disease, 192–201
aortic regurgitation and, 197–199
aortic stenosis with, 129, 149–150, 157, 195–197
coronary circulation physiology and, 192–195
management of, 199–200
mitral valve disease and, 93, 199
valve replacement surgery and, 10, 30
valvular heart disease interaction with, 192–201
Coronary bypass surgery
aortic stenosis surgery with, 157, 200
endocarditis and, 243
mitral regurgitation with, 222
Coumadin, 25
CT, *see* Computed tomography (CT)
Culture-negative endocarditis, 249, 254
Cyanosis, 26
Ebstein's anomaly with, 38
mitral valve disease with, 77, 78, 79
pulmonic stenosis with, 60, 61, 62–63

Diastole
left ventricular volume overload and, 19–21
mitral stenosis and, 97
muscle contractility and, 1, 2–3
pressure overload and, 5–6
Digitalis therapy
atrial fibrillation and, 105
congestive heart failure and, 252
mitral regurgitation with, 222

mitral stenosis with, 226
pregnancy and use of, 184
tricuspid regurgitation and, 55
Digitoxin
aortic regurgitation with, 218
aortic stenosis with, 224
pregnancy and use of, 184
Digoxin
mitral regurgitation with, 222
pregnancy and use of, 184, 188
Diltiazem hydrochloride, 226
Dipyridamole, with prosthetic valves, 272, 274, 277
Diuretics
aortic stenosis with, 224
congestive heart failure and, 252
mitral regurgitation with, 222
pregnancy and use of, 184, 189
tricuspid regurgitation and, 55
Dobutamine
aortic regurgitation with, 218
aortic stenosis with, 224
mitral regurgitation with, 222
Dopamine hydrochloride
aortic regurgitation with, 218
aortic stenosis with, 224
mitral regurgitation with, 222
Doppler ultrasonography
aortic insufficiency on, 162
aortic regurgitation on, 217–218
aortic stenosis on, 136, 224
Ebstein's anomaly on, 41
endocarditis on, 241, 243
evaluation in valvular heart disease with, 28–29
mitral insufficiency on, 111
mitral regurgitation on, 221
mitral stenosis on, 101–103, 225
mitral valve disease on, 77, 81–82
multivalvular heart disease on, 179
prosthetic valves on, 227, 268–269
pulmonic stenosis on, 66, 67–68
tricuspid regurgitation on, 52–53
tricuspid stenosis on, 53
Down's syndrome, 131
Drug therapy, *see* medications *and individual drugs*
Drug use and abuse, *see* Intravenous (IV) drug abuse
Dyspnea
aortic insufficiency and, 159
mitral stenosis and, 98, 105

Ebstein's anomaly, 37–43
cardiac catheterization and angiography in, 41–43
cineangiography of, 42
clinical features of, 38
echocardiography of, 40–41
electrocardiography of, 38–39
hemodynamics of, 38, 39
indications for surgery for, 43
natural history and management of, 43
pathophysiology of, 38
primary anatomical feature in, 38
pulmonic stenosis with, 58
radiographic features of, 39–40
ECG, *see* Electrocardiography (ECG)
Echocardiography
aortic insufficiency on, 162
aortic regurgitation on, 144, 217–218
aortic stenosis on, 133, 152–154
aortic valve congenital anomalies with, 131–132
congenital anomalies with, 144–145
endocarditis on, 241–243, 253
evaluation in valvular heart disease with, 28–29
follow-up after evaluation with, 29
mitral insufficiency on, 110–111, 113–114
mitral stenosis on, 100–101, 225
pregnancy and use of, 184
prosthetic valves on, 227, 268
pulmonic stenosis on, 66–68
tricuspid valve disease on, 51–52
see also M-mode echocardiography; Two-dimensional echocardiography
Edema
mitral stenosis and, 100
physical examination in valvular heart disease with, 27
Ehlers-Danlos syndrome, 107, 144–145
Eisenmenger syndrome, 33
Ejection click
aortic insufficiency with, 160
aortic stenosis with, 130, 151
Ejection fraction
aortic insufficiency and, 163
carotid pulse and, 27
echocardiography in, 28
exercise and, 205, 210, 211
pressure overload and, 6–7
volume overload and, 15
Elderly
aortic stenosis surgery in, 156–157
endocarditis and, 248–249
Electrocardiography (ECG)
aortic insufficiency on, 161
aortic regurgitation on, 217
aortic stenosis on, 133, 134–135, 138, 152, 223
Ebstein's anomaly on, 38–39
evaluation in valvular heart disease with, 28
mitral insufficiency on, 110, 113
mitral regurgitation and, 221
mitral stenosis on, 100
mitral valve disease on, 79
multivalvular heart disease on, 178
pregnancy and use of, 184
pulmonic stenosis on, 64–65
tricuspid atresia on, 34–35
tricuspid valve disease on, 51

Elfin facies, with left ventricular outflow tract disorders, 130
Embolism
endocarditis and, 238, 243, 245–246, 251, 254, 274
prosthetic valves and, 274
treatment of, 254
Emergencies
acute aortic regurgitation, 215–219
acute mitral regurgitation, 219–222
aortic stenosis, 222–225
mitral stenosis, 225–226
prosthetic heart valves, 226–229
Endocardial cushion defect
left ventricular outflow tract obstruction with, 88–89
mitral insufficiency and, 107
parachute mitral valve with, 86–87
Endocardial fibroelastosis, with mitral regurgitation, 78
Endocarditis, 234–257
catheterization in, 243
classification of, 234
clinical presentation in, 238–239
complications with, 243–247
congestive heart failure and, 243–244
culture-negative, 249, 254
definition of, 234
diagnosis of, 237–238
echocardiography of, 241–243
elderly and, 248–249
embolization and, 245–246
fungal, 253
general principles of management of, 240–241
history in evaluation of valvular heart disease and, 25
intravenous drug abusers and, 248
laboratory findings in, 239–240
pathogenesis of, 234–235
predisposing factors in, 235
pre-existing heart disease and, 235–237
prophylaxis for, 254–257
prosthetic valve, 247–248, 253–254, 263, 267, 268, 274
relapse and recurrent, 249–250, 254
rheumatic heart disease and, 235–236
splenomegaly in, 27
surgical therapy for, 251–254
tricuspid, 52, 56
see also Bacterial endocarditis; Infective endocarditis
Evaluation in valvular heart disease, 24–30
cardiac catheterization in, 29–30
chest film in, 28
Doppler ultrasonography in, 28–29
echocardiography in, 28–29
electrocardiography in, 28
follow-up after, 29
history in, 24–26
patient acceptance of condition and, 26
physical examination in, 26–27
questions to consider in, 24
radionuclide ventriculography in, 28–29
Exercise measurements, 204–213
aortic regurgitation with, 208–209
aortic stenosis with, 135–136, 204, 205, 207–208
exercise capacity in, 211–212
invasive hemodynamic measurements in, 206–210
mitral regurgitation with, 208
mitral stenosis with, 179, 206–207
multivalvular heart disease with, 179
noninvasive measurements in, 210–212
objectives of, 204
physiologic response and, 205–206
positional differences in, 206
prognostic information from, 204
radionuclide angiography with, 210–211
respiratory gas exchange in, 212
type of exercise performed and, 206
valve replacement evaluation with, 209–210
vasodilator therapy evaluation with, 210

Fibroelastosis, and mitral insufficiency, 107
Fibrosis, myocardial
cardiac muscle hypertrophy and, 4
left ventricular volume overload and, 21
pressure overload and, 2, 5
First heart sound
aortic insufficiency with, 160
aortic stenosis with, 151, 223
mitral regurgitation with, 79
mitral stenosis with, 97, 225
physical examination in valvular heart disease with, 27
pulmonic stenosis with, 63
Follow-up after evaluation in valvular heart disease, 29
Fontan procedure, tricuspid atresia on, 36
Fourth heart sound
aortic insufficiency with, 160
aortic stenosis with, 151, 223
Ebstein's anomaly with, 38
mitral insufficiency and, 113
mitral regurgitation and, 219
physical examination in valvular heart disease with, 27
Frank-Starling mechanism
aortic stenosis and, 150
exercise and, 205
left ventricular volume overload and, 13
mitral insufficiency and, 108, 116
Fungal endocarditis, 253
Fungemia, and endocarditis, 235
Furosemide
mitral regurgitation with, 222
pregnancy and use of, 184

Gas exchange, in exercise, 212

Gastrointestinal (GI) carcinoid tumors, 48
Genetic factors, and pulmonic stenosis, 61–62
Glenn shunt, and tricuspid atresia, 33, 34
Gorlin equation
  aortic stenosis with, 154
  mitral insufficiency with, 116
  mitral regurgitation with, 222
  mitral stenosis with, 96
  multivalvular heart disease with, 179
  prosthetic valve hemodynamics on, 269
  pulmonic stenosis with, 69–70
Graham-Steele murmur, 98

Hancock valve, 262
Heart sounds
  physical examination in valvular heart disease with, 27
  see also specific sounds
Hemodynamic abnormality
  assessment of, 25
  cardiac catheterization for, 29, 30
  pregnancy and, 186–187
  prosthetic valves and, 228, 269–270
Hemolytic anemia, and prosthetic valves, 276
Heparin, 25
  pregnancy and use of, 185
  prosthetic valves and, 273, 277
Hepatomegaly, in physical examination in valvular heart disease, 27
History
  aortic insufficiency and, 159
  evaluation in valvular heart disease with, 24–26
  multivalvular heart disease with, 177
  patient acceptance of condition and, 26
  pulmonic stenosis with, 61
  tricuspid regurgitation with, 49
  tricuspid stenosis with, 49
Hoarseness, in mitral stenosis, 98–99
Homocystinuria, 78
Hunter's syndrome, 144
Hurler's syndrome, 78, 144
Hydralazine hydrochloride
  aortic insufficiency with, 167
  aortic regurgitation with, 218
  mitral insufficiency with, 115
  mitral regurgitation with, 222
Hypereosinophlia, with endocarditis, 251
Hyperlipoproteinemia, and aortic stenosis, 147
Hyperthyroidism, 22
Hypertrophic cardiomyopathy
  mitral insufficiency and, 107
  mitral stenosis diagnosis and, 94
  Noonan's syndrome with, 62
  palpation of precordium in, 27
Hypertrophy, *see* Cardiac muscle hypertrophy; Left ventricular hypertrophy
Hypoplastic left ventricle, with mitral valve disease, 77
Hypoplastic right ventricle, with pulmonic stenosis, 58

Idiopathic hypertrophic subaortic stenosis (IHSS), 151, 152, 237, 276
Idiopathic mitral leaflet prolapse, 123
Immune complex disease, 239
Infant, and aortic stenosis, 132–133, 142–143
Infective endocarditis
  aortic insufficiency with, 157, 158, 164, 165
  aortic regurgitation with, 216, 218
  aortic stenosis with, 155
  categories of, 234
  intravenous (IV) drug abuse with, 46
  mitral insufficiency and, 107, 109, 111, 112, 113, 115, 117
  mitral stenosis and, 104
  mitral valve disease and, 93
  pathogenesis of, 234–235
  pregnancy and, 186
  prophylaxis for, 165, 186, 275, 277
  prosthetic valves and, 274–275
  quadricuspid aortic valve with, 127
  tricuspid regurgitation with, 46
  see also Endocarditis
Intravenous (IV) drug abuse
  aortic insufficiency with, 157
  endocarditis and, 234, 236–237, 248
  tricuspid regurgitation with, 46, 47–48, 52, 56, 190
Ionescu-Shiley pericardial xenograft, 227

Janeway lesions, 26, 238, 239
Jugular pulse
  physical examination in valvular heart disease with, 26
  pulmonic stenosis with, 63
  tricuspid atresia with, 34
  tricuspid valve disease with, 46, 49–50

Key-Hodgkin murmur, 216
Kidney embolization, with endocarditis, 245

Laryngeal nerve paralysis, and mitral stenosis, 98–99
Left atrial myxoma
  endocarditis and, 237, 244
  mitral insufficiency and, 107, 111, 115
  mitral valve disease and, 94, 107
Left atrium
  mitral insufficiency and, 110, 113, 114
  mitral regurgitation and, 208, 219
  mitral stenosis and enlargement of, 98, 99, 101
  pressure overload and, 7–8
  volume overload and, 13–15
Left ventricle
  aortic insufficiency and, 158–159, 166–167

aortic regurgitation and, 15, 178
aortic stenosis and, 133, 154, 156
chamber compliance in, 20
diastolic compliance and volume overload of, 19–21
mitral insufficiency and, 108, 110, 111–112, 113, 114, 115, 116
mitral regurgitation and, 15, 178
multivalvular heart disease and, 178, 179
muscle compliance in, 20
myocardial contractility and volume overload of, 15
pressure overload and, 8–9
volume overload and, 12, 13, 15, 19–21
Left ventricular end-diastolic pressure (LVEDP)
aortic stenosis and, 7
cardiac muscle hypertrophy and, 4
pressure overload and, 7
volume overload and, 16–19, 20
Left ventricular failure
aortic stenosis and, 149
mitral insufficiency with, 114
Left ventricular hypertrophy
aortic insufficiency and, 158, 160–161
aortic stenosis with, 5, 129, 149, 150, 154, 223
concentric, 13
echocardiography in, 28
electrocardiography (ECG) in, 28
fourth heart sound in, 27
multivalvular heart disease with, 178
volume overload effects on, 13
volume overload regression and, 21, 22
Left ventricular myxoma, and mitral insufficiency, 107
Lentiginosis, with left ventricular outflow tract disorders, 129, 130
Lillehei-Kaster valves, 262
Löeffler's endocarditis, 251
diagnosis of, 251
echocardiography in, 243
treatment of, 251
tricuspid regurgitation with, 48
tricuspid stenosis with, 48
Luetic disease, and aortic insufficiency, 157
Lupus erythematosus, and mitral insufficiency, 107

Marantic endocarditis, 250–251
diagnosis of, 250
echocardiography in, 243
Marfan's syndrome
aneurysmal dilatation of sinus of Valsalva in, 127, 144, 145
aortic insufficiency with, 157, 158
aortic regurgitation with, 144, 216, 217
biscuspid aortic valve with, 131
mitral insufficiency and, 107, 110, 111
mitral valve disease and, 78
multivalvular heart disease and, 174
tricuspid regurgitation with, 46, 48
Medications
history in evaluation of valvular heart disease and, 25
pregnancy and use of, 184–185
see also specific medications
MedTronic-Hall valve, 262
Methicillin, 240
Mitral insufficiency
acute, 112–114
afterload reduction in, 115
asymptomatic or mildly symptomatic, 117
catheterization and angiography in, 114–115
chest roentgenogram in, 110, 113
chronic, 106–118
clinical course of, 108–109, 112–113
congestive heart failure due to, 251–252
Doppler ultrasonography in, 111
echocardiography in, 110–111, 113–114
electrocardiography in, 110, 113
endocarditis and, 235, 250
etiology of, 106–107
mitral stenosis with, 96, 109
murmur in, 109–110
pathology of, 107
pathophysiology of, 107–108
physical findings in, 109–110
quantification of, 114–115
radioisotope evaluation in, 111–112
rheumatic carditis with, 97
treatment of, 115–118
valve replacement surgery in, 116–117
Mitral regurgitation
acquired, 78
acute, 219–222
aortic coarctation with, 85–86
aortic regurgitation with, 177–178
aortic stenosis with, 78, 176
cardiac catheterization in, 79–80
case reports of, 84–85
causes of, 24
chest roentgenography in, 79
chordal rupture in, 221
clinical signs in, 219
diagnosis and management of, 82
Doppler echocardiography in, 81–82, 179
electrocardiography in, 79
endocarditis and, 251
end-systolic stress-volume relation (ESSVR) in, 17, 19
etiology of, 219–221
exercise measurement in, 208, 211
heart sounds in, 27
left ventricular function in, 15, 178
multivalvular heart disease with, 175, 177–178, 179
murmur in, 79, 152
myocardial contractility and, 15–16
nuclear techniques in, 179
papillary muscle disorders and, 219–221
physical examination in, 79
pregnancy and, 188–189

radionuclide angiography in, 28, 54, 211
rheumatic, 144
symptoms in, 78
therapy for, 221–222
valve replacement in, 265
vasodilator therapy in, 181, 210
volume overload and, 12, 13, 15, 21, 22
Mitral stenosis, 93–106
aortic stenosis and, 177
atrial fibrillation with, 225
cardiac catheterization in, 79–80, 103–104
case report of, 82–84
chest roentgenogram in, 79, 99–100
clinical features of, 96–97, 225
congenital heart defects with, 83, 93–94
coronary arteriography in, 104
course of, 99
diagnosis and management of, 82
differential diagnosis of, 94, 96
Doppler echocardiography in, 82, 101–103, 225
echocardiography in, 100–101, 225
electrocardiography in, 79, 100
emergency with, 225–226
endocarditis and, 244
etiology of, 93–94
exercise measurement and, 179, 204, 205–207, 211
Gorlin equation in, 96
heart sounds in, 27
incidence of, 78
laboratory findings in, 225–226
mitral insufficiency with, 96, 109
multivalvular heart disease with, 178
murmur in, 97, 144, 160, 179
pathophysiology of, 94–96
physical examination in, 79, 97–98
pregnancy and, 187–188
pulmonary hypertension and, 94–96, 178
surgery for, 105–106
symptoms in, 78, 98–99
treatment of, 104–105, 187–188, 225–226
tricuspid regurgitation with, 49
tricuspid stenosis with, 50
valve replacement in, 106, 265
Mitral valve disease, 92–118
acquired, 78
anatomy of, 77–78, 92–93
cardiac catheterization in, 79–80
chest roentgenogram in, 79
classification of, 77–78
congenital, 77–90
difficulty of recognition of, 82
Doppler echocardiography in, 81–82
electrocardiography (ECG) in, 28, 79
fungal endocarditis and, 253
histologic structure of leaflet and, 93
incidence of, 78
medications for, 25
multivalvular heart disease with, 174, 176
physical examination in, 26, 79
surgery for, 83–84
symptoms in, 78–79
tricuspid regurgitation with, 47
tricuspid stenosis with, 49, 56
two-dimensional echocardiography in, 80–81, 88–89
Mitral valve prolapse, 93
endocarditis and, 237, 238
Marfan's syndrome with, 174
mitral insufficiency and, 106, 109, 110, 111, 115, 117
mitral regurgitation and, 221
symptoms in, 109
Mitral valve prostheses, 228, 229
M-mode echocardiography
aortic insufficiency on, 162
aortic regurgitation on, 217–218
aortic stenosis on, 136, 152
aortic valve congenital anomalies with, 131–132
Ebstein's anomaly on, 40–41
endocarditis on, 238, 241, 250
evaluation in valvular heart disease with, 29
mitral insufficiency on, 111, 117
mitral stenosis on, 100–101
prosthetic valves on, 227, 268
pulmonic stenosis on, 66–67
tricuspid atresia on, 36
tricuspid valve disease on, 52
Morguio's syndrome, 144
Multivalvular heart disease, 174–181
cardiac catheterization in, 179
chest roentgenography in, 178
chronicity of illness and sequence of events in, 177
echocardiography in, 178–179
electrocardiography in, 178
etiology of, 174
evaluation in, 177–179
history in, 177
multiple valve replacement in, 265–266
pathophysiology of, 174–177
physical examination in, 177–178
secondary lesions with, 174
surgical therapy for, 180
Multivariate analysis, in aortic stenosis diagnosis, 135
Murmur
aortic insufficiency with, 160
aortic regurgitation with, 144, 179, 216
aortic stenosis with, 123, 151–152, 177, 223
Austin-Flint, 144, 160, 179, 216
Ebstein's anomaly with, 38
endocarditis and, 237–238, 247, 248, 275
Graham-Steele, 98
Key-Hodgkin, 216
mitral insufficiency with, 109–110
mitral regurgitation with, 79, 152
mitral stenosis with, 79, 97, 144, 160, 177, 179
multivalvular heart disease with, 177–178, 179
prosthetic valves and, 226

pulmonary regurgitation with, 144
rheumatic heart disease and, 236
tricuspid regurgitation with, 178
Mycotic aneurysms, and endocarditis, 246–247
Myocardial abscess, and endocarditis, 244–245
Myocardial infarction
echocardiography in, 28
endocarditis and, 237, 238, 243, 253
mitral valve disease and, 93

Nafcillin sodium, 240
Neurologic deficit, evaluation of, 25
Nifedepine, 167
Nitroglycerine, with angina, 200
Nitroprusside
aortic insufficiency with, 167
mitral regurgitation with, 222
Noonan's syndrome
bicuspid aortic valve with, 131
pulmonic stenosis with, 62
Norepinephrine, and cardiac muscle hypertrophy, 4

Obstructive pulmonary vascular disease, 33
Ochronosis, with aortic stenosis, 147
Omniscience valve, 262
Ortner's syndrome, 98–99
Osler's nodes, 238, 239, 249
Oxygen consumption
aortic regurgitation and, 197, 198
aortic stenosis and, 195
autoregulation of, 193–194
exercise and, 205
factors determining, 192
pregnancy and, 186

Pacemakers, in pregnancy, 185
Pain, *see* Chest pain
Papillary muscle
contractility of, 1–2
mitral regurgitation and, 219–221
mitral valve disease and, 78, 80
parachute mitral valve and, 78, 80
volume overload and hypertrophy and, 15
Parachute mitral valve
cardiac catheterization in, 81, 83
endocardial cushion defect with, 86–87
mitral insufficiency and, 107
mitral regurgitation with, 85, 86
mitral stenosis diagnosis and, 94
papillary muscle abnormality and, 78
surgery for, 83–84
Parvus and tardus pulse, 151
Patent ductus arteriosus
endocarditis and, 237
volume overload and, 12
Patent foramen ovale, with Ebstein's anomaly, 38
Penicillin, with endocarditis, 239, 240, 241, 249
Pericardial effusion, on echocardiography, 28
Pericarditis, with endocarditis, 246
Peripheral pulse, in aortic stenosis, 134
Phonocardiography, with prosthetic valves, 267–268
Physical examination
aortic insufficiency with, 159–160
aortic stenosis with, 129–130, 150–152
auscultation of heart in multiple positions in, 26
evaluation in valvular heart disease with, 26–27
general appearance of patient in, 26
mitral regurgitation with, 79
mitral stenosis with, 79
multivalvular heart disease with, 177–178
as primary diagnostic test, 26
prosthetic valves and, 267
pulmonic stenosis with, 62–64
tricuspid regurgitation with, 49–51, 178
P-mitrale wave, 28
Pott's shunt, with tricuspid atresia, 33, 34, 36
Pregnancy, 183–190
aortic regurgitation and, 189–190
aortic valve stenosis and, 189
cardiac catheterization during, 184
cardiac therapy during, 184–185
cardiovascular diagnosis during, 183–184
drug therapy during, 184–185
echocardiography during, 184
electrocardiography during, 184
evaluation in valvular heart disease and, 25
general management of heart disease during, 185–186
hemodynamic changes during, 186–187
mitral regurgitation and, 188–189
mitral stenosis and, 98, 105, 187–188
prosthetic valves and, 277
pulmonic valve disease and, 190
radiation exposure during, 183–184
tricuspid valve disease and, 190
Premature atrial or ventricular beats, 161
Pressure overload, 1–10
arterial contribution in, 7–8
cardiac chamber changes in, 2–3
cardiac muscle hypertrophy in, 3–5
collagen deposition in, 1, 4–5
diastolic function in, 5–6
geometric considerations in, 1–3
multivalvular heart disease with, 174
muscle contractility in, 1–2, 7
regression of hypertrophy in, 9–10
right and left ventricular responses to, 8–9, 199
systolic function in, 6–7
Procainamide hydrochloride, 226
Propraolol hydrochloride, 226
Prostaglandins, and coronary regulation, 193
Prosthetic valves, 261–277
anticoagulation and, 272–273

aortic valve, 263–264
cardiac catheterization and, 227–228
categories of, 261
children and, 266
clinical examination in, 226–227
complications with, 263, 266
decision to use, 261
dysfunctional, 275–276
emboli and, 274
emergency with, 226–229
endocarditis and, 234, 236, 238, 240, 243, 247–248, 253–254, 274–275
evaluation of patient with, 266–269
general surgery and, 277
hemodynamics of, 228, 269–270
hemolytic anemia and, 276
mismatch with, 277
mitral valve, 264–265
mitral valve disease with, 84
multiple valve replacement with, 265–266
pregnancy and, 277
replacement of, 228–229
thromboembolism and, 270–272
thrombotic obstruction and, 273–274
unsatisfactory late results with, 276–277
valve failure rate for, 275
see also specific prostheses
Protein synthesis
cardiac muscle hypertrophy and, 4
volume overload and, 13
Pseudocoarctation, 125
Pulmonary artery
mitral stenosis and, 103
multivalvular heart disease and, 178
Pulmonary hypertension
aortic stenosis and, 140–141
endocarditis and, 244
mitral insufficiency with, 110, 113
mitral stenosis and, 94–96, 97, 98, 99, 105, 178
multivalvular heart disease with, 174, 176–177, 178
pregnancy and, 188
pulmonic stenosis with, 60
treatment of, 55
tricuspid atresia with, 33
tricuspid regurgitation with, 47, 51, 55, 176
Pulmonic insufficiency
mitral stenosis and, 96, 97–98
pregnancy and, 190
Pulmonic regurgitation
multivalvular heart disease with, 174, 176, 179
murmur in, 144
volume overload and, 12, 15
Pulmonic stenosis, 58–74
acquired, 60
angiocardiography in, 70–71
cardiac catheterization in, 68–71
chest roentgenogram in, 65–66
classification system for, 58–59
clinical features of, 61–68
course and prognosis in, 73–74
early work with, 58
echocardiography in, 66–68
electrocardiography (ECG) in, 28, 64–65
genetic factors in, 61–62
heart sounds in, 27
history in, 61
lesions associated with, 58
natural history of, 60–61
pathology of, 59–60
physical examination in, 62–64
pregnancy and, 190
severity of, 59
syndromes associated with, 62
treatment of, 71–73
tricuspid atresia with, 32, 33, 34, 35, 36
Pulmonic valve
intravenous drug abuse and, 248, 252
quadricuspid, 126

Quadricuspid aortic valve, 125–127
Quadricuspid pulmonic valve, 126
Quinidine, 25, 226

Radiography, *see* Chest radiography
Radioisotope evaluation, with mitral insufficiency, 111–112
Radionuclide angiography
aortic insufficiency on, 162–163
evaluation in valvular heart disease with, 28–29
exercise measurement in, 210–211
follow-up after evaluation with, 29
mitral regurgitation on, 54, 221
pregnancy and use of, 184
tricuspid regurgitation on, 54
Reiter's syndrome, 157, 161
Respiratory gas exchange, in exercise, 212
Reversed coarctation, in aortic stenosis, 130
Rheumatic heart disease
aortic insufficiency and, 157–158, 164, 165
aortic regurgitation and, 143–144
aortic stenosis and, 147, 148, 152
endocarditis and, 234, 235–236, 238, 243, 249, 250
history in evaluation of valvular heart disease and, 25
mitral insufficiency and, 106, 107, 110, 111, 115, 117
mitral regurgitation and, 144, 221
mitral stenosis and, 93, 96–97, 104–105, 117
mitral valve disease and, 78, 93, 117, 179
multivalvular heart disease and, 174
pregnancy and, 188
prophylaxis for, 104–105
pulmonic stenosis with, 60
tricuspid stenosis with, 48, 50, 52
tricuspid valve disease and, 46–47
Right atrial myxoma, with tricuspid stenosis, 48, 51

Right atrium
pressure overload and, 7–8
pulmonic stenosis with enlargement of, 64
volume overload and, 15
Right bundle-branch block, with Ebstein's anomaly, 38, 39
Right heart failure
chest roentgenography in, 178
hepatomegaly in, 27
mitral insufficiency and, 112
mitral stenosis and, 96, 98
multivalvular heart disease with, 177
prosthetic valves and, 265
tricuspid regurgitation with, 47
Right ventricle
Ebstein's anomaly displacement into, 38
pressure overload and, 8–9
tricuspid regurgitation and, 50
volume overload and, 15, 50, 199
Right ventricular hypertrophy
echocardiography in, 28
electrocardiography (ECG) in, 28
mitral valve disease with, 79
Roth's sports, 238, 239
Rubella, 61–62

St. Jude bileaflet valve, 262, 266, 267
Saphenous vein bypass graft, and valve replacement, 200, 224
Sarcomere
left ventricular volume overload and, 13, 21
muscle contractility and length of, 1–2
Scheie's syndrome, 144
Second heart sound
aortic insufficiency with, 160
aortic stenosis with, 151
mitral regurgitation with, 79
physical examination in valvular heart disease with, 27
Semilunar valve, and volume overload, 12
Septal defects, *see* Atrial septal defect; Ventricular septal defect
Shone's syndrome, 77
Sinus of Valsalva
aneurysmal dilatation of, 127
endocarditis and, 246, 253
Skin rash, 25, 26
Smeloff-Cutter prostheses, 261
Starling's law, 1
Starr-Edwards prostheses, 226, 261, 262, 266, 267, 271, 276
Streptokinase, 228
Streptomycin, 241
Stroke volume
aortic insufficiency and, 163
aortic stenosis and, 7
pregnancy and, 187
pressure overload and, 3
radionuclide ventriculography in, 28
Subacute bacterial endocarditis, 27, 274
Subvalvular aortic stenosis, 128
Sudden death
aortic insufficiency and, 159
aortic stenosis and, 139, 155
prosthetic valves and, 263, 264
Supravalvular aortic stenosis, 128, 129, 196
Supravalvular mitral ring, 94
Supraventricular tachyarrhythmia
pregnancy and treatment of, 185
pulmonic stenosis with, 61
Syncope
aortic stenosis with, 140, 149, 150, 156, 207, 208, 223
history in evaluation of valvular heart disease and, 25
mitral valve disease with, 78, 187
pulmonic stenosis with, 61
Syphilis, 158
Systole
cardiac muscle hypertrophy and, 4
coronary circulation regulation and, 192, 194
mitral insufficiency and, 112–113
mitral stenosis and, 97
mitral valve function and, 93
muscle contractility and, 1–2, 3, 6
pressure overload and, 6–7
prosthetic valves and, 269

Tachycardia
aortic regurgitation with, 216
mitral regurgitation with, 79, 219
mitral stenosis with, 225–226
Tetralogy of Fallot, 190, 236
Thiazide diuretics, in pregnancy, 184
Third heart sound
aortic regurgitation with, 216
Ebstein's anomaly with, 38
mitral regurgitation with, 79, 219
physical examination in valvular heart disease with, 27
pulmonic stenosis with, 63
tricuspid regurgitation with, 50
Thromboembolic phenomenon
mitral insufficiency and, 109
prosthetic valves and, 262, 263, 264, 266, 270–272
Thrombotic noninfective endocarditis, 234
Thyrotoxicosis, with tricuspid regurgitation, 48
Tissue valves, 262–263
Tobramycin, 240
Transposition of great arteries
pressure overload and, 8
pulmonic stenosis with, 58
tricuspid atresia with, 32, 33
Trauma, 25
aortic regurgitation with, 216
mitral insufficiency and, 107
Tricuspid aortic valve
aortic stenosis with, 129, 147
echocardiography in, 131

cusps of unequal size in, 125
pathophysiology of, 129
Tricuspid atresia, 32–37
cardiac catheterization and angiography in, 36
classification of, 32, 33
clinical features of, 33–34
echocardiography in, 36
electrocardiography (ECG) in, 34–35
hemodynamics of, 33
natural history and management of, 36–37
pathology and pathophysiology in, 32–33
radiographic features of, 35–36
terminology used with, 32
Tricuspid incompetence, 32, 37
Tricuspid insufficiency
mitral stenosis and, 96, 97
surgical treatment of, 55–56
Tricuspid regurgitation, 46–56
cardiac catheterization and angiography in, 42, 53–54
chest roentgenography in, 51
computed tomography (CT) in, 54–55
Doppler ultrasound in, 52–53, 179
Ebstein's anomaly associated with, 38
echocardiography in, 51–52
electrocardiography in, 51
etiology of, 46–48
exercise studies in, 179
hemodynamic effects of, 48
history in, 49
jugular venous pulse in, 26
laboratory findings in, 51
medical treatment of, 55
multivalvular heart disease with, 174, 175, 178, 179
pathophysiology of, 48–49
physical examination in, 49–51, 178
pregnancy and, 190
pulmonic stenosis with, 61
radioisotope evaluation in, 54
secondary, 48–49
surgical treatment of, 55–56
volume overload and, 12, 15
Tricuspid stenosis, 32, 37, 46–56
aortic valvular disease with, 56
cardiac catheterization in, 53–54
chest roentgenography in, 51
computed tomography (CT) in, 54–55
Doppler ultrasound in, 53
echocardiography in, 51–52
electrocardiography in, 51
etiology of, 48
hemodynamic effects of, 49
history in, 49
laboratory findings in, 51
medical treatment of, 55
mitral valvular disease with, 56
pathophysiology of, 49
physical examination in, 49–51
pregnancy and, 190
radioisotope evaluation in, 54
rheumatic, 48, 50, 52
surgical treatment of, 55–56
Tricuspid valve
endocarditis of, 52, 56, 238, 252
intravenous drug abuse and, 248
myxomatous degeneration of, 48
Tricuspid valve prostheses, 228, 266
Turner's syndrome
bicuspid aortic valve with, 131
pulmonic stenosis with, 62
Two-dimensional echocardiography
aortic insufficiency on, 158, 162
aortic regurgitation on, 217
aortic stenosis on, 136, 152–154, 223–224
aortic valve congenital anomalies with, 132
cleft mitral leaflet on, 88
cor triatriatum on, 80–81
Ebstein's anomaly on, 41
endocarditis on, 238, 241, 242
mitral insufficiency on, 110–111
mitral regurgitation on, 220, 221
mitral stenosis on, 101, 225
mitral valve disease on, 77, 80–81, 88–89
prosthetic valves on, 227, 268
pulmonic stenosis on, 67–68
tricuspid atresia on, 36
tricuspid valve disease on, 52

Ultrasonography, see Doppler ultrasonography
Unicommissural aortic valve, 125, 129, 144, 147
Univentricular heart with absence of right atrioventricular (AV) connection, 32; *see also* Tricuspid atresia
Urokinase, 228

Valve replacement surgery
aortic insufficiency and, 165, 166–167
aortic regurgitation and, 218–219
aortic stenosis and, 224–225
aortic valve, 263–264
bypass surgery with, 157, 200
cardiac muscle hypertrophy regression and, 9–10
congestive heart failure and, 251–252
coronary artery disease and, 30
endocarditis and, 56
evaluation in valvular heart disease and, 29–30
exercise measurement evaluation in, 209–210
hypothermic arrest of ventricle during, 10
mitral insufficiency with, 116–117
mitral stenosis with, 106
mitral valve disease with, 83, 84
mortality comparisons for, 180, 181
multivalvular heart disease with, 180
replacement of valve in, 228–229
tricuspid valve disease with, 46, 55–56, 180
see also Prosthetic valves
Vancomycin hydrochloride, 240
Vasodilator therapy

aortic insufficiency and, 167–168
exercise measurement evaluation in, 210
multivalvular heart disease with, 181
pregnancy and use of, 185
pulmonary hypertension in tricuspid regurgitation and, 55
Venereal disease, 25
Ventricles, *see* Left ventricle; Right ventricle
Ventricular hypertrophy, *see* Left ventricular hypertrophy; Right ventricular hypertrophy
Ventricular septal aneurysm, with tricuspid regurgitation, 48
Ventricular septal defect
aortic regurgitation with, 145
endocarditis and, 235, 236, 237
mitral regurgitation with, 220
pulmonic stenosis with, 58, 71
tricuspid atresia with, 33, 36
volume overload and, 12
Ventricular tachycardia, with mitral insufficiency, 109
Ventriculography, *see* Radionuclide angiography
Verapamil
mitral stenosis with, 226
pregnancy and use of, 185, 188
Volume overload, 12–22
cardiac chamber adaptations to, 12–15
causes of, 12
diastolic compliance and, 19–21
end-systolic stress-volume relation (ESSVR) in, 16–19, 22
heart sounds in, 27
left atrium and, 13–15
left ventricle and, 13, 22
multivalvular heart disease with, 174
myocardial contractility and hypertrophy in, 15–19
regression of myocardial adaptations after relief of, 21–22
right ventricle and right atrium and, 15, 199
tricuspid regurgitation and, 50

Warfarin
mitral stenosis and, 105
mitral valve disease surgery with, 84
pregnancy and use of, 185
prosthetic valves and, 266, 272, 273, 277
Waterston shunt, and tricuspid atresia, 33, 34, 35
Whipple's disease, 94, 157
Wolff-Parkinson-White syndrome, type B, 38, 39